Psychiatric Illness in Women

Emerging Treatments and Research

Psychiatric Illness in Women

Emerging Treatments and Research

Edited by

Freda Lewis-Hall, M.D.
Teresa S. Williams, B.Sc.
Jill A. Panetta, Ph.D.
John M. Herrera, Ph.D.

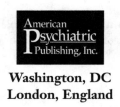

American Psychiatric Publishing, Inc.

Washington, DC
London, England

Note: Each individual author has worked to ensure that all information in this book concerning drug dosages, schedules, and routes of administration is accurate as of the time of publication and consistent with standards set by the U.S. Food and Drug Administration and the general medical community. As medical research and practice advance, however, therapeutic standards may change. For this reason and because human and mechanical errors sometimes occur, it is recommended that readers follow the advice of a physician who is directly involved in their care or the care of a member of their family. A product's current package insert should be consulted for full prescribing and safety information.

Books published by American Psychiatric Publishing, Inc., represent the views and opinions of the individual authors and do not necessarily represent the policies and opinions of APPI or the American Psychiatric Association.

A portion of proceeds from the sale of this book will be donated to the Lilly Center for Women's Health to support women's health programs.

Copyright © 2002 American Psychiatric Publishing, Inc.
ALL RIGHTS RESERVED

Manufactured in the United States of America on acid-free paper
06   05   04   03   02   5   4   3   2   1
First Edition

American Psychiatric Publishing, Inc.
1400 K Street, N.W.
Washington, DC 20005
www.appi.org

Library of Congress Cataloging-in-Publication Data
Psychiatric illness in women : emerging treatments and research / edited by Freda Lewis-Hall ... [et al.].-- 1st ed.
    p. ; cm.
Includes bibliographical references and index.
ISBN 1-58562-003-3 (alk. paper)
    1. Mentally ill women--Care. 2. Mental illness--Treatment. 3. Mentally ill women--Research. I. Lewis-Hall, Freda.
    [DNLM: 1. Mental Disorders--therapy. 2. Mental Disorders--epidemiology. 3. Sex Factors. 4. Women. WM 140 P9745 2002]
RC451.4.W6 P75 2002
616.89'0082--dc21   2001045810

British Library Cataloguing in Publication Data
A CIP record is available from the British Library.

Contents

I

Anxiety Disorders and Other
Related Disorders

II

Major Depressive Disorder and
Related Disorders

III

Schizophrenia and
Related Disorders

IV

Dementia and
Related Disorders

V

Other Psychiatric Illnesses and Special Topics

Contributors

Kathryn Abel, Ph.D., M.R.C.P., M.R.C.Psych., M.A.
Senior Lecturer, University of Manchester, Manchester, England

Nancy C. Andreasen, M.D., Ph.D.
Andrew H. Woods Chair of Psychiatry and Director of the Mental Health Clinical Research Center, University of Iowa College of Medicine, Iowa City, Iowa

Leslie Born, M.Sc.
Ph.D. Candidate, Institute of Medical Science, University of Toronto, Toronto; Women's Health Concerns Clinic, St. Joseph's Healthcare, Hamilton, Ontario, Canada

Elizabeth S. Bowman, M.D.
Clinical Professor, Department of Neurology, Indiana University School of Medicine, Indianapolis, Indiana

Kathleen T. Brady, M.D., Ph.D.
Professor of Psychiatry, Medical University of South Carolina, Department of Psychiatry and Behavioral Sciences, Center for Drug and Alcohol Programs, Charleston, South Carolina

Neil S. Buckholtz, Ph.D.
Chief, Dementias of Aging Branch, Neuroscience and Neuropsychology of Aging Program, National Institute on Aging, Bethesda, Maryland

Vivien K. Burt, M.D., Ph.D.
Director, Women's Life Center, and Professor of Psychiatry, University of California—Los Angeles School of Medicine and UCLA Neuropsychiatric Institute, Los Angeles, California

David J. Castle, M.Sc., M.D., M.R.C.P.
Clinical Director/Directorate of Mental Health Services, Fremantle Hospital and Health Service, Fremantle, Western Australia, Australia

Lee S. Cohen, M.D.
Director, Perinatal and Reproductive Psychiatry Clinical Research Program, Massachusetts General Hospital; and Associate Professor of Psychiatry, Harvard Medical School, Cambridge, Massachusetts

Christine Culhane, B.Pharm.
Drug Information Pharmacist, Mental Health Research Institute of Victoria, Parkville, Victoria, Australia

Bonnie S. Dansky, Ph.D.
Client Services Manager, CB Technologies, Landenberg, Pennsylvania

Ruth A. Dickson, M.D., F.R.C.P.C.
Associate Professor of Psychiatry, University of Calgary; and Associate Vice President of Clinical Research, Eli Lilly Canada, Calgary, Alberta, Canada

Rebecca M. Evans, M.D.
Assistant Professor of Psychiatry, Department of Neurology, Indiana University School of Medicine, Indianapolis, Indiana

Martin R. Farlow, M.D.
Professor and Vice Chairman for Research, Department of Neurology, Indiana University School of Medicine, Indianapolis, Indiana

Edyta J. Frackiewicz, Pharm.D.
Research Pharmacologist, California Clinical Trials, Beverly Hills, California

Steven Friedman, Ph.D.
Professor of Psychiatry, Department of Psychiatry, State University of New York Health Science Center at Brooklyn, Brooklyn, New York

William M. Glazer, M.D.
Associate Clinical Professor of Psychiatry, Department of Psychiatry, Harvard Medical School, Massachusetts General Hospital, Menemsha, Massachusetts

Shelly F. Greenfield, M.D., M.P.H.
Medical Director, Alcohol and Drug Abuse Ambulatory Treatment Program, McLean Hospital; and Assistant Professor of Psychiatry, Harvard Medical School, Belmont, Massachusetts

John M. Herrera, Ph.D.
Professor of Psychiatry, Howard University, Washington, D.C.

Anne L. Hoff, Ph.D.
Associate Professor of Psychiatry, University of California, Davis School of Medicine, Napa Psychiatric Research Center, Napa State Hospital, Napa, California

Judy Hope, M.B., B.S.
Research Clinician, Box Hill Hospital, Box Hill, Victoria, Australia

Amy L. Hostetter, B.A.
Emory University, Department of Psychiatry and Behavioral Sciences, Atlanta, Georgia

Dilip V. Jeste, M.D.
Estelle and Edgar Levi Chair in Aging and Professor of Psychiatry and Neuroscience, Department of Psychiatry, University of California, San Diego; and Director of the Division of Geriatric Psychiatry, VA San Diego Healthcare System, San Diego, California

Walter H. Kaye, M.D.
Professor of Psychiatry; and Director of Research, Eating Disorders Module, University of Pittsburgh School of Medicine, Department of Psychiatry, Western Psychiatric Institute and Clinic, Pittsburgh, Pennsylvania

Nicholas A. Keks, Ph.D., M.B.B.S., F.R.A.N.Z.C.P.
Professor of Psychiatry, Monash University and Box Hill Hospital, Box Hill, Victoria, Australia

Charlotte Kennedy, Ph.D.
Assistant Professor, University of Tennessee, Memphis, School of Medicine, Department of Psychiatry, UTMG Behavioral Health Center, Memphis, Tennessee

Cindy L. Kidner, M.A.
Student Research Assistant, Department of Psychiatry, University of Texas Southwestern Medical Center at Dallas, Dallas, Texas

Kelly L. Klump, Ph.D.
Postdoctoral Clinical Research Fellow, University of Pittsburgh School of Medicine, Department of Psychiatry, Western Psychiatric Institute and Clinic, Pittsburgh, Pennsylvania

Natalie Krapivensky, M.B.B.S., F.R.A.N.Z.C.P.
Consultant Psychiatrist, St. Vincent's Hospital, Fitzroy, Victoria, Australia

William S. Kremen, Ph.D.
Associate Professor of Psychiatry, University of California, Davis School of Medicine, Napa Psychiatric Research Center, Sacramento, California

Jonathan P. Lacro, Pharm.D.
Associate Clinical Professor of Psychiatry, Department of Psychiatry, University of California, San Diego, VA San Diego Healthcare System, San Diego, California

William B. Lawson, M.D., Ph.D.
Professor and Chair of Psychiatry, Howard University School of Medicine, Washington, D.C.

Richard Lewine, Ph.D.
Director of Schizophrenia Disorder Program and Department of Psychiatry and Behavioral Sciences, Emory University, Atlanta, Georgia

Freda Lewis-Hall, M.D.
Team Leader, Primary Care Product Team, Eli Lilly and Company, Indianapolis, Indiana

Keh-Ming Lin, M.D., M.P.H.
Professor of Psychiatry, University of California—Los Angeles, Research Center on the Psychobiology of Ethnicity and Department of Psychiatry, Harbor-UCLA Research and Education Institute, Torrance, California

Laurie A. Lindamer, Ph.D.
Assistant Adjunct Professor of Psychiatry, Department of Psychiatry, University of California, San Diego, VA San Diego Healthcare System, San Diego, California

Rachel Loewy, B.A.
Graduate student, Department of Psychology, Emory University, Atlanta, Georgia

Deborah Marin, M.D.
Director of Geriatric Psychiatry, Vice Chair of Psychiatry, and Associate Professor, Department of Psychiatry, Mount Sinai Medical School, New York, New York

Elaine McParland, M.D., J.D.
Research Consultant, Department of Geriatrics, Mount Sinai Medical School, New York, New York

Ricardo P. Mendoza, M.D.
Professor of Psychiatry, University of California—Los Angeles School of Medicine, Los Angeles, California

Scott D. Moffat, Ph.D.
National Institutes of Health Postdoctoral Fellow, Gerontology Research Center, National Institute on Aging, Baltimore, Maryland

Judith Neugroschl, M.D.
Assistant Clinical Professor, Department of Psychiatry, Mt. Sinai Medical School, New York, New York

Grace O'Leary, M.D.
Instructor in Psychiatry, Harvard Medical School; Medical Director, Partial Hospital Program, McLean Hospital, Belmont, Massachusetts

Jill A. Panetta, Ph.D.
Chief Scientific Officer, InnoCentive, Indianapolis, Indiana

Cheryl Paradis, Psy.D.
Associate Professor, Marymount Manhattan College; and Associate Clinical Professor, Department of Psychiatry, State University of New York Health Science Center at Brooklyn, Brooklyn, New York

Susan M. Resnick, Ph.D.
Senior Staff Fellow, Laboratory of Personality and Cognition, Gerontology Research Center, National Institute on Aging, Baltimore, Maryland

David A. Ruskin, M.D.
Assistant Clinical Professor of Psychiatry, University of California—Los Angeles School of Medicine, Los Angeles, California

Mary V. Seeman, M.D.C.M., F.R.C.P.C., F.A.C.P.
Emeritus Professor of Psychiatry, University of Toronto, Centre for Addiction and Mental Health, Toronto, Ontario, Canada

Lisa C. Smith, Ph.D.
Assistant Clinical Professor, Department of Psychiatry, State University of New York Health Science Center at Brooklyn, Brooklyn, New York

Michael W. Smith, M.D.
Associate Professor of Psychiatry, University of California—Los Angeles School of Medicine, Los Angeles, California

John J. Sramek, Pharm.D.
Director of Research, California Clinical Trials, Beverly Hills, California

Meir Steiner, M.D., Ph.D., F.R.C.P.C.
Professor of Psychiatry and Behavioral Neurosciences and Obstetrics and Gynecology, McMaster University; Director of Research, Department of Psychiatry; and Director, Women's Health Concerns Clinic, St. Joseph's Healthcare, Hamilton, Ontario, Canada

Zachary N. Stowe, M.D.
Associate Professor of Psychiatry, Emory University, Department of Psychiatry and Behavioral Sciences, Atlanta, Georgia

Michael Strober, Ph.D.
Professor of Psychiatry, Neuropsychiatric Institute and Hospital, School of Medicine, University of California at Los Angeles

Amgad Tanaghow, F.R.C.Psych. (U.K.), F.R.A.N.Z.C.P.
Director of Psychiatry, St. Vincent's Hospital, Fitzroy, Victoria, Australia

Adele C. Viguera, M.D.
Associate Director, Perinatal Psychiatry Program, Massachusetts General Hospital; and Instructor in Psychiatry, Harvard Medical School, Cambridge, Massachusetts

Deborah J. Walder, M.D.
Graduate student, Department of Psychology, Emory University, Atlanta, Georgia

Elaine F. Walker, Ph.D.
Samuel Candler Dobbs Professor of Psychology and Neuroscience, Department of Psychology, Emory University, Atlanta, Georgia

Teresa S. Williams, B.Sc.
Clinical Development Associate, Eli Lilly and Company, Indianapolis, Indiana

Cheryl M. Wong, M.D.
Assistant Professor of Psychiatry, Mount Sinai School of Medicine, Department of Psychiatry, Bronx Veterans Affairs Medical Center, Bronx, New York

Rachel Yehuda, Ph.D.
Professor of Psychiatry, Mount Sinai School of Medicine, Department of Psychiatry, Bronx Veterans Affairs Medical Center, Bronx, New York

Kimberly A. Yonkers, M.D.
Associate Professor, Department of Psychiatry, Yale University School of Medicine, New Haven, Connecticut

Foreword

Nancy C. Andreasen, M.D., Ph.D.

*F*or most of its history, medicine has assumed that the archetypal physician would be a man. Research studies of the treatment or natural history of diseases usually were done in men. Likewise, the "typical" patient that physicians were taught to interview or treat was also male. Medication dosages were taught in a "one size fits all" framework, without any recognition of possible sex differences in body size or drug metabolism. The reasons for the emphasis on the study of males are perhaps understandable. Women were excluded from leadership roles in everything—not just medicine. Their exclusion from research studies was partly done out of a genuine desire to protect them from exposure to unnecessary risk, and their cyclical endocrine changes could make the interpretation of research data more difficult as well.

However, women constitute 50% (or even slightly more) of the human race. It does seem only fair, therefore, that they should be represented in professions such as medicine and as subjects in the study of human diseases. Fortunately, we live in an era when "women's health" has become an important emphasis in medicine and when women have at last been admitted to the medical profession as equal partners. Both men and women are enjoying the benefits of this change.

As this book illustrates, our understanding of psychiatric illnesses in women has benefited substantially from these relatively recent efforts to understand sex differences in the onset, presentation, course, and treatment of mental illnesses. Epidemiological studies have shown that mental illnesses may sometimes have striking differences in prevalence, suggesting that biological and psychosocial factors may interact to produce important differences in pathophysiology and etiology. Why, for example, is schizophrenia more common in men, and why does it have an earlier onset and a more malignant course than in women? Why do women have higher rates of mood disorders? Do estrogens exert a protective effect in illnesses such as schizophrenia and Alzheimer's disease? Should premenstrual syndromes be considered a "normal" experience or an illness? Why did anorexia nervosa and bulimia nervosa become so prevalent in the late twentieth century? Why do these eating disorders occur primarily in young women? How do men and women differ in their response to traumatic experiences? Why do women have a lower rate of substance abuse than men do? Are there secular trends in the changing prevalence of various psychiatric disorders in men and women? If so, what do these mean?

These are all interesting questions. This book was assembled as an up-to-date summary of the answers. In addition, important issues concerning both psychological and pharmacological treatment of psychiatric illnesses in women are examined. It provides useful information about recent developments in psychopharmacology. A more sex-aware approach to choosing medication doses is replacing the old "one size fits all" approach. Physicians are increasingly aware that, in addition to body size, factors such as liver enzymes or neuroendocrine interactions may affect the metabolism and bioavailability of drugs. Furthermore, illnesses that manifest differently in women or are specific to women are described and discussed.

Psychiatric illnesses may have a very different effect on women and men because of their different social responsibilities and societal expectations. Despite the changes produced by the women's movement, women still play the major role in caring both for children and for older parents.

This book also provides a helpful guide to the most recent developments in our understanding of the interaction between social and biological factors in the manifestations and treatment of mental illnesses in women, and it examines their effect on psychosocial treatment as well as pharmacological treatment.

Psychiatric Illness in Women should fill an important niche by giving readers a comprehensive and up-to-date summary of this timely topic.

Preface

*T*his book represents a small piece of the accumulating scientific knowledge that has been documented for major differences in the brain anatomy, physiology, and epidemiology of psychiatric disease in women. Reading through this text, one may realize that some of the information has been discovered quite recently and through serendipity. We hope that this current information will help guide and support decisions toward a better possible way of diagnosing and managing psychiatric diseases in women.

It is our sincere hope that this collected body of information will provide stimulation for the development of a cohesive and strategic agenda centered on research on women and psychiatric illnesses in women's health. It is also our hope to see this agenda translate into the appropriate treatments for women in the clinical environment; consequently, this novel scientific knowledge will not only be "esoteric" but also add to the diagnosis and management of psychiatric illnesses in women.

ACKNOWLEDGMENTS

We would like to take this opportunity to extend our deepest appreciation to our contributing authors and American Psychiatric Publishing for their unquestioning confidence and unwavering support. We recognize Drs. John Sramek and Edyta Frackiweicz for their timely editorial comments and Mary Beth Moster for providing assistance in our hour of need. We also thank our families for their love and encouragement during the production of this text. We extend our gratitude to our senior medical editor,

Marjorie A. Remmo, whose skills and patience made a complex undertaking seem extremely uncomplicated. We would finally like to express our sincere admiration for Eli Lilly and Company's Neuroscience Therapeutic Area (NSTA) and the Lilly Centre for Women's Health (LCWH). This text would have never been completed without the devoted support and commitment of the NSTA to advance research and understanding in the psychiatric and neurologic fields and without the dedicated encouragement and sponsorship of the LCWH toward the continuing focus on women's health.

DEDICATION

This text is dedicated to Dr. John Naden and to his lovely wife, Yolanda. This dedication is done in appreciation for their most beloved hospitality to the late Micaela Morales Herrera and her immediate and extended family in their hour of need. Suffice it to say some personal debts can never be repaid.

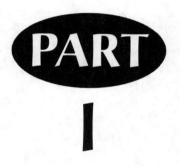

PART

1

Anxiety Disorders and Other Related Disorders

Introduction

*A*nxiety is considered a normal coping response, and for a person without an anxiety disorder, it can provide a means of arousal in response to a possible dangerous or unfamiliar situation. Symptoms such as increased heart rate, nervousness, and tension are included in this heightened awareness, and this sharpened attentiveness can lead to a positive outcome to the situation, such as being astute during a job interview. In contrast, *anxiety disorders* have negative effects on individuals, which can keep them from being able to cope with everyday life because of intense arousal in inappropriate situations. This illness of the nervous system is the most common type of mental disorder, with 15%–20% of the human population having some type of anxiety disorder. Additionally, sex differences have been found among anxiety disorders, with most of these disorders being more prevalent in women than in men.

In this part, the authors review sex differences in panic disorder and agoraphobia, posttraumatic stress disorder, and substance abuse disorder associated with posttraumatic stress disorder.

Although panic disorder with or without agoraphobia is more common in women than in men, the profile of symptoms does not differ between the sexes. A discussion of factors that affect women with panic disorder and comorbid psychiatric and medical disorders is presented within the first two chapters of this part. Included in this discussion are details about the effect of the reproductive life cycle, psychosocial variables, and treatment variables.

The third chapter includes recent epidemiological studies showing that women are affected by posttraumatic stress disorder more than men are, along with discussion about the differential vulnerability to trauma and the rate of development of posttraumatic stress disorder between the sexes.

This part features research that continues to uncover promising hypotheses for anxiety disorders. We hope that this research will further explain sex differences in prevalence rates and lead to more optimum therapies for anxiety disorders in the future.

1

Sex Differences in Anxiety Disorders

Kimberly A. Yonkers, M.D.
Cindy L. Kidner, M.A.

Sex differences exist in the prevalence and expression of many psychiatric disorders. For example, alcoholism and antisocial personality disorder are more common among men, whereas eating disorders and mood disorders are more common among women (Robins et al. 1984). Sex differences occur in the various anxiety disorders, both in prevalence and in the expression of the illness (Robins et al. 1984). This chapter is a review of the available information about sex differences in anxiety disorders and a discussion of hypothetical explanatory mechanisms. Sections of this chapter are an update of a previous review of the treatment of anxiety disorders in women (Yonkers and Gurguis 1995).

Approximately 10%–20% of the patients in general medical settings have an anxiety disorder, including phobias, panic disorder, generalized anxiety disorder (GAD), obsessive-compulsive disorder (OCD), and post-traumatic stress disorder (PTSD). Women are more likely to seek medical and psychiatric care for the distress associated with anxiety disorders, and women use more tranquilizers than do men (Verburgge and Steiner 1985). Significant sex differences are manifested in all of the anxiety disorders. An analysis of the causes of these sex differences could lead to a better understanding of the psychological and biological factors that underlie anxiety disorders. Unfortunately, as Cameron and Hill (1989) noted, little is known about sex-related features or mechanisms associated with anxiety disorders. Sex differences in the anxiety disorders have been attributed to genetics, to sex-role socialization, and to hormonal influences; all three elements are likely to play a role.

Regarding hormonal differences, ovarian hormones and their metabolites have bioactive effects and can directly contribute to the occurrence of or susceptibility to panic. The A-ring reduced progesterone metabolites allopregnenolone and tetrahydrodeoxycorticosterone bind to the γ-aminobutyric acid A (GABA$_A$) receptor in a partial agonist fashion (Majewska and Schwartz 1987). GABA agonists diminish anxiety, possibly by their inhibitory effects on adrenergic neurotransmission (Cameron et al. 1990). In a genetically prone individual, the repetitive binding and unbinding of these endogenous compounds may influence the biological propensity to develop panic and other forms of anxiety in women.

Other factors also are involved; for example, Jones and colleagues (1983) found menstrual cycle variations in the amount of adrenergic receptor binding. Furthermore, during the middle portion of the menstrual cycle, when estrogen levels peak and progesterone levels are low, noradrenergic sensitivity is increased, as shown by sensitivity to tyramine-induced blood pressure elevation (Ghose and Turner 1977; Hamilton 1991). Finally, if the neurotransmitter serotonin is involved in the expression of panic symptoms, progesterone may play a role in modulating serotonin neurotransmission. Progesterone receptors have been found on serotonin neurons in the dorsal and ventral raphe nuclei of primates (Bethea 1993).

PHOBIAS

The three major phobias are specific phobia (formerly known as simple phobia), social phobia, and agoraphobia. The sex ratio of each is shown in Table 1–1.

TABLE 1–1.   Lifetime prevalence of phobias in men and women in the Epidemiological Catchment Area survey

	Men (%)	Women (%)
Panic disorder with agoraphobia	2.9	7.7
Specific phobia	4.0	9.0
Social phobia	2.0	3.1

Source.   Rates taken from Robins et al. 1984 and Schneier et al. 1992.

Women experience a disproportionate number of all phobias compared with men. Several authors have proposed that developmental and sociological factors may be responsible and that the early onset of phobias and the longevity of these illnesses seem to implicate early developmental experiences. For example, one author suggested that women learn "helplessness, avoidance of mastery experiences, competition and lack of assertiveness" (Fodor 1974).

Specific Phobia

Description

Specific phobia is a marked and persistent fear of circumscribed objects or situations (Marks 1987). According to the DSM-IV-TR (American Psychiatric Association 2000) criteria for specific phobia (Table 1–2), the individual's fear of the phobic object or situation causes social or occupational impairment or significant emotional distress. More than 80% of the individuals who develop a specific phobia will do so before age 25 years (Bourdon et al. 1988).

Few individuals seek treatment for specific phobia, which may account for low prevalence rates in treatment settings. Specific phobias are more commonly detected when patients seek treatment for another disorder such as depression. A specific phobia may seriously affect a person's work or lifestyle, even if the individual does not seek treatment. For example, a person who would like to travel for work or pleasure may be inhibited or inconvenienced by a phobia about flying.

Sex Differences

Few studies have evaluated sex differences in phobias, and most researchers do not present their data in a way in which subgroups can be compared. The few available reports find that women are at three to four times greater risk of developing specific phobias than are men (Bourdon et al. 1988; Schneier et al. 1992). Even with functional impairment as a diagnostic restriction, community samples show 6-month prevalence rates of 9% in women and 4% in men (Bourdon et al. 1988).

The Fear Survey Schedule, developed by Wolpe and Lang (1964), is a common tool used in psychiatry and psychology to assess the severity of phobias. Thyer and colleagues (1985) reported that women tend to score higher on this instrument than do men, although the difference is not likely to be clinically significant. One study found that animal phobias are the most heritable phobias and appear to have the earliest onset in women (Kendler et al. 1992). Several groups have analyzed sex differences in the items identified as most fearful. Men and women identify similar fears,

---

TABLE 1–2.   DSM-IV-TR diagnostic criteria for specific phobia

---

A. Marked and persistent fear that is excessive or unreasonable, cued by the presence or anticipation of a specific object or situation (e.g., flying, heights, animals, receiving an injection, seeing blood).

B. Exposure to the phobic stimulus almost invariably provokes an immediate anxiety response, which may take the form of a situationally bound or situationally predisposed Panic Attack.   **Note:** In children, the anxiety may be expressed by crying, tantrums, freezing, or clinging.

C. The person recognizes that the fear is excessive or unreasonable.   **Note:** In children, this feature may be absent.

D. The phobic situation(s) is avoided or else is endured with intense anxiety or distress.

E. The avoidance, anxious anticipation, or distress in the feared situation(s) interferes significantly with the person's normal routine, occupational (or academic) functioning, or social activities or relationships, or there is marked distress about having the phobia.

F. In individuals under age 18 years, the duration is at least 6 months.

G. The anxiety, Panic Attacks, or phobic avoidance associated with the specific object or situation are not better accounted for by another mental disorder, such as Obsessive-Compulsive Disorder (e.g., fear of dirt in someone with an obsession about contamination), Posttraumatic Stress Disorder (e.g., avoidance of stimuli associated with a severe stressor), Separation Anxiety Disorder (e.g., avoidance of school), Social Phobia (e.g., avoidance of social situations because of fear of embarrassment), Panic Disorder With Agoraphobia, or Agoraphobia Without History of Panic Disorder.

Specify type:

   Animal Type
   Natural Environment Type (e.g., heights, storms, water)
   Blood-Injection-Injury Type
   Situational Type (e.g., airplanes, elevators, enclosed places)
   Other Type (e.g., fear of choking, vomiting, or contracting an illness; in children, fear of loud sounds or costumed characters)

---

although the way in which they rank the severity differs slightly (Bourdon et al. 1988; Thyer et al. 1985). Additionally, the physiological response to these sources of fear appears to be analogous in men and women (Katkin and Hoffman 1975).

Need for Future Research

Given the disproportionate risk for phobias in men and women, more work needs to be done exploring sex differences in the type of, severity of, and precipitants to specific phobias. Given the higher severity in women reported in one study, it is important to explore whether impairment differs in men and women.

Social Phobia

Description

According to DSM-IV-TR, the persistent fear of situations in which an individual may be open to scrutiny by others is known as social phobia. Social phobia has a greater effect on the quality of an individual's life than does a specific phobia (Table 1–3) in that avoidance may impair daily functioning, and individuals go to great lengths to evade the feared social situation. Social phobia differs from agoraphobia in that individuals do not fear large crowds per se; rather, they fear being observed or examined by either a crowd or an individual. The Epidemiologic Catchment Area (ECA) survey reported that 56% of the individuals with social phobia developed the disorder by age 15 years, and more than 85% developed the disorder by age 28 years (Schneier et al. 1992). Only 5% of the individuals with social phobia seek psychiatric treatment (Schneier et al. 1992).

Patients with social phobia frequently have comorbid conditions. The most common of these conditions are specific phobia, agoraphobia, major depressive disorder, and alcohol abuse (Schneier et al. 1992). In clinical populations, depression and suicidal ideation are found in more than 90% of the patients and alcohol abuse is seen in as many as 50% (Liebowitz et al. 1985; Uhde et al. 1991).

The disorder may be categorized into two types: generalized social phobia and limited social phobia. In the generalized form of the disorder, patients have global fears of social situations such as attending parties or classes where they may receive attention and be subject to scrutiny. Limited social phobia is the fear of embarrassment or negative criticism in specific situations, such as public speaking or playing an instrument in a performance. To be properly classified as social phobia, the fear must be significant enough to cause distress or impairment.

Sex Differences

Social phobia is less common in women than specific phobia or agoraphobia. However, social phobia occurs more frequently in women than in men. According to community data (Schneier et al. 1992), the lifetime prevalence rate for social phobia is about 2.4%, of which 70% are women. A logistic regression analysis showed social phobia is associated not only with being female but also with being single, of younger age, of lower socioeconomic status, and of lesser education (Schneier et al. 1992). More men than women are seen in clinical settings, perhaps because women experience relatively less social dysfunction associated with the illness (Marks 1987).

A specialty clinic–based study examined severity for a variety of social fears in men and women and found significant differences (Turk et al.

TABLE 1–3.   DSM-IV-TR diagnostic criteria for social phobia

A. A marked and persistent fear of one or more social or performance situations in which the person is exposed to unfamiliar people or to possible scrutiny by others. The individual fears that he or she will act in a way (or show anxiety symptoms) that will be humiliating or embarrassing. **Note:** In children, there must be evidence of the capacity for age-appropriate social relationships with familiar people and the anxiety must occur in peer settings, not just in interactions with adults.

B. Exposure to the feared social situation almost invariably provokes anxiety, which may take the form of a situationally bound or situationally predisposed Panic Attack. **Note:** In children, the anxiety may be expressed by crying, tantrums, freezing, or shrinking from social situations with unfamiliar people.

C. The person recognizes that the fear is excessive or unreasonable. **Note:** In children, this feature may be absent.

D. The feared social or performance situations are avoided or else are endured with intense anxiety or distress.

E. The avoidance, anxious anticipation, or distress in the feared social or performance situation(s) interferes significantly with the person's normal routine, occupational (academic) functioning, or social activities or relationships, or there is marked distress about having the phobia.

F. In individuals under age 18 years, the duration is at least 6 months.

G. The fear or avoidance is not due to the direct physiological effects of a substance (e.g., a drug of abuse, a medication) or a general medical condition and is not better accounted for by another mental disorder (e.g., Panic Disorder With or Without Agoraphobia, Separation Anxiety Disorder, Body Dysmorphic Disorder, a Pervasive Developmental Disorder, or Schizoid Personality Disorder).

H. If a general medical condition or another mental disorder is present, the fear in Criterion A is unrelated to it, e.g., the fear is not of Stuttering, trembling in Parkinson's disease, or exhibiting abnormal eating behavior in Anorexia Nervosa or Bulimia Nervosa.

Specify if:

>   **Generalized:**   if the fears include most social situations (also consider the additional diagnosis of Avoidant Personality Disorder)

1998). Women experienced greater difficulties with speaking to authority figures, public speaking, being observed while working or entering a room, being the center of attention, voicing disagreement, and giving a party. For men, fear was greater for using public bathrooms. Although this study did not find sex differences in the rates of comorbidity among men and women with social phobia, other studies diverge. In a clinic-based report, comorbidity with agoraphobia was higher among women, whereas men with social phobia were more likely to have an additional substance abuse diagnosis (Yonkers et al. 2001).

Potential sex differences in the course of social phobia have been examined (Yonkers et al. 2001). Likelihood of remission was equally poor between both sexes; after 8 years of longitudinal follow-up, only 38% of women and 32% of men had full remission. Particularly poor prognosis was found for subjects who had poor global functioning at study outset or had a history of suicide attempts. In both cases, the women from these subgroups were far less likely to experience remission than were the men.

Need for Future Research

The impairment associated with social phobia has only recently begun to receive recognition. Research should investigate why women with social phobia are less likely to be recognized and to seek treatment. More research on the course of social phobia is needed to identify and understand those with particularly poor prognoses. Treatments should be evaluated for relative efficacy in both men and women.

Agoraphobia

Description

Agoraphobia, derived from the Greek word *agora*, meaning marketplace, is a fear of public places, particularly crowded places (Marks 1987). Agoraphobia may or may not be associated with panic disorder (see "Panic Disorder" section later in this chapter). In DSM-III (American Psychiatric Association 1980), agoraphobia applied to patients who had phobic avoidance, with or without panic. DSM-III-R (American Psychiatric Association 1987) defined the following categories:

- Agoraphobia without history of panic disorder
- Panic disorder with agoraphobia
- Panic disorder without agoraphobia

DSM-IV-TR maintains this distinction (Tables 1–4A and 1–4B). This change reflects the view that agoraphobia may develop as a consequence of panic attacks (Klein and Gorman 1987), although some maintain that the phobia occurs first and that panic is simply a common manifestation of exposure to a feared object (Marks 1987). More than 70% of the patients with agoraphobia develop the illness before age 25 years, and 50% of the patients may develop it before age 15 years (Von Korff et al. 1985).

Sex Differences

Based on the DSM-III definition, the sex difference in prevalence rates for agoraphobia, with or without panic attacks, is striking. Nearly 8% of the

---

TABLE 1–4A. DSM–IV–TR diagnostic criteria for panic disorder with agoraphobia

A. Both (1) and (2):
  (1) recurrent unexpected Panic Attacks
  (2) at least one of the attacks has been followed by 1 month (or more) of one (or more) of the following:
    (a) persistent concern about having additional attacks
    (b) worry about the implications of the attack or its consequences (e.g., losing control, having a heart attack, "going crazy")
    (c) a significant change in behavior related to the attacks
B. The presence of Agoraphobia.
C. The Panic Attacks are not due to the direct physiological effects of a substance (e.g., a drug of abuse, a medication) or a general medical condition (e.g., hyperthyroidism).
D. The Panic Attacks are not better accounted for by another mental disorder, such as Social Phobia (e.g., occurring on exposure to feared social situations), Specific Phobia (e.g., on exposure to a specific phobic situation), Obsessive-Compulsive Disorder (e.g., on exposure to dirt in someone with an obsession about contamination), Posttraumatic Stress Disorder (e.g., in response to stimuli associated with a severe stressor), or Separation Anxiety Disorder (e.g., in response to being away from home or close relatives).

TABLE 1–4B. DSM–IV–TR diagnostic criteria for agoraphobia without history of panic disorder

A. The presence of Agoraphobia related to fear of developing panic-like symptoms (e.g., dizziness or diarrhea).
B. Criteria have never been met for Panic Disorder.
C. The disturbance is not due to the direct physiological effects of a substance (e.g., a drug of abuse, a medication) or a general medical condition.
D. If an associated general medical condition is present, the fear described in Criterion A is clearly in excess of that usually associated with the condition.

---

women in the ECA survey had agoraphobia, whereas only 3% of the men appeared to have the disorder (Bourdon et al. 1988). Men, however, were more likely to inform their physician about their illness than were women in one study (Bourdon et al. 1988). A disproportionate sex ratio was also discovered in the National Comorbidity Survey, which used DSM-IV (American Psychiatric Association 1994) criteria and found that 3.5% of the men and 7.0% of the women had a lifetime episode of agoraphobia (Kessler et al. 1994). Work from other countries, including Canada (Bland et al. 1988), Germany (Wittchen et al. 1992), and Taiwan (Hwu et al. 1989), also found a greater propensity for women to have agoraphobia, suggesting that this is a cross-cultural phenomenon.

Fodor (1974) suggested that women are not taught mastery and assertiveness, tools that are helpful in overcoming fears and phobias. She also speculated that for women in unequal marriages, economic concerns and the traditional fears that accompany the female marital role may lead to agoraphobia. However, because the age at onset may be quite early (see previous subsection), it is unlikely that unhappy marriages are the predominant cause of agoraphobia (Bourdon et al. 1988). Interestingly, the severity of agoraphobia in women is inversely correlated with their scores on masculinity scales, supporting the notion that sex-role socialization may be a factor in susceptibility to agoraphobia (Chambless and Mason 1986).

Although sex differences do not appear to be a factor in the average age at onset of agoraphobia (Bourdon et al. 1988), the peak years for illness onset are broader for women than for men (Eaton et al. 1994; Von Korff et al. 1985), suggesting a longer period of high risk for women. Ongoing work indicates that more than 80% of the patients are symptomatic for at least 1 year after their agoraphobia is detected, with men and women having about the same risk of remaining ill (Yonkers et al. 1998).

Need for Future Research

The age at onset of agoraphobia is early. Future work should include cohorts of children, adolescents, and young adults to better understand the sex differences in prevalence rates. After the illness begins, the clinical course appears equivalent in men and women. Nonetheless, treatment interventions should be evaluated for their efficacy in both men and women.

PANIC DISORDER

Description

Initially, a patient with a panic attack presents in medical or psychiatric settings with the fear that his or her symptoms are those of a heart attack or a life-threatening illness. The panic attack itself is a sudden paroxysm that comprises four or more of the following somatic symptoms: shortness of breath, sweating, trembling, choking, nausea, dizziness, chills or hot flushes, feelings of unreality, numbness or tingling, heart palpitations, and chest discomfort. Patients also feel out of control or fear that something catastrophic is about to occur. Symptom onset is acute, but symptoms dissipate gradually. To meet DSM-IV-TR criteria for panic disorder (Table 1–5), panic attacks must be recurrent, unprovoked, and followed by 1 month or more of persistent concern about having additional attacks or significant behavioral change related to the attacks. Men and women report the same profile of panic symptoms (Chambless and Mason 1986; Scheibe

TABLE 1–5.	DSM–IV–TR criteria for panic attack

Note: A Panic Attack is not a codable disorder. Code the specific diagnosis in which the Panic Attack occurs (e.g., 300.21 Panic Disorder With Agoraphobia).

A discrete period of intense fear or discomfort, in which four (or more) of the following symptoms developed abruptly and reached a peak within 10 minutes:

(1) palpitations, pounding heart, or accelerated heart rate
(2) sweating
(3) trembling or shaking
(4) sensations of shortness of breath or smothering
(5) feeling of choking
(6) chest pain or discomfort
(7) nausea or abdominal distress
(8) feeling dizzy, unsteady, lightheaded, or faint
(9) derealization (feelings of unreality) or depersonalization (being detached from oneself)
(10) fear of losing control or going crazy
(11) fear of dying
(12) paresthesias (numbness or tingling sensations)
(13) chills or hot flushes

and Albus 1992), but sex differences are seen, as noted in the following subsection.

Genetic studies indicate a heritable component to the etiology of panic disorder. First-degree relatives of probands with panic disorder are five times more likely to develop panic disorder with agoraphobia than are relatives of probands without panic disorder (Crowe et al. 1983).

Concurrent medical disorders, such as mitral valve prolapse and hyperthyroidism, also may be biological contributors to the onset of panic (Lohr et al. 1986).

Sex Differences

In women, frequency rates of uncomplicated panic are lower than rates for agoraphobia, but uncomplicated panic is still two to three times more common in women than in men, as reported below. The community rate for uncomplicated panic ranges from 16 to 21 per 1,000 women and 6 to 9 per 1,000 men (Eaton et al. 1991). In addition to frequent comorbidity with agoraphobia, panic disorder in women is commonly seen with specific phobia, GAD, and major depressive disorder (Scheibe and Albus 1992). Although concurrent alcohol abuse and dependence commonly occur in women with panic disorder (Nunes et al. 1988; Yonkers et al. 1998), this relation is stronger for men (Nunes et al. 1988; Yonkers et al. 1998).

Genetic studies indicate that female relatives of probands show a rate of panic disorder with agoraphobia that is three times higher than for male relatives, but male relatives are more likely to have alcoholism. Uncomplicated panic is also more prevalent in female relatives of probands than in male relatives (Crowe et al. 1983).

Mitral valve prolapse and hyperthyroidism, which have been associated with panic disorder, also occur more frequently in women than in men (Lohr et al. 1986). It is not clear whether the association is causal. Some have suggested that the somatic symptoms associated with these general medical conditions may be misinterpreted as catastrophic, forming the nidus of a panicogenic cognition (Clark 1986). If this is true, it may be a factor contributing to the higher rates of panic in women.

Sex differences in the duration of panic have been found in older studies that evaluated the course of illness retrospectively (Maier and Buller 1988; Noyes et al. 1980). In these studies, women had a more protracted course than did men. A more recent short-interval, prospective, follow-up study extended the results of these older studies by showing that women with uncomplicated panic were equally likely to experience a remission, but they were twice as likely to have a recurrence as their male colleagues (Yonkers et al. 1998). In addition, women were more likely to have agoraphobia with panic, and this comorbid condition decreased the likelihood of remitting from the illness (Yonkers et al. 1998). These two findings explain the earlier observations of a longer episode of illness for women with panic compared with men.

Premenstrual hormone changes also may play a role in panic disorder. For example, although men and women report the same profile of panic symptoms, many women complain of premenstrual worsening of panic. This phenomenon has been assessed in three small cohorts. Among women who retrospectively complained of premenstrual worsening, Cameron et al. (1988) found only a small increase in panic. Similarly, Cook et al. (1990) did not find an increase in panic but did find an increase in overall anxiety levels during the premenstrual phase. Among women with panic, Stein et al. (1989) did not find luteal phase worsening of panic, but among a comparison group of women with documented premenstrual dysphoric disorder, they did find greater anxiety premenstrually. Of note, women with premenstrual disorders are prone to develop panic after exposure to a variety of anxiogenic compounds, including lactate, carbon dioxide, CCK antagonists, and benzodiazepine antagonists (Facchinetti et al. 1992; Harrison et al. 1989; Le Melledo et al. 1995, 2000). Premenstrual increases in anxiety in some women and the sensitivity of those with premenstrual dysphoria to panic suggest a role for ovarian hormones in modulating vulnerability to anxiety and panic. Analogous mechanisms may be responsible for postpartum anxiety and panic in women (Metz et al. 1988).

Need for Future Research

The association of premenstrual hormone changes with panic disorder needs further exploration. Biological differences in vulnerability may influence the sex difference in prevalence of panic disorder. As noted in the beginning of this chapter, fluctuating levels of sex hormones may influence neurotransmitter systems or other physiological parameters and change the thresholds for symptom development. For example, progesterone causes a mild chronic hyperventilation (Damas-Mora et al. 1980). Carr and Sheehan (1984) suggested that this luteal phase increase in ventilation increases the likelihood of panic in susceptible people. On the other hand, Klein (1993), who maintains that panic develops from triggering of a "suffocation alarm," believes that the decrease in hyperventilation after progesterone withdrawal provokes panic. Provocation tests could investigate the role of gonadal steroids, endogenous hormonal fluctuations, and sex in the genesis of panic attacks.

GENERALIZED ANXIETY DISORDER

Description

The original conceptualization of GAD centered on the anxiety associated with panic and phobic disorders. GAD was meant to describe the anticipatory anxiety seen in panic and phobic states, the anxious prodrome that occurs before panic, and the residual anxiety that lingers after an attack. The DSM-IV-TR criteria for GAD include both physical and cognitive manifestations of anxiety (Table 1–6). The physical manifestations include fatigue, restlessness, muscle tension, and sleep disturbance. Cognitive features include worry and apprehension. Under DSM-III criteria, a hierarchy of all other anxiety disorders and depression had to be considered before a diagnosis of GAD could be given. DSM-III-R and DSM-IV retained the hierarchical exclusion of major depressive disorder and stipulated that the worry experienced not be restricted to concerns about phobias, panic, obsessions, or compulsions. The ECA survey reported that a diagnosis of GAD is not associated with greater comorbidity for panic and agoraphobia (Blazer et al. 1991), although others find a high association between GAD and depression (Kendler et al. 1992; Kessler et al. 1998; Merikangas et al. 1985).

Sex Differences

Based on the DSM-III criterion of 1 month of illness, the ECA survey reported that GAD occurs twice as often in women as in men. Depending on the exclusionary criteria used, 1-year prevalence rates ranged from 2.4% to

---

TABLE 1–6.   DSM-IV-TR diagnostic criteria for generalized anxiety disorder

A. Excessive anxiety and worry (apprehensive expectation), occurring more days than not for at least 6 months, about a number of events or activities (such as work or school performance).

B. The person finds it difficult to control the worry.

C. The anxiety and worry are associated with three (or more) of the following six symptoms (with at least some symptoms present for more days than not for the past 6 months).   **Note:** Only one item is required in children.

    (1) restlessness or feeling keyed up or on edge
    (2) being easily fatigued
    (3) difficulty concentrating or mind going blank
    (4) irritability
    (5) muscle tension
    (6) sleep disturbance (difficulty falling or staying asleep, or restless unsatisfying sleep)

D. The focus of the anxiety and worry is not confined to features of an Axis I disorder, e.g., the anxiety or worry is not about having a Panic Attack (as in Panic Disorder), being embarrassed in public (as in Social Phobia), being contaminated (as in Obsessive-Compulsive Disorder), being away from home or close relatives (as in Separation Anxiety Disorder), gaining weight (as in Anorexia Nervosa), having multiple physical complaints (as in Somatization Disorder), or having a serious illness (as in Hypochondriasis), and the anxiety and worry do not occur exclusively during Posttraumatic Stress Disorder.

E. The anxiety, worry, or physical symptoms cause clinically significant distress or impairment in social, occupational, or other important areas of functioning.

F. The disturbance is not due to the direct physiological effects of a substance (e.g., a drug of abuse, a medication) or a general medical condition (e.g., hyperthyroidism) and does not occur exclusively during a Mood Disorder, a Psychotic Disorder, or a Pervasive Developmental Disorder.

5.0% for women and from 1.0% to 2.4% for men (Blazer et al. 1991). An epidemiological study specifically investigating this disorder in female twins found a lifetime prevalence of 23.5% and 5.9% with a 1-month and a 6-month definition, respectively (Kendler et al. 1992). The ECA survey did not provide data regarding sex according to the duration of symptoms or the average age at onset (Blazer et al. 1991). Unlike panic disorder, the clinical course of GAD appears to be the same for men and women in that the risks for remission and relapse are approximately equivalent (Yonkers et al. 1996). The co-occurrence of GAD and dysthymia is common in women (Shores et al. 1992).

The genetic basis of panic disorder has been adequately substantiated, but the same is not true of GAD. However, Kendler and colleagues (1992) found that for women, genetic factors play a significant role in the etiology of GAD, regardless of whether the definition for length of illness is 1 or

6 months. This team found that major depressive disorder and GAD share genetic factors in women. They also noted the effect of individual life experiences on the genesis of GAD.

The clinical courses of GAD in men and women have been compared and found to be similar (Yonkers et al. 1996). Whereas Clusters B and C personality disorders are predictive of greater chronicity, patient sex is not (Yonkers et al. 2000). However, this is the case after only up to 5 years of follow-up, and, given the chronicity of the disorder, it is possible that sex differences may occur after longer intervals of evaluation.

Need for Future Research

GAD continues to be a controversial diagnostic category, although the stability of the syndromal criteria is becoming well established. It is still not known why there is a preponderance of the illness in women. The association between GAD and depression may at least in part explain why GAD is more common in women. Further investigations should explore the role of comorbidity in GAD.

OBSESSIVE-COMPULSIVE DISORDER

Description

Obsessions are recurrent ego-dystonic ideas or thoughts, and *compulsions* are behaviors that are repeated in an attempt to ward off anxiety (Table 1–7). Patients with OCD have either obsessions or compulsions or both. OCD ranks fourth in lifetime prevalence among all psychiatric disorders (Robins et al. 1984).

Sex Differences

The ECA survey found similar prevalence rates of OCD for men and women (Robins et al. 1984), contradicting the general belief that the disorder is more common in men (Insel 1990; Rasmussen and Tsuang 1984). The survey did show sex differences in the age at onset (Robins et al. 1984). Several significant features differentiate OCD in men compared with women (Yonkers and Ellison 1996). One study found that males develop OCD between ages 5 and 15 years, whereas females often develop the disorder between ages 26 and 35 years (Noshirvani et al. 1991). The later-onset type of OCD may begin with an episode of depression that improves, while the obsessions and compulsions remain (Welner et al. 1976). In contrast, a prospective study showed that the only subjects who recovered from

TABLE 1–7. DSM-IV-TR diagnostic criteria for obsessive-compulsive disorder

A. Either obsessions or compulsions:

Obsessions as defined by (1), (2), (3), and (4):

(1) recurrent and persistent thoughts, impulses, or images that are experienced, at some time during the disturbance, as intrusive and inappropriate and that cause marked anxiety or distress

(2) the thoughts, impulses, or images are not simply excessive worries about real-life problems

(3) the person attempts to ignore or suppress such thoughts, impulses, or images, or to neutralize them with some other thought or action

(4) the person recognizes that the obsessional thoughts, impulses, or images are a product of his or her own mind (not imposed from without as in thought insertion)

Compulsions as defined by (1) and (2):

(1) repetitive behaviors (e.g., hand washing, ordering, checking) or mental acts (e.g., praying, counting, repeating words silently) that the person feels driven to perform in response to an obsession, or according to rules that must be applied rigidly

(2) the behaviors or mental acts are aimed at preventing or reducing distress or preventing some dreaded event or situation; however, these behaviors or mental acts either are not connected in a realistic way with what they are designed to neutralize or prevent or are clearly excessive

B. At some point during the course of the disorder, the person has recognized that the obsessions or compulsions are excessive or unreasonable. **Note:** This does not apply to children.

C. The obsessions or compulsions cause marked distress, are time consuming (take more than 1 hour a day), or significantly interfere with the person's normal routine, occupational (or academic) functioning, or usual social activities or relationships.

D. If another Axis I disorder is present, the content of the obsessions or compulsions is not restricted to it (e.g., preoccupation with food in the presence of an Eating Disorder; hair pulling in the presence of Trichotillomania; concern with appearance in the presence of Body Dysmorphic Disorder; preoccupation with drugs in the presence of a Substance Use Disorder; preoccupation with having a serious illness in the presence of Hypochondriasis; preoccupation with sexual urges or fantasies in the presence of a Paraphilia; or guilty ruminations in the presence of Major Depressive Disorder).

E. The disturbance is not due to the direct physiological effects of a substance (e.g., a drug of abuse, a medication) or a general medical condition.

Specify if:

With Poor Insight: if, for most of the time during the current episode, the person does not recognize that the obsessions and compulsions are excessive or unreasonable

OCD were women with a dual diagnosis of OCD and depression. Others have noted that depression co-occurs with OCD more often in women than in men (Noshirvani et al. 1991).

Early-onset OCD is associated with a poor prognosis, and males may be more treatment resistant. Because men seek treatment for OCD over longer periods and have greater treatment resistance (Rasmussen and Tsuang 1984), the pre-ECA finding of male predominance is partially explained (Table 1–8). In addition to the length and severity of the disorder, other unique sex-related features include differences in symptoms expressed. Persons who compulsively wash tend to be women, and men are more likely to have checking rituals (Akhtar et al. 1975; Dawson 1977; Noshirvani et al. 1991). In addition, obsessions about food and weight, including diagnoses of anorexia, are more common in women (Kasvikis et al. 1986). A related disorder, trichotillomania, which is the compulsive pulling out of one's hair, also appears to be more prevalent in women (Swedo 1993).

TABLE 1–8.　Sex-divergent features of obsessive-compulsive disorder

Women	Men
Have older age at onset	Frequently engage in checking rituals
Frequently also experience depression and anorexia	Have longer and more severe illness
Engage in compulsive washing	
More often have the associated disorder of trichotillomania	

Need for Future Research

The sex differences in OCD are pronounced. Symptom profiles appear to differ between men and women, and men may have an earlier onset and more treatment resistance. Understanding the underlying psychobiology in these sex differences may be a window into understanding the causes of the illness in both men and women. As with GAD, there is a strong suggestion that the relation between the anxiety disorder and depressive disorder may bear on the sex differences detected. These and other leads should be investigated.

POSTTRAUMATIC STRESS DISORDER

Description

PTSD is a distinctive symptom cluster that develops after an individual experiences or witnesses a life-threatening event. PTSD is most often a sequela of combat exposure or natural disasters, although, particularly in women, PTSD may occur as a result of rape, incest, or childhood sexual abuse. The symptoms of PTSD fall into three categories: 1) reexperiencing of the traumatic event, 2) avoidance or general numbing of responsiveness, and 3) increased sympathetic arousal. Symptoms should be present for at least 1 month to satisfy DSM-IV-TR diagnostic criteria (Table 1–9). The age at onset of PTSD depends on when the traumatic event occurs. Being female, having neuroticism, and having a family history of anxiety or depression are risk factors for developing PTSD, based on a logistic regression model (Bresslau et al. 1991).

A report based on the ECA survey found a surprisingly low lifetime rate of 1% for PTSD (Helzer et al. 1987); the highest prevalence rates in the ECA survey were found among combat veterans (9%) and assault victims (3%). As described below, later studies indicated higher prevalence rates (Breslau and Davis 1992; Breslau et al. 1991).

Various disturbances, such as dissociative experiences, borderline personality disorder, and dissociative identity disorder, are associated with childhood trauma (Hamilton and Jensvold 1992; Herman et al. 1989; Putnam et al. 1986; Ross and Anderson 1988; Soloff and Millward 1983). The reported rate of physical and sexual abuse ranges from 60% to 80% among women with borderline personality disorder (Herman et al. 1989; Soloff and Millward 1983). The rate is at least as high in patients with dissociative identity disorder (Ross and Anderson 1988). Elevated rates of physical and/or sexual abuse are found among children with a diagnosis of borderline personality disorder (Famularo et al. 1991; Goldman et al. 1992). Based on these findings, the question is whether borderline personality disorder is better conceptualized as a variant of chronic PTSD (Hamilton and Jensvold 1992; Saunders and Arnold 1991). Childhood abuse is invasive and is experienced as shameful. The secretive nature of abuse limits a child's ability to seek help, protection, and validation that the abuse is not the child's fault. Furthermore, childhood abuse may occur during critical periods in development when the effect of the trauma can cause pervasive and lasting impairment. Because of this longevity, a patient may present with what seems to be a personality disorder when the true diagnosis actually is PTSD.

In addition to developmental theories, biological theories may be helpful in understanding PTSD. Neurobiological hypotheses on the mechanisms of PTSD invoke the role of various neurotransmitter systems in an attempt to understand the causes of PTSD. The most compelling theories focus on limbic system dysfunction and the interactions of catecholamines and endogenous opioid peptides. Chronic arousal, as manifested by a strong startle response and physical reactivity, is a hallmark of PTSD and

---

TABLE 1–9.   DSM-IV-TR diagnostic criteria for posttraumatic stress disorder

---

A. The person has been exposed to a traumatic event in which both of the following were present:

    (1) the person experienced, witnessed, or was confronted with an event or events that involved actual or threatened death or serious injury, or a threat to the physical integrity of self or others

    (2) the person's response involved intense fear, helplessness, or horror. **Note:** In children, this may be expressed instead by disorganized or agitated behavior

B. The traumatic event is persistently reexperienced in one (or more) of the following ways:

    (1) recurrent and intrusive distressing recollections of the event, including images, thoughts, or perceptions. **Note:** In young children, repetitive play may occur in which themes or aspects of the trauma are expressed.

    (2) recurrent distressing dreams of the event. **Note:** In children, there may be frightening dreams without recognizable content.

    (3) acting or feeling as if the traumatic event were recurring (includes a sense of reliving the experience, illusions, hallucinations, and dissociative flashback episodes, including those that occur on awakening or when intoxicated). **Note:** In young children, trauma-specific reenactment may occur.

    (4) intense psychological distress at exposure to internal or external cues that symbolize or resemble an aspect of the traumatic event

    (5) physiological reactivity on exposure to internal or external cues that symbolize or resemble an aspect of the traumatic event

C. Persistent avoidance of stimuli associated with the trauma and numbing of general responsiveness (not present before the trauma), as indicated by three (or more) of the following:

    (1) efforts to avoid thoughts, feelings, or conversations associated with the trauma

    (2) efforts to avoid activities, places, or people that arouse recollections of the trauma

    (3) inability to recall an important aspect of the trauma

    (4) markedly diminished interest or participation in significant activities

    (5) feeling of detachment or estrangement from others

    (6) restricted range of affect (e.g., unable to have loving feelings)

    (7) sense of a foreshortened future (e.g., does not expect to have a career, marriage, children, or a normal life span)

TABLE 1–9.   DSM-IV-TR diagnostic criteria for posttraumatic stress disorder *(continued)*

D. Persistent symptoms of increased arousal (not present before the trauma), as indicated by two (or more) of the following:
    (1) difficulty falling or staying asleep
    (2) irritability or outbursts of anger
    (3) difficulty concentrating
    (4) hypervigilance
    (5) exaggerated startle response

E. Duration of the disturbance (symptoms in Criteria B, C, and D) is more than 1 month.

F. The disturbance causes clinically significant distress or impairment in social, occupational, or other important areas of functioning.

Specify if:

Acute: if duration of symptoms is less than 3 months
Chronic: if duration of symptoms is 3 months or more

Specify if:

With Delayed Onset: if onset of symptoms is at least 6 months after the stressor

suggests overactivity of adrenergic and possibly dopaminergic systems (Charney et al. 1993). Noradrenergic supersensitivity occurs in the model of inescapable shock (van der Kolk et al. 1985). In this paradigm, an animal's repeated exposure to inescapable shock causes depletion of dopamine and serotonin, thus leading to noradrenergic and dopaminergic supersensitivity and autonomic hyperarousal. Repeated shock also leads to release of endogenous opiates, as seen in animal models of stress-induced analgesia (Charney et al. 1993). Again, after repeated administration of uncontrollable shock, the animals develop endogenous opiate-dependent analgesia to subsequent aversive stimuli. The stress response seen in these animals is believed to be similar to that experienced by humans exposed to trauma. In particular, reexperiencing the trauma of the pain of self-mutilation may lead to an increase in endogenous opiate activity; the soothing opiate response subsequently, perhaps, reinforces these behaviors (van der Kolk et al. 1985). Opioid (endogenous opioid peptides) secretion also may lead to certain dissociative phenomena.

Sex Differences

A large health maintenance organization–based study showed prevalence rates of 11% for women and 7% for men, with an overall rate nine times higher than the rate based on the ECA data (Breslau et al. 1991). Nearly 24% of the individuals exposed to trauma developed symptoms of PTSD (Breslau et al. 1991); 31% of the women and 19% of the men exposed to trauma developed PTSD (Breslau et al. 1991) (Table 1–10).

A subsequent report compared groups with chronic PTSD and those with acute PTSD. The investigators found that although women constituted 65% of the acute PTSD group, they constituted 85% of the chronic group, with symptoms lasting at least 1 year (Breslau and Davis 1992).

Women are less likely to be exposed to traumatic events (Breslau et al. 1991) but more likely to develop psychological distress following exposure to stressful events (Kessler and McLeod 1984). They are also exposed to a greater number of "network events" (e.g., events experienced by people who are intimate with the female subject). The combination of personal traumatic experiences and network events leads to higher psychological stress and greater cumulative stress. Findings by Kessler and McLeod (1984) support psychological theories regarding the importance of other individuals in a woman's emotional health. Miller and Stiver (1993) posit that women need to stay connected to others. The loss of these connections is the antecedent to anxiety and depressive reactions.

As noted earlier in this subsection, PTSD in women has some distinctive features and may occur as a result of trauma, sexual abuse, or incest. Worsening of PTSD symptoms, particularly dissociative episodes during the luteal phase of the menstrual cycle, has been reported (Hamilton 1991). Of note, levels of endogenous opioid peptides vary across a menstrual cycle such that levels increase during the follicular and early luteal phases and decrease just before menses (Chuong et al. 1985; Giannini et al. 1990). Whether fluctuations in the levels of endogenous opioid peptides correlate with PTSD symptoms or with symptoms of dissociation is unknown. The fluctuations in symptoms noted by some clinicians suggest that it does seem judicious to monitor women for menstrual cycle entrainment of symptoms.

TABLE 1–10.   Sex-related features of posttraumatic stress disorder

Community rate in women is 11%.

Community rate in men is 7%.

Chronic symptoms are more likely to develop in women.

Childhood sexual abuse is associated with borderline personality disorder in women.

Posttraumatic stress disorder symptoms may fluctuate across the menstrual cycle.

Need for Future Research

Putative menstrual cycle fluctuations in endogenous opioid peptides and the possible role of endogenous opioid peptides in PTSD are alluring. However, many studies investigating endogenous opioid peptides rely on peripheral measures that may or may not be relevant to brain activity. Future studies should use paradigms to investigate this system in the brain and to include hypotheses to test the role of the patient's sex in the analyses.

SUMMARY

Sex differences exist among the anxiety disorders, with most disorders being more prevalent in women. For panic disorder with agoraphobia and PTSD, the course of illness is longer in women than in men. For OCD, the course of illness is longer and the morbidity is greater in men than in women. Symptom profiles are similar in men and women for panic disorder, phobias, and PTSD, but they may vary for OCD. Ongoing research continues to uncover promising hypotheses for anxiety disorders. In the future, this research may explain sex differences in prevalence rates. It is hoped that research into these factors will provide increasing understanding of the biological, psychological, and developmental substrates for anxiety disorders.

REFERENCES

Akhtar S, Wig NN, Varma VK, et al: A phenomenological analysis of symptoms in obsessive-compulsive neurosis. Br J Psychiatry 127:342–348, 1975

American Psychiatric Association: Diagnostic and Statistical Manual of Mental Disorders, 3rd Edition. Washington, DC, American Psychiatric Association, 1980

American Psychiatric Association: Diagnostic and Statistical Manual of Mental Disorders, 3rd Edition, Revised. Washington, DC, American Psychiatric Association, 1987

American Psychiatric Association: Diagnostic and Statistical Manual of Mental Disorders, 4th Edition. Washington, DC, American Psychiatric Association, 1994

American Psychiatric Association: Diagnostic and Statistical Manual of Mental Disorders, 4th Edition, Text Revision. Washington, DC, American Psychiatric Association, 2000

Bethea CL: Colocalization of progestin receptors with serotonin in raphe neurons of macaque. Neuroendocrinology 57:1–6, 1993

Bland RC, Orn H, Newman SC: Lifetime prevalence of psychiatric disorders in Edmonton. Acta Psychiatr Scand 338(suppl):24–32, 1988

Blazer DG, Hughes D, George LK, et al: Generalized anxiety disorder, in Psychiatric Disorders in America. Edited by Robins LN, Regier DA. New York, Free Press, 1991, pp 181–203

Bourdon KH, Boyd JH, Rae DS, et al: Gender differences in phobias: results of the ECA community survey. J Anxiety Disord 2:227–241, 1988

Breslau N, Davis G: Posttraumatic stress disorder in an urban population of young adults: risk factors for chronicity. Am J Psychiatry 149:671–675, 1992

Breslau N, Davis GC, Andreski P, et al: Traumatic events and posttraumatic stress disorder in an urban population of young adults. Arch Gen Psychiatry 48:216–222, 1991

Cameron OG, Hill EM: Women and anxiety. Psychiatr Clin North Am 12:175–186, 1989

Cameron OG, Kuttesch D, McPhee K, et al: Menstrual fluctuation in the symptoms of panic anxiety. J Affect Disord 15:169–174, 1988

Cameron OG, Smith CB, Lee MA, et al: Adrenergic status in anxiety disorders: platelet alpha 2-adrenergic receptor binding, blood pressure, pulse, and plasma catecholamines in panic and generalized anxiety disorder patients and in normal subjects. Biol Psychiatry 28:3–20, 1990

Carr DB, Sheehan DV: Panic anxiety: a new biological model. J Clin Psychiatry 45:323–330, 1984

Chambless DL, Mason J: Sex, sex-role stereotyping and agoraphobia. Behav Res Ther 24:231–235, 1986

Charney DS, Deutch AY, Krystal JH, et al: Psychobiologic mechanisms of posttraumatic stress disorder. Arch Gen Psychiatry 50:295–305, 1993

Chuong CJ, Coulam CB, Kao PC, et al: Neuropeptide levels in premenstrual syndrome. Fertil Steril 44:760–765, 1985

Clark DM: A cognitive approach to panic. Behav Res Ther 24:461–470, 1986

Cook BL, Noyes R Jr, Garvey MJ, et al: Anxiety and the menstrual cycle in panic disorder. J Affect Disord 19:221–226, 1990

Crowe RR, Noyes R, Pauls DL, et al: A family study of panic disorder. Arch Gen Psychiatry 40:1065–1069, 1983

Damas-Mora J, Davies L, Taylor W, et al: Menstrual respiratory changes and symptoms. Br J Psychiatry 136:492–497, 1980

Dawson JH: The phenomenology of severe obsessive-compulsive neurosis. Br J Psychiatry 131:75–78, 1977

Eaton WW, Dryman A, Weissman MM: Panic and phobia: the diagnosis of panic disorder and phobic disorder, in Psychiatric Disorders in America: The Epidemiologic Catchment Area Study. Edited by Robins LN, Reiger DA. New York, Free Press, 1991, pp 155–203

Eaton WW, Kessler RC, Wittchen HU, et al: Panic and panic disorder in the United States. Am J Psychiatry 151:413–420, 1994

Facchinetti F, Romano G, Fava M, et al: Lactate infusion induces panic attacks in patients with premenstrual syndrome. Psychosom Med 54:288–296, 1992

Famularo R, Kinscherff R, Fenton T: Posttraumatic stress disorder among children clinically diagnosed as borderline personality disorder. J Nerv Ment Dis 179:428–431, 1991

Fodor IG: The phobic syndrome in women: implications for treatment, in Women in Therapy: New Psychotherapies for a Changing Society. Edited by Franks V, Burtle V. New York, Brunner/Mazel, 1974, pp 132–168

Ghose K, Turner P: The menstrual cycle and the tyramine pressor response test. Br J Clin Pharmacol 4:500–502, 1977

Giannini AJ, Martin DM, Turner CE: Beta-endorphin decline in late luteal phase dysphoric disorder. Int J Psychiatry Med 20:279–284, 1990

Goldman SJ, D'Angelo EJ, DeMaso DR, et al: Physical and sexual abuse histories among children with borderline personality disorder. Am J Psychiatry 149:1723–1726, 1992

Hamilton J: Forging a women's health research agenda (conference proceedings), in Clinical Pharmacology Panel Report. Edited by Blementhal SJ, Parry B, Sherwin B. Washington, DC, National Women's Health Resource Center, 1991, pp 1–27

Hamilton JA, Jensvold M: Personality, psychopathology and depression in women, in Personality and Psychopathology: Feminist Reappraisals. Edited by Blumenthal SJ, Parry B, Sherwin B. New York, Guilford, 1992, pp 116–143

Harrison W, Sandberg D, Gorman J, et al: Provocation of panic with carbon dioxide inhalation in patients with premenstrual dysphoria. Psychiatr Res 27:183–192, 1989

Helzer JE, Robins LN, McEvoy L: Post-traumatic stress disorder in the general population: findings of the Epidemiologic Catchment Area survey. N Engl J Med 317:1630–1634, 1987

Herman JL, Perry JC, van der Kolk BA: Childhood trauma in borderline personality disorder. Am J Psychiatry 146:490–495, 1989

Hwu HG, Yeh EK, Chang LY: Prevalence of psychiatric disorders in Taiwan defined by the Chinese Diagnostic Interview Schedule. Acta Psychiatr Scand 79:136–147, 1989

Insel TR: New pharmacologic approaches to obsessive compulsive disorder. J Clin Psychiatry 51(20 suppl):47–51, 1990

Jones SB, Bylund DB, Rieser CA, et al: Alpha 2-adrenergic receptor binding in human platelets: alterations during the menstrual cycle. Clin Pharmacol Ther 34:90–96, 1983

Kasvikis JG, Tsakiris F, Marks IM: Women with obsessive-compulsive disorder frequently report a past history of anorexia nervosa. Int J Eat Disord 5:1069–1075, 1986

Katkin ES, Hoffman LS: Sex differences in phobia and self-report of fear: a psychophysical assessment. J Abnorm Psychol 85:607–610, 1975

Kendler KS, Neale MC, Kessler RC, et al: Generalized anxiety disorder in women: a population-based twin study. Arch Gen Psychiatry 49:267–272, 1992

Kessler RC, McLeod JD: Sex differences in vulnerability to undesirable life events. A Sociological Review 49:620–631, 1984

Kessler RC, McGonagle KA, Zhao S, et al: Lifetime and 12-month prevalence of DSM-III-R psychiatric disorders in the United States: results from the National Comorbidity Survey. Arch Gen Psychiatry 51:8–19, 1994

Kessler R, Stang P, Wittchen H-U, et al: Lifetime panic-depression comorbidity in the National Comorbidity Survey. Arch Gen Psychiatry 55:801–808, 1998

Klein DF: False suffocation alarms and spontaneous panic: subsuming the CO_2 hypersensitivity theory. Arch Gen Psychiatry 50:306–317, 1993

Klein DF, Gorman JM: A model of panic and agoraphobic development. Acta Psychiatr Scand 76(suppl):87–95, 1987

Le Melledo J, Bradwejn J, Koszycki D, et al: Premenstrual dysphoric disorder and response to cholecystokinin-tetrapeptide. Arch Gen Psychiatry 52:605, 1995

Le Melledo J, Van Driel M, Coupland N, et al: Response to flumazenil in women with premenstrual dysphoric disorder. Am J Psychiatry 157:821–823, 2000

Liebowitz MR, Gorman JM, Fyer AJ, et al: Social phobia: review of a neglected anxiety disorder. Arch Gen Psychiatry 42:729–736, 1985

Lohr KN, Kamberg CJ, Keeler EB, et al: Chronic disease in a general adult population. West J Med 145:537–545, 1986

Maier W, Buller R: One year follow-up of panic disorder: outcome and prognostic factors. European Archives of Psychiatry and Neurological Sciences 238:105–109, 1988

Majewska MD, Schwartz RD: Pregnenolone-sulfate: an endogenous antagonist of the gamma-aminobutyric acid receptor complex in brain? Brain Res 404:355–360, 1987

Marks IM: Fears, Phobias and Rituals, 2nd Edition. Oxford, England, Oxford University Press, 1987

Merikangas KR, Weissman MM, Pauls DL: Genetic factors in the sex ratio of major depression. Psychol Med 15:63–69, 1985

Metz AM, Sichel DA, Goff DC: Postpartum panic disorder. J Clin Psychiatry 49:278–279, 1988

Miller JB, Stiver I: A relational approach to understanding women's lives and problems. Psychiatr Ann 23:424–431, 1993

Noshirvani HF, Kasvikis Y, Marks IM, et al: Gender-divergent aetiological factors in obsessive-compulsive disorder. Br J Psychiatry 158:260–263, 1991

Noyes R, Clancey J, Hoenk PR, et al: The prognosis of anxiety neurosis. Arch Gen Psychiatry 37:173–178, 1980

Nunes E, Quitkin F, Berman C: Panic disorder and depression in female alcoholics. J Clin Psychiatry 49:441–443, 1988

Putnam FW, Gurroff JJ, Silberman EK, et al: The clinical phenomenology of multiple personality disorder: review of 100 recent cases. J Clin Psychiatry 47:285–293, 1986

Rasmussen SA, Tsuang MT: The epidemiology of obsessive compulsive disorder. J Clin Psychiatry 45:450–457, 1984

Robins LN, Helzer JE, Weissman MM, et al: Lifetime prevalence of specific disorders in three sites. Arch Gen Psychiatry 41:949–958, 1984

Ross CA, Anderson G: Phenomenological overlap of multiple personality disorder and obsessive-compulsive disorder. J Nerv Ment Dis 176:295–299, 1988

Saunders EA, Arnold F: Borderline Personality Disorder and Childhood Abuse: Revisions in Clinical Thinking and Treatment Approach (Work in Process 59). Wellesley, MA, Stone Center, 1991

Scheibe G, Albus M: Age at onset, precipitating events, sex distribution, and co-occurrence of anxiety disorders. Psychopathology 25:11–18, 1992

Schneier FR, Johnson J, Hornig CD, et al: Social phobia: comorbidity and morbidity in an epidemiological sample. Arch Gen Psychiatry 49:282–288, 1992

Shores MM, Glubin T, Cowley DS, et al: The relationship between anxiety and depression: a clinical comparison of generalized anxiety disorder, dysthymic disorder, panic disorder, and major depressive disorder. Compr Psychiatry 33:237–244, 1992

Soloff PH, Millward JW: Developmental histories of borderline patients. Compr Psychiatry 24:574–588, 1983

Stein MB, Schmidt PJ, Rubinow DR, et al: Panic disorder and the menstrual cycle: panic disorder patients, healthy control subjects, and patients with premenstrual syndrome. Am J Psychiatry 146:1299–1303, 1989

Swedo SE: Trichotillomania. Psychiatr Ann 23:402–407, 1993

Thyer BA, Tomlin P, Curtis GC, et al: Diagnostic and gender differences in the expressed fears of anxious patients. J Behav Ther Exp Psychiatry 16:111–115, 1985

Turk C, Heimberg R, Orsillo S, et al: An investigation of gender differences in social phobia. J Anxiety Disord 12:209–223, 1998

Uhde TW, Tancer ME, Black B: Phenomenology and neurobiology of social phobia: comparison with panic disorder. J Clin Psychiatry 52(suppl):31–40, 1991

van der Kolk BA, Greenberg M, Boyd H: Inescapable shock, neurotransmitters, and addiction to trauma: toward a psychobiology of post traumatic stress. Biol Psychiatry 20:314–325, 1985

Verburgge LM, Steiner RP: Prescribing drugs to men and women. Health Psychol 4:79–98, 1985

Von Korff M, Eaton W, Keyl P: The epidemiology of panic attacks and panic disorder: results from three community surveys. Am J Epidemiol 122:970–981, 1985

Welner A, Reich T, Robin E: Obsessive-compulsive neurosis record, follow-up and family studies, 1: inpatient record study. Compr Psychiatry 17:577–589, 1976

Wittchen H-U, Essau CA, Von Zerssen D, et al: Lifetime and six-month prevalence of mental disorders in the Munich follow-up study. European Archives of Psychiatry and Neurological Sciences 241:247–258, 1992

Wolpe J, Lang P: Manual for the Fear Survey Schedule. San Diego, CA, EDITS, 1964

Yonkers KA, Ellison JM: Anxiety disorders in women and their pharmacological treatment, in Psychopharmacology and Women: Sex, Gender, and Hormones. Edited by Jensvold MF, Halbreich U, Hamilton A. Washington, DC, American Psychiatric Press, 1996, pp 262–285

Yonkers KA, Gurguis G: Gender differences in the prevalence and expression of anxiety disorders, in Gender Psychopathology. Edited by Seeman MV. Washington, DC, American Psychiatric Press, 1995, pp 113–130

Yonkers KA, Massion A, Warshaw M, et al: Phenomenology and course of generalised anxiety disorder. Br J Psychiatry 168:308–313, 1996

Yonkers KA, Zlotnick C, Allsworth J, et al: Is the course of panic disorder the same in women and men? Am J Psychiatry 155:596–602, 1998

Yonkers KA, Dyck I, Warshaw M, et al: Factors predicting the clinical course of generalised anxiety disorder. Br J Psychiatry 176:544–550, 2000

Yonkers KA, Dyck IR, Keller MB: An eight-year longitudinal comparison of clinical course and characteristics of social phobia among men and women. Psychiatr Serv 52:637–643, 2001

2

Panic Disorder With Agoraphobia

Women's Issues

Lisa C. Smith, Ph.D.
Steven Friedman, Ph.D.
Cheryl Paradis, Psy.D.

*A*nxiety disorders are among the most frequently occurring mental disorders, second only to substance abuse disorders (Robins et al. 1984). Panic disorder has been estimated to affect 1.5%–3% of the United States population, with 3%–4% experiencing a panic attack at some point in their lives (Kessler et al. 1994). The overwhelming majority of those with panic disorder are women. In this chapter, we summarize the research on factors that affect women who have panic disorder, such as comorbid psychiatric and medical disorders, psychosocial variables, the effect of the reproductive cycle, and treatment.

The DSM-IV-TR diagnostic criteria for panic disorder (American Psychiatric Association 2000) are recurrent unexpected panic attacks consisting of the sudden onset of a discrete period of intense fear or discomfort with a range of autonomic symptoms of arousal (e.g., heart palpitations, shortness of breath, light-headedness). At least one of the attacks has been followed by at least 1 month of persistent concern about having additional attacks, worry about the implications of the attack or its consequences, or a significant change in behavior related to the attacks. The panic attacks are not due to the direct physiological effects of a substance or a general medical condition and are not better accounted for by another mental disorder.

EPIDEMIOLOGY

In the Epidemiological Catchment Area (ECA) survey (Robins et al. 1984), the lifetime prevalence of panic disorder in women was double that in men (2% vs. 1%), and the rates for panic disorder with concurrent agoraphobia were even higher (8% in women vs. 4% in men). Similarly, in the National Comorbidity Survey (NCS; Kessler et al. 1994), the lifetime prevalence of panic disorder was 5% in women and 2% in men. A 2:1 sex ratio was maintained for panic disorder and agoraphobia in the NCS data. This sex difference in diagnosis is found across many cultures, as seen in studies from Canada; Europe; and Los Angeles, California (Mexican Americans) (Eaton et al. 1994).

Despite the sex difference in prevalence, most research indicates that the profile of symptoms does not differ between men and women (Chambless and Mason 1986; Feighner et al. 1972; Noyes et al. 1991; Oei et al. 1990; Scheibe and Albus 1992; Yonkers 1994). However, one study (Scheibe and Albus 1992) did find that women had more panic symptoms and higher use of medical services than did men. Some studies found that among patients with panic disorder, women endorsed slightly greater fear (Chambless and Mason 1986; Oei et al. 1990; Scheibe and Albus 1992), although Hafner (1981) found that men were more fearful, especially about somatic concerns. A troubling finding was reported by the Harvard/Brown Anxiety Disorders Research Project (HARP) (Yonkers et al. 1998) study. This study showed a higher incidence of suicidal thoughts reported by women, but this was the only symptom difference found. Dick et al. (1994) reported that the highest risk for panic disorder was found in women ages 25–44 who had a family history of panic disorder and were separated or divorced.

The HARP study (Yonkers et al. 1998), which consisted of 412 male and female patients with panic disorder with or without agoraphobia who were followed up for approximately 5 years, found no significant differences between men and women in terms of panic symptom level of severity at baseline. However, women were more likely to be given diagnoses of panic and agoraphobia (85% vs. 75%), and men were more likely to be given diagnoses of uncomplicated panic (25% vs. 15%). The rate of panic remission was similar for both groups after 5 years (approximately 39%). However, the recurrence of panic symptoms was higher in women than in men (82% vs. 51%) during the follow-up period, even when alcohol abuse and agoraphobia were statistically controlled. Overall, women were more likely to have panic with concurrent agoraphobia and were more likely to experience a recurrence of panic symptoms even after the initial remission of panic.

COMORBID PSYCHIATRIC CONDITIONS

The long-term sequelae for untreated panic disorder have been well studied. Obviously, one of the most common complications of panic disorder is the development of agoraphobia, which is characterized by marked phobic avoidance of "situations from which escape might be difficult (or embarrassing) or in which help may not be available in the event of having an unexpected or situationally predisposed Panic Attack or panic-like symptoms" (American Psychiatric Association 2000, p. 433).

Subjects with panic disorder frequently have a variety of comorbid conditions, primarily major depression (30%–80% of the patients with panic disorder experience at least one episode of depression in their lives) (Liebowitz and Fyer 1994) and alcohol and substance dependence or abuse (diagnosed in approximately 15%–25% of the patients with panic disorder) (Cox et al. 1990). Breier et al. (1984) found more severe anxiety disorder, greater levels of past impairment, and a longer duration of panic disorder in patients with comorbid depression. In the literature, a consistent finding is that the rate of comorbid alcoholism is higher in men than in women with panic disorder (Crowe et al. 1983). A history of alcohol abuse or dependence was more common in men than in women at intake (44% vs. 23%) and after remission (53% vs. 25%) (Yonkers et al. 1998). An analysis of data from the ECA survey (Leon et al. 1995) showed that the rate of current alcohol abuse or dependence was 13% for women compared with 40% for men.

Patients often have a host of other comorbid Axis I disorders as well, including somatization disorder, generalized anxiety disorder, and obsessive-compulsive disorder (OCD) (McNally 1994). Yonkers and Gurguis (1995) reported that the comorbidity of agoraphobia, generalized anxiety disorder, and specific phobia is higher in women with panic disorder and that a trend for longer duration of agoraphobia is seen in women. In this study, OCD occurred more often in men with panic disorder after remission, even though no sex differences in demographics, treatment, or remission rates for panic disorder were found.

Numerous studies (Brooks et al. 1989; McNally 1994) have found that patients with panic disorder, with or without agoraphobia, are often given diagnoses (40%–65%) of Axis II disorders primarily from Cluster B (dependent type) (Reich et al. 1987). In DSM-IV (American Psychiatric Association 1994), the category of mixed anxiety-depressive disorder was proposed to encompass disorders that are often considered subthreshold in psychiatric practice but are often seen in primary care settings and may be particularly more common in women; however, at this time, no data are available to support this hypothesis.

PSYCHOSOCIAL ISSUES

It has been suggested that anxiety disorders are diagnosed more often in females because of a biologically determined difference between the sexes. In one large study of adolescents that included 1,079 subjects who never met the criteria for any psychiatric disorder (Lewinsohn et al. 1998), 95 subjects who met criteria for an anxiety disorder, 47 subjects who had recovered from an anxiety disorder, and 47 subjects who had a current disorder, females were significantly more likely to have current and/or a history of anxiety disorders. This difference emerged early in life, and retrospective data collected indicated that by age 6 years, females experienced an anxiety disorder twice as often as males did.

In this study, psychosocial variables were examined and controlled. These variables included major life events, such as stress of daily hassles, self-consciousness, low self-esteem, low self-confidence, emotional reliance, poor coping skills, low social support, more physical illness, poor self-rated physical health, less obesity, less exercise, and a greater number of physical symptoms. Even controlling for all these psychosocial variables did not substantially reduce the magnitude of association between sex and anxiety disorders. The authors (Lewinsohn et al. 1998) concluded that "this finding did not support the hypothesis that gender differences and vulnerability of anxiety disorders are explained by different social roles and experiences, at least in adolescents" (p. 113).

An alternative hypothesis for the higher incidence of panic disorder with agoraphobia in women than in men is the sex difference in women's experiences and expectations regarding their upbringing and social roles. Clum and Knowles (1991) suggested that women may have learned avoidant behavior as part of their stereotypic sex-role behavior. It has been well noted that women are generally more likely to avoid fear and less likely to expose themselves to fear-inducing situations. Zuckerman et al. (1980) found that the trait of sensation seeking was higher in men and that harm avoidance was higher in women. Fodor (1974) reviewed the effects of sex-role social-ization, which fosters "extreme superhelplessness, avoidance of mastery ex-periences and competition and a lack of assertiveness" (p. 140) in women. In addition, women may be more likely to fear negative social conse-quences of panic, which is hypothesized to be a contributing factor to avoidance.

These propensities would increase the likelihood that a woman born with a genetic risk for panic, or any other anxiety disorder, would have a lifetime of avoidance behavior, which may increase the risk of developing full-blown panic disorder with agoraphobia. Similarly, when behavioral treatment requires confronting the feared object during exposure exercises, women may find the treatment more difficult to engage in than men do. It has been suggested frequently that men with phobias cope with their symp-toms by drinking (Yonkers and Gurguis 1995; Yonkers et al. 1998) rather than staying home and are therefore more likely to use alcohol as a strategy for coping with their panic and anxiety.

Another issue in the sex differences found in panic disorder is the valid-ity of the diagnosis itself. The general goal of psychiatric diagnosis is to make judgments about symptoms and behavior in a standardized manner. However, the sex of the complainant has long been shown to affect such clinical judgments. One of the most well-known studies of the effect of sex on judgments of mental health in the social psychiatry literature was con-ducted by Broverman et al. (1970). In this study, clinicians assigned healthy men the same qualities as healthy individuals in general, whereas stereotyp-ically healthy women were characterized by qualities similar to anxiety symptoms, such as being less independent and adventurous as well as more excitable and emotional in a minor crisis.

Padgett (1997) reviewed the literature on diagnostic sex bias in mental health. She cited the Fujita et al. (1991) study in which women were found to be generally more expressive of emotion than men while asserting equiv-alent levels of well-being. This finding points to the influence of sex on self-report data collection strategies. She also stated that the threshold for the diagnosis of a mental disorder is set lower and thus is more attainable for women than for men. Psychiatric symptoms may be more easily over-looked in men, especially by primary care practitioners who are the largest source of treatment providers for anxiety disorders. This diagnostic bias may be particularly relevant to panic disorder in that anxiety disorders have consistently been found among those psychiatric syndromes with the low-est diagnostic agreement (Zerbe 1995).

In summary, some question remains as to whether men and women have the same degree of anxiety symptoms or whether the difference lies in their likelihood of admitting to psychiatric symptoms. In addition, there may be some discrepancy in clinicians' abilities to detect anxiety symptoms in both sexes and to recognize them as a problem for both men and women.

Life Stressors

Stress, as it affects anxiety disorders, has several different aspects. Predisposing factors for panic disorder with agoraphobia that have been the focus of clinical research include childhood events and premorbid personality traits, as well as stressors that may precipitate the onset of the disorder. In addition, levels of stress as a part of the course of the disorder also have been investigated. Within this literature, the definition of stress itself has been conceptualized in three separate components: stressful life events, chronic stress conditions, and daily hassles (Anderson 1991; Wade et al. 1993).

Much attention has been devoted to identifying specific life events that may help precipitate the initial panic episode. Most of the research evidence shows that the onset of anxiety symptoms seems to occur following a period of high levels of background stress or an identifiable precipitant (Barlow 1998; Buglass et al. 1977; Doctor 1982; Faravelli 1985; Finlay-Jones and Brown 1981; Last et al. 1984; Pollard et al. 1989; Raskin et al. 1982; Roy-Byrne et al. 1986; Solyom et al. 1974). Finlay-Jones and Brown (1981) and Roy-Byrne et al. (1986) reported a high frequency of severe life events that connoted danger and threat at the time of onset of panic disorder, as well as a higher proportion of events that were uncontrollable and undesirable. Faravelli (1985) reported that events involving death and illness were the most frequent precipitating events. More specifically, interpersonal problems, separation or loss, and serious illness both in the individual and in a significant other have been named as precipitants to panic symptoms (Barlow 1998).

Chronic stressors during the course of the disorder predicted a poorer outcome, as indicated by a higher level of posttreatment symptoms, less improvement, and less likelihood of recovery (Wade et al. 1993). Wade et al. (1993) also reported that ongoing marital difficulty (15%) was the most frequently cited stressor. However, the chronicity of the stressor had more of an effect on the maintenance of agoraphobic symptoms than did the type of stressor. Overall, women seem to be more prone to experience a variety of these stressors.

Trauma

Several traumatic events occur significantly more often in women than in men and may be related to the development of panic attacks and agoraphobia. These include incest, childhood or adult sexual abuse, and marital violence. Zerbe (1995) stated that the research findings on trauma are "important not only for the challenging perspective they add to the etiology of anxiety and depression in women, but also for the revisionist picture they paint of contemporary neurobiological hypotheses related to anxiety" (p. A45). The predominant methodologies in the literature of psychological correlates of trauma are identifying victims of trauma and obtaining rates of psychopathology or recording the histories of trauma in patients with current diagnoses of panic disorder.

Levels of trauma in populations with panic disorder have been higher than those in nonclinical populations. Smith et al. (1999) found rates of history of trauma as high as 69% in a sample of predominantly minority female patients with panic disorder. Falsetti et al. (1995) found rates of history of lifetime trauma as high as 94% in a sample of subjects with panic disorder.

Resnick et al. (1994) found that 90% of the female rape victims studied had four or more panic symptoms during the assault. Pribor and Dinwiddie (1992) sampled female incest survivors from every center in the St. Louis, Missouri, area specializing in programs for sexually abused women. They found a significantly higher rate of panic disorder as well as agoraphobia in women with a history of abuse when compared with women in the general population. The relation between panic disorder and the severity of trauma also has been explored. Walker et al. (1992) sampled women scheduled for laparoscopy and found no diagnostic differences between women who reported either no abuse or less severe levels of abuse. However, when comparing these two groups with a group reporting more severe abuse, panic disorder was significantly more prevalent in the latter group.

Falsetti et al. (1995) proposed two complementary pathways through which trauma experiences could predispose individuals to later panic attacks. First, conditioned external and internal stimuli associated with the trauma could later trigger seemingly spontaneous panic reactions. Second, chronic levels of hyperarousal and hypervigilance following a posttraumatic stress reaction could leave the individual more vulnerable to subsequent panic triggers. Individuals who already have a heightened level of arousal will require less of a trigger to reach the threshold for panic. Falsetti and Resnick (1997) proposed that "panic attacks can become a conditioned response to trauma related cues and can also generalize in trauma victims with PTSD" (p. 684). These authors found that 69% of their sample of trauma victims reported experiencing panic attacks, regardless of sex.

Marital and Family Issues

As noted earlier in this chapter, a range of clinical reports suggest that agoraphobia typically is triggered by marital distress (Milton and Hafner

1979). The phobia, it is argued, resolves or at least contains an emerging marital conflict in a highly enmeshed family by binding the spouses in a "compulsory marriage" (Fry 1962). Also widely noted is the impression that the inadequacies and covert symptomatology of the spouse are obscured by the identified patient's phobia. In such a view, any effective treatment for the phobia poses a threat to the equilibrium that the symptom has purchased.

In their overview of marital functioning and the anxiety disorders, Emmelkamp and Gerlsma (1994) reviewed the available empirical evidence on the marital relationships of patients with agoraphobia. Overall, they concluded that few empirical data suggested that marriages of individuals with agoraphobia were different from those of nonphobic individuals. In addition, they indicated that three controlled studies (Agulnik 1980; Arrindell and Emmelkamp 1986; Buglass et al. 1977) did not support the view that partners of patients with agoraphobia had psychological disorders themselves. They also concluded that exposure therapy did not show adverse effects on the relationship; rather, limited evidence suggested that the relationship remained stable or improved. Finally, they concluded that partner-assisted therapy was no more effective than individual therapy.

Carter et al. (1994), in reviewing the evidence for the role of interpersonal relationships in patients with panic disorder with agoraphobia, arrived at a somewhat different conclusion. They stated that "there appears to be mixed evidence regarding the relationship difficulties theorized to be characteristic of the agoraphobia's interpersonal system" (p. 27–28). Because panic disorder with agoraphobia, by definition, involves urgent and characteristic efforts to enlist others in tasks of daily life, some clinicians (Friedman 1987) have argued that families (both of origin and current family) cannot avoid becoming involved. Although traditional family therapy, alone or adjunctively, has not been shown to improve symptoms noticeably, no controlled outcome studies have addressed this issue.

PANIC DISORDER AND THE REPRODUCTIVE CYCLE

Researchers also have investigated hormonal and biological factors in the role of panic disorder. Many studies have reported an association between panic disorder in women and hormonal changes caused by either physical maturation, the reproductive cycle, or menopause. Studies have focused on the effects of menstruation, contraceptive use, pregnancy, childbirth, and menopause on panic symptoms. Symptoms of panic may be the result of hormonal changes, particularly in women predisposed to panic disorder. A higher incidence of panic disorder in females postmenarche also has been attributed to these hormonal fluctuations. Anecdotally, many women report heightened feelings of anxiety during the week before menstruation.

Premenstrual Dysphoric Disorder

Premenstrual dysphoric disorder, also known as late luteal phase dysphoric disorder, is characterized by depressed mood, marked anxiety and affective instability, impaired sleep and concentration, physical symptoms of breast tenderness or swelling, sensations of "bloating" or weight gain, joint or muscle pain, and headaches. It is hypothesized that women with premenstrual dysyphoric disorder, like patients with panic disorder, are overly sensitive to somatic cues. In fact, Fava et al. (1992) reported that 59% of the 32 women seeking treatment for premenstrual dysphoric disorder had anxiety disorders alone or comorbid mood disorders. This oversensitivity to somatic cues can predispose patients to react with anxiety to physical symptoms of the menstrual cycle and the arousing effects of adrenaline. Women with premenstrual dysphoric disorder diagnoses have been found to have greater sensitivity to provocation of panic attacks and differences in serotonergic functions compared with women without premenstrual dysphoric disorder. These women are also hypothesized to be vulnerable to depressive symptoms (Halbreich 1997). For example, in one study (Sandberg et al. 1993), sodium lactate infusions were administered to 13 women seeking treatment for premenstrual dysphoric disorder. These women had no lifetime history of panic disorder. Fifty-eight percent of the women experienced a panic attack during sodium lactate infusion. This rate is similar to that of patients with a diagnosis of panic disorder who panic after sodium lactate infusion.

Researchers have found that women with premenstrual dysphoric disorder have a high rate of comorbid panic disorder, other anxiety disorders, and mood disorders (Facchinetti et al. 1992; Sandberg et al. 1993). It also has been reported that these women have significant clinical fluctuations of anxiety and depression during the premenstrual phase (Stein et al. 1989; Veeniga et al. 1994).

Contraceptive Use

Several case reports have suggested an association between the use of oral contraceptives, as well as levonorgestrel subdermal implants, and panic disorder. Deci et al. (1992) described two women who developed panic disorder with agoraphobia 6–8 months after starting triphasic oral contraceptives. This oral contraceptive regimen had doses of progesterone that increased over a 21-day period. At day 21, the progesterone abruptly ceased. These two women had their panic attacks during the premenstrual week when the progesterone level dropped abruptly. Both of these women stopped having panic attacks when they were switched to a constant-dose preparation of oral contraceptives.

Wagner and Berenson (1994) described two women who developed an onset of panic disorder and depression 1–2 months after the insertion of levonorgestrel capsules. Levonorgestrel is a long-acting subdural implant contraceptive system that releases a continuous dose of a synthetic progesterone. These women, who had no history of panic disorder, improved within 1 month after the removal of the levonorgestrel capsules. These case reports suggest that the hormones in oral contraceptives and levonorgestrel triggered panic symptoms in women who had preexisting vulnerability to panic disorder or depression.

Pregnancy

Pregnancy is a time of major physical and psychological changes. Hormonal changes are linked to drastic physical and emotional changes. In addition, women need to adjust psychologically and socially to the birth of a child. Rapid changes in identity to motherhood, family structures, and extra work and responsibilities occur during the pre- and postpartum period. For some women, this stressful period has been described as a period of well-being. For some vulnerable women who have a predisposition to panic symptoms or premenstrual dysphoric disorder (Halbreich 1997; Stein et al. 1989), pregnancy may lead to the initial onset of a panic disorder. Those women who already have symptoms of panic disorder may experience a worsening of panic symptoms.

Overall, the literature (Cohen et al. 1994, 1996; George et al. 1987; Northcott and Stein 1994; Sholomskas et al. 1993; Villeponteaux et al. 1992; Wisner et al. 1996) reports a variable effect of pregnancy on the development or course of panic disorder. Many case reports have described improved psychological health during pregnancy. Hormonal changes of pregnancy may prevent the onset of activity of the sympathetic nervous system. The increase in progesterone during pregnancy causes increased respiration and basal metabolic rate and lowers partial carbon dioxide pressure. For example, George et al. (1987) described three women with panic disorder who reported significant lessening in their panic symptoms during pregnancy. However, in more comprehensive studies, pregnancy had a more variable effect on anxiety. Retrospective surveys of women diagnosed with panic disorder during pregnancy (Cohen et al. 1996; Northcott and Stein 1994; Sholomskas et al. 1993; Villeponteaux et al. 1992) showed rates of worsening of panic symptoms during pregnancy ranging from 20% to 63%. Symptoms remained the same or improved in 56%–78% of the women.

Some authors (Cohen et al. 1996) have concluded that the variable course of panic disorder during pregnancy may be related to the severity of the panic symptoms. Women with milder symptoms before pregnancy were more likely to remain stable or experience a lessening of symptoms. Women with more severe panic symptoms prepregnancy were seen as at risk for increased severity of panic symptoms during pregnancy and postpartum. An interesting finding reported in both case reports and retrospective studies is that women who develop panic disorder associated with pregnancy may develop symptoms in their second or even subsequent pregnancies (Cohen et al. 1996; Northcott and Stein 1994; Sholomskas et al. 1993; Villeponteaux et al. 1992; Wisner et al. 1996).

Many of the hormonal fluctuations occurring during pregnancy change abruptly after childbirth. It is hypothesized that the onset or exacerbation of panic symptoms during the postpartum period results from the rapid decline of estrogen and progesterone, which lowers serotonin levels and respiratory rate. One retrospective study (Sholomskas et al. 1993) of 64 mothers with panic disorder found that 11% of the women reported a postpartum onset of their initial panic disorder within 12 weeks of their giving birth to their first child. A similarly high rate of postpartum onset of panic disorder has been reported in many other studies (Cohen et al. 1994, 1996; Northcott and Stein 1994; Sholomskas et al. 1993; Wisner et al. 1996).

Women who are at risk for panic reactions, as evidenced by a history of either panic attacks or premenstrual dysphoric symptoms, should be carefully monitored after delivery for signs of the onset of panic. Early intervention through education, or even possibly medication if the condition becomes severe, can make a meaningful difference in the resolution of panic symptoms.

Treatment of Panic Disorder During Pregnancy

A limited amount of controlled investigation into the treatment of panic disorder during pregnancy is available. The available studies are predominantly naturalistic in design. Robinson et al. (1992) recommended that four issues be considered to determine treatment of panic disorder for a pregnant woman: "the patient's preferences, the effects of withholding treatment, the effects of treatment on the child, and the effectiveness and availability of treatments" (p. 623). Many women are reluctant to use medication during pregnancy because of the potential vulnerability of the fetus. Only one study (Cohen et al. 1989) indicated adverse effects on the fetus of withholding treatment. In this study, panic-associated placental abruption was reported. Robinson et al. (1992) hypothesized that if the panic is left untreated, it could potentially interfere with appetite as a result of the effects of anxiety, foster exaggerated fears about the birth process and motherhood, increase the risk of self-medicating, or result in an unnecessary restriction of activity.

Both cognitive-behavioral interventions and pharmacological treatments have been reported to be effective in the treatment of panic disorder in pregnant women (Cohen et al. 1996; Robinson et al. 1992; Ware and DeVane 1990). Ware and DeVane (1990) reported successful imipramine treatment in two pregnant women. In both women, a dosage of 50 mg/day was effective in controlling panic attacks with no observable damage to the infant. However, in a study by Cohen et al. (1996), symptoms persisted in half the patients despite medication, and medication increases were often ineffective in further alleviating symptoms. In addition, the effects of psychoactive medications on breast-feeding are largely unknown. Ware and DeVane reported varying concentrations of antidepressants in breast milk and stated that it is prudent for women taking such medications to avoid breast-feeding.

Standard cognitive-behavioral therapy (CBT) includes giving information about panic and the fear of fear cycle; teaching symptom management skills, such as diaphragmatic breathing and relaxation training; cognitive restructuring of exaggerated, catastrophic fears; self-monitoring, typically in the form of symptom diaries; interoceptive and in vivo exposure to symptom sensations and avoided situations; and follow-up (Robinson et al. 1992; Rosenbaum et al. 1995). However, there is a lack of well-controlled studies in the application of this therapy to pregnant women. Robinson et al. (1992) reported a successful application of CBT in a single case-study format. They reported that CBT was at least as effective as alprazolam treatment, although the effects may take longer to obtain. However, CBT can result in greater long-term effects and prevention of relapse on withdrawal of active treatment.

In summary, some evidence suggests that both psychopharmacological and psychotherapeutic interventions can be effective in treating panic disorder during pregnancy. Treatment options should be discussed with patients and decisions made on an individual basis. CBT would appear to be the preferable first-line treatment given the potential hazards of medication. Several clinicians (Cohen et al. 1996; Rosenbaum et al. 1995; Ware and DeVane 1990) have suggested guidelines for the psychopharmacological treatment of panic disorder in pregnant women.

COMORBID MEDICAL CONDITIONS

Because panic symptoms are, by definition, somatic in nature, it is important to rule out potential medical conditions that may be directly causing, or at least contributing to, the anxiety disorder. Circumstances that suggest a likely organic contribution are late onset (after age 40), a lack of family history of anxiety disorders or substance abuse disorders, the absence of triggering events, and a poor response to typical panic treatments (Sanderson 1998). The following medical conditions are more prevalent in women than in men and should be ruled out when diagnosing panic disorder with agoraphobia.

Endocrine Disorders

Endocrine disorders involve the glands that secrete one or more specific chemicals or hormones that control and time the occurrence of processes essential to survival and reproduction. Examples of these glands include the pituitary, thyroid, parathyroid, and adrenal glands; ovaries; and pancreas. Endocrine disorders are the most common medical problems faced by women and are the most common medical codiagnosis to panic disorder (Norris 1998). Two hormones from the adrenal gland (epinephrine and cortisol) are important in the first phase of the stress response, the alarm phase. If stress persists, the resistance phase involves prolonged elevated secretion of cortisol but not epinephrine (Magliozzi et al. 1993). Magliozzi et al. (1993) found an inverse correlation between ratings of agoraphobic avoidance and the thyroid secreted chemical T_4 (thyroxine) in depressed women.

Of the patients with hyperthyroidism (excessive thyroid gland activity), 95% report nervousness or episodic anxiety as the primary complaint, and more than two-thirds report palpitations, tachycardia, and dyspnea. Hyperthyroidism is more common in women (1 of 1,000) than in men (1 of 3,000) partially because of the enhancement of thyroid hormones by estrogens (Jenkins 1998; Magliozzi et al. 1993; Norris 1998). One form of hyperthyroidism is Graves' disease, which is 20 times more common in women than in men. Symptoms of Graves' disease, which can be confused with an anxiety disorder, include restlessness, irritability, and anxiety (Jenkins 1998).

Hypoglycemia, an excessive secretion of insulin after ingesting carbohydrates, leading to rapid decline of blood sugar, gained popularity as a possible cause of panic attacks in the 1970s. Its symptoms include headache, mental dullness, confusion, anxiety, irritability, sweating, palpitations, tremor, and hunger. Subsequent research has not found hypoglycemia to be a common comorbid condition (Sanderson 1998), although in our clinical experience, many patients with panic disorder, both male and female, are convinced that their panic symptoms result from a hypoglycemic reaction.

Pheochromocytosis, tumors of catecholamine-secreting tissues that result in the secretion of excessive amounts of noradrenaline, is a rare condition with a prevalence rate of 0.01% that often has been mistaken for panic disorder. This condition is 20–50 times more common in women. Symptoms occur in episodes (paroxysmal attacks) lasting from minutes to 1 week. The most common symptoms are headache and hypertension but also include sweating, palpitations, dyspnea, restlessness, and anxiety. The possibility of this diagnosis should be considered when attacks are not as frequent or intense as typical, when somatic symptoms are more prominent than cognitive or affective symptoms, and when no avoidance behaviors are evident (Sanderson 1998).

Cardiovascular Disorders

One of the most common fears among persons with panic disorder is dying, usually from a "heart attack." This layperson's term actually consists of several possible medical conditions, such as arrhythmias, coronary artery disease, and valve disorders. Coronary heart disease (CHD) develops from atherosclerotic deposits inside the arteries. When arteries become blocked, angina pectoris, myocardial infarction, or coronary thrombosis can occur. The rate of CHD in women accelerates after menopause but never reaches the prevalence in men (Jenkins 1998). However, heart disease is the leading cause of death among women, and the clinical manifestations are most prevalent among postmenopausal women older than 60. During acute stress, women have smaller magnitude of blood pressure and vasoconstriction, as well as neuroendocrine and lipid responses to these stressors. Postmenopausal women experience larger physiological stress responses than do premenopausal women. African American women show greater vasoconstriction and attenuated heart rate to stress than do Caucasian women.

Among patients with chest pain referred for cardiac testing, patients with negative workups were younger and more likely to be female than male (Katon et al. 1988). Of 195 patients presenting with atypical or nonanginal chest pain, the patients with both coronary artery disease and panic disorder were primarily men with predominantly atypical angina, whereas those with panic disorder and no evidence of coronary artery disease were primarily women experiencing nonanginal chest pain.

Mitral valve prolapse results from the alteration or sagging in the connective tissue of the mitral heart valve. Mild conditions are often asymptomatic. Symptoms of a more severe condition may include chest pain, dyspnea, tachycardia, palpitations, light-headedness, fainting, fatigue, and anxiety. Conservative estimates of prevalence are 4%–7%, and the incidence is higher among women. The prevalence rate in women in their 30s can reach as high as 17%. Although no evidence indicates an increased rate of panic disorder in patients with mitral valve prolapse, mitral valve prolapse is a common codiagnosis with panic disorder. However, mitral valve prolapse has not been shown to affect the course or response to treatment of panic disorder (Sanderson 1998).

Hypertension, or high blood pressure, can cause damage to heart muscle, brain, kidneys, and other organs. It is a risk factor for cardiovascular accident (stroke), coronary artery disease, and myocardial infarction (heart attack). Hypertension is equally prevalent in women and men of European descent, but it is twice as common in African Americans, especially women. Hypertension does not present with detectable symptoms, thus earning the name "the silent killer." Stress has been shown to raise blood pressure over the short term but is not thought to create sustained hypertension (Jenkins 1998). Thus, patients' worries that increases in blood pressure caused by panic may result in an immediate dangerous medical situation are largely unfounded.

EFFECT OF PANIC DISORDER

For women with panic disorder in the ECA survey, 64%–69% were currently not employed, and 28% had not been employed in the past 5 years (Leon et al. 1995). Rates of financial dependence and receipt of welfare were elevated for all the anxiety disorders but highest in women with panic disorder (Leon et al. 1995). Only one-quarter to one-third of patients with panic disorder seek help from mental health establishments, but they are more likely to seek help in emergency departments and from primary care practitioners (Horwath et al. 1994). Borden et al. (1988) found that women were less likely to inform their physician about their anxiety symptoms than men were. Overall, it has been well established that people with anxiety have considerable social morbidity because of elevated rates of financial dependence on family, unemployment, and/or social services; substance abuse and dependence; and depressive disorders (Leon et al. 1995; McNally 1994). Unfortunately, single, divorced, or widowed women, in general, tend to have more financial problems, which are associated with an increased incidence of panic disorder and a poorer response to treatment.

TREATMENT

In the United States, although 20 million people have been estimated to have a 1-year prevalence of an anxiety disorder, only 6 million received treatment (Pennington 1997; Russo 1990). Russo (1990) reported that women make 58% of all visits to physicians but receive 73% of all psychotropic drug prescriptions. The prescription rate increases to 90% if the prescribing physician is not a psychiatrist. In addition, women are more likely than men to receive a prescription for an anxiolytic or antidepressant (Hohmann 1989). Padgett (1997) proposed several potential explanations for this difference in prescription patterns. She suggested that women may require medication more often, women have higher rates of use of all health care and thus have a greater opportunity to be prescribed medication, women may directly request such pharmacological treatments more often, or physicians may be predisposed to overmedicate women because of sex stereotypes.

Medication and Its Management

Our clinical impression is that many women who have panic disorder with agoraphobia tend to shy away from taking medication. They dislike putting "unknown substances" into their bodies and often make statements such as "I don't even like to take aspirin when I have a headache." This tendency can be viewed as a continued expression of phobic avoidance. Once swallowed, medication becomes interpreted as a dangerous substance that is no longer under their control. Patients often will stop taking medications if they experience common side effects that often actually mimic the anxiety symptoms that they wanted to eliminate in the first place.

Katon (1993) suggested several interventions to enhance medication compliance:

- Provide frequent support and be available.
- Use bibliotherapy, an alternative method of providing information and support.
- Be proactive and reframe the temporary discomfort of side effects as evidence that the medication is working.
- Educate the patient about the therapeutic dose range, and allow the patient to control how quickly the dose is raised. (A common mistake made by prescribing physicians is to stop short of a full therapeutic dose. Dosage should be raised until a patient is entirely free of acute panic attacks.)

Several classes of medications have been shown to be effective in addressing panic symptoms. These medications include monoamine oxidase inhibitors (MAOIs), tricyclic antidepressants (TCAs), selective serotonin reuptake inhibitors (SSRIs), and high-potency benzodiazepines. Rosenbaum et al. (1996) listed the goals of pharmacological treatment as being to block spontaneous panic attacks and correct disturbed physiological mechanisms. Encouragement to reenter phobic situations is then commonly advised.

SSRIs are currently considered the first-line treatment for panic disorder because of their therapeutic effectiveness, safety, and generally favorable side effect profiles (Welkowitz and Gorman 1994). However, it can be difficult to initiate the use of SSRIs because of a potentially aversive side effect of initial worsening of anxiety. Treatment should be initiated at a low dose and slowly titrated up to a therapeutic level. The length of time required to titrate the dose delays the onset of a therapeutic effect. Patients should be well informed of appropriate expectations concerning these side effects and the time needed to obtain therapeutic relief. In addition to their relatively low level of side effects, SSRIs have a benign cardiovascular profile, which may be more easily tolerated by patients with cardiac pathology.

One potential sex-related side effect is difficulty achieving orgasms during sexual intercourse in men and women and inability to ejaculate in men. This side effect may be addressed by applying greater amounts or longer duration of genital stimulation. In severe cases, medications such as yohimbine (5.4 mg) or cyproheptadine (4.0 mg) may be prescribed and taken as one tablet 1–2 hours before sexual activity will take place (Hollander and McCarley 1992).

TCAs were the first medications found to be effective in treating panic disorder (Klein 1964). Again, because of their potential for initially inducing increased jitteriness, low starting doses with gradual titration to a therapeutic level are recommended. TCAs have somewhat more intense side effects than SSRIs, consisting of cardiac disturbances, orthostatic hypotension, anticholinergic effects (dry mouth, blurred vision, constipation), weight gain, and sexual dysfunction.

MAOIs have been shown to affect the widest array of symptoms, including blocking panic attacks, relieving depression, and reducing social anxiety. However, MAOIs are less commonly prescribed because of their potential for adverse side effects (e.g., orthostatic hypotension, weight gain, and insomnia) in addition to strict dietary requirements prohibiting the intake of foods containing tyramine (Hollander and McCarley 1992).

High-potency benzodiazepines have been shown to be effective in blocking panic symptoms as well as controlling generalized and anticipatory anxiety (Rosenbaum et al. 1996; Welkowitz and Gorman 1994). The advantages of benzodiazepines are rapid onset of symptom relief and a safe, favorable side effect profile. However, the drawbacks to benzodiazepine use are interdose rebound anxiety, potential dependency and abuse, and withdrawal symptoms on sudden discontinuation. To address interdose rebound, or "watching the clock," patients typically require frequent dosing or should be prescribed one of the longer-acting drugs such as clonazepam.

The fear of drug dependency is often expressed and is almost always a concern of patients with panic disorder. Typically, women with panic disorder appear to underuse medication. Realistically, a patient's history of substance use should be taken into consideration, but the overwhelming majority of patients with panic disorder are at low risk for abusing medication (Welkowitz and Gorman 1994).

The achievement of a panic-free state ranges from 50% to 70% with either an antidepressant or a benzodiazepine in panic patients (Rosenbaum et al. 1996). In a meta-analysis, Gould et al. (1995) found that psychotropic medication effect sizes were significantly greater than those of placebo. Antidepressants resulted in a higher dropout rate. Unfortunately, 30%–75% of the patients continued to have panic attacks or residual phobic avoidance. Many patients require ongoing medication because relapse is common when medications are discontinued. Otto et al. (1993) found that the use of CBT increased the successful tapering of benzodiazepines in 76% of the patients with panic disorder, whereas only 25% were successful without adjunctive treatment.

Women may be at higher risk for developing side effects to traditional pharmacological treatments for panic because of a larger proportion of body fat, which potentially affects plasma levels (Zerbe 1995). Men tend to have faster clearance, resulting in lower plasma levels, whereas women have higher levels of medications available in their systems. Thus, therapeutic doses are often lower for women, with greater potential for side effects (Padgett 1997). Gender also affects rates of medication absorption and distribution throughout the body through factors such as lean body mass, endogenous and exogenous hormone levels, liver metabolism, gastric absorption and emptying, and cerebral blood flow.

Psychotherapy

CBT (Barlow 1998) for panic disorder emphasizes five key components: 1) information on panic disorder and the fear of fear cycle; 2) acquisition of symptom management skills, such as diaphragmatic breathing and progressive muscle relaxation; 3) cognitive restructuring, including elimination of catastrophic misinterpretation; 4) interoceptive exposure, so that desensitization to anxiety sensations occurs; and 5) in vivo exposure to eliminate avoidance of fear-inducing trigger situations.

In their review of the literature, Rosenbaum et al. (1995) found that successful CBT results in panic-free states ranging from 71% to 87% for short-term treatment. Treatment gains are also associated with long-term maintenance of gains. For example, 80% of the patients remained panic free at 2 years in a study by Craske et al. (1991). In literature reviews, it has been concluded that CBT trials and pharmacotherapy have similar efficacy (Clum et al. 1993; Otto et al. 1993). Some reviewers have concluded (Gould et al. 1995) that CBT has been associated with higher rates of retention in treatment and often has a superior cost–benefit ratio. Some evidence indicates that pharmacotherapy interferes with exposure-based interventions (Marks et al. 1993). However, Otto et al. (1994) found that under certain conditions, medications do not decrease the efficacy of CBT. In a recently completed multicenter trial (Barlow et al. 2000), the combination of imipramine and CBT had limited advantage acutely but more substantial benefit by the end of maintenance. However, CBT either alone or with placebo appeared durable in follow-up. Deciding which type of treatment to pursue should be made on a case-by-case basis, including the preference of the patient. CBT can facilitate recovery in patients receiving medication by teaching adaptive coping responses, aiding medication discontinuation, and addressing complications such as avoidance behavior (Otto et al. 1993, 1994).

Marital or family treatment is often clinically the most common adjunctive treatment suggested for panic disorder patients (Friedman 1987). In a meta-analysis of the effects of marital adjustment and involvement of the spouse in the behavioral treatment of agoraphobia, Dewey and Hunsley (1990) concluded that the better the pretreatment marital functioning of the patient, the greater the reduction in agoraphobia symptoms. This effect was maintained for up to 1 year after treatment. They also concluded that the effectiveness of spouse-involved exposure treatment was not significantly different from the effectiveness of not involving the spouse in the exposure treatment. However, the authors cautiously presented some data suggesting that involving the spouse may help lower the attrition rate from the typically high 25%–40% rate present in pharmacological treatments or the 12% rate typical in exposure-based treatments (Jansson and Ost 1982) to as low as 5% (Barlow et al. 1984).

CONCLUSION

It is a well-established finding in the epidemiological literature that panic disorder with or without agoraphobia is more common in women (Eaton et al. 1994; Kessler et al. 1994; Robins et al. 1984). The question is whether this difference in prevalence is the result of biological factors or is better attributed to experiential differences in social roles between the sexes. In many ways, the nature versus nurture distinction appears to be a false dichotomy. However, sex differences in the manifestation of panic disorder with agoraphobia may be useful in suggesting potential research directions, especially in terms of the physiological or biochemical underpinnings of panic.

Because of the marked sex difference in the prevalence of the disorder, study of treatments for panic disorder has been well investigated in women, who constitute most of the study subjects. Clinical research has resulted in a high rate of successful treatment outcomes (Clum et al. 1993; Craske et al. 1991; Otto et al. 1993; Rosenbaum et al. 1995). However, improvements in treatment are still required, especially for those treatment-resistant cases that appear to involve multiple coexisting conditions, personality characteristics, and personal histories of abuse and violence. To improve treatment outcome, Ackerman (1982) proposed that "Once an assessment of the behavioral limitations created by the phobia has been made and the characterological issues explored, the therapist should examine the patient's female role in family and society" (p. 157). Psychotherapy for women with panic disorder with agoraphobia may need to include attention to issues of self-esteem; assertiveness; acute and chronic life stresses, including sexual abuse and other traumas; family involvement in symptoms; discrimination and societal devaluation; and general attitudes toward mastery, competency, and dependency. Although untreated panic disorder is a chronic condition that can cause a host of complications, state-of-the-art treatment results in symptom reduction and improvement in the quality of life for patients.

REFERENCES

Ackerman R: Women's issues in the assessment and treatment of phobias, in Phobia: A Comprehensive Summary of Modern Treatments. Edited by DuPont L. New York, Brunner/Mazel, 1982, pp 153–160

Agulnik P: The spouse of the phobic patient. Br J Psychiatry 117:59–67, 1980

American Psychiatric Association: Diagnostic and Statistical Manual of Mental Disorders, 4th Edition. Washington, DC, American Psychiatric Press, 1994

American Psychiatric Association: Diagnostic and Statistical Manual of Mental Disorders, 4th Edition, Text Revision. Washington, DC, American Psychiatric Press, 2000

Anderson LP: Acculturative stress: a theory of relevance to black Americans. Clin Psychol Rev 11:685–702, 1991

Arrindell WA, Emmelkamp PM: Marital adjustment, intimacy, and needs in female agoraphobics and their partners: a controlled study. Br J Psychiatry 149:592–602, 1986

Barlow DH: Anxiety and Its Disorders: The Nature and Treatment of Anxiety and Panic. New York, Guilford, 1998

Barlow DH, O'Brien GT, Last CG: Couples treatment of agoraphobia. Behavior Therapy 15:41–58, 1984

Barlow DH, Gorman JM, Shear MK, et al: Cognitive-behavioral therapy, imipramine, or their combination for panic disorder: a randomized controlled trial. JAMA 283:2529–2536, 2000

Borden JW, Clum GA, Broyles SE, et al: Coping strategies and panic. J Anxiety Disord 2:339–352, 1988

Breier A, Charney DS, Heninger GR: Major depression in patients with agoraphobia and panic disorder. Arch Gen Psychiatry 41:1129–1135, 1984

Brooks RB, Baltazar PL, Munjack DJ: Co-occurrence of personality disorder with panic disorder, social phobia and generalized anxiety disorder: a review of the literature. J Anxiety Disord 3:259–285, 1989

Broverman IK, Broverman DM, Clarkson FE, et al: Sex-role stereotypes and clinical judgments of mental health. J Consult Clin Psychol 34:1–7, 1970

Buglass D, Clarke J, Henderson AS, et al: A study of agoraphobic housewives. Psychol Med 7:73–86, 1977

Carter MM, Turovsky J, Barlow DH: Interpersonal relationships in panic disorder with agoraphobia: a review of empirical evidence. Clinical Psychology Science and Practice 1:25–34, 1994

Chambless DL, Mason J: Sex, sex role stereotyping, and agoraphobia. Behav Res Ther 24:231–235, 1986

Clum GA, Knowles SL: Why do some people with panic disorders become avoidant? A review. Clin Psychol Rev 11:295–313, 1991

Clum GA, Clum GA, Surls R: A meta-analysis of treatments for panic disorder. J Consult Clin Psychol 61:317–326, 1993

Cohen LS, Rosenbaum JF, Heller VL: Panic attack–associated placental abruption: a case report. J Clin Psychiatry 50:266–267, 1989

Cohen LS, Sichel DA, Dimmock JA, et al: Postpartum course in women with preexisting panic disorder. J Clin Psychiatry 55:289–292, 1994

Cohen LS, Sichel DA, Faraone SV, et al: Course of panic disorder during pregnancy and the puerperium: a preliminary study. Biol Psychiatry 39:950–954, 1996

Cox BJ, Norton GR, Swinson RP, et al: Substance abuse and panic-related anxiety: a critical review. Behav Res Ther 28:385–393, 1990

Craske MG, Brown TA, Barlow DH: Behavioral treatment of panic disorder: a two-year follow-up. Behav Ther 22:289–304, 1991

Crowe RR, Noyes R, Pauls DL, et al: A family study of panic disorder. Arch Gen Psychiatry 40:1065–1069, 1983

Deci PA, Lydiard RB, Santos AB, et al: Oral contraceptives and panic disorder. J Clin Psychiatry 53:163–165, 1992

Dewey D, Hunsley J: The effects of marital adjustment and spouse involvement on the behavioral treatment of agoraphobia: a meta-analytic review. Anxiety Research 2:69–82, 1990

Dick CL, Bland RC, Newman SC: Epidemiology of psychiatric disorders in Edmonton: panic disorder. Acta Psychiatr Scand Suppl 376:45–53, 1994

Doctor RM: Major results of a large-scale pretreatment survey of agoraphobics, in Phobia: A Comprehensive Summary of Modern Treatments. Edited by Dupont RL. New York, Brunner/Mazel, 1982, pp 203–214

Eaton WW, Kessler RC, Wittchen HU, et al: Panic and panic disorder in the United States. Am J Psychiatry 151:413–420, 1994

Emmelkamp PM, Gerlsma C: Marital functioning and the anxiety disorders. Behavior Therapy 25:407–429, 1994

Facchinetti F, Romano G, Fava M, et al: Lactate infusion induces panic attacks in patients with premenstrual syndrome. Psychosom Med 54:288–296, 1992

Falsetti SA, Resnick HS: Frequency and severity of panic attack symptoms in a treatment seeking sample of trauma victims. J Trauma Stress 10:683–689, 1997

Falsetti SA, Resnick HS, Dansky BS, et al: The relationship of stress to panic disorder: cause or effect? in Does Stress Cause Psychiatric Illness? Edited by Mazure CM. Washington, DC, American Psychiatric Press, 1995, pp 11–147

Faravelli C: Life events preceding the onset of panic disorder. J Affect Disord 9:103–105, 1985

Fava M, Pedrazzi F, Guaraldi GP, et al: Comorbid anxiety and depression among patients with late luteal phase dysphoric disorder. J Anxiety Disord 6:325–335, 1992

Feighner JP, Robins E, Guze SB, et al: Diagnostic criteria for use in psychiatric research. Arch Gen Psychiatry 26:57–63, 1972

Finlay-Jones R, Brown GW: Types of stressful life events and the onset of anxiety and depressive disorders. Psychol Med 11:803–815, 1981

Fodor IG: The phobic syndrome in women: implications for treatment, in Women in Therapy: New Psychotherapies for a Changing Society. Edited by Franks V, Burtle V. New York, Brunner/Mazel, 1974, pp 132–168

Friedman S: Technical considerations in the behavioral-marital treatment of agoraphobia. American Journal of Family Therapy 15:111–122, 1987

Fry WF: The marital context of an anxiety syndrome. Fam Process 4:245–252, 1962

Fujita F, Diener E, Sandvik E: Gender differences in negative affect and well-being: the case for emotional intensity. J Pers Soc Psychol 61:427–434, 1991

George DT, Ladenheim JA, Nutt DJ: Effect of pregnancy on panic attacks. Am J Psychiatry 144:1078–1079, 1987

Gould RA, Otto MW, Pollack MH: A meta-analysis of treatment outcome for panic disorder. Clin Psychol Rev 15:819–844, 1995

Hafner RJ: Agoraphobia in men. Aust N Z J Psychiatry 15:243–249, 1981

Halbreich U: Premenstrual dysphoric disorders: a diversified cluster of vulnerability traits to depression. Acta Psychiatr Scand 95:169–176, 1997

Hohmann AA: Gender bias in psychotropic drug prescribing in primary care. Med Care 2:478–490, 1989

Hollander E, McCarley A: Yohimbine treatment of sexual side effects induced by serotonin reuptake blockers. J Clin Psychiatry 53:207–209, 1992

Horwath E, Johnson J, Hornig CD: Epidemiology of panic disorder, in Anxiety Disorders in African Americans. Edited by Friedman S. New York, Springer, 1994, pp 53–64

Jansson L, Ost L: Behavioral treatments for agoraphobia: an evaluative review. Clin Psychol Rev 2:311–336, 1982

Jenkins CD: Coronary heart disease, in Behavioral Medicine and Women: A Comprehensive Handbook. Edited by Blechman EA, Brownell KD. New York, Guilford, 1998, pp 609–614

Katon W: Panic Disorder in the Medical Setting (NIH Publ No 93-3482). Washington, DC, National Institute of Mental Health, 1993

Katon W, Hall ML, Russo J, et al: Chest pain: relationship of psychiatric illness to coronary arteriographic results. Am J Med 84:1–9, 1988

Kessler RC, McGonagle KA, Zhao S, et al: Lifetime and 12-month prevalence of DSM-III-R psychiatric disorders in the United States: results from the National Comorbidity Survey. Arch Gen Psychiatry 5:8–19, 1994

Klein D: Delineation of two-drug responsive anxiety syndromes. Psychopharmacologia 5:397–408, 1964

Last CG, Barlow DH, O'Brien GT: Precipitants of agoraphobia: role of stressful life events. Psychol Rep 54:567–570, 1984

Leon AC, Portera L, Weissman MM: The social costs of anxiety disorders. Br J Psychiatry Suppl 27:19–22, 1995

Lewinsohn PM, Gotlib IH, Lewinsohn M, et al: Gender differences in anxiety disorders and anxiety symptoms in adolescents. J Abnorm Psychol 107:109–117, 1998

Liebowitz MR, Fyer AJ: Diagnosis and clinical course of panic disorder with and without agoraphobia, in Treatment of Panic Disorder: A Consensus Development Conference. Edited by Wolf BE, Maser JD. Washington, DC, American Psychiatric Press, 1994, pp 19–30

Magliozzi JR, Maddock RJ, Gold AS, et al: Relationships between thyroid indices and symptoms of anxiety in depressed outpatients. Ann Clin Psychiatry 5:111–116, 1993

Marks IM, Swinson RP, Basoglu M, et al: Alprazolam and exposure alone and combined in panic disorder with agoraphobia: a controlled study in London and Toronto. Br J Psychiatry 162:776–787, 1993

McNally RJ: Panic Disorder: A Critical Analysis. New York, Guilford, 1994

Milton F, Hafner J: The outcome of behavior therapy for agoraphobia in relation to marital adjustment. Arch Gen Psychiatry 36:807–811, 1979

Norris DO: Endocrinology, in Behavioral Medicine and Women: A Comprehensive Handbook. Edited by Blechman EA, Brownell KD. New York, Guilford, 1998, pp 628–638

Northcott CJ, Stein MB: Panic disorder in pregnancy. J Clin Psychiatry 55:539–542, 1994

Noyes R Jr, Reich J, Christiansen J, et al: Outcome of panic disorder: relationship to diagnostic subtypes and comorbidity. Arch Gen Psychiatry 47:809–818, 1991

Oei TPS, Wanstall K, Evans L: Sex differences in panic disorder with agoraphobia. J Anxiety Disord 4:317–324, 1990

Otto M, Pollack M, Sachs G, et al: Discontinuation of benzodiazepine treatment: efficacy of cognitive-behavior therapy for patients with panic disorder. Am J Psychiatry 150:1485–1490, 1993

Otto M, Gould R, Pollack M: Cognitive-behavioral treatment of panic disorder: considerations for the treatment of patients over the long term. Psychiatric Annals 24:307–315, 1994

Padgett DK: Women's mental health: some directions for research. Am J Orthopsychiatry 67:522–534, 1997

Pennington A: Women's health: anxiety disorders. Prim Care 24:103–111, 1997

Pollard CA, Pollard HJ, Corn KJ: Panic onset and major events in the lives of agoraphobics: a test of contiguity. J Abnorm Psychol 98:318–321, 1989

Pribor EF, Dinwiddie SH: Psychiatric correlates of incest in childhood. Am J Psychiatry 149:52–56, 1992

Raskin M, Peeke HV, Dickman W, et al: Panic and generalized anxiety disorders: developmental antecedents and precipitants. Arch Gen Psychiatry 39:687–689, 1982

Reich J, Noyes R Jr, Troughton E: Dependent personality disorder associated with phobic avoidance in patients with panic disorder. Am J Psychiatry 144:323–326, 1987

Resnick HS, Falsetti SA, Kilpatrick DG, et al: Associations between panic attacks during rape assaults and follow-up PTSD or panic outcomes. Paper presented at the 10th annual meeting of the International Society for Traumatic Stress Studies, Chicago, IL, October 1994

Robins LN, Helzer JE, Weissman MM, et al: Lifetime prevalence of specific psychiatric disorders in three sites. Arch Gen Psychiatry 41:949–958, 1984

Robinson L, Walker JR, Andersen D: Cognitive-behavioural treatment of panic disorder during pregnancy and lactation. Can J Psychiatry 37:623–626, 1992

Rosenbaum JF, Pollock RA, Otto WM, et al: Integrated treatment of panic disorder. Bull Menninger Clin 59:A4–A26, 1995

Rosenbaum JF, Pollack RA, Jordan SK, et al: The pharmacotherapy of panic disorder. Bull Menninger Clin 60:A54–A75, 1996

Roy-Byrne PP, Vitaliano PP, Cowley DS, et al: Coping in panic and major depressive disorder: relative effects of symptom severity and diagnostic comorbidity. J Nerv Ment Dis 180:179–183, 1986

Russo NF: Overview: forging research priorities for women's mental health. Am Psychol 45:368–373, 1990

Sandberg D, Endicott J, Harrison W, et al: Sodium lactate infusion in late luteal phase dysphoric disorder. Psychiatry Res 46:79–88, 1993

Sanderson WC: Panic disorder, in Behavioral Medicine and Women: A Comprehensive Handbook. Edited by Blechman EA, Brownell KD. New York, Guilford, 1998, pp 737–740

Scheibe G, Albus M: Age at onset, precipitating events, sex distribution, and co-occurrence of anxiety disorders. Psychopathology 25:11–18, 1992

Sholomskas DE, Wickamaratne PJ, Dogolo L, et al: Postpartum onset of panic disorder: a coincidental event? J Clin Psychiatry 54:476–480, 1993

Smith LC, Friedman S, Nevid J: A clinical comparison of non-Hispanic European American and African American patients with panic disorder and agoraphobia. J Nerv Ment Dis 187:550–561, 1999

Solyom L, Beck P, Solyom C, et al: Some etiological factors in phobic neurosis. Canadian Psychiatric Association Journal 19:69–78, 1974

Stein MB, Schmidt PJ, Rubinow DR, et al: Panic disorder and the menstrual cycle: panic disorder patients, healthy control subjects, and patients with premenstrual syndrome. Am J Psychiatry 146:1299–1303, 1989

Veeniga AT, de Ruiter C, Kraaimaat FW: The relationship between late luteal phase dysphoric disorder and anxiety disorders. J Anxiety Disord 8:207–215, 1994

Villeponteaux VA, Lydiard RB, Laraia MT, et al: The effects of pregnancy on pre-existing panic disorder. J Clin Psychiatry 53:201–203, 1992

Wade SL, Monroe SM, Michelson LK: Chronic life stress and treatment outcome in agoraphobia with panic attacks. Am J Psychiatry 150:1491–1495, 1993

Wagner KD, Berenson AB: Norplant-associated major depression and panic disorder. J Clin Psychiatry 55:478–480, 1994

Walker EA, Katon WJ, Hansom J, et al: Medical and psychiatric symptoms in women with childhood sexual abuse. Psychosom Med 54:658–664, 1992

Ware MR, DeVane CL: Imipramine treatment of panic disorder during pregnancy. J Clin Psychiatry 51:482–484, 1990

Welkowitz LA, Gorman JM: An overview of anxiety disorders: focusing on panic disorder as a model, in Cultural Issues in the Treatment of Anxiety. Edited by Friedman S. New York, Guilford, 1994, pp 40–55

Wisner KL, Peindl KS, Hanusa BH: Effects of childbearing on the natural history of panic disorder with comorbid mood disorder. J Affect Disord 41:173–180, 1996

Yonkers KA: Panic disorder in women. J Womens Health 3:481–486, 1994

Yonkers KA, Gurguis G: Gender differences in anxiety disorders, in Gender and Psychopathology. Edited by Seeman MV. Washington, DC, American Psychiatric Press, 1995, pp 113–130

Yonkers KA, Zlotnick C, Allsworth J, et al: Is the course of panic disorder the same in women and men? Am J Psychiatry 155:596–602, 1998

Zerbe KJ: Anxiety disorders in women. Bull Menninger Clin 59:A38–A52, 1995

Zuckerman M, Buchsbaum MS, Murphy DL: Sensation seeking and its biological correlates. Psychol Bull 88:187–214, 1980

3

Sex Differences in Posttraumatic Stress Disorder

Cheryl M. Wong, M.D.
Rachel Yehuda, Ph.D.

*P*osttraumatic stress disorder (PTSD) was originally defined in 1980 to describe long-lasting symptoms that occur in response to trauma. The diagnosis revived psychiatry's long-standing interest in how stress results in behavioral and biological changes that ultimately lead to disorder. In 1980, the field of traumatology was heavily focused on when describing what happened to combat veterans of the Vietnam conflict. Therefore, most of what we know about the phenomenology and biology of PTSD is based on studies involving this patient population. Recently, attempts have been made to widen the focus by studying PTSD in women. Few studies to date have actually compared men and women. Therefore, many questions we may have with regard to sex differences cannot be answered by reviewing the literature. Most of what we know about this newly emerging field is based on very recent but scant evidence. Nonetheless, enough interesting findings exist to warrant a discussion of this issue and to formulate hypotheses to be tested in the future.

In this chapter, we review evidence from recent epidemiological studies that women are more affected by PTSD than are men. Women have a higher prevalence rate of PTSD and a higher rate of comorbidity associated with PTSD. Furthermore, PTSD in women may be qualitatively different because of the type of symptoms and time course of illness. What we infer from these observations is that a differential vulnerability to trauma and rate of development of PTSD are found between men and women. However, whether and to what extent these differences are associated with sex is still unclear. To help in an analysis of this issue, we present biological data from the important areas of neuroendocrinology and neuroimmunology, in which further study could help elucidate and tie together the many missing pieces in this puzzle. We then explore how this information might be used to further elucidate sex differences.

EPIDEMIOLOGY

Women Are at Higher Risk for Developing Posttraumatic Stress Disorder

In considering the prevalence of PTSD in men and women, the first observation is that PTSD is not an inevitable response to stress in either sex. What stands out from the data is that women develop PTSD twice as often as men do.

The range of prevalence rates of PTSD in trauma survivors in DSM-IV-TR (American Psychiatric Association 2000) is 3%–58%, which means that many individuals do not develop this condition in response to trauma exposure. The first major study of young adults found that of the 39% of the individuals exposed to trauma, only 23.6% developed PTSD at some point in their lives (Breslau et al. 1991). The prevalence rate of PTSD following a trauma appears to depend on the traumatic event. However, on the whole, PTSD is estimated to occur on average in 25% of the individuals who have been exposed to traumatic events (B.L. Green 1994), with rates considerably higher for life-threatening events than for those with lower impact (Kessler et al. 1995).

The lifetime prevalence of PTSD has consistently been shown to be twice as high in women as in men, regardless of the overall prevalence rate of the disorder found in each study sample (Table 3–1).

In addition, a community survey (Stein et al. 1997b) found that the prevalence of partial PTSD was 3.4% for women and 0.3% for men. These findings suggest a greater vulnerability of women compared with men to the development of PTSD after exposure to trauma.

TABLE 3–1. Lifetime prevalence of posttraumatic stress disorder, by sex

Study	Population	Trauma	Women/Girls (%)	Men/Boys (%)
Helzer et al. 1987	Adults	Mixed	1.3	0.5
Breslau et al. 1991	Adults	Mixed	11.3	6.0
J.R.T. Davidson et al. 1991	Adults	Mixed	1.7	0.9
B.L. Green et al. 1994	Adults	Buffalo Creek Disaster	12.0	0.0
Kessler et al. 1995	Adults	Mixed	10.4	5.0
Bromet et al. 1998	Adults	Mixed	19.4	7.6
B.L. Green et al. 1991	Children/Adults	Buffalo Creek Disaster	4.0	3.1
Garrison et al. 1993	Children/Adults	Hurricane Hugo	6.2 (white); 4.7 (black)	3.8 (white); 1.5 (black)
Brent et al. 1995	Children/Adults	Peer of suicide victim	5.5	0.0

Sex Differences in Rates of Trauma

One possible explanation for the higher prevalence of PTSD in women would be increased exposure to trauma. However, lifetime prevalence of exposure to at least one traumatic event also was found to be slightly higher in men than in women in some studies (60.7% in men and 51.2% in women—Kessler et al. 1995; 43.0% in men and 36.7% in women—Breslau et al. 1991) or did not vary by sex in others (Breslau et al. 1998). For example, 35.6% of the men and 14.5% of the women had witnessed someone being badly beaten or killed, 18.9% of the men and 15.2% of the women were involved in a natural disaster, and 25.0% of the men and 13.8% of the women were in a life-threatening accident (Kessler et al. 1995). In addition, the higher risk of PTSD in women was *not* accounted for by history of multiple traumatic events (Breslau et al. 1997b). In fact, the National Comorbidity Survey (NCS; Kessler et al. 1995) found that 10% of the men and 6% of the women were exposed to four or more types of trauma, some of which involved multiple occurrences. In an urban community, the mean number of distinct traumatic events was significantly greater in men compared with women (5.3 and 4.3, respectively, Breslau et al. 1998). Despite this, women had a higher prevalence of PTSD compared with men.

Sex Differences in Type of Trauma

Although men and women have comparable rates of overall trauma exposure, they may experience different types of life threats and trauma that explain the sex difference in PTSD. For example, men tend to be more exposed to war atrocities, violent crimes, being held captive, or being kidnapped, and women tend to experience higher rates of rape and physical abuse (Breslau et al. 1998). However, women had a higher probability of developing PTSD after exposure to a trauma compared with men, even *after* the type of trauma was controlled for (Breslau et al. 1997b, 1998; Kessler et al. 1995). For example, men in the NCS were twice as likely as women to report being seriously attacked or assaulted (11.1% vs. 6.9%; Kessler et al. 1995). However, this type of trauma was 15 times more likely to result in PTSD in women compared with men (21.3% vs. 1.8%). In a study of an urban population, the conditional risk of PTSD associated with trauma was 13.0% in females and 6.2% in males (Breslau et al. 1998). The sex difference was especially prominent following exposure to assaultive violence (36% in women vs. 6% in men).

Of particular interest was that the sex difference in PTSD was markedly greater if exposure occurred in childhood (before age 15 years) than later on (Breslau et al. 1997b).

Therefore, being a woman is a major risk factor for the development of PTSD.

Other Risk Factors and the Interaction With Sex

Risk factors for PTSD in both sexes include severity of trauma (Foy et al. 1984; March 1993; Yehuda et al. 1998); history of stress, abuse, or trauma (Bremner et al. 1997; Zaidi and Foy 1994); history of behavior or psychological problems (Helzer et al. 1987); preexisting psychiatric disorders (McFarlane 1989); family history of psychopathology (S. Davidson et al. 1985); genetic factors (True et al. 1993); subsequent exposure to reactivating environmental factors (Kluznick et al. 1986; March 1993; McFarlane 1989; Schnurr et al. 1993; S. Soloman and Smith 1994); initial psychological reaction to trauma, such as emotional numbing (Epstein et al. 1998; Feinstein and Dolan 1991; Mayou et al. 1993; Shalev et al. 1996); and early separation (Breslau et al. 1991; McFarlane 1988). Breslau et al. (1997a) found that preexisting anxiety and depressive disorders played only a small part in the observed sex difference in lifetime prevalence of PTSD. The observed role of preexisting anxiety and depressive disorders in the sex difference in PTSD was a function of the higher rate of preexisting anxiety and depressive disorders for women than for men (J.C. Anderson et al. 1995; Breslau et al. 1997a; Burke et al. 1990; Kessler et al. 1995). Parental PTSD also has been found to be a risk factor for the development of PTSD, which is a new idea introduced to the field (Yehuda et al. 1995c). Risk factors predicting exposure to trauma but not to onset of PTSD, controlling for type of trauma, were a history of affective disorder in women and a history of anxiety disorder and parental mental disorder in men (Breslau et al. 1998).

Interestingly, these risk factors interact with sex. For example, the effect of precombat abuse on PTSD symptoms was seen in female but not in male Desert Storm veterans. Specifically, the women describing precombat abuse reported much greater PTSD symptomatology than did the women denying precombat abuse (Engel et al. 1993). This once again highlights the increased vulnerability to the development of PTSD in women compared with men.

Women Are Also More Vulnerable to Comorbid Disorders

PTSD rarely occurs in the absence of other conditions. Approximately 50%–90% of the individuals with chronic PTSD have a comorbid psychiatric disorder (Freedy et al. 1992; Kulka et al. 1990). Kessler et al. (1995)

found that only 21% of the women and 12% of the men with PTSD had no other disorder. This reinforces the idea that PTSD is not randomly distributed throughout the population but rather that subgroups of people are more vulnerable to the development of PTSD and other psychiatric disorders.

In patients with PTSD, common comorbid disorders include major depressive disorder, alcoholism, drug abuse, personality disorder, anxiety disorders such as panic disorder and generalized anxiety disorder, and dissociative disorders (Friedman et al. 1987; Jordan et al. 1991; Kofoed et al. 1993; Kulka et al. 1990; Zlotnick et al. 1996).

Of particular interest is that women with PTSD tended to have higher rates of comorbid major depressive disorder and substance abuse compared with men (Blanchard et al. 1995; Clark et al. 1997; Silove et al. 1997; Wasserman et al. 1997). PTSD significantly increased the risk for the development of first-onset major depressive disorder and alcohol abuse and dependence in women (Breslau et al. 1997b).

Estimates of the rate of current PTSD in substance-abusing women ranged from 43% to 59% (Brown et al. 1995; Dansky et al. 1995). Women substance abusers were five times more likely than men to have PTSD, controlling for types of trauma in both groups (Wasserman et al. 1997). Moreover, "harder" substances such as cocaine and opioids have a higher association with trauma and PTSD than do substances such as marijuana and alcohol (Cottler et al. 1992; Schnitt and Nocks 1984).

This reinforces the need to study why certain subgroups of PTSD patients, especially women, develop certain other comorbid psychiatric conditions but other subgroups do not.

Sex Differences in Qualitative Experience of Posttraumatic Stress Disorder Symptoms

A recent study has reported sex differences in how PTSD is experienced (Breslau et al. 1998). Women tended to experience certain symptoms more frequently than men did: more intense psychological reactivity to stimuli that symbolize the trauma, restricted affect, and exaggerated startle response. This is also reflected in the higher mean number of PTSD symptoms after a violent assault experienced by women compared with men. Women also tended to have a longer course of illness than did men. The median duration of PTSD symptoms was 48.1 months in women and 12.1 months in men, with a median time to remission of PTSD symptoms of 35 months for women compared with 9 months for men. The results of this study underscore the necessity to delineate sex differences in the experience of PTSD.

BIOLOGICAL FINDINGS IN POSTTRAUMATIC STRESS DISORDER

Neuroendocrine Response: Hypothalamic–Pituitary–Adrenal Axis Dysregulation

Many aspects of the neuroendocrine responses observed in PTSD do not appear to resemble response patterns observed in acute stress studies in animals. However, some of this may be due to the time evaluated since onset of the stressor. Most studies of PTSD have been performed directly following the trauma, when the response to stress is usually evaluated acutely.

Studies have yielded important data with regard to neuroendocrine alterations in PTSD, showing hypersensitization of the hypothalamic-pituitary-adrenal (HPA) axis to stress, which is manifested by a decreased cortisol release and an increased negative feedback inhibition (Yehuda et al. 1995a, 1998). Hypersecretion of corticotropin-releasing factor (CRF) also has been described in PTSD (Bremner et al. 1993), as has blunting of corticotropin response to CRF (Smith et al. 1989). Other studies have reported lower 24-hour urinary cortisol excretion levels in PTSD patients compared with other psychiatric groups and nonpsychiatric control subjects (Mason et al. 1986; Yehuda et al. 1990, 1993c). PTSD subjects also have been shown to have lower plasma cortisol levels in the morning (Boscarino 1996) and at several time points throughout the circadian cycle (Yehuda et al. 1994) and to have a greater circadian signal-to-noise ratio compared with control subjects without PTSD (Yehuda et al. 1996a). In contrast, Pitman and Orr (1990) found elevated cortisol levels in combat veterans with PTSD compared with combat veterans who did not have PTSD.

In addition, PTSD subjects had an increased number of lymphocyte glucocorticoid receptors (which are needed for cortisol to exert its effects) compared with psychiatric and nonpsychiatric control groups (Yehuda et al. 1992a, 1993c, 1996b) and may have had enhanced suppression of cortisol in response to dexamethasone (Dinan et al. 1990; Halbreich et al. 1989; Kosten et al. 1990; Kudler et al. 1987; Olivera and Fero 1990; Yehuda et al. 1993a, 1995a). This response is distinctly different from that found in depression and other psychiatric disorders. In addition, administration of metyrapone, which blocks conversion of 11-deoxycortisol to cortisol and thereby attenuates the negative feedback effects of cortisol at the anterior pituitary, increased corticotropin release (Yehuda et al. 1996c). These observations support the hypothesis of enhanced negative feedback regulation of cortisol as an important feature of PTSD (Yehuda et al. 1993b, 1995a). Also, all the above studies were performed in male combat veterans, as shown in Table 3–2.

TABLE 3–2. Hypothalamus–pituitary–adrenal axis dysregulation in posttraumatic stress disorder

Study	Men/Boys	Women/Girls	Both sexes	Findings
Mason et al. 1986	Combat veterans	Not studied	Not studied	↓Cortisol
Kudler et al. 1987	Combat veterans	Not studied	Not studied	↑Suppression to DST
Halbreich et al. 1989	Combat veterans	Not studied	Not studied	↑Suppression to DST
Smith et al. 1989	Combat veterans	Not studied	Not studied	↓Corticotropin to corticotropin-releasing hormone
Dinan et al. 1990	Combat veterans	Not studied	Not studied	↑Suppression to DST
Kosten et al. 1990	Combat veterans	Not studied	Not studied	↑Suppression to DST
Olivera and Fero 1990	Combat veterans	Not studied	Not studied	↑Suppression to DST
Pitman and Orr 1990	Combat veterans	Not studied	Not studied	↑Cortisol
Yehuda et al. 1990	Combat veterans	Not studied	Not studied	↓Cortisol
Yehuda et al. 1993c	Combat veterans	Not studied	Not studied	↓Cortisol/↑Lymphocyte glucocorticoid receptor
Yehuda et al. 1993a	Combat veterans	Not studied	Not studied	↑Suppression to DST
Yehuda et al. 1994	Combat veterans	Not studied	Not studied	↓Cortisol
Yehuda et al. 1995a	Combat veterans	Not studied	Not studied	↑Lymphocyte glucocorticoid receptor/↑Suppression to DST
Boscarino 1996	Combat veterans	Not studied	Not studied	↓Cortisol
Yehuda et al. 1996a	Combat veterans	Not studied	Not studied	↓Cortisol
Yehuda et al. 1996b	Combat veterans	Not studied	Not studied	↑Lymphocyte glucocorticoid receptor
Yehuda et al. 1996c	Combat veterans	Not studied	Not studied	↑Corticotropin with metyrapone
Bremner et al. 1993	Combat veterans	Not studied	Not studied	↑Corticotropin-releasing factor
Jensen et al. 1997	Combat veterans	Not studied	Not studied	↓Cortisol
Kellner et al. 1997	Combat veterans	Not studied	Not studied	↓Cortisol
Lemieux and Coe 1995	Not studied	Childhood abuse	Not studied	↑Cortisol

TABLE 3–2. Hypothalamus–pituitary–adrenal axis dysregulation in posttraumatic stress disorder *(continued)*

Study	Men/Boys	Women/Girls	Both sexes	Findings
Resnick et al. 1995	Not studied	Rape victims	Not studied	↓Cortisol
Heim et al. 1997	Not studied	Sexual abuse	Not studied	↑Suppression to DST
Stein et al. 1997a	Not studied	Sexual/Physical abuse	Not studied	↑Lymphocyte glucocorticoid receptor/ ↑Suppression to DST
Bauer et al. 1994	Not studied	Not studied	East German refugees	↓Cortisol
Yehuda et al. 1995b	Not studied	Not studied	Holocaust survivors	↓Cortisol
Goenjian et al. 1996	Not studied	Not studied	Earthquake survivors	↓Cortisol/↑Suppression to DST

Note. DST=dexamethasone suppression test.

Only a few studies have evaluated women with PTSD who had traumatic stressors other than combat. Female patients with childhood-abuse-related PTSD had increased daily levels of cortisol and norepinephrine compared with female childhood-abuse victims without PTSD (Lemieux and Coe 1995). The norepinephrine-to-cortisol ratio was not significantly elevated in female patients with abuse-related PTSD, as in male combat veterans with PTSD. The authors wondered whether the discrepancy between their findings and others was caused by sex, an interaction between sex and age at onset, or physiological variation to phase of the disorder. Note, however, that most of the subjects in their study were obese, which is a significant factor because it affects HPA-axis function. Rape victims with a history of criminal victimization had lower plasma cortisol levels shortly after the rape compared with nontraumatized individuals (Resnick et al. 1995), as has been found in male combat veterans with PTSD. Sexually abused girls who were not evaluated for the presence of PTSD had normal cortisol levels with a decreased corticotropin response to corticotropin-releasing hormone (CRH), thereby showing HPA axis dysregulation (DeBellis et al. 1994a). Women with a history of physical or sexual abuse who have PTSD also had increased lymphocyte glucocorticoid receptors, as in male veterans with PTSD (Stein et al. 1997a). In addition, female adult PTSD patients with a history of sexual abuse have similar patterns of enhanced dexamethasone suppression of plasma cortisol when compared with male combat veterans with PTSD (Heim et al. 1997; Stein et al. 1997a).

In general, it seems that HPA axis dysregulation in women may resemble that in men, but only three studies to date have included both male and female subjects. Male and female Holocaust survivors with PTSD have been found to have lower 24-hour urinary cortisol excretion, as in male combat veterans with PTSD (Yehuda et al. 1995b). A study evaluated adolescent Armenian earthquake victims with PTSD from two towns; each town had a different trauma severity associated with it depending on distance from the epicenter. Adolescents who were exposed to greater trauma and had higher symptom severity had lower morning baseline cortisol levels and greater cortisol suppression by dexamethasone, which is consistent with most of the findings in adult patients with PTSD (Goenjian et al. 1996). A subset of 84 refugees from East Germany had a diagnosis of PTSD ($n=12$), and these subjects had lower cortisol levels than did healthy control subjects (Bauer et al. 1994). No sex differences were found in any of these three studies. However, more studies are needed before a conclusion can be drawn.

Catecholamine Alterations

The catecholamine system was the first biological system to be linked with trauma exposure. World War I veterans with shell shock had increased heart and respiratory rates in response to gunfire and increased levels of anxiety and blood pressure in response to epinephrine injections (Meakins and Wilson 1918). World War II veterans with this same clinical reaction were given diagnoses of *physioneurosis* (Kardiner 1941). These observations prompted many subsequent studies of psychophysiology. Some of these studies noted differences at baseline between combat veterans with PTSD and control subjects not exposed to any trauma (Blanchard et al. 1986; Brende 1982; Dobbs and Wilson 1960; Kardiner 1941; Malloy et al. 1983; Pitman et al. 1990).

Baseline catecholamine studies have yielded mixed results, however. Some studies noted increased baseline urinary catecholamine levels in patients with PTSD compared with control subjects (Kosten et al. 1987; Yehuda et al. 1992b). Other studies have not found differences between the two groups (Mellman et al. 1995; Perry et al. 1990), and one study found decreased catecholamine levels in subjects with PTSD compared with control subjects (Pitman RK, Orr SP, Yehuda R: "Ambulatory Monitoring of Heart Rate and Catecholamine Excretion in Vietnam Veterans With Post-Traumatic Stress Disorder," unpublished data). Studies of baseline plasma catecholamine levels and their metabolites also have been mixed. No differences between subjects with PTSD and control groups were found in some studies (Blanchard et al. 1991; McFall et al. 1990), another study found higher levels in PTSD patients (Yehuda et al. 1998), and yet another showed lower levels in patients with PTSD (Murburg et al. 1995).

Plasma catecholamine and metabolite levels were higher after neuroendocrine provocation (Southwick et al. 1993) or stress testing (Blanchard et al. 1991; McFall et al. 1990) in male combat veterans with PTSD compared with nonpsychiatric control subjects, showing hyperresponsiveness of the catecholamine system paralleling that of the HPA axis. Fewer α_2-adrenergic receptors have been found in subjects with PTSD (Perry et al. 1987, 1990), perhaps in response to chronic elevations of circulating catecholamines. Epinephrine caused faster degradation of α_2 receptors in patients with PTSD compared with control subjects, indicating that receptors of patients with PTSD are more sensitive (Perry et al. 1990). All of the above studies were done in male combat veterans, as shown in Table 3–3.

Among survivors of non-combat-related trauma with PTSD, very few studies have been done in women. The results also have been mixed. Women with PTSD who were sexually abused as children had higher baseline catecholamine levels (Lemieux and Coe 1995), as did girls who were sexually abused who were not evaluated for the presence of PTSD (DeBellis et al. 1994b) and showed increased physiological responses to traumatic imagery (Orr 1997). Studies involving mixed-sex samples found that Armenian children with PTSD who had survived an earthquake had increased

TABLE 3–3. Catecholamine alterations in posttraumatic stress disorder

Study	Men/Boys	Women/Girls	Both sexes	Findings
Meakins and Wilson 1918	Combat veterans	Not studied	Not studied	↑Blood pressure with epinephrine
Kardiner 1941	Combat veterans	Not studied	Not studied	↑Blood pressure with epinephrine
Dobbs and Wilson 1960	Combat veterans	Not studied	Not studied	↑Physiological response to challenge
Brende 1982	Combat veterans	Not studied	Not studied	↑Physiological response to challenge
Malloy et al. 1983	Combat veterans	Not studied	Not studied	↑Physiological response to challenge
Blanchard et al. 1986	Combat veterans	Not studied	Not studied	↑Physiological response to challenge
Kosten et al. 1987	Combat veterans	Not studied	Not studied	↑Baseline catecholamines
Perry et al. 1987	Combat veterans	Not studied	Not studied	↓α_2-Adrenergic receptors
McFall et al. 1990	Combat veterans	Not studied	Not studied	No difference in baseline catecholamines; ↑epinephrine to challenge
Perry et al. 1990	Combat veterans	Not studied	Not studied	No difference in baseline catecholamines
Pitman et al. 1990	Combat veterans	Not studied	Not studied	↑Physiological response to challenge
Blanchard et al. 1991	Combat veterans	Not studied	Not studied	No difference in baseline catecholamines; ↑heart rate and norepinephrine to challenge
Yehuda et al. 1992b	Combat veterans	Not studied	Not studied	↑Baseline catecholamines
Southwick et al. 1993	Combat veterans	Not studied	Not studied	↑Baseline catecholamines after challenge
Mellman et al. 1995	Combat veterans	Not studied	Not studied	No difference in baseline catecholamines
Murburg et al. 1995	Combat veterans	Not studied	Not studied	↓Baseline catecholamines
Yehuda et al. 1998	Combat veterans	Not studied	Not studied	↑Baseline catecholamines
Pitman et al., unpublished*	Combat veterans	Not studied	Not studied	↓Baseline catecholamines
Lemieux and Coe 1995	Not studied	Sexual abuse victims	Not studied	↑Baseline catecholamines
Orr 1997	Not studied	Sexual abuse victims	Not studied	↑Baseline catecholamines
Perry 1994	Not studied	Not studied	Noncombat trauma victims	↑Physiological response to challenge
Goenjian et al. 1996	Not studied	Not studied	Earthquake survivors	↓α_2-Adrenergic receptors; ↑Baseline catecholamines

Note. *Pitman RK, Orr SP, Yehuda R: "Ambulatory Monitoring of Heart Rate and Catecholamine Excretion in Vietnam Veterans With Post–Traumatic Stress Disorder," unpublished data baseline catecholamine metabolite levels (Goenjian et al. 1996). In contrast, Holocaust survivors with PTSD had lower baseline catecholamine levels (Yehuda 1999). Traumatized children had fewer α_2-adrenergic receptors, as was the case in combat veterans (Perry 1994). No sex differences were reported in these studies. Once again, no conclusions about sex differences can be inferred from the studies done to date because too few of them make a direct comparison between male and female patients with PTSD in the same study sample.

Immune Response

Very few studies of immune function in patients with PTSD have been done, but this is a relevant parameter to a discussion of sex differences because women generally have a more active immune response than do men and concomitantly have a higher incidence of autoimmune disease. In addition, the interactions between the immune and the neuroendocrine systems with regard to stress are highly interconnected. Moreover, the modulatory effects of sex hormones on both of these systems have been shown to be significant, although the exact relations have yet to be determined. How the body reacts to stress may determine its risk for the development of disease and illness. A deeper understanding of how the immune response in PTSD manifests itself is therefore a needed component for our understanding of the pathophysiology of the disorder. A more detailed discussion of immune function and response is addressed later in this chapter (see sections "Sex as a Modulating Factor in the Biological Response to Stress" and "Biological Response to Stress").

Studies involving subjects experiencing non-combat-related trauma have evaluated immune function acutely after the event. However, these patients were not given diagnoses of PTSD. No sex differences were found in most of the following studies. A study involving workers at an airline crash site found that those workers exposed to body parts had increased natural killer (NK) cell cytotoxicity 2 months after the crash, but this decreased to control levels 6 months later (Delahanty et al. 1997). Earthquake victims showed acute increases in multiple immune measures, which lessened over time (CD3$^+$, CD8$^+$, CD16$^+$, CD56$^+$ lymphocytic cells; T-cell blastogenesis; and NK cell cytotoxicity) (G. F. Solomon et al. 1997). Studies done in Israeli civilians during and after a period of Scud missile attacks during the Persian Gulf War found that during the war period, NK cell cytotoxicity and cell-mediated immunity were significantly elevated, as were plasma levels of corticotropin, neurotensin, and substance P (Weiss et al. 1996). Another study examined immune function in a community exposed to Hurricane Andrew (Ironson et al. 1997). Increased NK cell count and decreased NK cell cytotoxicity and CD4 and CD8 numbers were found in the community 4 months after the disaster. In this study, men had higher NK cell cytotoxicity and blood pressure levels than women did.

The following studies were performed in single-sex samples. Immune reactivity in men just released from a war prisoner camp in Bosnia was measured (Dekaris et al. 1993). Activated T and B lymphocytes and total human leukocyte antigen (HLA)-DR lymphocytes increased. The ratio of CD4 (helper T) to CD8 (suppressor T or cytotoxic) cells was decreased, as were NK cell cytotoxicity and phagocytic function. In addition, serum interferon, cortisol, and prolactin were significantly lowered with an increase in tumor necrosis factor. A sample of sexually abused girls showed a higher incidence of plasma antinuclear antibody titers compared with adult healthy female control subjects, but no difference in titer levels was seen when compared with healthy control girls (DeBellis et al. 1996).

Only four studies of immune response have involved subjects with PTSD, all of whom were male combat veterans (Table 3–4). One study found that proinflammatory serum interleukin (IL)-1β levels but not soluble IL-2 receptors (another proinflammatory cytokine measure) were significantly higher than those in control subjects (Spivak et al. 1997). The IL-1β levels did not correlate with cortisol levels, severity of PTSD, anxiety, or depressive symptoms. They did, however, correlate with duration of PTSD symptoms. Another study showed increased NK cell cytotoxicity in subjects with PTSD compared with control subjects, but no differences were found between subjects with PTSD and control subjects with regard to lymphocytic subtypes (CD2, CD3, CD8, CD16, CD20, and CD56) and endocrine measures (cortisol, prolactin, growth hormone, and DHEA-SO_4) (Laudenslager et al. 1998). The third study found that patients with PTSD had enhanced in vivo cell-mediated immunity based on the standardized CMI Multitest compared with control subjects (Watson et al. 1993). Another study showed that patients with PTSD had decreased in vitro NK cell cytotoxicity in response to methionine-enkephalin challenge compared with control subjects (Mosnaim et al. 1993).

These few studies showed that chronic PTSD increases cell-mediated immunity, which is the opposite of what is found in most chronic stress models in which cell-mediated immunity is suppressed. No studies have been done with female subjects with PTSD, however.

In light of the neuroendocrine and immune findings, there is support for the notion that an intimate relation exists between these two systems in PTSD. However, how they interact to give rise to these findings and psychopathology remains unclear. In addition, how sex functions as a modulator has not been well studied at all.

TABLE 3–4. Immune response in male combat veterans with posttraumatic stress disorder

Study	Findings
Mosnaim et al. 1993	↓NK cell cytotoxicity with MET
Watson et al. 1993	↑Delayed-type hypersensitivity
Spivak et al. 1997	↑Interleukin 1β
Laudenslager et al. 1998	↑NK cell cytotoxicity

Note. MET=methionine-enkephalin; NK=natural killer.

Response to Stress

Hans Seyle first described the stress syndrome produced by noxious stimuli in 1936 (Seyle 1956). The stress syndrome included three stages: the alarm reaction, resistance, and exhaustion. The major role of glucocorticoids was purportedly during the alarm reaction. The biological stress response includes involvement of the HPA axis, catecholamine system, and immunological system, with modulating factors such as gonadal hormones. The interactions among all these systems regulate the body's reaction to stress, and any dysfunction in response in any part of the cascade would give rise to pathology.

The importance of estrogens in the stress response is illustrated in the animal literature that shows sex differences in the response to stress.

Differences between responses to acute stress and responses to chronic stress also must be delineated. Much of the animal research has been done in acute stress situations; only a few studies have examined the effects of chronic stress on the organism. In contrast, most of the studies in human subjects have been done in subjects with chronic PTSD; very few, done only more recently, have examined the effects of acute trauma on the individual. Much more investigation is required to fully characterize each state.

Behavioral Response to Stress and Sex Differences

Different animal models of stress have been studied, including exposing rats to different stresses, such as intermittent tail shocks, forced swimming, immobilization, predatory stress (i.e., exposure to cats), and administration of medications such as insulin. Rats show several different behavioral responses to different types of stress. The animals respond to immobilization stress by a decrease in rearing behavior, decreased food intake, decreased exploration, and hypothermia (Plaznik et al. 1993). With inescapable tail shocks, the animals initially will struggle and attempt to escape but finally show a decrease in attempts or failure to escape (Chaouloff 1991). In the forced swimming stress test, rats will become immobile in response to the stress (Chaouloff 1991). This is in contrast to PTSD, in which the development of the disorder does not depend on the type of trauma a person is exposed to.

Response to chronic stress includes weight loss in response to prolonged immobilization. Chronic stress in rats also facilitated classical conditioning in males but impaired classical conditioning in females (Wood and Shors 1998). A comparison of intact male and female rats with ovariectomized females and with intact females who were administered tamoxifen (an estrogen antagonist) showed that stress-induced impairment in female conditioning was dependent on ovarian hormones. These findings underscored sex differences in long-term responses to chronic stress, such as associative learning and emotional responding, and implicated estrogen as the underlying mechanism.

Physical restraint in rodents has been found to increase susceptibility to herpes simplex virus infection (Rasmussen et al. 1957) and to Malony sarcoma virus (Levine et al. 1962) but to decrease susceptibility to allergic encephalomyelitis (Levine et al. 1962). Electric shock stimulation increases susceptibility to coxsackie B virus and decreases susceptibility to rodent malaria (Friedman et al. 1965). Apparently, the same stressor can have different effects on different pathophysiological processes and disease processes.

This finding parallels our observations in human beings, in which trauma exposure can result in the development of not only PTSD but also depression and other anxiety disorders. The effects of stress on people, much like in animals, include symptoms such as somatic complaints (e.g., decreased appetite), social withdrawal, attention problems, anxiety, and depression (Mollica et al. 1997). As already mentioned, exposure to trauma does not necessarily lead to the development of PTSD. In addition, no associations have been found between type of trauma and types of psychological distress experienced (Winje 1996). Female Southeast Asian refugees and female prison inmates have reported significantly higher levels of psychological distress compared with male counterparts in response to stress (Chung et al. 1998; Lindquist and Linquist 1997). Also, of those persons who handled the dead during disasters, inexperienced women had higher anticipated stress levels than did inexperienced men (McCarroll et al. 1993).

This again draws our attention to the greater vulnerability of women compared with men in regard to the development of greater psychological distress in response to stress and to the development of mental illnesses such as anxiety and depressive disorders. Much more knowledge must be elucidated before we can ascertain the reasons for these observations.

Sex as a Modulating Factor in the Biological Response to Stress

Estrogens, derived from the aromatization of testosterone in the brain, account for sex-specific organization of neural circuits controlling gonadotropin release and sexual behavior. Sex hormones also have organizing and activating effects on the HPA axis (Figure 3–1).

Organizing effects of estrogens refer to the effects of neonatal sex hormones on the sensitivity of the HPA axis to sex hormones in adulthood; these include sex differences in the gene expression of hypothalamic CRH, hippocampal and hypothalamic glucocorticoid receptors, and diurnal corticosterone secretion, as well as responsiveness of CRF and glucocorticoid receptor messenger RNA (mRNA) levels to exogenous estradiol (McCormick et al. 1998; Patchev et al. 1995).

Activating effects of estrogens refer to the elevating effects of estrogen on the HPA axis in the adult brain, including the influence of estrogen on CRH, arginine-vasopressin, and glucocorticoid receptor gene expression (Ansar Ahmed and Talal 1990; Bohler et al. 1990; Magiakou et al. 1997; Ogilvie and Rivier 1997; Peiffer et al. 1991). In contrast, androgens exert an inhibitory influence on the HPA axis. These gonadal effects may account for the induction of enhanced activity of the HPA axis at the period of late proestrus (Carey et al. 1995).

In rats, corticosterone and corticotropin levels as well as functional activity of the HPA axis were higher in females than in males under both basal conditions and stress conditions when basal levels were controlled for. In humans, greater activation of the neuroendocrine response (corticotropin and prolactin release) was seen during stress in women compared with men (Jezova et al. 1996). Whether sex steroids are in part responsible for these observations has not been conclusively shown; however, many supportive findings show the interaction between female hormones and neuroendocrine function.

Ovariectomized rats had reduced corticotropin and corticosterone responses to stress (Burgess and Handa 1993; Kitay 1963; Viau and Meaney 1991). Also, prenatal stress significantly increased plasma corticotropin and B levels in female rats but not males. In addition, differences were found in glucocorticoid receptor density in the septum, frontal cortex, and amygdala between females and males. As such, the effect of prenatal stress on HPA function is substantially more marked in females than in males (McCormick et al. 1995).

Sex steroids have been implicated in autoimmune processes (Ansar Ahmed and Talal 1990; Lahita 1990). Females have higher levels of immunoglobulin (Ig) G, IgG1, IgM, and IgA than do males in several species (Butterworth et al. 1967; Grossman 1985). Humoral responses to T-cell-

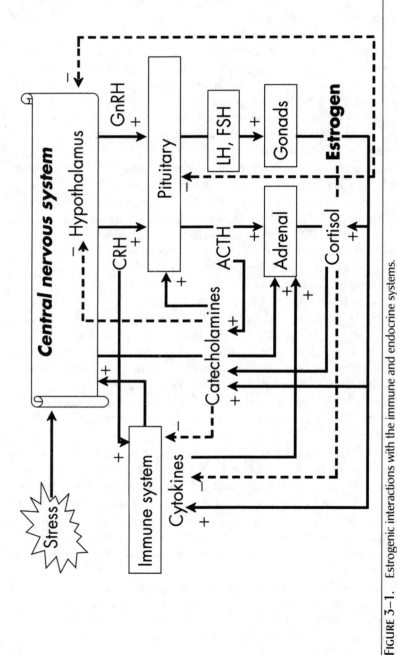

FIGURE 3–1. Estrogenic interactions with the immune and endocrine systems.

Note. ACTH=adrenocorticotropic hormone; CRH=corticotropin-releasing hormone; FSH=follicle-stimulating hormone; GnRH=gonadotropin-releasing hormone; LH=luteinizing hormone.

independent and T-cell-dependent antigens are greater in magnitude and more prolonged in females than in males (Eidinger and Garrett 1972; Terres et al. 1968). Estrogen may enhance antibody production, with specificity for foreign and self-antigens (Ansar Ahmed et al. 1989). Estrogens also alter the cytokines that alter B-cell antibody differentiation. In vitro, estrogen increased interferon-γ production (Fox et al. 1991), and dihydrotestosterone inhibited IL-4, IL-5, and interferon-γ production (antiinflammatory cytokines) (Daynes et al. 1990). These findings suggest that gonadal steroids act through regulation of T-cell cytokine production to alter B-cell production. In addition, T- and B-cell expression of androgen and estrogen receptors has been reported (Danel et al. 1983; Luster et al. 1984; Stimson 1988).

Females experience a higher incidence of autoimmune diseases such as systemic lupus erythematosus and rheumatoid arthritis (Duvic et al. 1978; Grossman et al. 1991; Masi and Kaslow 1978). Estrogen also has been found to enhance immune complex-mediated glomerulonephritis as a result of polyclonal B-cell activation.

Sex steroids also may influence the immune system via T-cell differentiation in the thymus. Estrogen has been found to decrease T-cell differentiation in the thymus (CD4, CD8, thymocytes) and increase in T-cell differentiation in the liver (Okuyama et al. 1992; Screpanti et al. 1989). T-cell differentiation in the liver has been associated with reactivity to self, including aging, infectious disease, autoimmunity, and athymia in animals.

How the Menstrual Cycle Affects the Hypothalamic-Pituitary-Adrenal Axis and the Response to Stress

Interaction of the stress hormone cortisol and gonadal female hormones has been examined. Cortisol slowed luteinizing hormone (LH) pulse frequency and, by interference, hypothalamic gonadotropin-releasing hormone secretion. LH pulse amplitude was unchanged. Mean estradiol levels were not affected, but LH and follicle-stimulating hormone levels were significantly reduced (Saketos et al. 1993). Cortisol is believed to exert a physiological role in oocyte maturation or ovulation (Fateh et al. 1989). An increase in total and free cortisol in the follicle during LH surge has been documented (Harlow et al. 1997). High levels of free cortisol in preovulatory follicular fluid may confine and reduce some of the inflammatory-like reactions that take place close to follicular rupture (C.Y. Anderson and Hornes 1994).

In humans, the follicular phase is the interval from menses to ovulation, and the luteal phase is the interval from ovulation to menses. During the follicular phase, LH and follicle-stimulating hormone levels decline. Estradiol and progesterone levels are also lower in the follicular phase compared with the luteal phase.

In rats, comparisons of proestrus and estrus have found that during estrus, the phase with lower estrogen and progesterone secretion, HPA axis reactivity is relatively reduced (Carey et al. 1995; Pollard et al. 1975; Viau and Meaney 1991), glucocorticoid receptor mRNA expression is increased (Peiffer et al. 1994), and hypothalamic CRH mRNA expression is reduced (Bohler et al. 1990; Peiffer et al. 1994; Viau and Meaney 1991).

Lactation suppressed the HPA response to stress (plasma cortisol, corticotropin, and glucose levels) (Altemus et al. 1995). In addition, basal norepinephrine levels were reduced in lactating women. These results indicate that the stress response of the neurohormonal system is blunted in lactating women. The effect of ovariectomy in premenopausal women on the HPA axis is characterized by reduced stimulated secretion of corticotropin and steroids but normal stimulated cortisol production (DeLeo et al. 1998).

Numerous studies in humans have documented stability of baseline cortisol levels across the menstrual cycle (Genazzani et al. 1975; Parker et al. 1981; Rabin et al. 1990; Rubinow et al. 1988; Schoneshofer and Wagner 1977), two studies have reported higher cortisol levels in the luteal phase (Gennazzani et al. 1975; Tersman et al. 1991), and no study has found higher cortisol levels in the follicular phase. Little has been done to study the changing sensitivity of tissues to glucocorticoids during the menstrual cycle.

Altemus et al. (1997) studied glucocorticoid feedback and glucocorticoid receptor mRNA expression during different phases of the menstrual cycle. The findings included a greater suppression of plasma cortisol in response to a 0.25-mg dose of dexamethasone in the follicular phase compared with the luteal phase of the menstrual cycle. In addition, expression of the type II glucocorticoid receptor gene in lymphocytes was increased in the follicular phase of the cycle. These results suggested that the luteal phase of the menstrual cycle in humans is associated with reduced sensitivity to glucocorticoid feedback. Enhanced cortisol suppression in the early follicular phase was noted in another study (Tandon et al. 1991). Two prior studies of dexamethasone suppression in nondepressed healthy women did not find any effect of cycle phase, most likely because the standard 1.0-mg dose of dexamethasone caused a complete or almost complete suppression of cortisol in both phases of the cycle (Parker et al. 1983; Roy-Byrne et al. 1986). Past studies that were consistent with the findings of Altemus et al. (1997) reported that cortisol responses to metoclopramide were enhanced in the luteal phase compared with the follicular phase (Seki 1989), cortisol responses to a psychological stress were enhanced in the luteal phase compared with the ovulatory phase (Marinari et al. 1976), and cortisol responses to exercise also were enhanced in the luteal phase (Lavoie et al. 1987). The finding of reductions in lymphocyte mRNA during the luteal phase suggests that changes in cortisol suppression in response to dexamethasone across the cycle are mediated in part by changes in the efficiency of dexamethasone feedback at glucocorticoid receptors.

How estrogen affects glucocorticoid receptor mRNA expression remains unclear. Estrogen may activate estrogen receptors in the hippocampus and paraventricular nucleus or the CRF gene, which increases glucocorticoid receptor mRNA expression. Estrogen also may modulate glucocorticoid receptor gene expression by activating or repressing transcriptional mechanisms (Cato and Ponta 1989; Green and Chambon 1987). Another alternative is that estrogen and progesterone may modulate the HPA axis by nongenomic, non-receptor-mediated mechanisms (McEwen 1994; Wong and Moss 1992). In addition, gonadal steroids may influence some neurotransmitters, such as the serotonergic and noradrenergic systems, which alter HPA axis responsivity (Feldman and Seidenfeld 1991; Maccari et al. 1992).

Biological Response to Stress

The neuroendocrine response to stress involves a cascade of secretory events initiated by CRH and arginine-vasopression produced by the hypothalamus and ultimately results in the release of glucocorticoids from the adrenal gland. The circulating glucocorticoids then regulate the HPA axis through feedback effects on the synthesis and secretion of hypothalamic and pituitary hormones, thereby controlling the basal activity level. The corticosteroid receptors in the hippocampus are very sensitive to this negative feedback system.

Animal models of stress have shown that restraint stress suppressed NK cell activity and the primary development of cytotoxic T cells of mice inoculated with the herpes simplex virus (Bonneau et al. 1991) (Table 3–5). Restraint and electric shocks also inhibited the activation of herpes simplex virus–specific memory cells (Ader 1980; Kuscenov et al. 1992). Forced swimming stress decreased NK activity and increased lung metastases in a tumor model (Ben-Eliyahu et al. 1991). In response to separation and/or early weaning, rodents had decreased lymphoproliferative responses to mitogenic stimulation and reduced response to subsequent antigenic challenge (Ackerman et al. 1988; Michaut et al. 1981). Repeated stress in laboratory animals led to recurrent endotoxemia, which decreased the reactivity of the HPA axis to a variety of stimuli and decreased the production of tumor necrosis factor (Hadid et al. 1996).

Acute stress responses in healthy men include increases in NK cells and their cytotoxic activity (Benschop et al. 1996; Schedlowski et al. 1993) (Table 3–6). Chronic psychological stress such as bereavement has been associated with changes in components of immunological reactivity, such as reduced lymphoproliferative responses to mitogenic stimulation (Barthrop et al. 1977; Benschop et al. 1996; Schleifer et al. 1983) and impaired NK cell activity (Irwin et al. 1987). Other reports have described similar

TABLE 3–5. Animal models of the biological response to stress

Study	Type of stress	Findings
Bonneau et al. 1991	Restraint stress	↓NK cell cytotoxicity and suppressor T-cell development
Ader 1980; Kuscenov et al. 1992	Restraint stress and electric shocks	↓Activation of memory T cells
Ben-Eliyahu et al. 1991	Forced swimming stress	↓NK cell cytotoxicity and ↑lung metastases in tumor model
Ackerman et al. 1988; Michaut et al. 1981	Separation and/or early weaning	↓Lymphoproliferative response to mitogenic stimulation; ↓response to antigenic rechallenge
Hadid et al. 1996	Repeated stress with variety of stimuli	Recurrent endotoxemia; ↓HPA axis reactivity; TNF-α production

Note. HPA=hypothalamic-pituitary-adrenal; NK=natural killer; TNF-α=tumor necrosis factor alpha.

changes in immune function associated with the affective response to other losses, such as marital separation and divorce (Kiecolt-Glaser and Glaser 1986). Medical student responses were studied before upcoming examinations; mitogenic responsiveness, NK cell activity, and percentage of helper T cells in the blood were decreased (Kiecolt-Glaser and Glaser 1986). These students also had decreased interferon production during the examination period. They had increased antibody titers to the Epstein-Barr virus during examination periods (Glaser et al. 1985), showing decreased cell-mediated control over the latent virus. Chronic psychological stress in subjects suppressed cellular immunity, resulting in increased severity of the common cold, accompanied by increased titers of cold-virus antibody (Cohen and Williamson 1991).

Glucocorticoids have immunosuppressive properties. They regulate cytokine production, inhibit responses to self-antigens, and limit inflammatory processes (Munck and Guyre 1991; Munck et al. 1984; Stam et al. 1983; Wick et al. 1993). They act by binding to cytosolic receptors on T and B cells and macrophages (Cupps and Fauci 1982; Werb et al. 1978) to initiate multiple immunoregulatory reactions. Glucocorticoids limit immune responsiveness by initiating programmed cell death, altering lymphocyte distribution and trafficking, and regulating lymphocyte cytokine production, all of which result in reduced immune reactivity. However, acute stress can result in trafficking of lymphocytes, which can increase antigen-specific cell-mediated immunity, as in the case of delayed-type hypersensitivity, in which exposure to a challenge stress results in trafficking of lymphocytes and macrophages to the site of acute challenge (Dhabhar 1996; Dhabhar and McEwen 1996a, 1996b). This immune-enhancing effect of acute stress

TABLE 3–6. Human models of the biological response to stress

Study	Stress	Findings
Benschop et al. 1996	Acute stress in healthy men	↑NK cell number and NK cell cytotoxicity
Schedlowski et al. 1993	Chronic psychological stress (e.g., bereavement)	↓CMI and ↑antibody titers to cold virus; ↓lymphoproliferative response to mitogenic stimulation; ↓NK cell cytotoxicity
Cohen and Williamson 1991		
Barthrop et al. 1977	Marital separation and divorce	↓Lymphoproliferative response to mitogenic stimulation; ↓NK cell cytotoxicity
Benschop et al. 1996		
Schleifer et al. 1983		
Irwin et al. 1987		
Kiecolt-Glaser and Glaser 1986		
Kiecolt-Glaser and Glaser 1986	Examination stress in medical students	↓Lymphoproliferative response to mitogenic stimulation; ↓NK cell cytotoxicity; ↓% helper T cells in blood; ↓interferon production
Glaser et al. 1985		↑Antibody titers to Epstein-Barr virus

Note. CMI=cell-mediated immunity; NK=natural killer.

involves an established immune "memory" (Dhabhar et al. 1996). However, *repeated* stress causes significant suppression of delayed-type hypersensitivity (Dhabhar and McEwen 1996a, 1996b) and suppression of cell-mediated immunity.

The anti-inflammatory and immunosuppressive effects of glucocorticoids are mediated in part by inhibition of macrophage production of proinflammatory cytokines such as IL-1, tumor necrosis factor, and IL-6 (Barber et al. 1993; Snyder and Unanue 1982; Van Den Bergh et al. 1994). Glucocorticoid-induced inhibition of T-cell proliferation was correlated with reduced IL-2 production (another proinflammatory cytokine) (Gillis et al. 1979; Pinkstone et al. 1987). In addition, glucocorticoids cause upregulation of the receptors for IL-1, IL-2, IL-6, and interferon-γ. Glucocorticoids also were found to enhance IL-4 (an anti-inflammatory cytokine) production by activated T cells (Daynes and Araneo 1989). This pattern of cytokine production leads to inhibition of cell-mediated responses and to enhanced antibody production. Therefore, the chances of acquiring an infection by a viral or bacterial pathogen that requires cell-mediated immunity for elimination are increased.

In contrast, long-term exposure to a stressor gives rise to a different profile of events compared with an acute response. Exposure to an acute stressor in animal models was immunosuppressive, with lower mitogen responsiveness, but chronic stress in one study led to an enhancement of immune function (Monjian and Collector 1977). Effects of long-term in vivo corticosterone treatment on T-cell function in rats were as follows: little effect on IL-2 levels and CD4 and CD8 cell numbers and significant decreases in B-cell populations (Sterzer et al. 1997), which is in contrast to acute effects of glucocorticoids. Also, decreased cytokine level does not necessarily lead to decreased cytokine activity because upregulation of the corresponding receptors also occurs, thereby increasing the sensitivity of the target cell to cytokines (Weigers et al. 1995). Therefore, if this biological response to decreased cytokine levels is interrupted or delayed, there might be a potentially dangerous effect on the organism. Thus, it would make sense to measure both cytokine and receptor levels to obtain a more global impression of a patient's immune status.

Corticotropin itself may have immunoregulatory properties. It reportedly reduced antibody (humoral) responses and interferon-γ production in vitro (Clarke and Bost 1989; Johnson et al. 1982, 1984). Corticotropin also may be capable of regulating immune cells locally; however, this remains controversial (Blalock 1989; Carr and Blalock 1991; Heijnen et al. 1991).

McEwen applied the notions of allostasis (the ability to achieve stability through change) (Sterling and Eyer 1988) and allostatic load (the long-term effect of the physiological response to stress) (McEwen and Stellar

1993) to the stress response. Allostatic systems enable us to respond to physical states and to a stressful challenge. The most common allostatic responses involve the sympathetic nervous system and the HPA axis (McEwen 1998). Activation of these systems by stress results in the release of catecholamines, corticotropin, and ultimately cortisol. Inactivation of these systems returns cortisol and catecholamine levels to baseline. However, an inefficient inactivation system overexposes the organisms to stress hormones, thereby increasing the allostatic load over time, resulting in pathophysiological consequences (McEwen 1998).

The failure to turn off the HPA axis and sympathetic systems efficiently after stress has been found to be age related in animal studies (McCarty 1985; McEwen 1992; Sapolsky 1992). The return to baseline levels of stress-induced cortisol has been shown to be slowed (Seeman and Robbins 1994) and the negative-feedback effects of cortisol are reduced in elderly human subjects (Wilkinson et al. 1997). It has been speculated that the allostatic systems have become exhausted with increasing allostatic loads. One could postulate that with enormous allostatic loads, as in the case of chronic PTSD, a similar pattern also might emerge (McEwen 1998).

Other Modulators of the Biological
Response to Stress: Circadian Rhythm

Apart from sex, another modulator of the HPA stress response is circadian rhythm. Ultradian patterns of circulating corticotropin and cortisol levels measured in the men and women were indicative of pulsatile secretory activity within the HPA axis (Gallagher et al. 1973; Lui et al. 1987; Veldhuis et al. 1989). More important, dynamic interactions have been observed between the ultradian rhythm of basal corticosterone release in the female rat and response to acute stress (Windle et al. 1998). This study found continuous, but variable, activity of the HPA axis throughout the day, suggesting alternate periods of secretion and inhibition, which had significant effects on the corticosterone responses to acute stress. When stress coincided with a rising, secretory phase of a pulse, corticosterone concentrations were increased. In contrast, when stress coincided with a falling, nonsecretory phase of a pulse, a response no greater than the basal pulse was evoked. Therefore, the alternate periods of secretion and inhibition HPA axis activity are important determinants of response to stress.

THE EFFECTS OF SEX ON POSTTRAUMATIC
STRESS DISORDER: A WORKING HYPOTHESIS

If estrogen facilitates the stress response, as reflected by increased cortisol, then low estrogen levels, such as in the follicular phase of the menstrual cycle in women, may favor a "PTSD-like" response to stress, and high estrogen levels, such as in the luteal phase, may favor more of a depression response. Women who are in their follicular phase during the time of exposure to trauma may be at greater risk for the development of a PTSD-like response to trauma. This could mean that HPA sensitization might be a risk factor for, rather than a consequence of, PTSD. This hypothesis could be tested. In the immediate aftermath of a trauma, cortisol levels are low in trauma survivors who will subsequently develop PTSD compared with those who will not develop PTSD. Lower cortisol levels appear to be present in individuals who are at risk for PTSD (e.g., children of Holocaust survivors). One possible reason for younger females to be more susceptible to the development of PTSD is that estrogen levels are extremely low in prepubescent girls, and this would favor a PTSD-like response to trauma. However, because this hypothesis explains increased vulnerability to trauma in only half of the menstrual cycle in women, other factors must play a part, possibly immune factors.

In PTSD, findings have been consistent with a hyperactive HPA axis, with increased CRF and decreased cortisol levels. It is not clear at this point which is the driving force and locus of change. In any case, increased CRF and decreased cortisol levels would both result in increased cell-mediated immunity, which has been found in the few studies done in men with PTSD. Whether this is in any way a compensatory effect or a detrimental one remains to be seen. In women, the modulatory effects of estrogen would come into play. One could postulate that in women, humoral responses would tend to be increased because of the estrogenic effect. However, estrogen results in decreased CRF and increased cortisol responses, which could result in a decrease in cell-mediated immunity. The combination of increased antibody response and decreased cell-mediated immunity could result in overproduction of antibodies and possibly autoantibodies. This would have a negative effect and could result in greater disease expression, thereby explaining in part why women are more vulnerable to the development of PTSD compared with men. It would therefore make sense to study whether there are indeed sex differences in the immune response of subjects with PTSD and to attempt to correlate this with neuroendocrine abnormalities, which could indicate a profile of increased risk in women with PTSD compared with men with the disorder.

CONCLUSION

Women have a higher prevalence of PTSD than do men. Women tend to have increased comorbidity with PTSD and have different qualitative symptomatic experiences and time courses of the illness. The biological differences between males and females have been discussed in relation to the psychoimmunoendocrinology and the stress response. Differences in response to stress in these highly interactive systems between males and females are apparent, and there is every reason to believe that some of these differences may be expressed in PTSD. However, this needs to be empirically determined.

REFERENCES

Ackerman SH, Keller SE, Schleifer SJ, et al: Premature maternal separation and lymphocyte function. Brain Behav Immun 2:161–165, 1988

Ader R: Presidential address: psychosomatic and psychoimmunologic research. Psychosom Med 42:307–321, 1980

Altemus M, Deuster PA, Gallivan E, et al: Suppression of the hypothalamic-pituitary-adrenal axis responses to stress in lactating women. J Clin Endocrinol Metab 80:2954–2959, 1995

Altemus M, Redwine L, Leong Y-M, et al: Reduced sensitivity to glucocorticoid feedback and reduced glucocorticoid receptor mRNA expression in the luteal phase of the menstrual cycle. Neuropsychopharmacology 17:100–109, 1997

American Psychiatric Association: Diagnostic and Statistical Manual of Mental Disorders, 4th Edition, Text Revision. Washington, DC, American Psychiatric Association, 2000

Anderson CY, Hornes P: Intrafollicular concentration of free cortisol close to follicular rupture. Hum Reprod 9:1944–1949, 1994

Anderson JC, Williams S, McGee R, et al: DSM-III disorders in preadolescent children. Arch Gen Psychiatry 58:1–12, 1995

Ansar Ahmed S, Talal N: Sex hormones and the immune system—part 2: animal data. Baillieres Clin Rheumatol 4:13–31, 1990

Ansar Ahmed S, Dauphinee MJ, Montoya AI, et al: Estrogen induces normal murine CD5+ B cells to produce autoantibodies. J Immunol 142:2647–2653, 1989

Barber AE, Coyle SM, Marano MA, et al: Glucocorticoid therapy alters hormonal and cytokine responses to endotoxin in man. J Immunol 150:1999–2006, 1993

Bartrop RW, Luckhurst E, Lazarus L, et al: Depressed lymphocyte function after bereavement. Lancet 1:834–836, 1977

Bauer M, Priebe S, Graf K-J, et al: Psychological and endocrine abnormalities in refugees from East Germany, part II: serum levels of cortisol, prolactin, luteinizing hormone, follicle stimulating hormone, and testosterone. Psychiatry Res 51:75–85, 1994

Ben-Eliyahu S, Yirmiya R, Liebeskind JC, et al: Stress increases metastatic spread of a mammary tumor in rats: evidence for mediation by the immune system. Brain Behav Immun 5:193–205, 1991

Benschop RJ, Jacobs R, Sommer B, et al: Modulation of the immunologic response to acute stress in humans by beta-blockade or benzodiazepines. FASEB J 10:517–524, 1996

Blalock JE: A molecular basis for bidirectional communication between the immune and neuroendocrine systems. Physiol Rev 69:1–32, 1989

Blanchard EB, Kolb LC, Pallmayer TP, et al: A psychophysiological study of posttraumatic stress disorder in Vietnam veterans. Behav Res Ther 24:645–652, 1986

Blanchard EB, Kolb LC, Prins A, et al: Changes in plasma norepinephrine to combat-related stimuli among Vietnam veterans with PTSD. J Nerv Ment Dis 179:371–373, 1991

Blanchard EB, Hickling EJ, Taylor AE, et al: Psychiatric morbidity associated with motor vehicle accidents. J Nerv Ment Dis 183:495–504, 1995

Bohler HCL, Zoeller T, King JC, et al: Corticotropin releasing hormone mRNA is elevated on the afternoon of proestrus in the parvocellular paraventricular nuclei of the female rat. Mol Brain Res 8:259–262, 1990

Bonneau RH, Sheridan JF, Feng N, et al: Stress-induced suppression of herpes simplex virus (HSV)-specific cytotoxic T lymphocyte and natural killer cell activity and enhancement of acute pathogenesis following local HSV infection. Brain Behav Immun 5:170–192, 1991

Boscarino JA: Posttraumatic stress disorder, exposure to combat, and lower plasma cortisol among Vietnam veterans: findings and clinical implications. J Consult Clin Psychol 64:191–201, 1996

Bremner JD, Southwick SM, Johnson DR, et al: Childhood physical abuse and combat-related post-traumatic stress disorder. Am J Psychiatry 150:234–239, 1993

Bremner J, Licinio J, Darnell A, et al: Elevated CSF corticotropin releasing factor. Am J Psychiatry 154:624–629, 1997

Brende J: Electrodermal responses in post-traumatic syndromes. J Nerv Ment Dis 170:352–361, 1982

Brent DA, Perper JA, Moritz G, et al: Posttraumatic stress disorder in peers of adolescent suicide victims: predisposing factors and phenomenology. J Am Acad Child Adolesc Psychiatry 34:209–215, 1995

Breslau N, Davis GC, Andreski P, et al: Traumatic events and posttraumatic stress disorder in an urban population of young adults. Arch Gen Psychiatry 48:216–222, 1991

Breslau N, Schultz L, Peterson SL: Sex differences in depression: a role for preexisting anxiety. Psychiatry Res 44:69–76, 1997a

Breslau N, Davis GC, Andreski P, et al: Sex differences in posttraumatic stress disorder. Arch Gen Psychiatry 54:1044–1048, 1997b

Breslau N, Kessler RC, Chilcoat HD, et al: Trauma and posttraumatic stress disorder in the community. Arch Gen Psychiatry 55:626–632, 1998

Bromet E, Sonnega A, Kessler RC: Risk factors for DSM-III-R posttraumatic stress disorder: findings from the National Comorbidity Survey. Am J Epidemiol 147:353–361, 1998

Brown PJ, Recupero PR, Stout R: PTSD substance abuse comorbidity and treatment utilization. Addict Behav 20:251–254, 1995

Burgess LH, Handa RJ: Estrogen-induced alterations in the regulation of mineralocorticoid and glucocorticoid receptor messenger RNA expression in the female rat anterior pituitary gland and brain. Mol Cell Neurosci 4:191–198, 1993

Burke JD Jr, Wittchen H-U, Regier DA, et al: Extracting information from diagnostic interviews on co-occurrence of symptoms of anxiety and depression, in Comorbidity of Mood and Anxiety Disorders. Edited by Maser JD, Cloninger CR. Washington, DC, American Psychiatric Press, 1990, pp 649–667

Butterworth M, McClellan B, Allansmith M: Influence of sex on immunoglobulin levels. Nature 214:1224–1225, 1967

Carey MP, Deterd CH, de Koning J, et al: The influence of ovarian steroids on hypothalamic-pituitary-adrenal regulation in the female rat. J Endocrinol 144:311–321, 1995

Carr DJJ, Blalock JE: Neuropeptide hormones and receptors common to the immune and neuroendocrine systems: bidirectional pathway of intersystem communication, in Psychoneuroimmunology—II. Edited by Ader R, Felten DL, Cohen N. San Diego, CA, Academic Press, 1991, pp 573–588

Cato ACB, Ponta H: Different regions of the estrogen receptor are required for synergistic action with the glucocorticoid and progesterone receptors. Mol Cell Biol 9:5324–5330, 1989

Chaouloff F: Behavioral adaptation to stress: improvement by tianeptine. Presse Med 20:1817–1822, 1991

Chung RC, Bemak F, Kagawa-Singer M, et al: Gender differences in psychological distress among Southeast Asian refugees. J Nerv Ment Dis 186:112–119, 1998

Clark DB, Pollock N, Bukstein OG, et al: Gender and comorbid psychopathology in adolescents with alcohol dependence. J Am Acad Child Adolesc Psychiatry 36:1195–1203, 1997

Clarke BL, Bost KL: Differentiation expression of functional adrenocorticotropic hormone receptors by subpopulations of lymphocytes. J Immunol 143:464–469, 1989

Cohen S, Williamson GM: Stress and infectious disease in humans. Psychol Bull 109:5–24, 1991

Cottler LB, Compton WM III, Mager D, et al: Posttraumatic stress disorder among substance users from the general population. Am J Psychiatry 149:664–670, 1992

Cupps TR, Fauci AS: Corticosteroid-mediated immunoregulation in man. Immunol Rev 65:133–135, 1982

Danel L, Souwine G, Monier JC, et al: Specific estrogen binding sites in human lymphoid cells and thymic cells. J Steroid Biochem Mol Biol 18:559–563, 1983

Dansky B, Saladin M, Brady K, et al: Prevalence of victimization and posttraumatic stress disorder among women with substance use disorders: a comparison of telephone and in-person assessment samples. International Journal of the Addictions 4:297–305, 1995

Davidson JRT, Hughes D, Blazer DG: Posttraumatic stress disorder in the community: an epidemiological study. Psychol Med 21:713–721, 1991

Davidson S, Schwartz M, Storck M, et al: A diagnostic and family study of posttraumatic stress disorder. Am J Psychiatry 142:90–93, 1985

Daynes RA, Araneo BA: Contrasting effects of glucocorticoids on the capacity of T cells to produce growth factors interleukin 2 and interleukin 4. Eur J Immunol 19:2319–2325, 1989

Daynes RA, Araneo BA, Dowell TA, et al: Regulation of murine lymphokine production in vivo, III: the lymphoid tissue microenvironment exerts regulatory influences over T helper cell function. J Exp Med 171:979–996, 1990

DeBellis MD, Chrousos GP, Dorn LD, et al: Hypothalamic-pituitary-adrenal axis dysregulation in sexually abused girls. J Clin Endocrinol Metab 78:249–255, 1994a

DeBellis MD, Lefter L, Trickett PK, et al: Urinary catecholamine excretion in sexually abused girls. J Am Acad Child Adolesc Psychiatry 33:320–327, 1994b

DeBellis MD, Burke L, Trickett PK, et al: Antinuclear antibodies and thyroid function in sexually abused girls. J Trauma Stress 9:369–378, 1996

Dekaris D, Sabioncello A, Mazuran R, et al: Multiple changes of immunologic parameters in prisoners of war. JAMA 270:595–599, 1993

Delahanty DL, Dougall AL, Craig KJ, et al: Chronic stress and natural killer cell activity after exposure to traumatic death. Psychosom Med 59:467–476, 1997

DeLeo V, ma Larca A, Talluri B, et al: Hypothalamo-pituitary-adrenal axis and adrenal function before and after ovariectomy in premenopausal women. Eur J Endocrinol 138:430–435, 1998

Dhabhar FS: Stress-Induced Enhancement of Antigen-Specific Cell-Mediated Immunity: The Role of Hormones and Leukocyte Trafficking. New York, Rockefeller University, 1996

Dhabhar FS, McEwen BS: Moderate stress enhances and chronic stress suppresses cell-mediated immunity in vivo (abstract). Society for Neuroscience Abstracts 22:1250, 1996a

Dhabhar FS, McEwen BS: Stress-induced enhancement of antigen-specific cell-mediated immunity. J Immunol 156:2608–2615, 1996b

Dhabhar FS, Miller AH, McEwen BS, et al: Stress-induced changes in blood leukocyte distribution: role of adrenal steroid hormones. J Immunol 157:638–644, 1996

Dinan TG, Barry S, Yatham LN, et al: A pilot study of a neuroendocrine test battery in post-traumatic stress disorder. Biol Psychiatry 28:665–672, 1990

Dobbs D, Wilson WP: Observations on the persistence of neurosis. Disorders of the Nervous Systems 21:40–46, 1960

Duvic M, Steinberg AD, Klassen LW: Effect of the anti-estrogen nafoxidine on NZB/W autoimmune disease. Arthritis Rheum 21:414–417, 1978

Eidinger D, Garrett TJ: Studies of the regulatory effects of the sex hormones on antibody formation and stem cell differentiation. J Exp Med 136:1098–1116, 1972

Engel CC Jr, Engel AL, Campbell SJ, et al: Posttraumatic stress disorder symptoms and precombat sexual and physical abuse in Desert Storm veterans. J Nerv Ment Dis 181:683–688, 1993

Epstein RS, Fullerton CS, Ursano RJ: Posttraumatic stress disorder following an air disaster: a prospective study. Am J Psychiatry 155:934–938, 1998

Fateh M, Ben-Rafael Z, Benadiva CA, et al: Cortisol levels in human follicular fluid. Fertil Steril 51:538–541, 1989

Feinstein A, Dolan R: Predictors of post-traumatic stress disorder following physical trauma: an examination of the stressor criterion. Psychol Med 21:85–91, 1991

Feldman S, Seidenfeld J: Depletion of hypothalamic norepinephrine and serotonin enhances the dexamethasone negative feedback effect on adrenocortical secretion. Psychoneuroendocrinology 16:397–405, 1991

Fox HS, Bons BL, Parslow TG: Estrogen regulates the IFN-gamma promoter. J Immunol 146:4362–4367, 1991

Foy DW, Sipprelle RC, Rueger DB, et al: Etiology of post-traumatic stress disorder in Vietnam veterans. J Consult Clin Psychol 40:1323–1328, 1984

Freedy JR, Shaw DL, Jarrell MP: Towards an understanding of the psychological impact of natural disasters: an application of the conservation resources stress model. J Trauma Stress 5:441–454, 1992

Friedman MK, Kolb L, Arnold A, et al: Chief Medical Director's Special Committee on PTSD: Third Annual Report. Washington, DC, Department of Veterans Affairs; 1987, pp 17–119

Friedman SB, Ader R, Glasgow LA: Effects of psychological stress in adult mice inoculated with coxsackie B virus. Psychosom Med 27:361–368, 1965

Gallagher TF, Yoshida K, Roffwarf HD, et al: ACTH and cortisol secretory patterns in man J Clin Endocrinol Metab 36:1058–1068, 1973

Garrison CZ, Weinrich MW, Hardin SB, et al: Post-traumatic stress disorders in adolescents after a hurricane. Am J Epidemiol 138:522–530, 1993

Genazzani AR, Lemarchand-Beraud TH, Aubert ML, et al: Pattern of plasma ACTH, hGH, and cortisol during menstrual cycle. J Clin Endocrinol Metab 41:431–437, 1975

Gillis S, Crabtree GR, Smith KA: Glucocorticosteroid induced inhibition of T cell growth factor production, I: effect on mitogen-induced lymphocyte proliferation. J Immunol 123:1624–1631, 1979

Glaser R, Thorn BE, Tarr KL, et al: Effects of stress on methyltransferease synthesis: an important DNA repair enzyme. Health Psychol 4:403–412, 1985

Goenjian AK, Yehuda R, Pynoos RS, et al: Basal cortisol and dexamethasone suppression of cortisol among adolescents after the 1988 earthquake in Armenia. Am J Psychiatry 153:929–934, 1996

Green BL: Psychosocial research in traumatic stress: an update. J Trauma Stress 7:341–362, 1994

Green BL, Korol M, Grace MC, et al: Children and disaster: age, gender, and parental effects on PTSD symptoms. J Am Acad Child Adolesc Psychiatry 30:945–951, 1991

Green BL, Grace MC, Vary MG, et al: Children of disaster in the second decade: a 17-year follow-up of Buffalo Creek survivors. J Am Acad Child Adolesc Psychiatry 33:71–79, 1994

Green S, Chambon P: Oestradiol induction of a glucocorticoid-responsive gene by a chimeric receptor in hypothalamus. Nature 325:75–78, 1987

Grossman CJ: Interactions between the gonadal steroids and the immune system. Science 227:257–261, 1985

Grossman CJ, Roselle GA, Mendenhall CL: Sex steroid regulation of autoimmunity. J Steroid Biochem Mol Biol 40:649–659, 1991

Hadid R, Spinedi E, Giovambattista A, et al: Decreased hypothalamic-pituitary-adrenal axis response to neuroendocrine challenge under repeated endotoxemia. Neuroimmunomodulation 3:62–68, 1996

Halbreich U, Olympia J, Carson S, et al: Hypothalamo-pituitary-adrenal activity in indigenously depressed post-traumatic stress disorder patients. Psychoneuroendocrinology 14:365–370, 1989

Harlow CR, Jenkins JM, Winston RM: Increased follicular fluid total and free cortisol levels during the luteinizing hormone surge. Fertil Steril 68:48–53, 1997

Heijnen CJ, Kavelaars A, Ballieux RE: β-Endorphin: cytokine and neuropeptide. Immunol Rev 119:41–63, 1991

Heim C, Ehlert U, Rexhausen J, et al: Psychoendocrinological observations in women with chronic pelvic pain. Ann N Y Acad Sci 821:456–458, 1997

Helzer J, Robins L, McEvoy L: Post-traumatic stress disorder in the general population: findings of the Epidemiologic Catchment Area survey. N Engl J Med 317:1630–1634, 1987

Ironson G, Wynings C, Schneiderman N, et al: Posttraumatic stress symptoms, intrusive thoughts, loss, and immune function after Hurricane Andrew. Psychosom Med 59:128–141, 1997

Irwin M, Daniels M, Smith TL, et al: Impaired natural killer cell activity during bereavement. Brain Behav Immun 1:98–104, 1987

Jensen CF, Keller TW, Peskind ER, et al: Behavioral and neuroendocrine responses to sodium lactate infusion in subjects with posttraumatic stress disorder. Am J Psychiatry 154:266–268, 1997

Jezova D, Jurankova E, Mosnarova A, et al: I: Neuroendocrine response during stress with relation to gender differences. Acta Neurobiol Exp (Warsz) 56:779–785, 1996

Johnson HM, Smoth EM, Torres BA, et al: Regulation of the in vitro antibody responses by neuroendocrine hormones. Proc Natl Acad Sci U S A 79:4171–4174, 1982

Johnson HM, Torress BA, Smith EM, et al: Regulation of lymphokine (gamma-interferon) production by corticotropin. J Immunol 132:246–250, 1984

Jordan K, Schlenger W, Hough R, et al: Lifetime and current prevalence of specific psychiatric disorders among Vietnam veterans and controls. Arch Gen Psychiatry 48:207–215, 1991

Kardiner A: The Traumatic Neurosis of War. New York, Hoeber, 1941

Kellner M, Baker DG, Yehuda R: Salivary cortisol and PTSD symptoms in Persian Gulf War combatants. Ann N Y Acad Sci 821:442–443, 1997

Kessler RC, Sonnega A, Bromet E, et al: Posttraumatic stress disorder in the National Comorbidity Survey. Arch Gen Psychiatry 52:1048–1060, 1995

Kiecolt-Glaser JK, Glaser R: Psychological influences on immunity. Psychosomatics 27:621–624, 1986

Kitay JL: Pituitary-adrenal function in the rat after gonadectomy and gonadal replacement. Endocrinology 73:253–260, 1963

Kluznick JC, Speed N, Van Valkenberg C, et al: Forty-year follow-up of United States prisoners of war. Am J Psychiatry 143:1443–1446, 1986

Kofoed L, Friedman MJ, Peck R: Alcoholism and drug abuse in patients with PTSD. Psychiatr Q 64:151–171, 1993

Kosten TR, Mason JW, Giller EL, et al: Sustained urinary norepinephrine and epinephrine levels in post-traumatic stress disorder. Psychoneuroendocrinology 12:13–20, 1987

Kosten TR, Wahby V, Giller E, et al: The dexamethasone suppression test and thyrotropin-releasing hormone stimulation test in post-traumatic stress disorder. Biol Psychiatry 28:657–664, 1990

Kudler H, Davidson J, Meador K, et al: The DST and post-traumatic stress disorder. Am J Psychiatry 144:1068–1071, 1987

Kulka RA, Schlenger WE, Fairbank JA, et al: Trauma and the Vietnam War Generation: Report of Findings From the National Vietnam Veterans Readjustment Study. New York, Brunner/Mazel, 1990

Kuscenov AV, Grota LJ, Schmidt SG, et al: Decreased herpes simplex viral immunity and enhanced pathogenesis following stressor administration in mice. J Neuroimmunol 88:129–138, 1992

Lahita RG: Sex hormones and the immune system, part 1: human data. Baillieres Clin Rheumatol 4:1–12, 1990

Laudenslager ML, Aasal R, Adler L, et al: Elevated cytotoxicity in combat veterans with long-term post-traumatic stress disorder: preliminary observations. Brain Behav Immun 12:74–79, 1998

Lavoie JM, Dionne N, Helie R, et al: Menstrual cycle phase dissociation of blood glucose homeostasis during exercise. J Appl Physiol 62:1084–1089, 1987

Lemieux AM, Coe CL: Abuse-related posttraumatic stress disorder: evidence for chronic neuroendocrine activation in women. Psychosom Med 57:105–115, 1995

Levine S, Strebel R, Wenk EJ, et al: Suppression of experimental allergic encephalomyelitis by stress. Proc Soc Exp Biol Med 109:294–298, 1962

Lindquist CH, Linquist CA: Gender differences in distress: mental health consequences of environmental stress among jail inmates. Behav Sci Law 15:503–523, 1997

Lui JH, Kazer RR, Ramussen DD: Characterization of the twenty-four hour secretion patterns of adrenocorticotropin and cortisol in normal women and patients with Cushing's disease. J Clin Endocrinol Metab 64:1027–1035, 1987

Luster MI, Hayes HT, Korach K, et al: Estrogen immunosuppression is regulated through estrogenic responses in the thymus. J Immunol 133:110–116, 1984

Maccari S, Mormede P, Piazza PV, et al: Hippocampal type I and type II corticosteroid receptors are modulated by central noradrenergic systems. Psychoneuroendocrinology 17:103–112, 1992

Magiakou MA, Mastorakos G, Webster E, et al: The hypothalamic-pituitary-adrenal axis and the female reproductive system. Ann N Y Acad Sci 816:42–56, 1997

Malloy PE, Fairbanks JA, Keane TM: Validation of a multimethod assessment of post-traumatic stress disorder in Vietnam veterans. J Clin Consult Psychol 51:488–494, 1983

March JS: What constitutes a stressor? The "criterion A" issue, in Posttraumatic Stress Disorder: DSM-IV and Beyond. Edited by Davidson JRT, Foa EB. Washington, DC, American Psychiatric Press, 1993, pp 37–54

Marinari KT, Leshner AI, Doyle MP: Menstrual cycle status and adrenocortical reactivity to psychological stress. Psychoneuroendocrinology 1:213–218, 1976

Masi AT, Kaslow RA: Sex effects in systemic lupus erythematosus: a clue to pathogenesis. Arthritis Rheum 21:480–483, 1978

Mason JW, Giller EL, Kosten TR, et al: Urinary-free cortisol in posttraumatic stress disorder. J Nerv Ment Dis 174:145–149, 1986

Mayou R, Bryant B, Duthie R: Psychiatric consequences of road traffic accidents. BMJ 307:647–651, 1993

McCarroll JE, Ursano RJ, Ventis WL, et al: Anticipation of handling the dead: effects of gender and experience. Br J Clin Psychol 32:466–468, 1993

McCarty R: Sympathetic-adrenal medullary and cardiovascular responses to acute cold stress, I: adult and aged rats. J Auton Nerv Syst 12:15–22, 1985

McCormick CM, Smythe JW, Sharma S, et al: Sex-specific effects of prenatal stress on hypothalamic-pituitary-adrenal responses to stress and brain glucocorticoid receptor density in adult rats. Brain Res Dev Brain Res 84:55–61, 1995

McCormick CM, Furey BF, Child M, et al: Neonatal sex hormones have "organizational" effects on the hypothalamic-pituitary-adrenal axis of male rats. Brain Res Dev Brain Res 105:295–307, 1998

McEwen BS: Reexamination of the glucocorticoid hypothesis of stress and aging, in Progress in Brain Research, Vol 93: The Human Hypothalamus in Health and Disease. Edited by Swaab DF, Hofman MA, Mirmiran M, et al. Amsterdam, The Netherlands, Elsevier Science, 1992, pp 365–383

McEwen BS: Steroid hormone actions on the brain: When is the genome involved? Horm Behav 28:396–405, 1994

McEwen BS: Protective and damaging effects of stress mediators. N Engl J Med 338:171–179, 1998

McEwen SB, Stellar E: Stress and the individual: mechanisms leading to disease. Arch Intern Med 153:2093–2101, 1993

McFall M, Murburg M, Ko G, et al: Autonomic response to stress in Vietnam combat veterans with post-traumatic stress disorder. Biol Psychiatry 27:1165–1175, 1990

McFarlane AC: The longitudinal course of posttraumatic morbidity: the range of outcomes and their predictors. J Nerv Ment Dis 176:30–39, 1988

McFarlane AC: The aetiology of post-traumatic morbidity: predisposing, precipitating and perpetuating factors. Br J Psychiatry 54:221–228, 1989

Meakins JC, Wilson RM: The effect of certain sensory stimulation on the respiratory rate in cases of so-called "irritable heart." Heart 7:17–22, 1918

Mellman TA, Adarsh K, Kulik-Bell R, et al: Nocturnal/daytime urine noradrenergic measures and sleep in combat-related PTSD. Biol Psychiatry 38:174–179, 1995

Michaut RJ, Decahmbre RP, Doumere S, et al: Influences of early maternal deprivation on adult humoral immune response in mice. Physiol Behav 26:189–191, 1981

Mollica RF, Poole C, Son L, et al: Effects of war trauma on Cambodian refugee adolescents' functional health and mental health state. J Am Acad Child Adolesc Psychiatry 36:1098–1106, 1997

Monjian AA, Collector MI: Stress-induced modulation of the immune response. Science 196:307–308, 1977

Mosnaim AD, Wolf ME, Maturana P, et al: In vitro studies of natural killer cell activity in post-traumatic stress disorder patients: response to methionine-enkephalin challenge. Immunopharmacology 25:107–116, 1993

Munck A, Guyre PM: Glucocorticoids and immune function, in Psychoneuroimmunology—II. Edited by Ader R, Felten DL, Cohen N. San Diego, CA, Academic Press, 1991, pp 447–474

Munck A, Guyre PM, Holbrook NJ: Physiological functions of glucocorticoids in stress and their relation to pharmacological actions. Endocrinol Rev 5:25–44, 1984

Murburg MM, McFall ME, Lewis N, et al: Plasma norepinephrine kinetics in patients with post-traumatic stress disorder. Biol Psychiatry 38:819–825, 1995

Ogilvie KM, Rivier C: Gender differences in hypothalamo-pituitary-adrenal axis response to alcohol in the rat: activational roles of gonadal steroid. Brain Res 766:19–28, 1997

Okuyama R, Abo T, Seki S, et al: Estrogen administration activates extrathymic T cell differentiation in the liver. J Exp Med 175:661–669, 1992

Olivera AA, Fero D: Affective disorders, DST, and treatment in PTSD patients: clinical observations. J Trauma Stress 3:407–414, 1990

Orr SP: Psychophysiologic reactivity to trauma-related imagery in PTSD: diagnostic and theoretical implications of recent findings. Ann N Y Acad Sci 821:114–124, 1997

Parker CR, Winkel CA, Rush M, et al: Plasma concentrations of 11-deoxycorticosterone in women during the menstrual cycle. Obstet Gynecol 58:26–30, 1981

Parker CR, Rush M, MacDonald PC: Stress concentrations of deoxycortisterone in women during the luteal phase of the ovarian cycle are not suppressed by dexamethasone treatment. Journal of Steroid Biochemistry 19:1313–1317, 1983

Patchev VK, Hayashi S, Orikasa C, et al: Implications of estrogen-dependent brain organization for gender differences in hypothalamic-pituitary-adrenal regulation. FASEB J 9:419–423, 1995

Peiffer A, LaPointe B, Barden N: Hormonal regulation of type II glucocorticoid receptor messenger ribonucleic acid in rat brain. Endocrinology 129:2166–2174, 1991

Peiffer A, Morale MC, Barden N, et al: Modulation of glucocorticoid receptor gene expression in the thymus by the sex steroid hormone milieu and correlation with sexual dimorphism of immune response. Endocr J 2:181–192, 1994

Perry BD: Neurobiological sequelae of childhood trauma: PTSD in children, in Catecholamine Function in PTSD. Edited by Murburg M. Washington, DC, American Psychological Association Press, 1994, pp 233–255

Perry BD, Giller EL, Southwick SM: Altered platelet alpha2-adrenergic binding sites in post-traumatic stress disorder. Am J Psychiatry 144:1511–1512, 1987

Perry BD, Southwick SM, Yehuda R, et al: Adrenergic receptor regulation in post-traumatic stress disorder, in Biological Assessments and Treatment of Post-Traumatic Stress Disorder. Edited by Giller EL. Washington, DC, American Psychiatric Press, 1990, pp 87–114

Pinkstone P, Saltini C, Muller-Quernheim J, et al: Corticosteroid therapy suppresses spontaneous interleukin 2 release and spontaneous proliferation of lung T lymphocytes of patients with active pulmonary sarcoidosis. J Immunol 139:755–760, 1987

Pitman RK, Orr SP: Twenty-four hour urinary cortisol and catecholamine excretion in combat-related post-traumatic stress disorder. Biol Psychiatry 27:245–247, 1990

Pitman RK, Orr SP, Forgue DF, et al: Psychophysiologic response to combat imagery of Vietnam veterans with posttraumatic stress disorder versus other anxiety disorders. J Abnorm Psychol 99:49–54, 1990

Plaznik A, Palejko W, Stefanski R, et al: Open field behavior of rats reared in different social conditions: the effects of stress and imipramine. Pol J Pharmacol 45:243–252, 1993

Pollard I, White B, Banett JR, et al: Plasma glucocorticoid elevation and desynchronization of the estrous cycle following unpredictable stress in the rat. Behavioral Biology 14:103–108, 1975

Rabin DS, Schmidt PJ, Campbell G, et al: Hypothalamic-pituitary-adrenal function in patients with the premenstrual syndrome. J Clin Endocrinol Metab 71:1158–1162, 1990

Rasmussen AF, Marsh JT, Brill NQ: Increased susceptibility to herpes simplex in mice subjected to avoidance-learning stress or restraint. Proc Soc Exp Biol Med 96:183–189, 1957

Resnick HS, Yehuda R, Pitman RK, et al: Effect of previous trauma on acute plasma cortisol level following rape. Am J Psychiatry 152:1675–1677, 1995

Roy-Byrne PP, Rubinow DR, Gwirtsman H, et al: Cortisol response to dexamethasone in women with premenstrual syndrome. Neuropsychobiology 16:61–63, 1986

Rubinow DR, Hoban MC, Grover GN, et al: Changes in plasma hormones across the menstrual cycle in patients with menstrually related mood disorder and in control subjects. Am J Obstet Gynecol 158:5–11, 1988

Saketos M, Sharma N, Santoro NF: Suppression of the hypothalamic-pituitary-ovarian axis in normal women by glucocorticoids. Biol Reprod 49:1270–1276, 1993

Sapolsky RM: Stress, the Aging Brain and the Mechanisms of Neuron Death. Cambridge, MA, MIT Press, 1992

Schedlowski M, Jacobs R, Stratman G, et al: Changes of natural killer cells during acute psychological stress. J Clin Immunol 12:119–126, 1993

Schleifer SJ, Keller SE, Camerino M, et al: Suppression of lymphocyte stimulation following bereavement. JAMA 250:374–377, 1983

Schnitt JM, Nocks JJ: Alcoholism treatment of Vietnam veterans with post-traumatic stress disorder. J Subst Abuse Treat 1:179–189, 1984

Schnurr PP, Friedman MJ, Rosenberg SD: Preliminary MMPI scores as predictors of combat-related PTSD symptoms. Am J Psychiatry 150:479–483, 1993

Schoneshofer M, Wagner GG: Sex differences in corticosteroids in man. J Clin Endocrinol Metab 45:814–817, 1977

Screpanti I, Morrone S, Meco D, et al: Steroid sensitivity of thymocyte subpopulations during intrathymic differentiation. J Immunol 142:3378–3383, 1989

Seeman TE, Robbins RJ: Aging and hypothalamic-pituitary-adrenal response to challenge in humans. Endocr Rev 15:233–260, 1994

Seki K: Variability of cortisol and adrenocorticotropic hormone responses to metoclopramide during menstrual cycle. Gynecol Obstet Invest 27:201–203, 1989

Seyle H: The Stress of Life. New York, McGraw-Hill, 1956

Shalev AY, Peri T, Cannetti L, et al: Predictors of PTSD in injured trauma survivors: a prospective study. Am J Psychiatry 153:219–225, 1996

Silove D, Sinnerbrink I, Field A, et al: Anxiety, depression and PTSD in asylum-seekers: associations with pre-migration trauma and post-migration stressors. Br J Psychiatry 170:351–357, 1997

Smith MA, Davidson J, Ritchie JC, et al: The corticotropin releasing hormone test in patients with posttraumatic stress disorder. Biol Psychiatry 26:349–355, 1989

Snyder DS, Unanue ER: Corticosteroids inhibit macrophage 1a expression and interleukin 1 production. J Immunol 129:1803–1805, 1982

Solomon GF, Segerstrom SC, Grohr P, et al: Shaking up immunity: psychological and immunologic changes after a natural disaster. Psychosom Med 59:114–127, 1997

Solomon S, Smith E: Social support and perceived controls as moderators of responses in dioxin and flood exposure, in Individual and Community Responses to Trauma and Disaster: The Structure of Human Chaos. Edited by Ursano RJ, McCaughy BG, Fullteron CS. New York, Cambridge University Press, 1994

Southwick SM, Krystal JH, Morgan CA, et al: Abnormal noradrenergic function in post-traumatic stress disorder. Arch Gen Psychiatry 50:266–274, 1993

Spivak B, Shohat B, Mester R, et al: Elevated levels of serum interleukin-1β in combat-related posttraumatic stress disorder. Biol Psychiatry 42:345–348, 1997

Stam WB, Van Oosterhout AJM, Nijkamp FP: Pharmacologic modulation of TH1 and TH2-associated lymphokine production. Life Sci 53:1921–1934, 1993

Stein MB, Yehuda R, Koverola C, et al: Enhanced dexamethasone suppression of plasma cortisol in adult women traumatized by childhood sexual abuse. Biol Psychiatry 42:680–686, 1997a

Stein MB, Walker JR, Hazen AL, et al: Full and partial posttraumatic stress disorder: findings from a community survey. Am J Psychiatry 154:1114–1119, 1997b

Sterling P, Eyer J: Allostasis: a new paradigm to explain arousal pathology, in Handbook of Life Stress, Cognition and Health. Edited by Fisher S, Reason J. New York, Wiley, 1988, pp 629–649

Sterzer P, Wiegers GJ, Reul JMHM: Effects of long-term in vivo corticosterone treatment on T-cell function and splenocyte subsets in the rat. Max Planck Institute of Psychiatry: Scientific Report, 1994–1997. Edited by Fischer F, Burkart-Lauer B. Munich, Germany, Clinical Institute, 1997

Stimson WH: Oestrogen and human T lymphocytes: presence of specific receptors in the T-suppressor/cytotoxic subset. Scand J Immunol 28:345–350, 1988

Tandon R, Haskett RF, Cardona D, et al: Menstrual cycle effects on the dexamethasone suppression test in major depression. Biol Psychiatry 29:485–488, 1991

Terres G, Morrison SL, Habicht GS: A quantitative difference in the immune response between male and female mice. Proc Soc Exp Biol Med 127:664–667, 1968

Tersman Z, Collins A, Eneroth P: Cardiovascular responses to psychological and physiological stressors during the menstrual cycle. Psychosom Med 53:185–197, 1991

True W, Rice J, Eisen S, et al: A twin study of genetic and environmental contributions to liability for post-traumatic stress symptoms. Arch Gen Psychiatry 50:257–264, 1993

Van Den Bergh P, Dobber R, Ramlal R, et al: Role of opioid peptides in the regulation of cytokine production by murine CD4+ T cells. Cell Immunol 154:109–122, 1994

Veldhuis JB, Iranmanesh A, Lizzalde G, et al: Amplitude modulation of a burst-like mode of cortisol secretion subserves the circadian glucocorticoid rhythm. J Clin Endocrinol Metab 71:452–463, 1989

Viau V, Meaney MJ: Variations in the hypothalamic-pituitary-adrenal response to stress during the estrous cycle in the rat. Endocrinology 129:2503–2511, 1991

Wasserman DA, Havassy BE, Boles SM: Traumatic events and post-traumatic stress disorder in cocaine users entering private treatment. Drug Alcohol Depend 46:1–8, 1997

Watson IPB, Muller HK, Jones IH, et al: Cell-mediated immunity in combat veterans with post-traumatic stress disorder. Med J Aust 159:513–516, 1993

Weigers GJ, Labeur MS, Stec I, et al: Glucocorticoid hormones accelerate anti-T-cell receptor-stimulated T-cell growth. J Immunol 155:1893–1902, 1995

Weiss DW, Hirt T, Tarcie N, et al: Studies in psychoneuroimmunology: psychological, immunological, and neuroendocrinological parameters in Israeli civilians during and after a period of Scud missiles attacks. Behav Med 22:5–14, 1996

Werb S, Foley R, Munck A: Interaction of glucocorticoids with macrophages: identification of glucocorticoid receptors in monocytes and macrophages. J Exp Med 147:1684–1694, 1978

Wick G, Hu Y, Kroemer G: Immunoendocrine communications via the hypothalamus-pituitary-adrenal axis in autoimmune diseases. Endocr Rev 14:539–563, 1993

Wilkinson CW, Peskind ER, Raskind MA: Decreased hypothalamic-pituitary-adrenal axis sensitivity to cortisol feedback inhibition in human aging. Neuroendocrinology 65:79–90, 1997

Windle RJ, Wood SA, Shanks SL, et al: Ultradian rhythm of basal corticosterone release in the female rat: dynamic interaction with the response to acute stress. Endocrinology 139:443–450, 1998

Winje D: Long-term outcome of trauma in adults: the psychological impact of a fatal bus accident. J Consult Clin Psychol 64:1037–1043, 1996

Wong M, Moss RL: Long-term and short-term electrophysiological effects of estrogen on the synaptic properties of hippocampal CA1 neurons. J Neurosci 12:3217–3225, 1992

Wood GE, Shors TJ: Stress facilitates classical conditioning in males, but impairs classical conditioning in females through activational effects of ovarian hormones. Proc Natl Acad Sci U S A 95:4066–4071, 1998

Yehuda R: Parental PTSD as a risk factor for PTSD, in Risk Factors for Posttraumatic Stress Disorder (Progress in Psychiatry Series). Edited by Yehuda R. Washington, DC, American Psychiatric Press, 1999, pp 93–124

Yehuda R, Southwick SM, Nussbaum G, et al: Low urinary cortisol excretion in PTSD. J Nerv Ment Dis 178:366–369, 1990

Yehuda R, Lowy MT, Southwick SM, et al: Lymphocyte glucocorticoid receptor number in posttraumatic stress disorder. Am J Psychiatry 148:499–504, 1992a

Yehuda R, Southwick SM, Ma X, et al: Urinary catecholamine excretion and severity of symptoms in PTSD. J Nerv Ment Dis 180:321–325, 1992b

Yehuda R, Southwick SM, Krystal JH, et al: Enhanced suppression of cortisol following dexamethasone administration in posttraumatic stress disorder. Am J Psychiatry 150:83–86, 1993a

Yehuda R, Giller EL, Mason JW: Psychoneuroendocrine assessment of posttraumatic stress disorder: current progress and new directions. Prog Neuropsychopharmacol Biol Psychiatry 17:541–550, 1993b

Yehuda R, Boiseneau D, Mason JW, et al: Relationship between lymphocyte glucocorticoid receptor number and urinary-free cortisol excretion in mood, anxiety, and psychotic disorder. Biol Psychiatry 34:18–25, 1993c

Yehuda R, Teicher MH, Levengood RA, et al: Circadian regulation of basal cortisol levels in posttraumatic stress disorder. Ann N Y Acad Sci 746:378–380, 1994

Yehuda R, Giller EL Jr, Levengood RA, et al: Hypothalamic-pituitary-adrenal functioning in post-traumatic stress disorder: expanding the concept of the stress response spectrum, in Neurobiological and Clinical Consequences of Stress: From Normal Adaptation to Post-Traumatic Stress Disorder. Edited by Friedman MJ, Charney DS, Deutch AY. Hagerstown, MD, Lippincott-Raven, 1995a, pp 351–366

Yehuda R, Kahana B, Schmeidler J, et al: Impact of cumulative lifetime trauma and recent stress on current posttraumatic stress disorder symptoms in Holocaust survivors. Am J Psychiatry 152:1815–1818, 1995b

Yehuda R, Kahana B, Binder-Byrnes K, et al: Low urinary cortisol excretion in Holocaust survivors with posttraumatic stress disorder. Am J Psychiatry 152:982–986, 1995c

Yehuda R, Teicher MH, Trestman RL, et al: Cortisol regulation in post-traumatic stress disorder and major depression: a chronobiological analysis. Biol Psychiatry 40:79–88, 1996a

Yehuda R, Boiseneau D, Lowy MT, et al: Dose-response changes in plasma cortisol and lymphocyte glucocorticoid receptors following dexamethasone administration in combat veterans with and without posttraumatic stress disorder. Arch Gen Psychiatry 52:583–593, 1996b

Yehuda R, Levengood RA, Schmeidler J, et al: Increased pituitary activation following metyrapone administration in post-traumatic stress disorder. Psychoneuroendocrinology 21:1–16, 1996c

Yehuda R, Siever L, Teicher MH, et al: Plasma norepinephrine and MHPG concentrations and severity of depression in combat PTSD and major depressive disorder. Biol Psychiatry 44:56–63, 1998

Zaidi LY, Foy DW: Childhood abuse and combat-related PTSD. J Trauma Stress 7:33–42, 1994

Zlotnick C, Zakriskie AL, Shea MT, et al: The long-term sequelae of sexual abuse: support for a complex posttraumatic stress disorder. J Trauma Stress 9:195–205, 1996

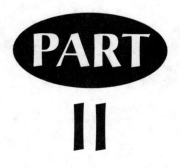

PART

II

Major Depressive
Disorder and Related
Disorders

Introduction

Mood disorders trouble both men and women; however, sex-related differences exist not only in the lifetime prevalence but also in the expression, comorbidity, and course of the illness. For example, unipolar depressive disorders, dysthymia, and seasonal affective disorder are more common in women than in men, and women are more likely to have comorbid psychiatric disorders (anxiety, panic disorders, eating disorders). Prevalence rates for bipolar affective disorder remain nearly equal for men and women; however, women are more prone to rapid mood cycling, and they are the only of the two sexes who can experience firsthand premenstrual syndromes.

In this part, the authors review sex differences in major mood disorders. They focus on female-specific aspects of mood disorders, such as the role of a woman's reproductive life cycle.

The effect of sex on the psychopharmacology of antidepressants is presented. The efficacy and side-effect profile of tricyclic antidepressants and selective serotonin reuptake inhibitors are discussed, as well as female-specific factors, such as pregnancy and oral contraceptive use, that affect the disposition and dose requirements of psychotropic medications. A review of the role of environmental-based factors (e.g., exposure to xenobiotics, alcohol, cigarette smoke) and hormonal variables on psychopharmacology and the mechanisms surrounding cross-ethnic differences in drug effectiveness are provided.

Substantial epidemiological evidence indicates that the postpartum period is a time of increased vulnerability for women to develop mood disorders. Among other symptoms, women may develop feelings of exhaustion, hopelessness, guilt, fear, and sadness during this time. It is important to identify and treat these symptoms quickly. Postpartum illness, including early identification, risk factors, treatment options, and prevention and treatment strategies, with an emphasis on the potential effect on infant well-being, is examined within this part.

Finally, this part includes a chapter on sex differences in the epidemiology, course of illness, medical consequences, and psychiatric comorbidity. Also included in this chapter is information on treatment outcome as seen in premenstrual syndromes.

Women and Depression

Special Considerations in Assessment and Management

Vivien K. Burt, M.D., Ph.D.

Mood disorders affect both women and men, and when they occur, their effect is felt profoundly by both sexes. Nevertheless, increasing data suggest that for women, several sex-specific issues deserve special consideration in terms of assessment, management, and prophylaxis against future recurrence.

A LIFE CYCLE VIEW OF MOOD DISORDERS IN WOMEN

Several large epidemiological studies (Kessler et al. 1994; Weissman et al. 1991) have reported that the prevalence of unipolar depressive disorders is at least twice as high in women as in men. Women have a particularly increased vulnerability to depressive disorders during the childbearing years, approximately between ages 18 and 44; in these years, women shoulder myriad roles and responsibilities, are more likely to experience sexual and domestic violence, and are frequently disadvantaged in terms of both social and financial status. Also, during these years, many women experience both pregnancy and the postpartum (Table 4–1).

TABLE 4–1.　Reproductive junctures as times for affective monitoring in vulnerable women

Pregnancy
Postpartum
Miscarriage
Premenstruum
Assisted reproductive technology
Perimenopause

Increasingly, as women postpone pregnancy and approach the later child-bearing years, they experience difficulty achieving pregnancy and then resort to the newer modalities offered by assisted reproductive technology. Because women with histories of depression are at increased risk for subsequent depressive episodes, treatment of depression may be needed in the setting of pregnancy, in the postpartum period, or when undergoing procedures to induce pregnancy (Hynes et al. 1992; Trantham 1996). In some cases, women who experience miscarriage also are at risk for depressive disorders (Janssen et al. 1996, 1997; Neugebauer et al. 1997). In addition, the premenstrual days, occurring during the luteal phase of the menstrual cycle, are times of affective vulnerability for some women, as exemplified by both premenstrual dysphoric disorder and premenstrual exacerbation of other psychiatric disorders (Hendrick et al. 1996a).

As women move into the years beyond those of reproductive capability, they enter the perimenopause, a transition that appears to represent further affective vulnerability, particularly for women with premenstrual complaints or a lengthy perimenopause with prominent vasomotor symptoms (Avis and McKinlay 1991, 1995; Burt et al. 1998; Soares et al. 2001). The hormonal changes characteristic of postmenopausal women do not appear to precipitate depressive disorders in women. Nevertheless, a robust history of affective episodes is a risk factor for recurrent affective illness over the life span (Post 1992).

SEX-SPECIFIC FEATURES OF MOOD DISORDERS

Unipolar Depressive Disorders

Two longitudinal studies have suggested that women may have longer episodes of depression than men do and also may be more likely than men to have chronic and recurring illness (Sargeant et al. 1990; Winokur et al. 1993) (Table 4–2). Certainly, for women with chronic, recurring depressive illness, reproductive life events may predict recurrence and chronicity (Pajer 1995). Additionally, it appears that for women, severely adverse life events before the onset of depression are the strongest and most consistent predictors of slow time to recovery from major depression (Kendler et al. 1997). Major depression in men and women is generally similar in both characteristics and severity; however, in patients treated with a combination of antidepressants and interpersonal psychotherapy, women tended to report more atypical symptoms (e.g., appetite and weight increase) and were inclined to report more somatic symptoms than men did (Frank et al. 1988). The same study also found that men responded to treatment more quickly than women did.

TABLE 4–2.   Sex-specific features of mood disorders

Unipolar depression
   Longer duration of depression
   Chronicity linked to reproductive events
   Atypical symptoms
   More somatic symptoms
   Delayed response to treatment
   Seasonal susceptibility
   Comorbidity (psychiatric and medical)
Bipolar disorder
   More depression
   More rapid cycling
   More mixed (dysphoric) manias
   Chronicity linked to postpartum decompensation

Women also are more susceptible to depressive episodes in relation to the annual seasons. Seasonal affective disorder is four to six times more prevalent in women than in men and is characterized by depressive symptoms, hypersomnia, hyperphagia, and weight gain localized to the winter months (Rosenthal et al. 1984, 1992).

Several studies have suggested that women who are depressed are more likely to have comorbid anxiety disorders, including panic disorder, phobias, and obsessive-compulsive disorder (Rapaport et al. 1995). Eating disorders predominate in women, and women with eating disorders are more likely to have concurrent depression (Kendler et al. 1991). Women with depression also have a high degree of medical comorbidity. Thus, depressed women are more likely to have migraine headaches (Breslau et al. 1994; Merikangas et al. 1990) and chronic fatigue syndrome (Hickie et al. 1995).

Bipolar Affective Disorder

Unlike unipolar depression, bipolar affective disorder shows no overall difference in prevalence rates (Kessler et al. 1994; Robins et al. 1984). Nevertheless, there are a number of clinically significant sex-specific differences with regard to bipolar affective disorder. Women with bipolar disorder are more likely to experience depression (Angst 1978; Bland and Orn 1978; Clayton 1983; Roy-Byrne et al. 1985; Winokur and Clayton 1967) and are at increased risk for rapid cycling (Leibenluft 1996). Also, some data suggest that the predisposition of women for depression is seen as a sex-specific phenomenon in bipolar disorder, such that women may be more likely to experience mixed (dysphoric) manias (Leibenluft 1996). Women with a history of bipolar disorder are at increased risk for postpartum decompensation, particularly postpartum psychosis (Cohen et al. 1995), and they appear to more readily experience premenstrual relapse or symptom exacerbation (Hendrick et al. 1996a).

SEX-SPECIFIC MANAGEMENT OF MOOD DISORDERS

Pharmacokinetics

Sex differences in the pharmacokinetics of medications account for several clinically important differences in the way medications are absorbed, distributed, metabolized, and eliminated. Estrogen regulates cytochrome P450 3A3/3A4 activity in the liver, altering rates of hepatic metabolism of certain medications (Fazio 1991; Greenblatt et al. 1980; Hamilton et al. 1996; Hendrick et al. 1996a; Yonkers and Hamilton 1995). Progesterone appears to influence drug absorption by delaying gastric emptying time. Both estrogen and progesterone may compete with psychotropic medications for protein binding sites, thus affecting their bioavailability as a function of hormonal levels. The clinical relevance of these effects is unclear, and further studies are needed to shed light on the ways in which they alter treatment response.

By inducing clearance and metabolism of estrogen, carbamazepine appears to impair oral contraceptive efficacy. Postmenopausal women taking carbamazepine may require higher doses of hormone replacement therapy for adequate relief of vasomotor symptoms associated with estrogen depletion (Burt and Hendrick 1999). Nevertheless, there is some indication that serum levels of antidepressants vary with the menstrual cycle (Hendrick et al. 1996a) and are affected by the administration of oral contraceptives (Kimmel et al. 1992). There are reports of changing serum lithium levels in association with times in the menstrual cycle (Conrad and Hamilton 1986; Kukopoulos et al. 1985). Studies are needed to address whether lithium levels vary with either a particular menstrual cycle phase or oral contraceptive administration in women with bipolar disorder (Leibenluft 1996).

Nonconventional Psychoactive Agents

The addition of an augmenting agent to an antidepressant regimen, particularly when partial efficacy has been shown, is an approach that is used in both men and women. Triiodothyronine enhancement of antidepressant effectiveness appears to be more effective in women than in men (Coppen et al. 1972; Prange et al. 1969).

The significance of estrogen and progesterone as psychoactive substances has recently become a subject of interest (Arpels 1996; Halbreich et al. 1995; Stahl 1998). Estrogen is antidopaminergic (Seeman and Lang 1990) and serotonergic (Sherwin and Suranyi-Cadotte 1990), and metabolites of progesterone also may have anxiolytic effects (Freeman et al. 1993; Rapkin et al. 1997). Preliminary studies have suggested that estrogen may play a role in the treatment of depression in perimenopausal women (Schmidt et al. 2000; Soares et al. 2001) and in postmenopausal women (Schneider et al. 1997), in the prevention of recurrent postpartum psychosis and postpartum depression (Sichel et al. 1995), and in the treatment of postpartum depression (Gregoire et al. 1996).

TREATMENT CUSTOMIZED TO REPRODUCTIVE LIFE EVENTS

Pregnancy

The treatment of depression or bipolar disorder in pregnancy presents very specific issues necessarily pertinent to women only. Thus, although it is generally presumed that it is best to refrain from medications in pregnancy if possible, it is also true that known risks are associated with disabling depression or bipolar disorder during pregnancy (Altshuler et al. 1996; Steer et al. 1992). Similarly, decompensated bipolar women may be at particularly increased risk for several adverse outcomes (Burt and Hendrick 1999). Thus, carefully constructed risk–benefit analyses must be made to formulate efficacious approaches to the management of mood disorders in pregnant women.

A recent meta-analysis of the use of antidepressants in pregnancy suggested that, for the most part, tricyclic antidepressants and fluoxetine are relatively safe during pregnancy (Altshuler et al. 1996; Nulman et al. 1997), and a recent small study suggested that the same may be true for some of the newer selective serotonin reuptake inhibitors (Kulin et al. 1998), citalopram (Ericson et al. 1999), and venlafaxine (Einarson et al. 2001). Because both carbamazepine and valproic acid pose serious teratogenic risks, lithium—despite increasing the risk of congenital cardiovascular anomalies such as Ebstein's anomaly (from 1 in 20,000 to 1 in 1,000)—is now considered the safest mood stabilizer for use during pregnancy in severely decompensated bipolar women or women whose history indicates that they are likely to decompensate on discontinuation of mood-stabilizing pharmacotherapy (Altshuler et al. 1996; Cohen et al. 1994).

Postpartum

Because postnatal women are at risk for mood disorders when compared with women at any other time in their lives (Kendell et al. 1987), special consideration should be given to the treatment of mood disorders in this population. The postpartum period is a time of especially heightened risk for mood disorders when compared with other times in women's lives (Kendell et al. 1987), and the issue of treatment decision making is particularly complicated when the patient is breast-feeding an infant. A recent analysis of the literature on the use of psychiatric medications by nursing mothers suggested that the selective serotonin reuptake inhibitors do not appear to cause adverse effects in exposed infants (Burt et al. 2001). Antidepressants may be efficacious for the prevention of recurrent postpartum major depression in women with histories of postpartum mood disorders (Wisner and Wheeler 1994). Similarly, women with bipolar disorder appear to benefit from postpartum prophylaxis with mood stabilizers (Cohen et al. 1995).

Approximately half of new mothers breast-feed their infants. Unfortunately, the data regarding the degree of drug passage to the infant and the subsequent effects of exposure on infant growth and development are limited. In general, drugs that are less protein bound and more lipophilic are passed more easily into breast milk. There is a growing, albeit still small, literature on the use of antidepressants and mood stabilizers by nursing mothers. Because breast milk offers major advantages to a developing infant, physicians and new mothers with postpartum mood disorders are often faced with the difficult decision of whether to abandon breast-feeding before psychopharmacological intervention, refrain from using psychotropic medication while breast-feeding, or continue to breast-feed while taking one or more psychoactive agents. Clinicians and patients should sort out the pertinent issues as a prelude to finalizing the recommendation regarding psychotropic treatment by the nursing mother. These issues include understanding the risks of exposure of a particular medication (and its active metabolites), respecting the wishes of the parents with regard to the issue of breast-feeding, and evaluating the risk of not using medication to treat an active postpartum mood disorder. Of note, it is important for infants who ingest breast milk from a depressed mother taking a psychopharmacological agent to be assessed at baseline (before the onset of treatment) and at regular, frequent intervals over the course of the treatment (Burt et al. 2001). Other safeguards that are sometimes used are to direct mothers to time breast-feeding so that drug levels are likely to be lowest in breast milk (i.e., just prior to the longest nap time in an infant) and to monitor infant drug levels and clinical changes in the infant (Hendrick et al. 1996b).

Menopause

Because for some women, the transition to menopause (i.e., perimenopause) may be associated with depressive symptoms, although not necessarily major depression (Avis and McKinlay 1991, 1995; Burt et al. 1998; Soares and Almeida 2001; Stewart and Boydell 1993), the evaluation of depression in a middle-aged woman should be addressed in the context of relevant sex-specific physiological and hormonal changes. Thus, for women between ages 42 and 55 who complain of depressive symptoms, assessment should include not only a full psychiatric examination but also an evaluation of somatic symptoms and changes in the menstrual pattern. A comprehensive characterization of somatic complaints comprises a description of vasomotor symptoms, such as hot flushes or cold sweats (even if menstrual cycling is regular), and a characterization of sleep pattern. Questions about changes in libido or sexual responsiveness are essential because such changes may reflect hormonal changes and/or dyspareunia associated with vaginal dryness and atrophy. Thyroid assessment is particularly important as women age because thyroid disease in women increases with age and may be associated with depression.

For women who present with depression and who are experiencing symptoms of the menopausal transition (menstrual cycle irregularity, vasomotor symptoms, changes in sexual desire or responsiveness, and dyspareunia), measuring serum follicle-stimulating hormone and estradiol levels on day 2 or 3 of the cycle may provide helpful information. A follicle-stimulating hormone level greater than 25 IU/L with an estradiol concentration less than 40 pg/mL suggests perimenopause, even if menstrual cycle irregularity is not reported (Burt et al. 1998). Perimenopausal women presenting with depressive symptoms but not major depression may be given estrogen in replacement doses because alleviating vasomotor symptoms may restore normal sleep architecture and secondarily improve dysphoric mood, irritability, decreased concentration, and poor memory. Furthermore, preliminary studies have suggested that transdermal estrogen may alleviate depressive symptoms in perimenopausal women, independent of its effect on vasomotor symptoms (Schmidt et al. 2000; Soares et al. 2001). If psychiatric complaints do not improve after several weeks, the addition of standard antidepressant therapy (usually involving the implementation of antidepressant medications) is appropriate. For middle-aged women who present with major depression, regardless of whether they are perimenopausal, the standard of care at this time suggests that antidepressants are the appropriate treatment. Such women still may benefit from estrogen replacement, because effective removal of vasomotor symptoms often restores sleep cycle regularity and, secondarily, an improvement in irritability, dysphoria, and cognitive function is likely (Burt et al. 1998). An additional benefit of estrogen replacement is a decreased risk of osteoporosis (American College of Physicians 1992; Greendale and Judd 1993).

CONCLUSION

To effectively treat mood disorders in women and to prevent the recurrence of illness in vulnerable women, clinicians must understand the female-specific aspects of mood disorders. Increasing data suggest that women's reproductive life events may precipitate or exacerbate mood instability, particularly in patients with personal and family histories of mood disorder. Endogenous and exogenous hormonal vacillations appear to affect mood in women and, in some cases, may alter response to treatment with psychoactive agents. Although preliminary data suggest that estrogen and other reproductive hormonal agents may be useful in the treatment of mood disorders in women, this remains a subject for rigorous research. Finally, it is clear that in order to effectively manage mood disorders in women, psychiatrists and other clinicians who treat mental illness in women must fully understand the medical and psychological aspects of women's health over the longitudinal course of their lives.

REFERENCES

Altshuler LL, Cohen L, Szuba MP, et al: Pharmacologic management of psychiatric illness during pregnancy: dilemmas and guidelines. Am J Psychiatry 153:592–606, 1996

American College of Physicians: Guidelines for counseling postmenopausal women about preventive hormone therapy. Ann Intern Med 117:1038–1041, 1992

Angst J: The course of affective disorders, II: typology of bipolar manic-depressive illness. Archiv fur Psychiatrie und Nervenkrankheiten 226:65–73, 1978

Arpels JC: The female brain hypoestrogenic continuum from the premenstrual syndrome to menopause: a hypothesis and review of supporting data. J Reprod Med 41:633–639, 1996

Avis NE, McKinlay SM: A longitudinal analysis of women's attitudes toward the menopause: results from the Massachusetts Women's Health Study. Maturitas 13:65–79, 1991

Avis NE, McKinlay SM: The Massachusetts Women's Health Study: an epidemiologic investigation of the menopause. J Am Med Womens Assoc 50:45–49, 1995

Bland RC, Orn H: 14-year outcome in early schizophrenia. Acta Psychiatr Scand 58:327–338, 1978

Breslau N, Merikangas K, Bowden CL: Comorbidity of migraine and major affective disorders. Neurology 44(suppl 7):S17–S22, 1994

Burt VK, Hendrick VC: Psychiatric assessment of female patients, in The American Psychiatric Press Textbook of Psychiatry. Edited by Hales RE, Yudofsky SC, Talbott JA. Washington, DC, American Psychiatric Press, 1999, pp 1429–1445

Burt VK, Altshuler LL, Rasgon N: Depressive symptoms in the perimenopause: prevalence, assessment, and guidelines for treatment. Harv Rev Psychiatry 6:121–132, 1998

Burt VK, Suri R, Altshuler L, et al: The use of psychotropic medications during breast feeding. Am J Psychiatry 158:1001–1009, 2001

Clayton PJ: The prevalence and course of the affective disorders, in The Affective Disorders. Edited by Davis JM, Maas JW. Washington, DC, American Psychiatric Press, 1983, pp 193–201

Cohen LS, Friedman JM, Jefferson JW, et al: A reevaluation of risk of in utero exposure to lithium. JAMA 271:146–150, 1994

Cohen LS, Sichel DA, Robertson LM, et al: Postpartum prophylaxis for women with bipolar disorder. Am J Psychiatry 152:1641–1645, 1995

Conrad CD, Hamilton JA: Recurrent premenstrual decline in serum lithium concentration: clinical correlates and treatment implications. Journal of the American Academy of Child Psychiatry 26:852–853, 1986

Coppen A, Whybrow P, Noguera R, et al: The comparative antidepressant value of L-tryptophan and imipramine with and without attempted potentiation by liothyronine. Arch Gen Psychiatry 26:234–241, 1972

Einarson A, Fatoye B, Sarkur M, et al: Pregnancy outcome following gestational exposure to venlafaxine: a multicenter prospective controlled study. Am J Psychiatry 158:1728–1730, 2001

Ericson A, Kallen B, Wilholm BE: Delivery outcome after the use of antidepressants in early pregnancy. Eur J Clin Pharmacol 55:503–508, 1999

Fazio A: Oral contraceptive drug interactions: important considerations. South Med J 84:997–1002, 1991

Frank E, Carpenter LL, Kupfer DJ: Sex differences in recurrent depression: are there any that are significant? Am J Psychiatry 145:41–45, 1988

Freeman EW, Purdy RH, Coutifaris C, et al: Anxiolytic metabolites of progesterone: correlation with mood and performance measures following oral progesterone administration to healthy female volunteers. Clinical Neuroendocrinology 58:478–484, 1993

Greenblatt DJ, Allen MD, Harmatz JS, et al: Diazepam disposition determinants. Clin Pharmacol Ther 27:301–312, 1980

Greendale GA, Judd JL: The menopause: health implications and clinical management. J Am Geriatr Soc 41:426–436, 1993

Gregoire AJ, Kumar R, Everitt B, et al: Transdermal oestrogen for treatment of severe postnatal depression. Lancet 347:930–933, 1996

Halbreich U, Rojansky N, Palter S, et al: Estrogen augments serotonergic activity in postmenopausal women. Biol Psychiatry 37:434–441, 1995

Hamilton JA, Grant M, Jensvold MF: Sex and treatment of depressions: when does it matter? in Psychopharmacology and Women: Sex, Gender, and Hormones. Edited by Jensvold MF, Halbreich U, Hamilton JA. Washington, DC, American Psychiatric Press, 1996, pp 241–255

Hendrick V, Altshuler LL, Burt VK: Course of psychiatric disorders across the menstrual cycle. Harv Rev Psychiatry 4:200–207, 1996a

Hendrick V, Burt VK, Altshuler LL: Psychotropic guidelines for breast-feeding mothers (letter). Am J Psychiatry 153:1236–1237, 1996b

Hickie IB, Lloyd AR, Wakefield D: Chronic fatigue syndrome: current perspectives on evaluation and management. Med J Aust 163:314–318, 1995

Hynes GJ, Callan VJ, Terry DJ, et al: The psychological well-being of infertile women after a failed IVF attempt: the effects of coping. Br J Med Psychol 65:269–278, 1992

Janssen HJEM, Cuisinier MCJ, Hoogduin KAL, et al: Controlled prospective study on the mental health of women following pregnancy loss. Am J Psychiatry 153:226–230, 1996

Janssen HJEM, Cuisinier MC, Kees deGraaw PHM, et al: A prospective study of risk factors predicting grief intensity following pregnancy loss. Arch Gen Psychiatry 54:56–61, 1997

Kendell RE, Chalmers JC, Platz C: Epidemiology of puerperal psychoses. Br J Psychiatry 150:662–673, 1987

Kendler KS, MacLean C, Neale M, et al: The genetic epidemiology of bulimia nervosa. Am J Psychiatry 148:1627–1637, 1991

Kendler KS, Walters EE, Kessler RC: The prediction of length of major depressive episodes: results from an epidemiological sample of female twins. Psychol Med 27:107–117, 1997

Kessler RC, McGonagle KA, Zhao S, et al: Lifetime and 12-month prevalence of DSM-III-R psychiatric disorders in the United States: results from the National Comorbidity Survey. Arch Gen Psychiatry 51:8–19, 1994

Kimmel S, Gonzalves L, Youngs D, et al: Fluctuating levels of antidepressants. J Psychosom Obstet Gynaecol 2:109–115, 1992

Kukopoulos A, Minnai G, Muller-Oerlinghausen B: The influence of mania and depression on the pharmacokinetics of lithium: a longitudinal single-case study. J Affect Disord 8:159–166, 1985

Kulin NA, Pastuszak A, Sage SR, et al: Pregnancy outcome following maternal use of the new selective serotonin reuptake inhibitors: a prospective controlled multicenter study. JAMA 279:609–610, 1998

Leibenluft E: Women with bipolar illness: clinical and research issues. Am J Psychiatry 153:163–173, 1996

Merikangas KR, Angst J, Isler H: Migraine and psychopathology: results of the Zurich cohort study of young adults. Arch Gen Psychiatry 47:849–853, 1990

Neugebauer R Kline J, Shrout P, et al: Major depressive disorder in the 6 months after miscarriage. JAMA 277:383–388, 1997

Nulman I, Rovet J, Stewart DE, et al: Neurodevelopment of children exposed in utero to antidepressant drugs. N Engl J Med 336:258–262, 1997

Pajer K: New strategies in the treatment of depression in women. J Clin Psychiatry 56(suppl 2):30–37, 1995

Post RM: Transduction of psychosocial stress into the neurobiology of recurrent affective disorder. Am J Psychiatry 149:999–1010, 1992

Prange AJ Jr, Wilson IC, Rabon AM, et al: Enhancement of imipramine antidepressant activity by thyroid hormone. Am J Psychiatry 126:457–469, 1969

Rapaport MH, Thompson PM, Kelsoe JR Jr, et al: Gender differences in outpatient research subjects with affective disorder: a comparison of descriptive variables. J Clin Psychiatry 56:67–72, 1995

Rapkin AJ, Morgan M, Goldman L, et al: Progesterone metabolite allopregnanolone in women with premenstrual syndrome. Obstet Gynecol 90:709–714, 1997

Robins LN, Helzer JE, Weissman MM, et al: Lifetime prevalence of specific psychiatric disorders in three sites. Arch Gen Psychiatry 41:949–958, 1984

Rosenthal NE, Sack DA, Gillin JC, et al: Seasonal affective disorder: a description of the syndrome and preliminary findings with light therapy. Arch Gen Psychiatry 41:72–80, 1984

Rosenthal NE, Sack DA, Gillin JC et al: Seasonal affective disorder: a description of the syndrome and preliminary findings with light therapy. Arch Gen Psychiatry 53:289–292, 1992

Roy-Byrne P, Post RM, Uhde TW, et al: The longitudinal course of recurrent affective illness: life chart data from research patients at the NIMH. Acta Psychiatr Scand Suppl 317:2–34, 1985

Sargeant JK, Bruce ML, Florio LP, et al: Factors associated with 1-year outcome of major depression in the community. Arch Gen Psychiatry 47:519–526, 1990

Schmidt PJ, Nieman L. Danaceau RN, et al: Estrogen replacement in perimenopause-related depression: a preliminary report. Am J Obstet Gynecol 183:414–420, 2000

Schneider LS, Small GW, Hamilton SH, et al: Estrogen replacement and response to fluoxetine in a multicenter geriatric depression trial. Am J Geriatr Psychiatry 5:97–106, 1997

Seeman MV, Lang M: The role of estrogens in schizophrenia gender differences. Schizophr Bull 16:185–194, 1990

Sherwin BB, Suranyi-Cadotte BE: Up-regulatory effect of estrogen on platelet 3H-imipramine binding sites in surgically menopausal women. Biol Psychiatry 28:339–348, 1990

Sichel DA, Cohen LS, Robertson LM, et al: Prophylactic estrogen in recurrent postpartum affective disorder. Biol Psychiatry 38:814–818, 1995

Soares CN, Almeida OP: Depression during the perimenopause (letter). Arch Gen Psychiatry 58:306, 2001

Soares CN, Almeida OP, Joffe H, et al: Efficacy of estradiol for the treatment of depressive disorders in perimenopausal women. Arch Gen Psychiatry 58:529–534, 2001

Stahl SM: Basic psychopharmacology of antidepressants, part 2: estrogen as an adjunct to antidepressant treatment. J Clin Psychiatry 59(suppl 4):15–24, 1998

Steer RA, Scholl TO, Hediger ML, et al: Self-reported depression and negative pregnancy outcomes. J Clin Epidemiol 45:1093–1099, 1992

Stewart DE, Boydell KM: Psychologic distress during menopause: associations across the reproductive life cycle. Int J Psychiatry Med 23:157–162, 1993

Trantham P: The infertile couple. Am Fam Physician 54:1001–1010, 1996

Weissman MM, Bruce MI, Leaf PJ, et al: Affective disorders, in Psychiatric Disorders in America. Edited by Robins LN, Regier DA. New York, Free Press, 1991, pp 53–80

Winokur G, Clayton P: Family history studies, II: sex differences and alcoholism in primary affective illness. Br J Psychiatry 113:973–979, 1967

Winokur G, Coryell W, Keller M, et al: A prospective follow-up of patients with bipolar and unipolar affective disorders. Arch Gen Psychiatry 50:457–465, 1993

Wisner KL, Wheeler SB: Prevention of recurrent postpartum major depression. Hosp Community Psychiatry 45:1191–1196, 1994

Yonkers KA, Hamilton JA: Psychotropic medications, in American Psychiatric Press Review of Psychiatry, Vol 14. Edited by Oldham JM, Riba MB. Washington, DC, American Psychiatric Press, 1995, pp 307–332

5

Effect of Sex on Psychopharmacology of Antidepressants

John J. Sramek, Pharm.D.
Edyta J. Frackiewicz, Pharm.D.

*W*omen's health issues in all areas, including mental health, have gained increasing awareness over the past decade. Sex differences in depression may result from the interaction of multiple factors, including social and environmental factors, genetics, and organizational and activational effects of hormones on the central nervous system (Halbreich and Lumley 1993). Several studies indicate that sex affects the pharmacokinetic profiles of certain antidepressants (see Table 5–1); however, these results need to be validated by larger, well-controlled trials.

SEX DIFFERENCES IN PREVALENCE RATES AND COURSE OF DEPRESSION

Being female is a major risk factor for depression; women with depression outnumber men by a 2:1 ratio (Kornstein 1997; Weissman and Klerman 1977). Epidemiological studies have consistently shown that the lifetime prevalence of major depression in women in the United States is 21.3%

TABLE 5–1.   Studies examining pharmacokinetic sex differences in patients taking antidepressants

Reference	Subjects	Sex	Intervention	Results
Barbhaiya et al. 1996	12 healthy elderly (>65 years) 12 healthy young (18–40 years)	6 M, 6 F 6 M, 6 F	300 mg of single-dose nefazodone (for evaluation of single-dose pharmacokinetics) 300 mg of nefazodone bid for 8 days for evaluation of steady state	Steady-state exposure to nefazodone and its metabolite was approximately 50% greater in elderly women relative to elderly men, young women, or young men ($P<0.05$).
Dahl et al. 1996	21 depressed patients with cytochrome P450 2D6 genotype Genotype determined 20 EM and 1 PM	8 M (7 EM, 1 PM) 13 F (13 EM)	50–150 mg/day of nortriptyline for 3 weeks	Female EM significantly higher levels of nortriptyline than male EM (3.8 ± 1.1 vs. 2.1 ± 0.5, $P<0.01$)
Gex-Fabry et al. 1990	150 depressed patients	64 M, 86 F	Clomipramine at individualized doses for 3 weeks	Significantly lower hydroxylation clearance of clomipramine by women ($P<0.05$)
Glassman et al. 1977	60 patients with primary affective disorder requiring hospitalization	42 M, 18 F	3.5 mg/kg of imipramine for 28 days (average dose females = 200 mg/day; average dose males = 250 mg/day)	Female response rate to imipramine higher; difference limited to the unipolar group
Greenblatt et al. 1987	25 healthy young (18–40 years) 18 healthy elderly (60–76 years)	12 M, 13 F 7 M, 11 F	Single-dose two-way crossover 50 mg of trazodone single dose and 25 mg of trazodone intravenously	Greater volume of distribution (1.5 vs. 1.27 L/kg, $P<0.001$) and half-life (7.6 vs. 5.9 hours, $P<0.05$) in elderly women than in young women; reduced clearance in elderly men (1.15 vs. 0.89 L/kg, $P<0.05$)

TABLE 5–1. Studies examining pharmacokinetic sex differences in patients taking antidepressants *(continued)*

Reference	Subjects	Sex	Intervention	Results
Klamerus et al. 1996	18 healthy young (21–44 years) 18 healthy elderly (60–80 years)	9 M, 9 F 9 M, 9 F	50 mg of venlafaxine, then 50 mg every 8 hours for 5 days	Venlafaxine and its metabolite disposition not significantly affected by sex
Moody et al. 1967	24 depressed patients	17 M, 7 F	50–150 mg/day of imipramine for at least 4 weeks and up to 2.5 years	Nonsignificant higher plasma levels in women
Preskorn and Mac 1985	110 depressed inpatients	Not stated	Clinically determined doses of amitriptyline	Higher plasma levels of amitriptyline in women older than 50 years than in age-matched men (2.03±0.59 ng/mL/mg vs. 1.76±0.78 ng/mL/mg, $P<0.05$)
Ronfeld et al. 1997	22 healthy young (18–45 years) 22 healthy elderly (>65 years)	11 M, 11 F 11 M, 11 F	50 mg/day of sertraline titrated to 200 mg/day for 9 days, then 200 mg/day for 21 days	Terminal elimination half-life of sertraline shorter in the young males (22.4 hours vs. 32.1–36.7 hours); maximum concentration and area under the curve (24 hours) approximately 25% lower in the males than in young females and elderly men and women

Note. EM=extensive metabolizer; F=female; M=male; PM=poor metabolizer.

compared with 12.7% in men, with a female-to-male relative risk of 1.7 (Kessler et al. 1993). Women are more likely to have an earlier age at onset than men and often become symptomatic in their mid-teenage years, whereas men more often become symptomatic in their 20s (Pajer 1995).

Longitudinal studies have reported that women have longer depressive episodes that are more likely to develop into a chronic and recurrent course of illness (Kornstein 1997). The sex difference in suicide rates among depressed individuals also has been studied, and although women are more likely to attempt suicide, the rate of completed suicide is higher in men, most likely because they use more lethal methods and are less likely to seek help for depression (Roy 1995).

Depressed women have higher rates of comorbid psychiatric disorders (e.g., anxiety, panic disorder, somatization, eating disorder) than do depressed men and more frequently recurring episodes of depression (Hamilton et al. 1996). Several explanations have been postulated to explain sex differences in the prevalence of depression (Gove and Tudor 1973; Nolen-Hoeksema 1987; Pugliesi 1992; Radloff 1975; Weissman and Klerman 1977). These reasons have encompassed artifactual, psychosocial, and biological aspects; we briefly discuss these theories before the discussion of sex differences in psychopharmacology (Nolen-Hoeksema 1987; Weissman and Klerman 1977).

Artifact Theories

Artifact theories have focused on sex differences in help-seeking behavior and symptom reporting and the possibility of diagnostic bias (Kornstein 1997). Studies have shown that women are more likely to seek treatment for psychological problems (Almqvist 1986) and use outpatient mental health services more frequently than men do (Greenley et al. 1987; Horgan 1985; Wells et al. 1986). The higher level of use by women may be explained by the help-seeking behavior process, which states that women are more likely to recognize a mental problem in its early stages and are more willing to seek outside help (Kessler et al. 1981).

Women more often have atypical symptoms, such as increased appetite and weight gain (Frank et al. 1988; Kornstein 1997; Young et al. 1990), and report a greater number of individual depressive symptoms than men do on self-rating scales (Hamilton et al. 1996). The greater propensity of symptom reporting by women has been proposed to be caused by various factors, including selection of information through attention and distraction, attribution of somatic sensations, and personality factors such as somatization and negative affectivity (Van Wijk and Kolk 1997).

Studies have shown that women receive and use more prescriptions for psychotropic drugs (Balter et al. 1974; Cafferata et al. 1983; Cooperstock

1971, 1979; Mant et al. 1983; Trinkoff et al. 1990) and are about twice as likely to receive a prescription for a psychotropic drug as men are (Cafferata et al. 1983). One explanation may be that physicians are influenced by sex stereotypes that prompt them to overreact to female symptoms of distress and underreact to male symptoms of distress (Padgett 1997). Other researchers have speculated that depression may be misdiagnosed in 30%–50% of female patients. This may be because other physical diseases have symptoms or certain medical treatments cause side effects that mimic depressive symptoms.

Psychosocial Theories

Psychosocial explanations for the higher rates of depression in women include the effects of sex-specific socialization, low social status, role and life stress, victimization, and maladaptive coping styles. Recent explanations also have focused on social changes that accompany adolescence because the 2:1 female-to-male ratio of depression appears during adolescence by age 15, whereas in childhood, rates of depression either do not differ or even show a slight excess in boys (Angold and Worthman 1993; Guyer et al. 1989; McGee et al. 1990; Rutter et al. 1976; Velez et al. 1989).

Certain sex differences in personality or behavioral styles have been found to be risk factors for increased susceptibility to depression in females (Nolen-Hoeksema and Gigus 1994). Women have been found to endure more suffering from the life events that take place because they invest their emotions in their personal relationships (Seeman 1997), internalize their feelings to a greater degree than men do, and tend to blame themselves for failure (Seeman 1997). Therefore, they are more prone to developing depression following stressful life events (Kornstein 1997). Women also react more poorly to stressors than men do because they have different coping styles that cause them to ruminate over distressing events, whereas men are more likely to distract themselves (Nolen-Hoeksema 1987).

Women who have experienced childhood sexual victimization, battery, sexual harassment, and rape are more likely to have depression than are women without such a history (Browne 1993; Finkelhor and Browne 1985; Mirowsky and Ross 1995). Research suggests that the increase in sexual abuse that occurs in early adolescence directly leads to more depression in females and to the sex difference in depression that emerges at that time (Nolen-Hoeksema and Gigus 1994).

Women are more likely to be affected by chronic stress associated with lower wages, job tedium, restricted upward mobility, and conflicts in domestic and labor force roles (Belle 1990; McLanahan et al. 1989). Women experience increased social and parental pressure to marry and have children earlier and to pursue sex-stereotyped activities and occupations. Those who adopt these sex-stereotyped roles, activities, and occupations often find themselves in low-status and low-paying jobs with restricted upward mobility, which can lead to hopelessness and despair. Marital status also affects depression rates; married women reported higher rates of mental illness than unmarried women (Paykel 1991).

Biological Theories

Biological theories of depression have focused on differences in brain structure and function, including neurotransmitter, neuroendocrine, and circadian systems; genetic transmission; and reproductive function (Kornstein 1997). Evidence from twin studies showed that depression has a genetic component (Paykel 1991). Because differences in the prevalence of depression between men and women apply only to adults and do not emerge until adolescence (Buchanan et al. 1992), there is speculation that the biological changes that occur during adolescence predispose females to developing depression (Angold and Rutter 1992; Brooks-Gunn and Ruble 1983; Crockett and Petersen 1987). The development of secondary sex characteristics at puberty may influence the emotional development of males and females (Brooks-Gunn 1988). It has been shown that girls value the physical changes that occur with puberty much less than boys do because of the inconvenience of menstruation, the weight gain in fat, and the loss of the prepubescent figure that is idealized by modern society (Greif and Ulman 1982). Males, on the other hand, like the pubertal changes their bodies undergo, such as increased body muscle mass (Dornbusch et al. 1984; Koff et al. 1990; Petersen 1979). Researchers have argued that both men and women who are dissatisfied with their bodies are more likely to be depressed; however, because women are more likely than men to be dissatisfied with their bodies, women are more prone to depression (Brooks-Gunn 1988). The chronic dieting that women often resort to because of negative body image may contribute to a sense of helplessness and depression (McCarthy 1990).

Researchers also have observed sex differences in the neurostructural aspects of the brain, including gross volume of the brain, neuronal morphology, and type and number of synapses. These sex differences are very prominent in structural areas that have been suggested to be involved in regulation of normal and abnormal mood and behaviors, such as the hypothalamus, amygdala, and cortex, and could contribute to the different rates of depression between the sexes (Halbreich and Lumley 1993).

The most popular biological theory of females' greater vulnerability to depression is based on the dysregulation of the ovarian hormones estrogen

TABLE 5–2. Studies examining adverse-effect sex differences in patients taking antidepressants

Reference	Subjects	Sex	Intervention	Results
Piazza et al. 1997	25 chronically depressed	14 F, 11 M	6-week course of sertraline or paroxetine	Desire, psychological arousal, overall sexual functioning significantly improved in women; orgasm delay, orgasm satisfaction, overall sexual functioning significantly worsened in men
Shen and Hsu 1995	110 outpatients treated with selective serotonin reuptake inhibitors (SSRIs)	Female	Clinic records retrospectively reviewed for loss of or decrease in libido, orgasmic disturbance	21 fluoxetine- and 9 paroxetine- and sertraline-treated patients with female sexual inhibition; SSRI-associated female sexual dysfunction occurs at a high rate.

example, because the societal emphasis on thinness is greater for women, they may not be willing to tolerate antidepressant weight gain (Hamilton et al. 1996). To ensure patient compliance, patients should be routinely monitored for the emergence of undesirable adverse effects, which can then be managed by waiting for spontaneous remission, reducing the dose, or substituting another antidepressant.

IMPLICATIONS FOR RESEARCH

The previously reviewed studies lend credence to the clinical observation that women show a differential response to antidepressant medication. These results, however, come from relatively small studies and need to be validated by larger, well-designed studies. Preclinical and early clinical sex data are vital for the optimal design of Phase II and III clinical trials and to assess whether special studies are needed to define sex-related differences in medication response ("Gender Studies in Product Development" 1995). Potential sex differences can easily be identified early in Phase I with the inclusion of sufficient numbers of females. Clinical data from Phase II and Phase III should be analyzed by sex to assess potential pharmacokinetic and pharmacodynamic differences. The data can then be used to design population pharmacokinetic modeling. In Phase III trials, sex can be used as a covariant in the analysis to examine for differences in response, adverse events, and electrocardiogram and laboratory data. If indicated, special additional studies in women should be conducted during the clinical development of therapeutic agents.

Side effects also should be examined more carefully because certain side effects may be sex specific. For example, the female vascular system differs from the male vascular system, and females thus may experience light-headedness, nausea, and headaches more frequently than men do. Certain side effects that may be overlooked when drug effect is considered include changes in the menstrual cycle ("Gender Studies in Product Development" 1995). Prospective studies, in order to ensure valid results, must control for factors such as comorbid psychiatric and medical disorders, concomitant psychotherapy, exogenous and endogenous hormones, and concomitant medications, all of which can affect antidepressant pharmacokinetics and pharmacodynamics. Male and female subjects participating in these studies will need to be matched for age and body weight because these also may affect the pharmacokinetics of the medication.

For years, women were not systematically included in early clinical research trials of medications, including antidepressants (LaRosa and Pinn 1993). The litigious atmosphere has reinforced conservatism in including women of childbearing potential in clinical trials (Dawkins and Potter 1991), and some Phase I protocols exclude women because of the known hormonal fluctuations that may interfere with obtaining consistent pharmacokinetic results (Dawkins and Potter 1991). These reasons may justify excluding women of childbearing potential from certain studies, but few compelling reasons have been presented for excluding women from clinical trials in general (LaRosa and Pinn 1993). Policies that exclude women from clinical trials to protect them and their unborn children are now considered paternalistic and discriminatory (Wright and Cew 1996). Furthermore, when clinical data obtained from men are extrapolated to women, they ignore potential sex differences in response to treatment, and current principles of clinical practice strive to optimize therapeutic benefit and minimize risk by individualizing treatment (Wright and Cew 1996). Data obtained from clinical trials could be beneficial in promoting health and treating and controlling disease in women (LaRosa and Pinn 1993), especially as they become major consumers of antidepressants in the market (Kinney et al. 1981).

The U.S. Food and Drug Administration (FDA) guidelines have until recently excluded "women of childbearing potential" from Phase I and early Phase II studies (Wright and Cew 1996). Now, the FDA has published updated expectations for including women in the clinical development programs of drugs, biologics, and medical devices (Department of Health and Human Services 1993). Recent events prompted the 103rd Congress to mandate specific National Institutes of Health (NIH) action concerning women as subjects in NIH-supported clinical research. In response to the mandate, the NIH revised its existing policy under the NIH Revitalization Act of 1993 and specified that women shall be included as subjects in clinical research and that in clinical trials, they shall be included so that valid analysis can be performed to assess differences among participating groups. Furthermore, this statute mandates that the NIH must engage in special efforts to recruit women into clinical research studies (LaRosa et al. 1995) because a clinical trial without appropriate numbers of women may be scientifically flawed, as would be a clinical trial without an appropriate control group or one with a serious methodological weakness. Therefore, the inclusion of women as research subjects is viewed as an issue of scientific merit (Hayunga et al. 1997). Preliminary analysis of the first available year of the NIH-wide demographic data indicated that substantial numbers of female subjects have been included as research subjects. The goal, however, of the NIH policy is not to satisfy any quotas for proportional representation but rather to conduct biomedical and behavioral research so that scientific knowledge acquired will be more generalizable to the population of the United States (Hayunga et al. 1997).

Finally, medical and scientific journals need to be more amenable to publishing not only studies that report sex differences but also studies that report no sex differences. Research findings on sex differences may be more interesting than findings on sex similarities because, psychologically and biologically, the survival of the human race has depended on men and women recognizing each other as different. However, medical and scientific journals should not reject research reporting no sex differences to present a more balanced and clearer view of the similarities and differences that may exist between the two sexes (Andreasen 1997).

CONCLUSION

Sex differences in depression prevalence, course, and treatment have been established, yet more research needs to be conducted in order to fully elucidate these phenomena. An increase in the number of women participating in early clinical trials may provide the impetus necessary to validate these findings in studies that are carefully designed and well-controlled. Until then, clinicians need to be aware that potential sex differences exist, and they need to take into account patient sex when diagnosing and treating depression (Table 5–3). Clinicians diagnosing depression in women must realize that women may not always present with the usual neurovegetative symptoms and may present with a comorbid psychiatric disorder(s) and greater functional impairment. Female patients also should be queried about sex-specific triggers of episodes, such as stressful life events, psychosocial factors such as history of sexual abuse and rape, seasonal patterns, reproductive events, and exogenous hormone therapy. Clinicians also should inquire about premenstrual worsening of depression and assess whether any fluctuations in symptoms are related to the menstrual cycle. When choosing medication, factors such as history of antidepressant response and side-effect profile should be considered, and female patients should be questioned regularly about the emergence of undesirable adverse events that may necessitate a change in treatment. Each of the above-mentioned individual factors must be carefully considered by clinicians to formulate the optimum treatment that would ensure favorable drug response, patient compliance, and decreased incidence of undesirable adverse events.

TABLE 5–3.   Clinical implications of sex differences in antidepressant pharmacokinetics and pharmacodynamics

Upward dosage adjustment of certain antidepressants may be necessary in the following cases:
  Pregnancy (if clinically indicated and benefits outweigh risks)
  Oral contraceptive users
  Male and female extensive metabolizers
Downward dosage adjustment of certain antidepressants may be necessary in the following cases:
  Elderly men
  Females
  Males and females experiencing undesirable medication side effects

REFERENCES

Abernethy DR, Greenblatt DJ, Shader RI: Imipramine disposition in users of oral contraceptive steroids. Clin Pharmacol Ther 35:792–797, 1984

Almqvist F: Sex differences in adolescent psychopathology. Acta Psychiatr Scand 73:295–306, 1986

Andreasen NC: What shape are we in? Gender, psychopathology, and the brain (editorial). Am J Psychiatry 154:1637–1639, 1997

Angold A, Rutter M: Effects of age and pubertal status on depression in a large clinical sample. Dev Psychopathol 4:5–28, 1992

Angold A, Worthman CW: Puberty onset of gender differences in rates of depression: a developmental, epidemiologic and neuroendocrine perspective. J Affect Disord 29:145–158, 1993

Balter MB, Levine J, Manheimer DI: Cross-national study of the extent of antianxiety/sedative drug use. N Engl J Med 290:769–774, 1974

Barbhaiya RH, Buch AB, Greene DS: A study of the effect of age and gender on the pharmacokinetics of nefazodone after single and multiple doses. J Clin Psychopharmacol 16:19–25, 1996

Barry P: Gender as a factor in treating the elderly. NIDA Res Monogr 65:65–69, 1986

Belle D: Poverty and women's mental health. Am Psychol 45:385–389, 1990

Brooks-Gunn J: Antecedents and consequences of variations in girls' maturational timing. Journal of Adolescent Health Care 9:365–373, 1988

Brooks-Gunn J, Ruble DN: Dysmenorrhea in adolescence, in Menarche. Edited by Golub S. Lexington, MA, Lexington Books, 1983, pp 251–262

Browne A: Family violence and homelessness: the relevance of trauma histories in the lives of homeless women. Am J Orthopsychiatry 63:370–384, 1993

Buchanan CM, Eccles J, Becker J: Are adolescents the victims of raging hormones? Evidence for activational effects on hormones on moods and behavior at adolescence. Psychol Bull 111:62–107, 1992

Cafferata GL, Kasper J, Bernstein A: Family roles, structure and stressors in relation to sex differences in obtaining psychotropic drugs. J Health Soc Behav 24:132–143, 1983

Cooperstock R: Sex differences in the use of mood-modifying drugs: an explanatory model. J Health Soc Behav 12:238–244, 1971

Cooperstock R: A review of women's psychotropic drug use. Can J Psychiatry 24:29–34, 1979

Crockett LJ, Petersen AC: Pubertal status and psychosocial development: findings from the early adolescence study, in Biological Psychosocial Interaction in Early Adolescence. Edited by Lerner RM, Foch TT. Hillsdale, NJ, Lawrence Erlbaum, 1987, pp 173–188

Dahl M, Bertilsson L, Nordin C: Steady-state plasma levels of nortriptyline and its 10-hydroxy metabolite: relationship to the CYP2D6 genotype. Psychopharmacology (Berl) 123:315–319, 1996

Dawkins K, Potter WZ: Gender differences in pharmacokinetics and pharmacodynamics of psychotropics: focus on women. Psychopharmacol Bull 27:417–426, 1991

Department of Health and Human Services: Guideline for the study and evaluating of gender differences in the clinical evaluation of drugs (notice). Federal Register 58:39406, 1993

Dornbusch SM, Carlsmith JM, Duncan PD, et al: Sexual maturation, social class, and the desire to be thin among adolescent females. J Dev Behav Pediatr 5:308–314, 1984

Edeki TI: Clinical importance of genetic polymorphism of drug oxidation. Mt Sinai J Med 63:291–300, 1996

Finkelhor D, Browne A: The traumatic impact of child sexual abuse: a conceptualization. Am J Orthopsychiatry 55:530–541, 1985

Frank E, Carpenter LL, Kupfer DJ: Sex differences in recurrent depression: are there any that are significant? Am J Psychiatry 145:41–45, 1988

Gender Studies in Product Development: Scientific Issues and Approaches Workshop. Washington, DC, November 6–7, 1995

Gex-Fabry M, Balant-Gorgia AE, Balant LP, et al: Clomipramine metabolism: model-based analysis of variability factors from drug monitoring data. Clin Pharmacokinet 19:241–255, 1990

Glassman AH, Perel JM, Shostak M, et al: Clinical implications of imipramine plasma levels for depressive illness. Arch Gen Psychiatry 34:197–204, 1977

Gove WR, Tudor JF: Adult sex roles and mental illness. American Journal of Sociology 78:812–835, 1973

Greenblatt DJ, Friedman H, Burstein ES, et al: Trazodone kinetics: effects of age, gender and obesity. Clin Pharmacol Ther 42:193–200, 1987

Greenley JR, Mechanic D, Cleary PD: Seeking help for psychologic problems: a replication and extension. Med Care 25:1113–1128, 1987

Greif EB, Ulman KJ: The psychological impact of menarche on early adolescent females: a review of the literature. Child Dev 53:1413–1430, 1982

Guyer B, Lescohier I, Gallagher SS, et al: Intentional injuries among children and adolescents in Massachusetts. N Engl J Med 321:1584–1589, 1989

Halbreich U, Lumley LA: The multiple interactional biological processes that might lead to depression and gender differences in its appearance. J Affect Disord 29:159–173, 1993

Hamilton JA, Jensvold MF: Sex and gender as critical variables in feminist psychopharmacology research and pharmacotherapy. Women and Therapy 16:9–30, 1995

Hamilton JA, Grant M, Jensvold MF: Sex and treatment of depressions: when does it matter? in Psychopharmacology and Women. Edited by Jensvold MF, Halbreich U, Hamilton JA. Washington, DC, American Psychiatric Press, 1996, pp 241–257

Hayunga EG, Costello MD, Pinn VW: Demographics of study populations. Applied Clinical Trials 9:41–45, 1997

Heitkemper M, Jarrett M, Bond EF, et al: GI symptoms, function, and psychophysiological arousal in dysmenorrheic women. Nurs Res 40:20–26, 1991

Horgan C: Specialty and general ambulatory mental health services: comparison of utilization and expenditures. Arch Gen Psychiatry 42:565–572, 1985

Hudson WR, Roehrkasse RL, Wald A: Influence of gender and menopause on gastric emptying and motility. Gastroenterology 96:11–17, 1989

Kessler RC, Brown RL, Broman CL: Sex differences in psychiatric help-seeking: evidence from four large-scale surveys. J Health Soc Behav 22:49–64, 1981

Kessler RC, McGonagle KA, Swartz M, et al: Sex and depression in the National Comorbidity Survey, I: lifetime prevalence, chronicity, and recurrence. J Affect Disord 29:85–96, 1993

Kinney EL, Trautmann J, Gold JA, et al: Underrepresentation of women in new drug trials: ramification and remedies. Ann Intern Med 95:495–499, 1981

Klamerus KJ, Parker VD, Rudolph RL, et al: Effects of age and gender on venlafaxine and O-desmethylvenlafaxine pharmacokinetics. Pharmacotherapy 16:915–923, 1996

Koff E, Rierdan J, Stubbs ML: Gender, body image and self-concept in early adolescence. Journal of Early Adolescence 10:56–68, 1990

Kornstein SG: Gender differences in depression: implications for treatment. J Clin Psychiatry 58(suppl 15):12–18, 1997

LaRosa JH, Pinn VW: Gender bias in biomedical research. J Am Med Womens Assoc 48:145–151, 1993

LaRosa JH, Seto B, Caban CE, et al: Including women and minorities in clinical research. Applied Clinical Trials 4:31–38, 1995

Legato MJ: Gender-specific physiology: how real is it? How important is it? Int J Fertil Womens Med 42:19–29, 1997

MacLeod SM, Soldin JJ: Determinants of drug disposition in man. Clin Biochem 19:67–71, 1986

Mant A, Broom DH, Duncan-Jones P: The path to prescription: sex differences in psychotropic drug prescribing for general practice patients. Social Psychiatry 18:185–192, 1983

McCarthy M: The thin ideal: depression and eating disorders in women. Behav Res Ther 28:205–215, 1990

McGee R, Feehan M, Williams S, et al: DSM-III disorders in a large sample of adolescents. J Am Acad Child Adolesc Psychiatry 29:611–619, 1990

McLanahan SS, Sorensen A, Watson D: Sex differences in poverty, 1950–1980. Signs: A Journal of Women in Culture and Society 15:102–144, 1989

Mirowsky J, Ross C: Sex differences in distress: real or artifact? American Sociological Review 60:449–468, 1995

Moody JP, Tait AC, Todrick A: Plasma levels of imipramine and desmethylimipramine during therapy. Br J Psychiatry 113:183–193, 1967

Nolen-Hoeksema S: Sex differences in unipolar depression: evidence and theory. Psychol Bull 101:259–282, 1987

Nolen-Hoeksema S: Sex Differences in Depression. Stanford, CA, Stanford University Press, 1990

Nolen-Hoeksema S, Gigus JS: The emergence of gender differences in depression during adolescence. Psychol Bull 115:424–443, 1994

Padgett DK: Women's mental health: some directions for research. Am J Orthopsychiatry 67:522–534, 1997

Pajer K: New strategies in the treatment of depression in women. J Clin Psychiatry 56(suppl 2):30–37, 1995

Parry BL: Reproductive factors affecting the course of affective illness. Psychiatr Clin North Am 12:207–220, 1989

Patkai P, Johansson G, Post B: Mood, alertness and sympathetic-adrenal medullary activity during the menstrual cycle. Psychosom Med 36:503–512, 1974

Paykel ES: Depression in women. Br J Psychiatry 158:22–29, 1991

Perel JM, Mendlewicz J, Shostak M, et al: Plasma levels of imipramine in depression: environmental and genetic factors. Neuropsychobiology 2:193–202, 1976

Petersen AC: Female pubertal development, in Female Adolescent Development. Edited by Sugar M. New York, Brunner/Mazel, 1979, pp 93–115

Piazza LA, Markowitz JC, Kocsis JH, et al: Sexual functioning in chronically depressed patients treated with SSRI antidepressants: a pilot study. Am J Psychiatry 154:1757–1765, 1997

Preskorn SH, Mac DS: Plasma levels of amitriptyline: effects of age and sex. J Clin Psychiatry 46:276–277, 1985

Pugliesi K: Women and mental health: two traditions of feminist research. Womens Health 19:43–68, 1992

Radloff LS: Sex differences in depression: the effects of occupation and marital status. Sex Roles 1:249–265, 1975

Ronfeld RA, Tremaine LM, Wilner KD: Pharmacokinetics of sertraline and its N-demethyl metabolite in elderly and young male and female volunteers. Clin Pharmacokinet 32(suppl 1):22–30, 1997

Roy A: Suicide, in Comprehensive Textbook of Psychiatry, VI. Edited by Kaplan HI, Sadock BJ. Baltimore, MD, Williams & Wilkins, 1995, pp 1739–1751

Rutter M, Graham P, Chadwick OF, et al: Adolescent turmoil: fact or fiction? J Child Psychol Psychiatry 17:35–56, 1976

Seeman MV: Psychopathology in women and men: focus on female hormones. Am J Psychiatry 154:1641–1647, 1997

Shen WW, Hsu JH: Female sexual side effects associated with selective serotonin reuptake inhibitors: a descriptive clinical study of 33 patients. Int J Psychiatry Med 25:239–248, 1995

Sutfin TA, Perini GI, Molan G, et al: Multiple-dose pharmacokinetics of imipramine and its major active and conjugated metabolites in depressed patients. J Clin Psychopharmacol 8:48–53, 1988

Tang MX, Jacobs D, Stern Y, et al: Effect of estrogen during menopause on risk and age at onset of Alzheimer's disease. Lancet 348:429–432, 1996

Trinkoff AM, Anthony JC, Munoz A: Predictors of the initiation of psychotherapeutic medicine use. Am J Public Health 80:61–65, 1990

Van Wijk CM, Kolk AM: Sex differences in physical symptoms: the contribution of symptom perception theory. Soc Sci Med 45:231–246, 1997

Velez CN, Johnson J, Cohen P: A longitudinal analysis of selected risk factors for childhood psychopathology. J Am Acad Child Adolesc Psychiatry 28:861–864, 1989

Wald A, Van Thiel DH, Hoechstetter L, et al: Gastrointestinal transit: the effect of the menstrual cycle. Gastroenterology 80:1497–1500, 1981

Weissman MM, Klerman GL: Sex differences in the epidemiology of depression. Arch Gen Psychiatry 34:98–111, 1977

Wells KB, Manning WG, Duan N: Sociodemographic factors and the use of outpatient mental health services. Med Care 24:75–85, 1986

Wilson K: Sex-related differences in drug disposition in man. Clin Pharmacokinet 9:189–202, 1984

Wisner KL, Perel JM, Wheeler SB: Tricyclic dose requirements across pregnancy. Am J Psychiatry 150:1541–1542, 1993

Wright DT, Cew NJ: Women as subjects in clinical research. Applied Clinical Trials 5:44–52, 1996

Yonkers KA, Kando JC, Cole JO, et al: Gender differences in pharmacokinetics and pharmacodynamics of psychotropic medication. Am J Psychiatry 149:587–595, 1992

Young MA, Scheftner WA, Fawcett J, et al: Gender differences in the clinical features of unipolar depressive disorder. J Nerv Ment Dis 178:200–203, 1990

Zuspan FP, Zuspan KJ: Ovulatory plasma amine (epinephrine and norepinephrine) surge in the woman. Am J Obstet Gynecol 117:654–661, 1973

6

Postpartum Mood Disorders

Identification and Treatment

Amy L. Hostetter, B.A.
Zachary N. Stowe, M.D.

*F*ew strides have been made in understanding the complexities of postpartum onset mental illness since its earliest documentation by Hippocrates in 400 B.C. and Tortula in the first century. Still others such as Marce and Hamilton are credited with the initial forays into the etiopathogenesis of these psychiatric disorders. To date, much of the literature and most patient support groups continue to support the hypothesis that biological aberrations herald the onset of psychiatric illness during the postpartum period; however, a burgeoning series of investigations have failed to confirm such biological associations. Although the etiology remains obscure, the epidemiological evidence that the childbearing years, particularly the postpartum period, represent a time of increased vulnerability for women to develop mood disorders is substantial.

It has been reported that "of all psychiatric hospital admissions of women, 6%–12.5% occur during the postpartum period" (Duffy 1983, p. 11). Whether or not this rise in psychiatric hospitalization after childbirth (Duffy 1983; Kendell et al. 1987) provides evidence for a distinct set of disorders or enhanced acuity of preexisting conditions continues to stimulate zealous discussion. Uniqueness or etiology seems a trivial debate in light of more than four decades of repeated clinical and laboratory evidence that maternal mental illness and separation have the propensity to adversely affect offspring. The prevalence and potential effect of postpartum mood disorders underscore the need for effective identification and treatment. In this chapter, we provide a brief review of postpartum illness, emphasizing the potential effect on infant well-being, early identification, risk factors, treatment options, and prevention strategies.

HISTORY AND EVOLUTION OF POSTPARTUM MENTAL ILLNESS

Although the connection between the postpartum period and psychiatric disturbance was described 24 centuries ago by Hippocrates, the events of the nineteenth century provided the foundation for questions that remain unanswered today. In 1845, Esquirol described a variety of mood disturbances associated with the postpartum period and disputed their relation with lactation. Subsequently, a French physician named Marce published *Insanity in Pregnant, Puerperal and Lactating Women* (1858). In this work, he detailed and discussed pertinent issues in the cases of 44 women. Marce proposed that postpartum mood disorders encompassed a variety of symptoms, which were not unique but could be found in nonpuerperal disorders as well. The combination of these symptoms, Marce proposed, formed a distinct syndrome that could be classified into two groups: those with early onset (increased confusion or delirium) and those with late onset (more physical symptoms). At the beginning of the twentieth century, distinguishing disorders based on the time of onset and whether postpartum disorders represented unique syndromes was being disputed. The American Psychiatric Association ruled to officially remove the term *postpartum* from the classification system, with diagnosis then based on the symptoms that were most apparent at the time of clinical presentation (Parry and Hamilton 1999). Following this, puerperal illnesses often were labeled as schizophrenic, affective, or toxic disorders (Purdy and Frank 1993). The introduction of antibiotics and sterile precautions reduced infection-induced psychosis following childbirth; consequently, the diagnosis of toxic insanity decreased (Purdy and Frank 1993).

Research on postpartum depression (PPD) has found conflicting results on whether symptoms of PPD differ from those of non-PPD. Pitt's (1968) studies described PPD as a distinct "atypical" depression with milder symptoms, a lack of neurovegetative symptoms and suicidal ideation, and a higher level of anxiety and irritability. In contrast, other studies that used standard psychiatric rating scales and structured interviews did not show significant differences in symptoms (Affonso et al. 1990; Cooper et al. 1988; Wisner et al. 1994). The "distinct diagnosis" debate has evolved in the DSM diagnostic classification system as well. The American Psychiatric Association (1968) first briefly acknowledged postpartum affective disorders in DSM-II. "Psychosis associated with childbirth" was listed as a psychosis caused by organic conditions. In DSM-III and DSM-III-R (American Psychiatric Association 1980, 1987), postpartum psychosis was noted only as an example of atypical psychosis. Currently, DSM-IV-TR (American Psychiatric Association 2000) lists "with postpartum onset" as a specifier for mood disorders and brief psychotic disorder. If symptom onset meeting diagnostic criteria for major depressive, manic, or mixed episode in major depressive disorder, bipolar I disorder, bipolar II disorder, or brief psychotic disorder is within 4 weeks of the birth of a child, the specifier "with postpartum onset" may be applied to diagnosis. The alterations in the diagnostic issues are not the only point of contention but are readily apparent in the etiological theories proposed.

The purported temporal association with childbirth has contributed to the contention that postpartum illnesses are biologically derived. However, the studies that have investigated potential biological alterations are notably negative or lack replication (Wisner and Stowe 1997). In addition, nonbiological theories involving intrapsychic conflict (Zilboorg 1943), personality structure, and psychosocial adaptability also have been postulated (Jansson 1963). Boyd was the first to propose a multifactorial etiology emphasizing individual vulnerability or predisposition to illness. He posed the question, "Is the patient's psychic reserve (hereditary constitution, training, personal psychologic organization) sufficient to resist the factors producing mental disorder (toxicity, endocrine imbalance, psychologic conflicts engendered by pregnancy)?" (Jansson 1963, p. 23).

Regardless of specific diagnostic recognition and etiological debate, considerable data underscore the potential adverse effect of maternal mental illness on infants.

EFFECT OF MATERNAL PSYCHIATRIC ILLNESS ON INFANT WELL-BEING

The adverse effect of maternal separation and maternal mental illness on offspring well-being has been established in both the animal and the human literature, respectively. Initial laboratory observations, starting in the early 1960s, showed adverse effects on socialization in maternally deprived offspring of primates (Harlow and Harlow 1966). Animal models of maternal separation have found persistent alterations in the offspring that persist into adulthood. These changes are widespread and include (but are not limited to) alteration in neuroendocrine axes (Plotsky and Meaney 1993), in neurotransmitter systems (Matthew et al. 1996), in behavior (Statham 1998), in central nervous system cytoarchitecture and receptors (McEwen et al. 1992; Sutanto et al. 1996), and in neuronal firing patterns (Stowe et al. 1998a). Whether or not such laboratory investigations of maternal separation are germane to clinical care is debatable; yet, the clinical evidence predates the earliest animal studies.

It has been more than five decades since the World Health Organization presentation showed the deleterious effects of prolonged maternal separation on human infants (Bowlby 1951). Another example of a severe form of maternal separation was described in a documentary that illustrated the profound effect of limited emotional contact in orphaned refugee infants. It has been said that "if normal maternal communication is experimentally disrupted for even brief periods, infants as young as 6 weeks respond with distress and avoidance" (L. Murray 1992, p. 544). The literature is replete with studies specific to maternal mental illness during the postpartum period, indicating its adverse effect on infants. These investigations have shown negative effects on maternal–infant attachment, infant cognitive competence, and child development and behavior (Avant 1981; Brazelton 1975; Campbell et al. 1995; Cogill et al. 1986; Cradon 1979; Cutrona and Troutman 1986; L. Murray and Cooper 1996; Teti et al. 1995; Whiffen and Gotlib 1989; Zahn-Waxler et al. 1984). Another series of studies with depressed mothers found a decrease in mother–infant behavioral and electrocardiogram synchrony (Field 1990; Field et al. 1989) as well as depressed infant behavior (Field et al. 1988). Remarkably, these effects were observed when the entry criterion for the depressed mothers was a Beck Depression Inventory (BDI) score greater than 12 (a score representing only mild to moderate depression). Depression may affect not only how the mother interacts with her infant but also how the mother perceives her infant. Depressed mothers have been shown to perceive their infant in a more negative manner and as more difficult to care for than do nondepressed control subjects (L. Murray et al. 1996; Whiffen and Gotlib 1989). Such data indicate that across a spectrum of severity, maternal mental illness may adversely affect the infant and the mother–infant interaction.

The clinical research alone warrants intervention, and if laboratory data are included, then identification, treatment planning, and prevention of maternal mental illness are mandated. Thus, clinicians must be familiar with the postpartum illness categories that encompass most of the research. The primary categories that most researchers agree on include postpartum blues, PPD, and postpartum psychosis.

POSTPARTUM BLUES (MATERNITY BLUES)

Postpartum blues, also known as maternity blues, occurs more frequently than the other postpartum disorders, affecting between 50% and 80% of mothers (Kennerley and Gath 1989; O'Hara 1991). The maternity blues is not typically considered a "disorder" warranting professional intervention. Postpartum blues usually has an onset within the first 2 weeks after delivery and can last from a few hours to a few days. Various symptoms have been described, including mild depression, irritability, confusion, mood instability, anxiety, headache, fatigue, and forgetfulness.

The cause of postpartum blues is unknown; however, much research has examined the dramatic biological changes occurring during labor, delivery, and the immediate postpartum period as well as psychosocial and personality factors (Condon and Watson 1987; A.J. George and Wilson 1981; Kennerley and Gath 1989; O'Hara et al. 1991b). In a study of 89 women, Condon and Watson (1987) investigated the causes and predictors of postpartum blues and found that the most prevalent predictor was having a sense of pessimism in late pregnancy about the delivery and the period immediately following delivery. They also noted three other risk factors associated with the blues: severity of premenstrual tension, ambivalent feelings toward the pregnancy, and viewing the pregnancy as emotionally difficult.

In another study of 182 women, O'Hara et al. (1991b) examined both the biological and the psychosocial factors of the blues. A personal and family history of depression, poor social adjustment, stressful life events, premenstrual depression, and levels of free and total estriol were associated with the blues. Anxiety and depressed mood during pregnancy, fear of labor, poor social adjustment, and retrospective evaluation of premenstrual tension were associated with the blues in another study that used a maternity blues questionnaire (Kennerley and Gath 1989).

Being able to identify the factors associated with the blues is important because data suggest that experiencing the blues places one at elevated risk for PPD (Hapgood et al. 1988). It is reported that approximately 20% of women with the blues experience major depression in the first postnatal year (Campbell et al. 1992; O'Hara 1991). These findings warrant careful observation of symptom progression during pregnancy and the postpartum period.

POSTPARTUM DEPRESSION

PPD is a major depressive episode with clinical symptoms that may include anxiety, irritability, anhedonia, fatigue, and sleep disturbance. Symptom onset of PPD generally is within 6 weeks postpartum (Stowe and Nemeroff 1995), and severity and duration vary (Wolkind et al. 1988). Rates of PPD are reportedly between 7% and 17% in adult women (Gotlib et al. 1989; Pitt 1968) and approximately 26% in adolescent mothers (Troutman and Cutrona 1990) in the first postpartum year. A review of 17 major studies examining the rates of PPD reported prevalence rates ranging from 5% to 22% (Richards 1990). This wide variance in prevalence shows the difficulty in determining the incidence of PPD with different assessment methods and diagnostic criteria, including definition of the duration of the postpartum period. Distinguishing between depressive symptoms and the supposed "normal" sequelae of childbirth, such as changes in weight, sleep, and energy, is a challenge that further complicates clinical diagnosis. Further confounding the determination of prevalence of PPD is a neglect to examine possible physical causes (including anemia, diabetes, and thyroid dysfunction) that could potentially contribute to depressive symptoms (Pedersen et al. 1993).

To address some of these confounds, rating scales have been developed specifically for this population. The Edinburgh Postnatal Depression rating scale, a 10-item scale that has evolved into a self-rated measure and has been translated into more than a dozen different languages, seems to be highly correlated with physician-rated depression measures (Cox et al. 1987). The Postpartum Depression Checklist was developed for health professionals as a tool to screen for PPD (Beck 1995). These scales are for use in the postpartum period; however, identification of women, prior to delivery, at high risk for postpartum-onset illness is the emerging standard of care.

The factors contributing to PPD have undergone considerable scrutiny (Duffy 1983; Gotlib et al. 1991; Marks et al. 1992; Stowe and Nemeroff 1995). Briefly, a personal and/or family history of a mood disorder (Playfair and Gowers 1981; Richards 1990), a previous episode of PPD (O'Hara 1991), depression or anxiety during pregnancy, and the maternity blues increase susceptibility to developing PPD (Gotlib et al. 1991; O'Hara 1986, 1991; O'Hara et al. 1991a). In addition, psychosocial issues, including marital discord, infant medical problems, unwanted or unplanned pregnancies, lack of social support, and stressful life events during pregnancy, are all predisposing factors that have been noted in the literature (Gotlib et al. 1991; Graff et al. 1991; Marks et al. 1992; O'Hara et al. 1991a; Unterman et al. 1990). In contrast, no association between demographic factors and onset of illness has been consistently found (Bagedahl Strindlund 1986; Marks et al. 1992). Identification of these risk factors, most of which are present before childbirth, provides caregivers with awareness of the potential for illness, making early identification, intervention, and prevention possible.

POSTPARTUM PSYCHOSIS

The previously cited investigations have noted the increased rate of admission to psychiatric hospitals with psychotic symptoms during the postpartum period (Kendell et al. 1987). Postpartum psychosis is the most severe postpartum mood disorder. It is relatively rare, reported to occur in only 1 or 2 of every 1,000 women (Kendell et al. 1987). This psychosis appears quickly after birth, within a few days, and in most cases within the first 3 weeks (Brockington et al. 1981). The majority (>70%) of these psychoses are either bipolar disorder or major depression with psychotic features. Brief reactive psychosis and schizophrenia also occur but more infrequently (McGorry and Connell 1990). Symptoms of this disorder include delusions, hallucinations, an impaired concept of reality, rapid mood swings ranging from depression to elation, insomnia, and abnormal or obsessive thoughts about the infant. This disorder has an estimated 5% rate of suicide and a 4% rate of infanticide (Knopps 1993). Postpartum psychosis constitutes a psychiatric emergency, and a presumptive diagnosis of psychosis warrants hospitalization.

The prognostic investigations of recurrent psychotic symptoms following an index episode during the postpartum period vary, although most studies agree that approximately 65% of these women will experience subsequent nonpuerperal psychotic episodes (Benvenuti et al. 1992; Schopf and Rust 1994; Videbech and Gouliaev 1995). It is noteworthy that investigations have indicated that up to two-thirds of these women experienced symptom relapse in subsequent pregnancies (Benvenuti et al. 1992; Schopf and Rust 1994). However, compared with women who experienced psychosis not precipitated by childbirth, those who experience affective postpartum psychosis are less likely to be readmitted to psychiatric hospitals, and if they are, they spend less time in them (Platz and Kendell 1988). Studies examining the characteristics of women who experience postpartum psychosis have found that they have a higher than average history of personal and familial psychiatric disorders.

OBSESSIVE-COMPULSIVE DISORDER AND PANIC DISORDER

The bulk of the extant literature has focused predominantly on the depressive disorders and psychosis during the postpartum period; however, evidence that anxiety disorders such as obsessive-compulsive disorder (OCD) and panic disorder may have their initial episodes during either pregnancy or the postpartum period has begun to accumulate. A retrospective study of 59 women with OCD found that 39% experienced symptom onset during pregnancy. Symptom onset also was reported during pregnancy in another four of five women in this study who had an abortion or miscarriage (Neziroglu et al. 1992). Other findings have indicated that preexisting OCD is exacerbated during pregnancy (Brandt and Mackenzie 1987; Williams and Koran 1997). Symptoms of OCD have been reported to develop or worsen during the postpartum period as well (Williams and Koran 1997). The obsessions experienced during these times often become centered on the fetus or the infant, and they are often accompanied by depression (Brandt and Mackenzie 1987; Williams and Koran 1997).

Early reports suggested that pregnancy might confer some sort of protection against panic attack (D. T. George et al. 1987), followed by an increase in panic symptoms during the postpartum period (Klein et al. 1995; Metz et al. 1988). Subsequent studies have reported a more complicated and variable course of panic disorder across gestation and the puerperium. A retrospective study of 49 women with panic disorder found similar rates of clinical improvement and symptom worsening during pregnancy (Cohen et al. 1994a). In contrast, in the postpartum period, out of a sample of 40 women, only 3 (7.5%) reported symptom improvement, whereas 14 (35.0%) had worsened symptoms, and 23 (57.5%) reported no change (Cohen et al. 1994b).

The presence of anxiety and obsessions in postpartum-onset disorders has been noted in DSM-IV (American Psychiatric Association 1994), and epidemiological data suggest a very high rate of comorbidity of depression and anxiety disorders in women (Kessler et al. 1994).

TREATMENT

Women of reproductive age typically have not been included in clinical trials, and the number of treatment studies specific to postpartum psychiatric illness is sparse. The National Institutes of Health and the U.S. Food and Drug Administration have emphasized the inclusion of women of reproductive age in future studies. This, of course, is of particular importance for postpartum psychiatric illness. Effective treatment planning for women with postpartum mood disorders or at high risk for such disorders must include the following: 1) professional and community education; 2) identification of women at risk; 3) antenatal and postnatal screening procedures; and 4) treatment options, including risk–benefit assessment for the use of psychotropic medications during breast-feeding.

Education

There are a variety of information sources such as Depression After Delivery (1-800-944-4PPD), a national support group providing information, volunteer contacts, and a Web site on the Internet. In addition, Postpartum Support International (1-805-967-7636) is a support group with international connections. More general information about mood disorders can be obtained from the National Depressive and Manic Depressive Association (1-800-826-3632), one of the largest patient-operated support and information systems in the United States. Several books about postpartum mental illness are available. *This Isn't What I Expected*, by Kleiman and Raskin (1994), provides a reasonable overview. These sources provide not only a knowledge base but also local resources for the professional, patient, and family.

Identification of Women at Risk

Most risk factors that predispose women to the development of postpartum mood disorders are present before delivery. The potential relation between postpartum blues and later PPD and the fact that more than 70% of the postpartum psychoses represent mood disorders underscore the need to reiterate the most commonly cited risk factors in order of their typical appearance during pregnancy and childbirth (Table 6–1).

High-risk populations identified before childbirth can be screened more closely for additional risk factors that are detectable on standardized depression rating scales.

Antenatal and Postnatal Screening

Routine obstetrical documentation of mood or anxiety complaints during pregnancy seldom occurs; however, data indicate that many women who experience postpartum illness had symptom or illness onset during pregnancy. For example, our group found that of 181 women presenting with complaints of depression during the postpartum period, 17% reported symptom onset during pregnancy (Hostetter et al. 1999). As noted earlier, more than one-third of the women with OCD also reported onset of illness during pregnancy (Neziroglu et al. 1992). These retrospective studies are not conclusive, but mounting data suggest that depression and/or anxiety during pregnancy is a risk factor for PPD (O'Hara et al. 1991a). The use of a depression rating scale, such as the Edinburgh Postnatal Depression Scale or the BDI, in early pregnancy establishes a baseline for comparison and subsequent assessment. Screening should include documentation of other risk factors such as marital discord and social support.

Evaluation during the first 2 weeks after childbirth may identify cases of postpartum blues. Screening for depression and anxiety at 6 weeks postpartum will identify more than 50% of the cases. Education, early identifica-

TABLE 6–1.   Risk factors for developing postpartum mood disorders

Time	Postpartum blues	Postpartum depression	Postpartum psychosis
Antenatal	Personal history of depression	Personal history of depression	History of postpartum psychosis
	Family history of depression	Family history of depression	Personal history of bipolar disorder
	Premenstrual depression	Premenstrual depression	Family history of bipolar disorder
	Poor social adjustment	Lack of social support	
	Stressful life events	Marital discord	
	Fear of labor	Stressful life events	
	Ambivalent feelings about pregnancy	Unwanted pregnancy	
	Pessimism in late pregnancy	Depression and/or anxiety during pregnancy	
Postnatal	Viewing pregnancy as emotionally difficult	Infant medical problems	
		Postpartum blues	

tion, and screening provide the foundation for effective individualized treatment planning.

Treatment Options

Despite the incidence of postpartum mood disorders and their potential detrimental consequences, surprisingly few treatment studies have been conducted. In community-derived samples, a variety of psychotherapeutic treatments (Rogerian, cognitive-behavioral, and psychodynamic), as well as individual counseling (Wickberg and Hwang 1996), have proven efficacious in treating PPD (O'Hara 1994). The best documented form of psychotherapy for women with PPD is interpersonal psychotherapy (IPT) (Stuart and O'Hara 1995). The premise behind IPT is that women with PPD typically experience a disruption in their interpersonal relationships; therefore, a therapy that targets these problems would be beneficial. A second community-based sample (N=61) showed the effectiveness of both cognitive-behavioral therapy (CBT) and fluoxetine monotherapy for the treatment of PPD (Appleby et al. 1997). Additional studies with CBT have reported efficacy comparable with that of alprazolam for the treatment of panic disorder during pregnancy and postpartum (Klosko et al. 1990; L. Robinson et al. 1992), although with a more delayed response. In contrast to more formal psychotherapy, social support groups were not effective in alleviating symptoms of maternal depression (Fleming et al. 1992).

The first pharmacological trial (N=21) conducted at a tertiary referral center showed a dramatic response in 20 women by 8 weeks of treatment with sertraline (Stowe et al. 1995). Another group reported successful treatment with the tricyclic antidepressant nortriptyline (Wisner and Perel 1991). The use of gonadal hormones in the treatment of postpartum mood disorders has included reports of progesterone treatment in postpartum psychosis (Schmidt 1943) and both sublingual and transdermal estrogen in the treatment of PPD (Ahokas et al. 1998; Gregoire et al. 1994, 1996; D. Murray 1996). The largest hormone study (N=34 active) showed a positive response that was sustained at 3-month follow-up, and no evidence of endometrial hyperplasia was found (D. Murray 1996). It is noteworthy that depressive symptoms as measured by the Edinburgh Postnatal Depression Scale were only modestly decreased, and more than one-third of these women were taking antidepressants during the study (Table 6–2).

A total of 186 women were actively treated in these case reports and studies. It is difficult to compare the efficacy of the various treatment modalities used because diagnostic entry criteria, depression rating scales, and sample recruitment were not consistent across studies. Clearly, further study is needed to compare the efficacy of treatment. Our group recently

TABLE 6–2. Treatment and prevention studies for postpartum depression (PPD)

	Active treatment				
	Design	N	Results	Comment	Reference
Antidepressants					
Fluoxetine	Prospective case series	4 active	All 4 patients made complete recovery with 20 mg/day. Final CGI=1.	All 4 patients had history of treatment for depression.	Roy et al. 1993
Sertraline	Prospective, open label	21 active	In 20 women, >50% reduction in depression scores; in 14 women, complete recovery.	Highly efficacious and well tolerated for women with PPD	Stowe et al. 1995
Fluoxetine and CBT	Double blind, placebo controlled, randomized	61 active	Significant symptom improvement with fluoxetine vs. placebo and with 6 sessions of CBT vs. 1.	Both fluoxetine and CBT are effective for PPD; no advantage in combining these therapies.	Appleby et al. 1997
Venlafaxine	Prospective, open label	15 active	Significant reduction in depression and anxiety scores.	Clinical improvement seen by 4 weeks of treatment.	Cohen et al. 2001
Psychotherapeutic					
Social support group	Prospective, controlled	44 social support, 15 information, 83 control	Eight social support sessions did not improve mood more than no intervention or information by mail.	Did not alleviate maternal depression; did increase mother's attention to infant.	Fleming et al. 1992
Interpersonal psychotherapy (IPT)	Prospective	6 active, 2 also taking medication	Significant reduction in multiple depression measures after 12 weeks of IPT.	Alternative to medication, focus on changes in interpersonal relationships postpartum.	Stuart and O'Hara 1995
Counseling	Prospective, controlled	15 active, 16 control	After 6 visits with health nurse, 12 of 15 women with PPD recovered; only 4 of 16 control subjects recovered.	Swedish health care system: counseling by health nurses is useful in treating PPD.	Wickberg and Hwang 1996

TABLE 6–2. Treatment and prevention studies for postpartum depression (PPD) *(continued)*

	Design	N	Results	Comment	Reference
			Active treatment		
Other					
Sublingual estrogen	Case report	2 active	Significant reduction in MADRS score within first 2 weeks of treatment.	ICD-10 diagnosis and only 4-week follow-up	Ahokas et al. 1998
Transdermal estrogen	Double blind, placebo controlled	34 active, 27 control	Estrogen subjects improved rapidly in the first month and significantly greater than control subjects.	Transdermal estrogen effective treatment; dose and duration of treatment guidelines needed.	Gregoire et al. 1996
			Prevention		
Antidepressants					
Antidepressants	Prospective, open label, controlled	15 active, 8 control	6.7% on antidepressant prophylaxis had recurrence compared with 62.5% without medication.	Antidepressant treatment effective prophylactic for PPD; 43% of the women were taking medications during pregnancy.	Wisner and Wheeler 1994
Psychotherapeutic					
Antenatal education classes	Prospective, controlled	85 active, 76 control	Only 15% of the subjects who took classes had postpartum upset compared with 37% of the control subjects.	Women who had their husbands attend class with them did better than those who did not.	Gordon and Gordon 1960
Other					
Progesterone	Prospective, controlled	94 active, 221 control	Women with a history of PPD given progesterone prophylactically; only 9 had PPD recurrence.	Progesterone effective only for prophylaxis; once symptomatic, it is ineffective.	Dalton 1985

Note. CBT=cognitive-behavioral therapy; CGI=Clinical Global Impression Scale; ICD-10=*International Statistical Classification of Diseases and Related Health Problems*, 10th Revision; MADRS=Montgomery-Åsberg Depression Rating Scale.

reported a dramatic treatment response (>90% by 8 weeks) to monotherapy with a selective serotonin reuptake inhibitor combined with education, supportive psychotherapy, and behavioral modification (Strader et al. 1997). Our group and several other academic centers specializing in women's mental health use a similar treatment model to prevent illness in women at high risk for recurrent episodes. Active prevention has become the standard of care.

PREVENTION STRATEGIES

It is imperative that health practitioners who come into contact with pregnant and postpartum women (obstetricians, midwives, nurses, pediatricians) be able to identify high-risk groups. Prophylactic treatment should be considered in women at high risk for recurrence of symptoms, particularly if the history indicates significant functional impairment.

Few prophylactic treatment studies have been conducted; those that have confirm its success. Wisner and Wheeler (1994) examined prophylactic treatment of women with a history of PPD. Two groups of women were compared: 1) those who chose postpartum monitoring and prophylactic treatment with an antidepressant ($n=15$) and 2) those who chose postpartum monitoring alone ($n=8$). Five of the monitoring-only group relapsed compared with only one of the medication group. These findings should be interpreted with caution, however; a possible confound is that 10 of the subjects in the study had depressive symptoms and were taking medication for some period during their pregnancy, suggesting active treatment rather than prevention. Progesterone therapy has shown success in preventing postnatal depression although not in treating symptoms once they have started (Dalton 1985); however, these results have not been duplicated. One group that administered intravenous estrogen to a select group of women ($n=11$) with severe mood disorders reported effectiveness in preventing recurrence (Sichel et al. 1995). For women with histories of postpartum psychosis or bipolar disorder, prophylactic lithium administration has been found to decrease the recurrence and severity of the illness (Cohen et al. 1995; Stewart 1988; Stewart et al. 1991). Psychosocial intervention, such as support during labor and psychoeducation of parents and children, may benefit some women in preventing recurrent PPD (Beardslee et al. 1997; Wolman et al. 1993).

The data on active treatment of postpartum mood disorders and the prevention of recurrent episodes in high-risk populations have shown considerable efficacy; however, somatic intervention often is complicated by a woman's decision to breast-feed.

ANTIDEPRESSANTS AND BREAST-FEEDING

The number of women planning to breast-feed has increased considerably in the past 20 years, with more than 60% planning to nurse (Briggs et al. 1998). It is beyond the scope of this review to discuss the benefits of breast-feeding, although most professional groups support breast milk as the ideal source of nutrition for infants (American Academy of Pediatrics 1993). The use of psychotropic medication, and specifically antidepressants, during lactation has been reviewed by numerous groups (Baum and Misri 1996; Buist et al. 1990; Llewellyn and Stowe 1998; Misri and Sivertz 1991; Mortola 1989; G.E. Robinson et al. 1986; Stowe et al. 1998b; Wisner and Perel 1988; Wisner et al. 1996). The studies of antidepressants in breast-feeding are typically limited to groups of fewer than 10. The literature includes reports on 49 women treated with tricyclic antidpressants, with the largest data set on nortriptyline ($N=17$) (Birnbaum et al. 1999; Wisner and Perel 1988; Wisner et al. 1996). The information on selective serotonin reuptake inhibitors now exceeds the available data on any other class of medications in the *Physicians' Desk Reference*. Reports with infant serum monitoring total 83 for the selective serotonin reuptake inhibitors, with the largest data sets for fluoxetine ($N=33$) and sertraline ($N=31$). Direct comparison of the breast-feeding studies is difficult because of variation in methodology and assay sensitivity. Our group completed a detailed study of both the pharmacokinetics of excretion and the infant serum measures for sertraline; we found that the maximum calculated infant dose is typically less than 1/500th the maternal dose (Stowe et al. 1997). Although the infant follow-up data are limited, any acute adverse effects on infants are limited to isolated case reports (Llewellyn and Stowe 1998). The selective serotonin reuptake inhibitor data are summarized in Table 6–3.

It is important to conduct with the patient and any significant others a thorough risk–benefit assessment, in which all treatment options, as well as the risk of not treating maternal mental illness, are discussed. If the decision to use an antidepressant is made, a medication that was effective in treating previous episodes of depression, data on the medication during breast-feeding, and possible side effects are the primary determinants.

How long to continue pharmacological treatment of postpartum mood disorders depends on each particular case; however, the recommendations based on the treatment of nonpuerperal major depression support treatment for 12 months following symptom resolution. At our program, we strongly encourage tapering the treatment over 1–2 months or longer.

These studies and the information noted earlier in this chapter raise several issues in the treatment of PPD:

TABLE 6–3.   Selective serotonin reuptake inhibitors in breast-feeding

Medication	Infant serum (n)	Infant follow-up	Reference
Citalopram	1		Jensen et al. 1997
Fluoxetine	1		Lester et al. 1993
	6		Kim et al. 1997
	4	4	Yoshida et al. 1998
	15		Birnbaum et al. 1999
Paroxetine	2		Birnbaum et al. 1999
	16		Stowe et al. 2000
Sertraline	1		Altshuler et al. 1995
	3		Mammen et al. 1997
	4		Eppersen et al. 1997
	12		Stowe et al. 1997
		12	Llewellyn et al. 1997
	8		Wisner et al. 1998
	4		Kristensen et al. 1998
	3		Birnbaum et al. 1999

- If exposure to maternal mental illness constitutes a risk for the infant, should the treatment with the most rapid symptom remission always be recommended?
- With the documented efficacy of IPT, should this be the treatment of choice to avoid infant exposure to medication in women who choose to continue breast-feeding?
- Should supraphysiological doses of gonadal hormones be used to treat psychiatric illness in women in their reproductive years in the absence of data on their safety and long-term effect?

SUMMARY

Despite the prevalence of postpartum mood disorders, for most of the twentieth century women have experienced them in silence or with little assistance. Determining whether these disorders are distinct entities is a debate best left to research and is of minimal clinical utility. The postnatal environment and presence of a newborn represent a unique clinical, neuroendocrine, and psychosocial situation that warrants increased professional attention. Only recently has research begun to focus on the treatment of disorders occurring during this time. Data now support the efficacy of both psychological and pharmacological treatment and prevention measures. However, such data are of little use if we fail to identify the illness. Awareness of the prevalence, risk factors, and potential adverse effects of these disorders will provide the foundation to address many of the questions pending. Until further studies are completed, postpartum mood disorders represent a heterogeneous group of disorders of multifactorial etiology that can be effectively treated, once identified.

REFERENCES

Affonso DD, Lovett S, Paul SM, et al: A standardized interview that differentiates pregnancy and postpartum symptoms from perinatal clinical depression. Birth 17:21–30, 1990

Ahokas AJ, Turtiainen S, Aito M: Sublingual oestrogen treatment of postnatal depression (letter). Lancet 351:109, 1998

Altshuler LL, Burt VK, McMullen M, et al: Breastfeeding and sertraline: a 24-hour analysis. J Clin Psychiatry 56:243–245, 1995

American Academy of Pediatrics, Committee on Nutrition: Pediatric Nutrition Handbook, 3rd Edition. Elk Grove Village, IL, American Academy of Pediatrics, 1993

American Psychiatric Association: Diagnostic and Statistical Manual of Mental Disorders, 2nd Edition. Washington, DC, American Psychiatric Association, 1968

American Psychiatric Association: Diagnostic and Statistical Manual of Mental Disorders, 3rd Edition. Washington, DC, American Psychiatric Association, 1980

American Psychiatric Association: Diagnostic and Statistical Manual of Mental Disorders, 3rd Edition, Revised. Washington, DC, American Psychiatric Association, 1987

American Psychiatric Association: Diagnostic and Statistical Manual of Mental Disorders, 4th Edition. Washington, DC, American Psychiatric Association, 1994

American Psychiatric Association: Diagnostic and Statistical Manual of Mental Disorders, 4th Edition, Text Revision. Washington, DC, American Psychiatric Association, 2000

Appleby L, Warner R, Whitten A, et al: A controlled study of fluoxetine and cognitive-behavioral counseling in the treatment of postnatal depression. BMJ 314:932–936, 1997

Avant K: Anxiety as a potential factor affecting maternal attachment. J Obstet Gynecol Neonatal Nurs 10:416–419, 1981

Bagedahl Strindlund M: Parapartum mental illness: timing of illness onset and its relation to symptoms and sociodemographic characteristics. Acta Psychiatr Scand 74:490–496, 1986

Baum AL, Misri S: Selective serotonin-reuptake inhibitors in pregnancy and lactation. Harv Rev Psychiatry 4:117–125, 1996

Beardslee WR, Salt P, Versage EM, et al: Sustained change in parents receiving preventive interventions for families with depression. Am J Psychiatry 154:510–555, 1997

Beck CT: Screening methods for postpartum depression. J Obstet Gynecol Neonatal Nurs 24:308–312, 1995

Benvenuti P, Cabras PL, Servi P, et al: Puerperal psychoses: a clinical case study with follow-up. J Affect Disord 26:25–30, 1992

Birnbaum CS, Cohen LS, Bailey JW, et al: Serum antidepressant concentrations of antidepressants and benzodiazepines in nursing infants: a case series. Pediatrics 104:E11, 1999

Bowlby J: Maternal Care and Mental Health (WHO Monogr Series 2). Geneva, Switzerland, World Health Organization, 1951

Brandt KR, Mackenzie TB: Obsessive-compulsive disorder exacerbated during pregnancy: a case report. Int J Psychiatry Med 17:361–367, 1987

Brazelton TB: Mother infant reciprocity, in Maternal Attachment and Mothering Disorders: A Roundtable. Edited by Klaus MH, Leger T, Trause MA. North Brunswick, NJ, Johnson & Johnson, 1975, pp 49–54

Briggs GG, Freeman RK, Yaffe SJ: Drugs in Pregnancy and Lactation, 5th Edition. Baltimore, MD, Williams & Wilkins, 1998

Brockington IF, Cernik KF, Schofield EM, et al: Puerperal psychosis: phenomena and diagnosis. Arch Gen Psychiatry 38:829–833, 1981

Buist A, Norman TR, Dennerstein L: Breastfeeding and the use of psychotropic medication: a review. J Affect Disord 19:197–206, 1990

Campbell SB, Cohn JF, Flanagan C, et al: Course and correlates of postpartum depression during the transition to parenthood. Dev Psychopathol 4:29–47, 1992

Campbell SB, Cohn JF, Meyers T: Depression in first-time mothers: mother–infant interaction and depression chronicity. Dev Psychol 31:349–357, 1995

Cogill SR, Caplan HL, Alexandra H, et al: Impact of maternal postnatal depression on cognitive development of young children. BMJ 292:1165–1167, 1986

Cohen LS, Sichel DA, Dimmock JA, et al: Impact of pregnancy on panic disorder: a case series. J Clin Psychiatry 55:284–288, 1994a

Cohen LS, Sichel DA, Dimmock JA, et al: Impact of pregnancy on panic disorder: a case series. J Clin Psychiatry 55:289–292, 1994b

Cohen LS, Sichel DA, Robertson LM, et al: Postpartum prophylaxis for women with bipolar disorder. Am J Psychiatry 152:1641–1645, 1995

Cohen LS, Viguera AC, Bouffard SM, et al: Venlafaxine in the treatment of postpartum depression. J Clin Psychiatry 62:592–596, 2001

Condon JT, Watson TL: The maternity blues: exploration of a psychological hypothesis. Acta Psychiatr Scand 76:164–171, 1987

Cooper PJ, Cambell EA, Day A, et al: Non-psychotic psychiatric disorder after childbirth: a prospective study of prevalence, incidence, course and nature. Br J Psychiatry 152:799–806, 1988

Cox JL, Holden JM, Sagovsky R: Detection of postnatal depression. Br J Psychiatry 150:782–786, 1987

Cradon AJ: Maternal anxiety and neonatal wellbeing. J Psychosom Res 23:113–115, 1979

Cutrona CE, Troutman BR: Social support, infant temperament, and parenting self-efficacy: a mediational model of postpartum depression. Child Dev 57:1507–1518, 1986

Dalton K: Progesterone prophylaxis used successfully in postnatal depression. Practitioner 229:507–508, 1985

Duffy CL: Postpartum depression: identifying women at risk. Genesis Jun/July:11, 21, 1983

Epperson CN, Anderson GM, McDougle CJ: Sertraline and breast-feeding (letter to the editor). N Engl J Med 336:1189–1190, 1997

Esquirol E: Des Maladies Mentales, Considerees Sous les Rapports Medical, Hygienique et Medico-Legal. Philadelphia, PA, Lea & Blanchard, 1845

Field T: Behavior-state matching and synchrony in mother-infant interactions of nondepressed versus depressed dyads. Dev Psychol 26:7–14, 1990

Field T, Healy B, Goldstein S, et al: Infants of depressed mothers show "depressed" behavior even with nondepressed adults. Child Dev 59:1569–1579, 1988

Field T, Healy B, LeBlanc WG: Sharing and synchrony of behavior states and heart rate in nondepressed versus depressed mother-infant interactions. Infant and Behavior Development 12:357–376, 1989

Fleming AS, Klein E, Corter C: The effects of a social support group on depression, maternal attitudes and behavior in new mothers. J Child Psychol Psychiatry 33:685–698, 1992

George AJ, Wilson KC: Monoamine oxidase activity and the puerperal blues syndrome. J Psychosom Res 25:409–413, 1981

George DT, Ladenheim JA, Nutt DJ: Effect of pregnancy on panic attacks. Am J Psychiatry 144:1078–1079, 1987

Gordon RE, Gordon KK: Social factors in prevention of postpartum emotional problems. Obstet Gynecol 15:433–438, 1960

Gotlib I, Whiffen VE, Mount JH, et al: Prevalence rates and demographic characteristics associated with depression in pregnancy and postpartum. J Consult Clin Psychol 57:269–274, 1989

Gotlib IH, Whiffen VE, Wallace PM, et al: Prospective investigation of postpartum depression: factors involved in onset and recovery. J Abnorm Psychol 100:122–132, 1991

Graff LA, Syck DG, Schallow JR: Predicting postpartum depressive symptoms: a structural modeling analysis. Percept Mot Skills 73:1137–1138, 1991

Gregoire AJP, Henderson A, Kumar R, et al: A controlled trial of oestradiol therapy for postnatal depression (abstract). Neuropsychopharmacology 10:901S, 1994

Gregoire AJ, Kumar R, Everitt B, et al: Transdermal oestrogen for treatment of severe postnatal depression. Lancet 347:930–933, 1996

Hapgood CC, Elkind GS, Wright JJ: Maternity blues: phenomena and relationship to later postpartum depression. Aust N Z J Psychiatry 22:299–306, 1988

Harlow HF, Harlow MK: Social deprivation of monkeys. Sci Am 207:136–146, 1966

Hostetter AL, Baugh CL, Stowe ZN: Postpartum depression: distinct entity or coincidence? American Psychiatric Association 152nd Annual Meeting, Washington, DC, May 15–20, 1999

Jansson B: Psychic insufficiencies associated with childbirth. Acta Psychiatr Scand 39(suppl), 1963

Jensen PN, Olesen OV, Bertelsen A, et al: Citalopram and desmethylcitalopram concentrations in breast milk and in serum of mother and infant. Ther Drug Monit 19:236–239, 1997

Kendell RE, Chalmers JC, Platz C: Epidemiology of puerperal psychosis. Br J Psychiatry 150:662–673, 1987

Kennerley H, Gath D: Maternity blues associations with obstetric, psychological, and psychiatric factors. Br J Psychiatry 155:367–373, 1989

Kessler RC, McGonagle KA, Zhao S, et al: Lifetime and 12 month prevalence of DSM-III-R psychiatric disorders in the United States. Arch Gen Psychiatry 51:8–19, 1994

Kim J, Misri S, Riggs KW, et al: Steroselective excretion of fluoxetine and norfluoxetine in breast milk and neonatal exposure. American Psychiatric Association 150th Annual Meeting, San Diego, CA, May 17–22, 1997

Kleiman K, Raskin VD: This Isn't What I Expected: Overcoming Postpartum Depression. New York, Bantam Books, 1994

Klein DF, Skrobala AM, Garfinkel RS: Preliminary look at the effects of pregnancy on the course of panic disorder. Anxiety 1:227–232, 1995

Klosko JS, Barlow DH, Tassinari RB, et al: A comparison of alprazolam and cognitive behavior therapy in the treatment of panic disorder. J Consult Clin Psychol 58:77–84, 1990

Knopps GG: Postpartum mood disorders a startling contrast to the joy of birth. Postgrad Med 93:103–116, 1993

Kristensen JH, Ilett KF, Dusci LJ, et al: Distribution and excretion of sertraline and N-desmethylsertraline in human milk. Br J Clin Pharmacol 45:453–457, 1998

Lester BM, Cucca J, Andreozzi L, et al: Possible association between fluoxetine hydrochloride and colic in an infant. J Am Acad Child Adolesc Psychiatry 32:1253–1255, 1993

Llewellyn A, Stowe ZN: Invited review: "psychotropic medications during lactation." J Clin Psychiatry 59(suppl 2):41–52, 1998

Llewellyn A, Stowe ZN, Nemeroff CB: Outcome after sertraline exposure. American Psychiatric Association 150th Annual Meeting, San Diego, CA, May 17–22, 1997

Mammen OK, Perel JM, Rudolph G, et al: Sertraline and norsertraline levels in three breastfed infants. J Clin Psychiatry 58:100–103, 1997

Marce LV: Traite de la Folie des Femmes Enceintes: Des Nouvelles Accouchées et des Norrices et Considerations Medico-Legales Qui Se Rattachent a Ce Sujet. Paris, France, JB Baillieres, 1858

Marks MN, Wieck A, Checkley SA, et al: Contribution of psychological and social factors to psychotic and non-psychotic relapse after childbirth in women with previous histories of affective disorder. J Affect Disord 29:253–263, 1992

Matthew K, Scott HF, Wilkinson LS, et al: Retarded acquisition and reduced expression of conditional locomotor activity in adult rats following repeated early maternal separation: effects of prefeeding, D-amphetamine, dopamine antagonists, and clonidine. Psychopharmacology 126:75–84, 1996

McEwen BS, Gould EA, Sakai RR: The vulnerability of the hippocampus to protective and destructive effects of glucocorticoids in relation to stress. Br J Psychiatry 15:18–23, 1992

McGorry P, Connell S: The nosology and prognosis of puerperal psychosis: a review. Compr Psychiatry 31:519–534, 1990

Metz A, Sichel DA, Goff DC: Postpartum panic disorder. J Clin Psychiatry 49:278–279, 1988

Misri S, Sivertz K: Tricyclic drugs in pregnancy and lactation: a preliminary report. Int J Psychiatry Med 21:157–171, 1991

Mortola JF: The use of psychotropic agents in pregnancy and lactation. Psychiatr Clin North Am 12:69–87, 1989

Murray D: Oestrogen and postnatal depression. Lancet 347:918–919, 1996

Murray L: The impact of postnatal depression on infant development. J Child Psychol Psychiatry 33:543–561, 1992

Murray L, Cooper PJ: The impact of postpartum depression on child development. International Review of Psychiatry 8:55–63, 1996

Murray L, Fiori-Cowley A, Hooper R: The impact of postnatal depression and associated adversity on early mother-infant interactions and later infant outcome. Child Dev 67:2512–2526, 1996

Neziroglu F, Anemone R, Yaryura-Tobias JA: Onset of obsessive-compulsive disorders in pregnancy. Am J Psychiatry 149:947–950, 1992

O'Hara MW: Social support, life events and depression during pregnancy and the puerperium. Arch Gen Psychiatry 43:569–573, 1986

O'Hara MW: Gynecology and obstetrics, in Postpartum Mental Disorders. Edited by Droegemeuller N, Sciarra J. Philadelphia, PA, JB Lippincott, 1991, pp 1–13

O'Hara MW: Psychosocial therapies in the postpartum period. Paper presented at National Institute of Mental Health Workshop on Mental Disorders During Pregnancy and Postpartum, Washington, DC, June 1994

O'Hara MW, Schlechte JA, Lewis DA, et al: Controlled prospective study of postpartum mood disorders: psychological, environmental, and hormonal variables. J Abnorm Psychol 100:63–73, 1991a

O'Hara MW, Schlechte JA, Lewis DA, et al: Prospective study of postpartum blues: biologic and psychosocial factors. Arch Gen Psychiatry 48:801–806, 1991b

Parry BL, Hamilton JA: Postpartum Psychiatric Syndromes: The Art of Psychopharmacology. New York, Guilford, 1999

Pedersen CA, Stern RA, Pate J, et al: Thyroid and adrenal measures during late pregnancy and the puerperium in women who have been major depressed or who become dysphoric postpartum. J Affect Disord 29:201–211, 1993

Pitt B: "Atypical" depression following childbirth. Br J Psychiatry 114:1325–1335, 1968

Platz C, Kendell RE: A matched-control follow-up and family study of "puerperal" psychoses. Br J Psychiatry 153:90–94, 1988

Playfair HR, Gowers JI: Depression following childbirth: a search for predictive signs. Journal of the Royal College of General Practitioners 31:201–208, 1981

Plotsky PM, Meaney MJ: Early, postnatal experience alters hypothalamic corticotropin-releasing factor (CRF) mRNA, median eminence CRF content and stress-induced release in adult rats. Brain Res Mol Brain Res 18:195–200, 1993

Purdy D, Frank E: Should post-partum mood disorders be given a more prominent or distinct place in the DSM-IV? Depression 1:59–79, 1993

Richards JP: Postnatal depression: a review of recent literature. Br J Gen Pract 40:472–476, 1990

Robinson GE, Stewart DE, Flak E: The rational use of psychotropic drugs in pregnancy and postpartum. Can J Psychiatry 31:183–190, 1986

Robinson L, Walker JR, Anderson D: Cognitive-behavioral treatment of panic disorder during pregnancy and lactation. Can J Psychiatry 37:623–626, 1992

Roy A, Cole K, Goldman Z, et al: Fluoxetine treatment of postpartum depression (letter). Am J Psychiatry 150:1273, 1993

Schmidt HJ: The use of progesterone in the treatment of postpartum psychosis. JAMA 121:190–193, 1943

Schopf J, Rust B: Follow-up and family study of postpartum psychoses. Eur Arch Psychiatry Clin Neurosci 244:101–111, 1994

Sichel DA, Cohen LS, Robertson LM, et al: Prophylactic estrogen in recurrent postpartum affective disorder. Biol Psychiatry 38:814–818, 1995

Statham A: Current evidence from animal investigations of a role for early mother-infant relationships in the aetiology of major depressive illness. Neurosciences in Psychiatry 1:40–44, 1998

Stewart DE: Prophylactic lithium in postpartum affective psychosis. J Nerv Ment Dis 176:485–489, 1988

Stewart DE, Klompenhouwer JL, Kendall RE, et al: Prophylactic lithium in postpartum affective psychosis: the experience of three centers. Br J Psychiatry 158:393–397, 1991

Stowe ZN, Nemeroff CB: Women at risk for postpartum-onset major depression. Am J Obstet Gynecol 173:639–645, 1995

Stowe ZN, Casarella J, Landry J, et al: Sertraline in the treatment of women with postpartum major depression. Depression 3:49–55, 1995

Stowe ZN, Owens MJ, Landry JC, et al: Sertraline and desmethylsertraline in human breast milk and nursing infants. Am J Psychiatry 154:1255–1260, 1997

Stowe ZN, Tang Z, Plotsky PM: Impact of neonatal stress on neuronal activity. American Psychiatric Association 151st Annual Meeting, Toronto, ON, Canada, May 30–June 4, 1998a

Stowe ZN, Strader JR, Nemeroff CB: Psychopharmacology during pregnancy and lactation, in The American Psychiatric Press Textbook of Psychopharmacology, 2nd Edition. Edited by Schatzberg AF, Nemeroff CB. Washington, DC, American Psychiatric Press, 1998b, pp 979–996

Stowe ZN, Cohen LS, Hostetter A, et al: Paroxetine in human breast milk and nursing infants. Am J Psychiatry 157:185–189, 2000

Strader JR, Llewellyn A, Stowe ZN, et al: Predictors of treatment response in postpartum depression. American Psychiatric Association 150th Annual Meeting, San Diego, CA, May 17–22, 1997

Stuart S, O'Hara MW: Interpersonal psychotherapy for postpartum depression: a treatment program. J Psychother Pract Res 4:18–29, 1995

Sutanto W, Rosenfeld P, de Kloet ER, et al: Long-term effects of neonatal maternal deprivation and ACTH on hippocampal mineralocorticoid and glucocorticoid receptors. Dev Brain Res 92:156–163, 1996

Teti DM, Messinger DS, Gelfand DM, et al: Maternal depression and the quality of early attachment: an examination of infants, preschoolers, and their mothers. Dev Psychol 31:364–376, 1995

Troutman B, Cutrona C: Nonpsychotic postpartum depression among adolescent mothers. J Abnorm Psychol 99:69–78, 1990

Unterman RR, Posner NA, Williams KN: Postpartum depressive disorders: changing trends. Birth 17:131–137, 1990

Videbech P, Gouliaev G: First admission with puerperal psychosis: 7–14 years of follow up. Acta Psychiatr Scand 91:167–173, 1995

Whiffen VE, Gotlib IH: Infants of postpartum depressed mothers: temperament and cognitive status. J Abnorm Psychol 98:274–279, 1989

Wickberg B, Hwang CP: Counseling of postnatal depression: a controlled study on a population based Swedish sample. J Affect Disord 39:209–216, 1996

Williams KE, Koran LM: Obsessive-compulsive disorder in pregnancy, the puerperium, and the premenstruum. J Clin Psychiatry 58:330–334, 1997

Wisner KL, Perel JM: Psychopharmacologic agents and electroconvulsive therapy during pregnancy and the puerperium, in Psychiatric Consultation in Childbirth Settings: Parent- and Child-Oriented Approaches. Edited by Cohen RL. New York, Plenum Medical Book, 1988, pp 165–206

Wisner KL, Perel JM: Serum nortriptyline levels in nursing mothers and their infants. Am J Psychiatry 149:1234–1236, 1991

Wisner KL, Stowe ZN: Psychobiology of postpartum mood disorders. Semin Reprod Endocrinol 15:77–89, 1997

Wisner KL, Wheeler SB: Prevention of recurrent postpartum major depression. Hosp Community Psychiatry 45:1191–1196, 1994

Wisner KL, Peindl K, Hanusa BH: Symptomatology of affective and psychotic illnesses related to childbearing. J Affect Disord 30:77–87, 1994

Wisner KL, Perel JM, Findling RL: Antidepressant treatment during breastfeeding. Am J Psychiatry 153:1132–1137, 1996

Wisner KL, Perel JM, Blumer J: Serum sertraline and N-desmethylsertraline levels in breast-feeding mother–infant pairs. Am J Psychiatry 155:690–692, 1998

Wolkind S, Zajicek-Colean E, Ghodsian J: Continuities in maternal depression. Int J Fam Psychol 1:167–181, 1988

Wolman W, Chalmers B, Hofmeyr GJ, et al: Postpartum depression and companionship in the clinical birth environment: a randomized, controlled study. Am J Obstet Gynecol 168:1388–1393, 1993

Yoshida K, Smith B, Craggs M, et al: Fluoxetine in breast milk and developmental outcome of breast-fed infants. Br J Psychiatry 172:175–179, 1998

Zahn-Waxler C, Cummings EM, Lonoff RJ, et al: Young offspring of depressed patients: a population of risk for affective problems and childhood depression, in Childhood Depression. Edited by Cichette D, Schneider-Rosen K. San Francisco, CA, Jossey-Bass, 1984, pp 81–105

Zilboorg G: Mind, Medicine, and Man. New York, Harcourt Brace, 1943

7

Premenstrual Syndromes

Meir Steiner, M.D., Ph.D., F.R.C.P.C.
Leslie Born, M.Sc.

Perhaps the most startling revelation in the burgeoning research on pre-menstrual syndromes is a recent agreement among many renowned women's health researchers on the diagnostic entity of the more severe form of premenstrual syndrome (PMS), premenstrual dysphoric disorder (PMDD) (Endicott et al. 1999). In addition, a plethora of new research findings on etiological factors and treatments for PMS and PMDD has become available in the past several years. The purpose of this chapter, therefore, is to provide health practitioners with current information on premenstrual syndromes, including their epidemiology, etiology, diagnosis, and treatment.

PMS can be defined as a pattern of emotional, behavioral, and physical symptoms that occur premenstrually and remit after menses. These symptoms typically include minor mood changes, breast tenderness, bloating, and headache (World Health Organization 1996). More than 100 physical and psychological symptoms have been attributed to the premenstruum (Budeiri et al. 1994). The premenstrual syndromes include the more com-

We would like to thank Janice Rogers and Carol Ballantyne for their assistance in the preparation of this manuscript.

mon PMS, the less prevalent PMDD, a condition known as premenstrual exacerbation, and menstrual psychosis.

PMDD, which usually comprises extremely distressing emotional and behavioral symptoms (irritability, dysphoria, tension, mood lability), first appeared in the appendix of DSM-III-R (American Psychiatric Association 1987) as late luteal phase dysphoric disorder; it was later renamed and incorporated into Appendix B of DSM-IV (American Psychiatric Association 1994).

EPIDEMIOLOGY

Prevalence

Epidemiological surveys have estimated that as many as 75% of women with regular menstrual cycles experience some symptoms of PMS (S.R. Johnson 1987). Most of these women do not require medical or psychiatric interventions. Since the emergence of the term *premenstrual syndrome* in the 1950s (Greene and Dalton 1953), PMS has become an increasingly discussed topic in popular media sources. Thus, the more effective self-management techniques are easily accessed by women through the media or through their peers. Women who feel they are unable to self-manage their PMS are most often seen in primary care settings and by gynecologists.

PMDD affects only 3%–8% of women in this age group (Andersch et al. 1986; Angst et al. 2001; Haskett et al. 1987; Johnson et al. 1988; Merikangas et al. 1993; Ramacharan et al. 1992; Rivera-Tovar and Frank 1990). These women report premenstrual symptoms, primarily mood symptoms, that are severe enough to seriously interfere with their lifestyle and relationships (Freeman et al. 1985; O'Brien et al. 1995). Women with PMDD usually do not respond to conservative and conventional interventions

A high proportion of women presenting with PMDD have a history of previous episodes of mood disorders, and women with continuing mood disorders report premenstrual magnification of symptoms and an emergence of new symptoms (Bancroft et al. 1994; Endicott 1993; Fava et al. 1992; Graze et al. 1990; Halbreich and Endicott 1985; Harrison et al. 1989; Kaspi et al. 1994; McLeod et al. 1993). For example, a lifetime history of major depressive disorder among PMDD patients has been reported in the range of 30%–70% (Yonkers 1997b). In prospective studies, 14%–16% of the women with PMDD had a lifetime history of anxiety disorder, whereas comorbid anxiety diagnoses have been reported as high as 32% (Yonkers 1997a). Thus, it is important to exclude the possibility that the presentation is of a different major psychiatric or medical problem with premenstrual onset.

Age and Parity

Women from menarche to menopause may report clinically significant menstrually related symptoms, and in general, the literature supports this finding (Endicott et al. 1999). However, age may be associated with the reporting of premenstrual symptoms (S.R. Johnson 1987) and the clinical presentation of PMS or PMDD. Onset of distressing symptoms is typically when women are in their late 20s to mid 30s (Freeman et al. 1995b).

Some evidence indicates that premenstrual symptoms worsen following childbirth (S.R. Johnson 1987), although this association has yet to be prospectively assessed over time.

Sociocultural Considerations

Research on PMS has occurred mostly in the United States but also in Europe, the Mediterranean, the Middle East, Southeast Asia, and Africa. Some broad cultural patterns regarding the nature and frequency of reported premenstrual symptoms can be delineated. For example, in a comparative analysis of population studies conducted in the United States, Bahrain, and Italy, affective symptoms (irritability, mood swings, tension) and weight gain were more prevalent among the United States women, whereas somatic symptoms (swelling, breast pain, backache) were more prevalent in the Italian and Bahrain groups (Dan and Monagle 1994). A higher frequency of somatic symptoms also has been reported in Swiss, Indian, and Chinese samples (Chandra and Chaturvedi 1989; Chang et al. 1995; Merikangas et al. 1993). In a recent prospective study of Icelandic women, a significantly lower percentage (2.4%) of women had a premenstrual symptom pattern as compared with prospective data of United States women; the authors suggested that "menstrual socialization" influences symptom expectation and reporting (Sveindóttir 1998).

A positive association between educational level and *severity* of premenstrual symptoms has been suggested (Marvan and Escobedo 1999), and an association between education and *type* of premenstrual symptomatology (i.e., the more highly educated group reporting a greater prevalence of psychological symptoms) can be delineated in multinational comparative analyses (Dan and Monagle 1994). Therefore, it is important to consider that cultural context, even level of education, may influence women's premenstrual experiences and thus the nature of what is relayed to health clinicians or research investigators.

Yet, specific conclusions about cultural differences in premenstrual symptomatology are hampered by differences in study methodology, such as mode of data collection and validity of translated instruments (Chang et al. 1999; Yu et al. 1996). Notwithstanding, the various theoretical approaches that underlie the study of PMS heavily influence interpretation of research findings. For example, PMS is still conceptualized by some as a biopsychosocial phenomenon and by others as a sociocultural phenomenon specific to Western culture (Anson 1999; T.M. Johnson 1987).

Risk Factors

Some factors that may increase the risk for PMS and PMDD have been pinpointed, although in most instances, more explicit evidence is required.

Age

Some evidence suggests that women are most likely to present with PMDD during the late 20s to the mid 30s (Freeman et al. 1995b), but there is increasing evidence that in many women symptoms started at menarche or shortly thereafter.

Menstrual Cycle Characteristics

There are mixed reports on the association of menstrual cycle characteristics with severity of premenstrual symptoms. One study found a higher prevalence of PMS in women whose menses lasted longer than 6 days (Deuster et al. 1999). Others have found an association between PMS symptoms and shorter menstrual cycle length, specifically in women with purely depressive symptoms (Hargrove and Abraham 1982).

Past or Current Psychiatric Illness

A high proportion of women presenting with PMDD have a history of previous episodes of major depression (Yonkers 1997b), minor depression (Pearlstein et al. 1990), postpartum depression (Pearlstein et al. 1990), seasonal affective disorder (Parry 1995), and bipolar disorder (Pearlstein et al. 1990), and some women with PMDD have a history of suicide attempts (Harrison et al. 1989), anxiety disorders (panic disorder, generalized anxiety disorder, phobia) (Yonkers 1997a), personality disorders, and/or substance abuse (Pearlstein et al. 1990). Women with an ongoing mood disorder report premenstrual magnification of symptoms and an emergence of new symptoms (Bancroft et al. 1994; Endicott 1993; Fava et al. 1992; Graze et al. 1990; Halbreich and Endicott 1985; Harrison et al. 1989; Kaspi et al. 1994; McLeod et al. 1993).

Family History

At least two population-based twin studies have determined that PMS is heritable (Condon 1993; Kendler et al. 1998).

Psychosocial Stressors

Life stressors involving major life events, relationships with significant others, work, social support (Fontana and Palfai 1994), or history of sexual abuse (Paddison et al. 1990) have been positively associated with PMS symptoms.

PATHOPHYSIOLOGY

The etiology of PMS and PMDD is still largely unknown. That PMS and PMDD are primarily biological phenomena (as opposed to just psychological or psychosocial events) is underscored by recent, convincing evidence of the heritability of premenstrual symptoms (Kendler et al. 1998) and the elimination of premenstrual complaints with suppression of ovarian activity (Schmidt et al. 1998) or surgical menopause (Casper and Hearn 1990; Casson et al. 1990). The current consensus seems to be that normal ovarian function rather than simple hormonal imbalance (Roca et al. 1996) is the cyclic trigger for PMDD-related biochemical events within the central nervous system and other target tissues. A psychoneuroendocrine mechanism triggered by the normal endocrine events of the ovarian cycle seems the most plausible explanation (Rubinow and Schmidt 1995; Schmidt et al. 1998). This viewpoint is attractive in that it encourages investigation of the neuroendocrine-modulated central neurotransmitters and the role of the hypothalamic-pituitary-gonadal axis in PMDD. Notwithstanding, a surge of recent research has encompassed other etiological influences, including female biological rhythms (sleep, body temperature) and psychosocial factors.

Ovarian Steroids

The role of the female sex hormones in premenstrual symptomatology has been considered of central importance, yet in women with PMDD, the ovarian axis is functioning normally with normal estrogen and progesterone levels (Schmidt et al. 1998). Recently, attention has shifted from a focus on estrogen and progesterone to the role of androgens in premenstrual dysphoria.

Early investigations of androgens in women suggested that elevated levels of serum testosterone in the luteal phase may contribute to severe premenstrual irritability (often a primary complaint) in women with PMDD. This hypothesis of increased androgenicity is backed by both animal and human studies of androgens and irritability and/or aggression and the successful treatment of PMS with androgen antagonists (Eriksson et al. 2000). One recent study, however, reported significantly *lower* total and free testosterone plasma levels in a sample of 10 women with PMS (Bloch et al. 1998). Further comparative studies of women with PMS and PMDD are therefore required.

Several studies have examined the role of allopregnanolone, the metabolite of progesterone, in the manifestation of premenstrual symptoms. Treatment studies have suggested that progesterone and progestogens actually may provoke, rather than ameliorate, the cyclical symptom changes of PMDD (Hammarback et al. 1985). Allopregnanolone, however, is thought to modulate γ-aminobutyric acid (GABA) receptor functioning and produce an anxiolytic effect (Rapkin et al. 1997). Quantitative differences in progesterone and allopregnanolone levels between PMS subjects and control subjects have been examined; the findings, however, are contradictory (Bicikova et al. 1998; Monteleone et al. 2000; Rapkin et al. 1997; Schmidt et al. 1994; Wang et al. 1996).

The serum concentrations of ionized magnesium and ionized calcium have been studied across the menstrual cycle in association with levels of estrogen, progesterone, and testosterone. Investigators have suggested that changes in the levels of magnesium or calcium or dramatic change in the calcium-to-magnesium ratio may underlie the premenstrual syndromes (Muneyvirci-Delale et al. 1998). However, significant fluctuations of total and ionized calcium during the menstrual cycle occur in women both with and without documented PMS (Thys-Jacobs and Alvir 1995).

Endocrine Abnormalities

An alternative strategy to measuring various hormone plasma levels in an attempt to discern the etiology of PMDD has been to search for endocrine abnormalities that have been repeatedly associated with various other forms of psychopathology. The main advantage of this approach is its potential to help further our understanding of PMDD as well as its relation to other psychiatric disorders. The current literature suggests that thyroid dysfunction may be found in a small group of women with PMS but that PMDD should not be viewed as a masked form of hypothyroidism (Korzekwa et al. 1996; Nikolai et al. 1990; Schmidt et al. 1993).

A dysregulation of cardiovascular (Girdler et al. 1998) and neuroendocrine responses (Cahill 1998; Girdler et al. 1998; Woods et al. 1998) to stress has been suggested in women with premenstrual symptoms.

Neurotransmitters

Of the neurotransmitters studied to date, increasing evidence suggests that serotonin may be important in the pathogenesis of PMDD (Rapkin 1992;

Rojansky et al. 1991; Steiner 1992; Steiner et al. 1997b; Yatham 1993). PMDD shares many features of other mood and anxiety disorders linked to serotonergic dysfunction (Endicott 1993; Pearlstein et al. 1990; Wurtman 1993). In addition, reduction in brain serotonin neurotransmission is thought to lead to poor impulse control, depressed mood, irritability, and increased carbohydrate craving—all mood and behavioral symptoms associated with PMDD (Meltzer 1989).

The serotonergic system is in close reciprocal relationship with gonadal hormones (Eriksson et al. 1994; Tuiten et al. 1995). In the hypothalamus, estrogen induces a diurnal fluctuation in serotonin (Cohen and Wise 1988), whereas progesterone increases the turnover rate of serotonin (Ladisich 1977).

Several studies concluded that serotonin *function* may be altered in women with PMDD. Some studies used models of neuronal function (such as whole blood serotonin levels, platelet uptake of serotonin, and platelet tritiated imipramine binding) and found altered serotonin function during all phases of the menstrual cycle (Ashby et al. 1988; Rapkin et al. 1987; Rojansky et al. 1991; Steege et al. 1992; Taylor et al. 1984). Other studies that used challenge tests (with L-tryptophan, fenfluramine, buspirone, *m*-chlorophenylpiperazine) suggested abnormal serotonin function in symptomatic women but differed in their findings as to whether the response to serotonin is blunted or heightened (Bancroft and Cook 1995; Bancroft et al. 1991; FitzGerald et al. 1997; Menkes et al. 1994; Steiner et al. 1999b; Su et al. 1997; Yatham 1993). In addition, powerful evidence implicating the serotonergic system has emerged from treatment studies: drugs facilitating serotonergic neurotransmission, such as selective serotonin reuptake inhibitors (SSRIs), are very effective in reducing premenstrual symptoms (Steiner et al. 1997c). These studies imply, at least in part, a possible change in 5-hydroxytryptamine type 1A ($5\text{-}HT_{1A}$) receptor sensitivity in women with premenstrual dysphoria.

The current consensus is that women with premenstrual dysphoria may be behaviorally or biochemically sub- or supersensitive to biological challenges of the serotonergic system (Halbreich and Tworek 1993; Leibenluft et al. 1994). It is not yet clear whether these women present with a trait or state marker (alternatively, both conditions could be possible) of premenstrual syndromes (Kouri and Halbreich 1997).

The GABA, adrenergic, and opioid neurotransmitter systems also have been implicated in the pathophysiology of PMS and PMDD. Investigators found reduced $GABA_A$ receptor sensitivity in the late luteal phase in patients with PMS (Sundstrom et al. 1998), and reduced plasma levels of GABA in the late luteal phase have been noted in women with PMDD (Halbreich et al. 1996).

Abnormal α_2-adrenergic receptor function is implicated in anxiety and depressive disorders. In a recent, controlled study of patients with PMDD, α_2-adrenergic receptor density positively correlated with symptom severity during the luteal phase; moreover, high follicular phase α_2-adrenergic receptor density predicted luteal phase symptom severity (Gurguis et al. 1998).

The role of endogenous opioids in the pathophysiology of PMDD—that is, that the sharp decline in opiate levels ("withdrawal") during the late luteal phase may lead to increased irritability, anxiety, tension, and aggression—has been the target of some investigation (Chuong et al. 1988; Mortola 1996; Rapkin et al. 1996). Preliminary investigation found that women with PMS have decreased luteinizing hormone response to naloxone during the midluteal phase, indicating a loss of central opioid tone (Rapkin et al. 1996). A small sample of women with PMS had a significant reduction in symptoms following treatment with an oral opiate antagonist (Chuong et al. 1988), which supports this hypothesis as an etiological factor.

Circadian Rhythms

Desynchronized circadian rhythms can induce mood disorders. Women with premenstrual syndromes frequently experience nocturnal sleep disturbance and daytime sleepiness. Patients with PMDD have decreased concentrations of nocturnal melatonin (serotonin is converted to melatonin in the pineal gland) compared with those of normal control subjects. An altered neuroendocrine response to light has been found in subjects with PMDD during the symptomatic luteal phase but not the asymptomatic follicular phase. In related studies, significant alterations of circadian changes in body temperature during the luteal phase have been documented in subjects with PMDD (Nakayama et al. 1997). Taken together, these findings portend that the biological rhythm of females is intrinsically unstable in the luteal phase, although this rhythm is stable in the follicular phase. Compared with normal control subjects, women with PMDD may be more sensitive to the acute suppressive effects of light on melatonin secretion and have an increased resistance to light-induced phase-shift responses (Parry and Newton 2001).

Genetic Predisposition

In a recent, longitudinal, population-based twin study of 1,312 menstruating female twins, researchers estimated the heritability of premenstrual symptoms at 56%, with negligible influence from family environmental factors and minimal influence related to genetic and environmental risk factors for lifetime major depression (Kendler et al. 1998). These data are congruent with the results of previous twin studies of genetic factors (Condon 1993; Kendler et al. 1992). A twin study of genetic and environmental variation in the menstrual cycle suggested that the age at menarche and menstrual cycle regularity, as well as propensity for premenstrual symptom reporting, may be inherited (van den Akker et al. 1987).

Sociocultural Factors

Menstruation and premenstrual symptoms have been referred to as the "curse," contributing to a negative perception of a natural cyclical event. The importance of subjective perception in the experience of menstrual events has been underscored in a recent report on the significant reduction of negative symptoms in a sample of women who met criteria for late luteal phase dysphoric disorder following a psychosocially based intervention that emphasized positive reframing (positive connotation) (G. Morse 1999). Social beliefs about menstruation, however, vary among different cultures and can influence both expectations about the menstrual cycle and the reporting of symptoms (e.g., see Sveindóttir 1998).

SCREENING AND DIAGNOSIS

Women with premenstrual syndromes are most often seen in primary care or by their obstetricians/gynecologists. The results of a recent United States study on the experience of women with PMS who sought medical attention suggested a high rate of missed diagnoses (Kraemer and Kraemer 1998). Because no objective diagnostic tests are available for PMS or PMDD, a complete medical and psychiatric history must be elicited. In addition to a retrospective history of the premenstrual symptoms, this interview should include a complete review of physical systems (including gynecological, endocrinological, and allergies), medical disorders, and family history of mental illness. Because the symptoms of anemia and thyroid disease often mirror those of PMS or PMDD, the patient should undergo laboratory investigations if any hints of an underlying medical cause for the symptoms arise. A high prevalence of past sexual abuse (40%) has been found among women seeking treatment for premenstrual symptoms (Paddison et al. 1990); therefore, screening for domestic violence is an essential aspect of the assessment.

Prospective daily rating of symptoms is essential in making a diagnosis of PMS or PMDD. To date, there is no consensus among investigators as to the best instruments for confirming prospectively the diagnosis of PMDD or the instruments most appropriate to measure treatment effects in clinical trials.

PMS has, in the past, been defined as a diversity of symptoms that appear during the week before menstruation and that resolve within a week of onset of menstruation. A diagnosis of PMS differs from that of PMDD in that neither a minimum number of symptoms nor functional impairment is required (World Health Organization 1996).

PMDD, as defined by DSM-IV-TR (American Psychiatric Association 2000), is much stricter in its delineation. To apply the DSM-IV-TR criteria, women must chart symptoms daily for two cycles, and their chief complaints must include 1 of 4 core symptoms (irritability, tension, dysphoria, and affective lability) and at least 5 of the 11 total symptoms. The symptoms should have occurred with most menstrual cycles during the past year and have interfered with social or occupational roles.

Some women may report significant seasonal variation in premenstrual symptoms (Maskall et al. 1997). In addition, the charting of troublesome symptoms should show clear worsening premenstrually and remit within a few days after the onset of menstruation ("on-offness"). A change in symptoms from the follicular to the luteal phase of at least 50% is suggested for a diagnosis of PMDD (Steiner et al. 1995). The within-cycle percent change is calculated by subtracting the follicular score from the luteal score, dividing by the luteal score, and multiplying by 100 (Steiner and Yonkers 1998). Functional impairment is a requirement for most Axis I/DSM-IV diagnostic categories.

Two examples of daily calendars that are useful in a clinical setting and aid in the required prospective measurement of symptoms include the Prospective Record of the Impact and Severity of Menstruation (Reid 1985) and the Calendar of Premenstrual Experiences (Mortola et al. 1990). These prospective tools allow respondents to rate a variety of physical and psychological symptoms, indicate negative and positive life events, record concurrent medications, and track menstrual bleeding and cycle length. These instruments contain the core symptoms and most of the additional symptoms considered for the DSM-IV-TR diagnosis of PMDD.

In a detailed study of three prospective symptom rating scales (used to establish severity of premenstrual mood symptoms and measure efficacy during a multicenter, controlled treatment trial for premenstrual dysphoria) (Steiner et al. 1995), researchers found that single-item visual analogue scales (for irritability, tension, and depression) and the Premenstrual Tension Syndrome Observer (PMTS-O) and Self-Rating (PMTS-SR) scales (Steiner et al. 1980) were sensitive to premenstrual symptoms worsening and sensitive to change over time. Furthermore, premenstrual mood symptoms as measured by visual analogue scales significantly correlated with PMTS-O and PMTS-SR scale scores, denoting an easy-to-administer, reliable, and valid method of data collection (Steiner et al. 1999a).

Given the sometimes close resemblance between PMDD and rapid-cycling bipolar II disorder (Hendrick and Altshuler 1998), and when faced with an unclear clinical case, Macmillan and Young (1999) have recommended the Bipolar Mood Diary in conjunction with a PMS daily record.

After completion of the two-cycle prospective diagnostic assessment phase, women may qualify for one of five diagnostic categories:

1. *PMS:* Women who receive this diagnosis meet ICD-10-CM (World Health Organization 1996) criteria for PMS, which include mild psychological discomfort and mostly feelings of bloating and weight gain, breast tenderness and swelling, swelling of hands and feet, various aches and pains, poor concentration, sleep disturbance, and change in appetite. Only one of these symptoms is required for this diagnosis, although the symptoms must be restricted to the luteal phase of the menstrual cycle, reach a peak shortly before menstruation, and cease with the menstrual flow or soon after.

2. *PMDD:* Women who receive this diagnosis meet DSM-IV-TR criteria for PMDD. *"Pure-pure" PMDD:* Women who receive this diagnosis meet DSM-IV-TR criteria for PMDD and have no other past or present psychiatric disorder. *"Pure" PMDD:* Women who receive this diagnosis meet DSM-IV-TR criteria for PMDD, have no other concurrent psychiatric disorder, but have a history of a past psychiatric disorder (Steiner and Wilkins 1996).

3. *PMS or PMDD and another medical or psychiatric illness:* Women who receive this diagnosis may meet criteria for PMS or PMDD but also have a current major psychiatric disorder or an unstable medical condition. Women meeting DSM-IV-TR criteria for major depressive disorder, cyclothymic disorder, dysthymic disorder, bipolar disorder (especially rapid-cycling type), anxiety disorders, schizophrenia, bulimia nervosa, or substance abuse may fall into this category. The cyclical nature of their symptoms may or may not match the phases of their menstrual cycle.

4. *Premenstrual exacerbation of an underlying medical or psychiatric illness:* Menstrual cycle–related exacerbation of common medical conditions such as migraine, epilepsy, asthma, irritable bowel syndrome, and diabetes as well as any psychiatric recurring/episodic illness is a well-recognized phenomenon (Case and Reid 2001).

5. *Menstrual psychosis:* In some women, transient psychotic symptoms may appear in sync with the menstrual cycle. This proposed classification can incorporate a broad range of phenomena, which may be grouped according to onset within the menstrual cycle (premenstrual, catamenial, paramenstrual, or mid-cycle) or according to stage in the repro-

ductive life cycle (prepubertal, postpartum, amenorrhea, menopause) (Brockington 1998). These relatively rare phenomena have been the focus of much debate, although the literature is, for the most part, confined to case reports. Several features delineate menstrual psychosis (as cited in Brockington 1998): acute or sudden onset, against a background of normality; brief duration, with full recovery; psychotic features (i.e., confusion, delusions, hallucinations, stupor, and mutism, or a manic syndrome); and a circa-menstrual (approximately monthly) periodicity, in regular relation with the menstrual cycle.

6. *No diagnosis:* None of the symptoms are severe enough to warrant a diagnosis, although the patient may subjectively sense disruptive symptoms, especially at times of increased psychosocial stress.

Applying these diagnostic criteria to women who seek help for premenstrual complaints will help the clinician plan treatment interventions.

PREMENSTRUAL DYSPHORIC DISORDER: A DISTINCT CLINICAL ENTITY

PMDD appears in Appendix B of DSM-IV-TR under the heading of depressive disorder not otherwise specified. Yet questions remain about its diagnostic entity, likely stemming from the high rates of comorbidity between PMDD and other mood or anxiety disorders. Researchers have attempted to resolve this, for the most part, by summing up similarities in features between PMDD and other mood disorders (Halbreich 1997; Odber et al. 1998; Yonkers 1997b) or between PMDD and anxiety disorders (Facchinetti et al. 1998; Yonkers 1997a). Other researchers have concentrated on the measurement of PMDD—in particular, the methods (Ekholm et al. 1998; Steiner et al. 1999a) and items (Gehlert et al. 1997, 1999) that easily delineate individuals with PMDD.

Recently, a group of experts reached a consensus that PMDD is a distinct clinical entity (Endicott et al. 1999). The findings are summarized as follows:

- PMDD has a distinct clinical picture with characteristic symptoms of irritability, anger, and internal tension.
- The onset and offset of its symptoms are closely linked to the luteal phase of the menstrual cycle.
- The genetic component of PMDD does not seem to be related to that of other depressive disorders.
- In PMDD, the hypothalamic-pituitary-adrenal axis functions normally, unlike its functioning in major depression.

- PMDD differs in response to treatment in comparison with other mood disorders (i.e., the specificity of drugs facilitating serotonergic neurotransmission, efficacy of intermittent dosing, rapid onset of response, maximal response at low doses, and rapid recurrence of symptoms with discontinuation of treatment).
- Eliminating the menstrual cycle will cure women with PMDD but not those with other mood disorders (after pregnancy, symptoms return once cycles have been reestablished).

Additional evidence regarding the distinctness of PMDD compared with major depression in biochemical markers (Rapkin et al. 1998) and circadian variables (Parry et al. 1999) also has come to light.

TREATMENT

Therapeutic interventions for premenstrual syndromes range from the conservative (lifestyle and stress management) to treatment with psychotropic medications and, for the more extreme cases, hormonal therapy or surgical procedures to eliminate ovulation or ovarian function. These treatments are successful in relieving symptoms for most women treated for PMDD, but to date, no one intervention has proven to be effective for all.

Most pharmacological therapies are now being tested in randomized controlled trials. The interpretation and generalization of results from many studies to date of complementary medicines or alternative therapies for the treatment of premenstrual syndromes are hindered by methodologic shortcomings (Pearlstein and Steiner 2000; Stevinson and Ernst 2001). Some treatments commonly perceived as a remedy for PMS (e.g., evening primrose oil) have not been found to be effective in controlled studies (Stevinson and Ernst 2001). Notwithstanding, a variety of well-studied nonpharmacologic and pharmacologic treatment options exist for the milder and more severe premenstrual syndromes.

For women who do not meet criteria for PMDD or other physical and psychological disorders but still have mild to moderate symptoms of PMS, conservative treatments are appropriate, and management without pharmacological interventions should be encouraged. Stressful life events should be queried and monitored. These patients may best respond to individual or group psychotherapy in combination with diet and lifestyle changes. Patients also should be taught to review their own monthly diaries and identify triggers to symptom exacerbation.

Women who manifest severe physical symptoms or a psychiatric disorder with premenstrual magnification should be treated for their primary condition. Premenstrual symptoms usually remit considerably with successful treatment of the primary condition, and residual symptoms can be treated as indicated.

Nonpharmacological Approaches

Lifestyle and stress management is a necessary adjunct to any therapeutic intervention, and patients should be educated and encouraged to practice these principles. The nonpharmacological approaches should be tried as first-line therapy, especially for milder symptoms.

Diet and Exercise

The elimination or reduction of caffeine (especially coffee), alcohol, chocolate, and tobacco and adherence to a diet composed of frequent high-protein and low-refined-sugar meals are strongly recommended. Patients should be encouraged to decrease sodium in the diet when edema or fluid retention occurs and, if possible, to reduce weight to within 20% of their ideal. Regular exercise (including aerobic exercise) is important and particularly effective when combined with the regular practice of stress management techniques.

Nutritional Supplements

- **Vitamin B$_6$:** Limited evidence suggests that daily doses of vitamin B$_6$, 50–100 mg/day, are likely to be beneficial in treating overall premenstrual symptoms and of some benefit in treating premenstrual depression. No conclusive evidence has been found of neurological side effects at this dose range; however, women receiving vitamin B$_6$ should be monitored for muscle weakness, numbness, clumsiness, and paresthesia (Wyatt et al. 1999).
- **Calcium:** A daily supplement of calcium carbonate containing 1,200 mg of elemental calcium effectively reduced overall luteal phase symptoms in a large sample of women with confirmed PMS (Thys-Jacobs et al. 1998), suggesting a link between calcium deficiency and PMS. Symptom reduction occurred by the third treatment cycle.
- **Magnesium:** Some evidence suggests that a daily supplement of 200 mg of magnesium for a minimum of 2 months is of benefit in treating premenstrual symptoms of fluid retention (weight gain, swelling of extremities, breast tenderness, abdominal bloating) (Walker et al. 1998).

Psychotherapy

Individual psychotherapy can aid women's psychological and social functioning, particularly for women who have endured distressing premenstrual symptoms for an extended length of time. Some evidence from controlled studies indicates that women with PMS may benefit from individual cognitive therapy (Blake et al. 1998) or coping skills training (Morse et al. 1991) in the reduction of premenstrual symptoms. The benefits of group treatment—with education, cognitive strategies, and peer support—in the management of PMS have been shown in several studies (Morse 1999; Seideman 1990; Taylor 1999; Walton and Youngkin 1987).

Light Therapy

Two studies have shown that bright-white light therapy is an effective intervention for late luteal phase dysphoric disorder, with, for example, a minimum of 2,500-lux cool-white fluorescent light for 2 hours in the morning (6:30 A.M.–8:30 A.M.) or in the evening (7:00 P.M.–9:00 P.M.) (Parry 1998; Parry et al. 1993) and 10,000-lux cool-white fluorescent light for 30 minutes in the evening (7:00 P.M.–9:00 P.M.) (Lam et al. 1999) during the symptomatic days in the luteal phase. Significant reductions in depression, irritability, and physical symptoms were observed. Furthermore, Parry (1998) found that the benefits of bright-light therapy were maintained in patients who completed at least 12 months of treatment.

Pharmacological Approaches

Pharmacological approaches include psychotropic medications and hormonal interventions. The newer antidepressants in particular, including many of the SSRIs, clomipramine (a tricyclic antidepressant with major serotonin reuptake inhibiting properties), and L-tryptophan, have shown excellent efficacy and minimal side effects in women with PMS and PMDD. Two anxiolytics also have been successful in the reduction of psychological symptoms; however, side effects and possible dependence inhibit their use. There is also evidence of success with estradiol implants, gonadotropin-releasing hormone analogues, danazol (a synthetic androgen), and oral contraceptives; however, many women are unable to tolerate the side effects of these interventions. A summary of suggested pharmacological approaches is shown in Table 7–1.

Selective Serotonin Reuptake Inhibitors

Consistent scientific evidence has confirmed the efficacy and tolerability of many of the SSRIs in the treatment of PMDD (both emotional and somatic symptoms); therefore, the SSRIs should be considered as the first-line pharmacological treatment for premenstrual mood symptoms (Dimmock et al. 2000; Eriksson 1999; Steiner et al. 1997c). More recently, several studies have indicated that intermittent (premenstrually only) treatment

TABLE 7–1. Pharmacological therapies[a]

Type	Recommended dose	References	Comments
Antidepressants			
Fluoxetine	20 mg/day	Steiner et al. 1995	Selective serotonin reuptake inhibitors are the first-line treatment for premenstrual mood symptoms
		Su et al. 1997	Highly efficacious and tolerable
		Pearlstein et al. 1997	Intermittent use (luteal phase only) offers decreased costs and lower side-effect burden
	20 mg/day 14 days before menses	Steiner et al. 1997a[b]	
	10 mg/day	Diegoli et al. 1998 (PMS)	
Sertraline	50–150 mg/day	Yonkers et al. 1997	
		Freeman et al. 1999a	
		Halbreich and Smoller 1997	
	50–150 mg/day luteal phase only	Young et al. 1998	
		Freeman et al. 1999b (PMS)	
		Jermaine et al. 1999	
Paroxetine	10–30 mg/day	Eriksson et al. 1995	
	5–30 mg/day late luteal phase only	Sundblad et al. 1997b	
Citalopram	20±10 mg/day from ovulation to day 2	Wikander et al. 1998	
Clomipramine	25–75 mg/day	Sundblad et al. 1992	
	25–75 mg/day 14 days before menses	Sundblad et al. 1993	
Venlafaxine	50–200 mg/day	Freeman et al. 2001b	
L-Tryptophan	6 g/day from ovulation to day 3	Steinberg et al. 1999	

TABLE 7–1. Pharmacological therapies[a] *(continued)*

Type	Recommended dose	References	Comments
Anxiolytics			
Alprazolam	0.25–2 mg/day (0.25–0.05 up to 4 times daily)	Smith et al. 1987	Dependence and tolerance can develop
		Harrison et al. 1990 Diegoli et al. 1998	Withdrawal symptoms can occur during menses Mixed reports on improvement of psychological symptoms
Buspirone	0.25–2 mg/day, 6–14 days before menses	Berger and Presser 1994 Freeman et al. 1995a	
	25–60 mg/day 12 days before menses	Rickels et al. 1989 Landén et al. 2001	
Ovulation suppression			
Danazol	200–400 mg/day during symptomatic days only	Sarno et al. 1987	Efficacious treatment for premenstrual migraines and mastalgia
		Hahn et al. 1995	At lower dose (200 mg/day), ovulation is not suppressed (i.e., fewer side effects)
		O'Brien and Abukhalil 1999	

TABLE 7–1.   Pharmacological therapies[a] (*continued*)

Type	Recommended dose	References	Comments
Leuprolide	3.75–7.5 mg intramuscular injection monthly	Brown et al. 1994	Potential risk for osteoporosis, cardiovascular disease with long-term use
		Freeman et al. 1997	Several months of use to reach full treatment effect
	7.5 mg intramuscular injection monthly with add-back conjugated estrogen 0.625 mg/day (Monday–Saturday) and 10 mg medroxyprogesterone acetate orally for 10 days during every fourth cycle	Mezrow et al. 1994	Add-back estrogen plus progestin reduced physical and psychological symptoms. Add-back estrogen or progesterone alone was associated with recurrence of PMS.
	3.75 mg/month with add-back transdermal estradiol 0.1 mg or progesterone vaginal suppository 200 mg twice daily	Schmidt et al. 1998	Lower dose relieved premenstrual depression and irritability and some physical complaints.
	3.75 mg intramuscular injection monthly with add-back tibolone 2.5 mg/day orally at the onset of vasomotor symptoms	DiCarlo et al. 2001	Add-back tibolone significantly reduced hot flashes.

TABLE 7–1. Pharmacological therapies[a] *(continued)*

Type	Recommended dose	References	Comments
Buserelin	400–900 μg/day intranasally	Bancroft et al. 1987[b]	Not available in the United States
	100 μg/day intranasally	Sundström et al. 1999	Low dose improved psychological symptoms, swelling, and headache.
	400–900 μg/day intranasally	Hammarback and Bäckström 1988	
Goserelin	3.6 mg subcutaneous injection monthly	West and Hillier 1994	Significant physical but not psychological relief
	3.6 mg implant—monthly	Leather et al. 1999	
Estradiol	100 g twice weekly patch with add-back dyrogesterone 10 mg or medroxyprogesterone 5 mg from days 17–26 of each cycle	Smith et al. 1995 Watson et al. 1989	

Note. [a]Double-blind, randomized, placebo-controlled studies, assessed prospectively for at least two complete cycles, in women with late luteal phase dysphoric disorder/premenstrual dysphoric disorder are quoted unless otherwise noted.
[b]Prospective case studies of premenstrual dysphoric disorder.

with SSRIs (Freeman et al. 1999a; Halbreich and Smoller 1997; Jermain et al. 1999; Steiner et al. 1997a; Sundblad et al. 1997; Wikander et al. 1998; Young et al. 1998), clomipramine (Sundblad et al. 1993), and L-tryptophan (Steinberg et al. 1999) is equally effective in alleviating PMDD and may offer a cheaper, easier to tolerate, and more attractive treatment option for a disorder that is itself intermittent. Severe PMS and PMDD respond to relatively low doses of SSRIs (e.g., 10–20 mg/day of fluoxetine or 50–100 mg/day of sertraline) (Diegoli et al. 1998; Freeman et al. 1999b; Jermain et al. 1999; Steiner et al. 1995). In addition, strong evidence indicates that response to treatment with SSRIs or clomipramine will be relatively immediate (within the first month of treatment); therefore, if no change in symptomatology occurs (even after several dosing increases), an alternative therapy should be considered within two to three menstrual cycles. SSRI treatment for women taking oral contraceptives is not contraindicated (Brown et al. 2000; Freeman et al. 2001a)

Anxiolytics

The efficacy of alprazolam (Berger and Presser 1994; Diegoli et al. 1998; Freeman et al. 1995a; Harrison et al. 1990; Smith et al. 1987) and buspirone (Landén et al. 2001; Rickels et al. 1989) in the reduction of premenstrual psychological symptoms also has been reported in randomized controlled trials; however, the effect is much smaller than that with the SSRIs. Intermittent dosing is also effective with both of these medications. The possibility of withdrawal symptoms with alprazolam portends a gradual taper during menses in some women. Dependence and tolerance are also a concern with alprazolam. Weight gain is a possible side effect of alprazolam (Evans et al. 1999).

Hormonal Interventions

The suppression of ovulation eliminates the symptoms of PMS and PMDD, implying the involvement of ovarian hormones in the etiology of premenstrual syndromes. The gonadotropin-releasing hormone agonists leuprolide (Brown et al. 1994; DiCarlo et al. 2001; Freeman et al. 1997; Mezrow et al. 1994; Schmidt et al. 1998), buserelin (Bancroft et al. 1987; Hammerback and Bäckström 1988; Sundström et al. 1999), and goserelin (Leather et al. 1999; West and Hillier 1994) are effective, as is danazol (Hahn et al. 1995; O'Brien and Abukhalil 1999; Sarno et al. 1987) and estradiol (Smith et al. 1995; Watson et al. 1989), in reducing physical and psychological premenstrual symptoms. In general, the gonadotropin-releasing hormone agonists are less effective in relieving mood symptoms compared with physical ones. Danazol (200–400 mg/day) has shown efficacy in the relief of premenstrual migraine and premenstrual mastalgia; the troublesome side effects are significantly reduced with lower doses (Hahn et al. 1995; O'Brien and Abukhalil 1999). Preliminary evidence suggests that "add-back" therapy with low-dose estrogen and progesterone replacement therapy may prevent some of the side effects (Mezrow et al. 1994; Schmidt et al. 1998). Intranasal buserelin or intramuscular leuprolide are the most appropriate gonadotropin-releasing hormone agonist treatments for clinical use.

Oral contraceptives suppress ovulation while maintaining menstruation through periodic steroid withdrawal. Premenstrual symptoms have been documented in women taking oral contraceptives (Freeman et al. 2001a; Sveindóttir and Bäckström 2000). Clinical trials on the use of oral contraceptives for the treatment of PMS are few in number. The more recent findings are, at best, suggestive of some benefit, mostly for the physical symptoms (increased appetite, cravings, and acne) (Freeman et al. 2001c; Graham and Sherwin 1992). Until additional research has been done, the use of oral contraceptives is not recommended for the treatment of PMS or PMDD.

Progesterone and progestogens are among the most widely prescribed treatments for PMS in the United States. Current evidence suggests that they are not likely to be effective in the management of premenstrual syndromes (Wyatt et al. 2001).

Surgical Approach

The last resort and line of treatment for women with PMDD should be a surgical approach. Two studies have reported the effectiveness of ovariectomy in the complete relief of severe premenstrual symptoms (Casper and Hearn 1990; Casson et al. 1990).

SUMMARY

The etiology of premenstrual syndromes has yet to be clarified in a comprehensive fashion; notwithstanding, the current consensus is that PMDD is a distinct clinical entity. We are now able to identify and classify those women who present with severe psychological symptoms and to determine whether these symptoms are attributable to only the premenstruum or are a magnification of a physical or psychiatric disorder. Women who do not have a concurrent disorder and who meet criteria for PMS but not PMDD should be treated conservatively. Women who meet criteria for PMDD can be successfully treated with low-dose SSRIs or clomipramine on an intermittent (luteal phase only) or daily basis.

Some evidence exists for the efficacy of calcium, magnesium, vitamin B_6, and bright artificial light, but further replication studies with these interventions are still needed.

Although pharmacological or surgical methods to abolish the menstrual cycle are very effective in eliminating symptoms of PMS and PMDD, these methods pose an ethical dilemma because they create a state of early menopause for young women, with all its potential ramifications.

REFERENCES

American Psychiatric Association: Diagnostic and Statistical Manual of Mental Disorders, 3rd Edition, Revised. Washington, DC, American Psychiatric Association, 1987, pp 367–369

American Psychiatric Association: Diagnostic and Statistical Manual of Mental Disorders, 4th Edition. Washington, DC, American Psychiatric Association, 1994, pp 717–718

American Psychiatric Association: Diagnostic and Statistical Manual of Mental Disorders, 4th Edition, Text Revision. Washington, DC, American Psychiatric Association, 2000

Andersch B, Wendestam C, Hahn L, et al: Premenstrual complaints, I: prevalence of premenstrual symptoms in a Swedish urban population. J Psychosom Obstet Gynaecol 5:39–49, 1986

Angst J, Sellaro R, Merikangas KR, et al: The epidemiology of perimenstrual psychological symptoms. Acta Psychiatr Scand 104:110–116, 2001

Anson O: Exploring the bio-psycho-social approach to premenstrual experiences. Soc Sci Med 49:67–80, 1999

Ashby CR Jr, Carr LA, Cook CL, et al: Alteration of platelet serotonergic mechanisms and monoamine oxidase activity in premenstrual syndrome. Biol Psychiatry 24:225–233, 1988

Bancroft J, Cook A: The neuroendocrine response to D-fenfluramine in women with premenstrual depression. J Affect Disord 36:57–64, 1995

Bancroft J, Boyle H, Warner P, et al: The use of an LHRH agonist, buserelin, in the long-term management of premenstrual syndromes. Clin Endocrinol 27:171–182, 1987

Bancroft J, Cook A, Davidson D, et al: Blunting of neuroendocrine responses to infusion of L-tryptophan in women with perimenstrual mood change. Psychol Med 21:305–312, 1991

Bancroft J, Rennie D, Warner P: Vulnerability to perimenstrual mood change: the relevance of a past history of depressive disorder. Psychosom Med 56:225–231, 1994

Berger CP, Presser B: Alprazolam in the treatment of two subsamples of patients with late luteal phase dysphoric disorder: a double-blind, placebo-controlled crossover study. Obstet Gynecol 84:379–385, 1994

Bicikova M, Dibbelt L, Hill M, et al: Allopregnanolone in women with premenstrual syndrome. Horm Metab Res 30:227–230, 1998

Blake F, Salkovskis P, Gath D, et al: Cognitive therapy for premenstrual syndrome: a controlled trial. J Psychosom Res 45:307–318, 1998

Bloch M, Schmidt PJ, Su TP, et al: Pituitary-adrenal hormones and testosterone across the menstrual cycle in women with premenstrual syndrome and controls. Biol Psychiatry 43:897–903, 1998

Brockington I: Menstrual psychosis. Archives of Women's Mental Health 1:3–13, 1998

Brown CS, Ling FW, Andersen RN, et al: Efficacy of depot leuprolide in premenstrual syndrome: effect of symptom severity and type in a controlled trial. Obstet Gynecol 84:779–786, 1994

Brown CS, Parker N, Ling F, et al: Sertraline in contraceptive users with premenstrual dysphoric disorder. Obstet Gynecol 95(suppl):29S, 2000

Budeiri DJ, LiWanPo A, Dornan JC: Clinical trials of treatments of premenstrual syndrome: entry criteria and scales for measuring treatment outcomes. Br J Obstet Gynaecol 101:689–695, 1994

Cahill CA: Differences in cortisol, a stress hormone, in women with turmoil-type premenstrual symptoms. Nurs Res 47:278–284, 1998

Case AM, Reid RL: Menstrual cycle effects on common medical conditions. Comprehensive Therapy 27:65–71, 2001

Casper RF, Hearn MT: The effect of hysterectomy and bilateral oophorectomy in women with severe premenstrual syndrome. Am J Obstet Gynecol 162:105–109, 1990

Casson P, Hahn PM, Van Vugt DA, et al: Lasting response to ovariectomy in severe intractable premenstrual syndrome. Am J Obstet Gynecol 162:99–105, 1990

Chandra PS, Chaturvedi SK: Cultural variations in premenstrual experiences. Int J Soc Psychiatry 35:343–349, 1989

Chang AM, Holroyd E, Chau JP: Premenstrual syndrome in employed Chinese women in Hong Kong. Health Care for Women International 16:551–561, 1995

Chang AM, Chau JP, Holroyd E: Translation of questionnaires and issues of equivalence. J Adv Nurs 29:316–322, 1999

Chuong CJ, Coulam CB, Bergstralh EJ, et al: Clinical trial of naltrexone in premenstrual syndrome. Obstet Gynecol 72:332–336, 1988

Cohen IR, Wise PM: Effects of estradiol on the diurnal rhythm of serotonin activity in microdissected brain areas of ovariectomized rats. Endocrinology 122:2619–2625, 1988

Condon JT: The premenstrual syndrome: a twin study. Br J Psychiatry 162:481–486, 1993

Dan AJ, Monagle L: Sociocultural influences on women's experiences of perimenstrual symptoms, in Premenstrual Dysphorias: Myths and Realities. Edited by Gold JH, Severino SK. Washington, DC, American Psychiatric Press, 1994, pp 201–211

Deuster PA, Adera T, South Paul J: Biological, social, and behavioral factors associated with premenstrual syndrome. Arch Fam Med 8:122–128, 1999

DiCarlo C, Palomba S, Tommaselli GA, et al: Use of leuprolide acetate plus tibolone in the treatment of severe premenstrual syndrome. Fertil Steril 75:380–384, 2001

Diegoli MSC, da Fonseca AM, Diegoli CA, et al: A double-blind trial of four medications to treat severe premenstrual syndrome. Int J Gynaecol Obstet 62:63–
67, 1998

Dimmock PW, Wyatt KM, Jones PW, et al: Efficacy of selective serotonin-reuptake
inhibitors in premenstrual syndrome: a systematic review. Lancet 356:1131–
1136, 2000

Ekholm UB, Ekholm NO, Backstrom T: Premenstrual syndrome: comparison between different methods to diagnose cyclicity using daily symptom ratings.
Acta Obstet Gynecol Scand 77:551–557, 1998

Endicott J: The menstrual cycle and mood disorders. J Affect Disord 29:193–200,
1993

Endicott J, Amsterdam J, Eriksson E, et al: Is premenstrual dysphoric disorder a
distinct clinical entity? Journal of Women's Health and Gender-Based Medicine 8:663–679, 1999

Eriksson E: Serotonin reuptake inhibitors for the treatment of premenstrual dysphoria. Int Clin Psychopharmacol 14:S27–S33, 1999

Eriksson E, Alling C, Andersch B, et al: Cerebrospinal fluid levels of monoamine
metabolites: a preliminary study of their relation to menstrual cycle phase, sex
steroids, and pituitary hormones in healthy women and in women with premenstrual syndrome. Neuropsychopharmacology 11:201–213, 1994

Eriksson E, Hedberg MA, Andersch B, et al: The serotonin reuptake inhibitor paroxetine is superior to the noradrenaline reuptake inhibitor maprotiline in the
treatment of premenstrual syndrome. Neuropsychopharmacology 12:167–
176, 1995

Eriksson E, Sundblad C, Landén M, et al: Behavioural effects of androgens in
women, in Mood Disorders in Women. Edited by Steiner M, Yonkers K,
Eriksson E. London, United Kingdom, Martin Dunitz, 2000, pp 233–245

Evans SM, Foltin RW, Fischman MW: Food "cravings" and the acute effects of alprazolam on food intake in women with premenstrual dysphoric disorder. Appetite 32:331–349, 1999

Facchinetti F, Tarabusi M, Nappi G: Premenstrual syndrome and anxiety disorders:
a psychobiological link. Psychother Psychosom 67:57–60, 1998

Fava M, Pedrazzi F, Guaraldi GP, et al: Comorbid anxiety and depression among
patients with late luteal phase dysphoric disorder. J Anxiety Disord 6:325–335,
1992

FitzGerald M, Malone K, Li S, et al: Blunted serotonin response to fenfluramine
challenge in premenstrual dysphoric disorder. Am J Psychiatry 154:556–558,
1997

Fontana AM, Palfai TG: Psychosocial factors in premenstrual dysphoria: stressors,
appraisal, and coping processes. J Psychosom Res 38:557–567, 1994

Freeman EW, Sondheimer S, Weinbaum PJ, et al: Evaluating premenstrual symptoms in medical practice. Obstet Gynecol 65:500–505, 1985

Freeman EW, Rickels K, Sondheimer SJ, et al: A double-blind trial of oral progesterone, alprazolam, and placebo in the treatment of severe premenstrual syndrome. JAMA 274:51–57, 1995a

Freeman EW, Rickels K, Schweizer E, et al: Relationships between age and symptom severity among women seeking medical treatment for premenstrual symptoms. Psychol Med 25:309–315, 1995b

Freeman EW, Sondheimer SJ, Rickels K: Gonadotropin-releasing hormone agonist in the treatment of premenstrual symptoms with and without ongoing dysphoria: a controlled study. Psychopharmacol Bull 33:303–309, 1997

Freeman EW, Rickels K, Sondheimer SJ, et al: Differential response to antidepressants in women with premenstrual syndrome/premenstrual dysphoric disorder: a randomized controlled trial. Arch Gen Psychiatry 56:932–939, 1999a

Freeman EW, Rickels K, Arredondo F, et al: Full- or half-cycle treatment of severe premenstrual syndrome with a serotonergic antidepressant. J Clin Psychopharmacol 19:3–8, 1999b

Freeman EW, Rickels K, Sondheimer SJ, et al: Concurrent use of oral contraceptives with antidepressants for premenstrual syndromes [letters to the editors]. J Clin Psychopharmcol 21:540–542, 2001a

Freeman EW, Sondheimer SJ, Rickels K, et al: Efficacy and safety of venlafaxine for premenstrual dysphoric disorder. Obstet Gynecol 97(suppl):S9–S10, 2001b

Freeman EW, Kroll R, Rapkin A, et al: Evaluation of a unique oral contraceptive in the treatment of premenstrual dysphoric disorder. J Womens Health Gend Based Med 10:561–569, 2001c

Gehlert S, Chang CH, Hartlage S: Establishing the diagnostic validity of premenstrual dysphoric disorder using rasch analysis. J Outcome Meas 1:2–18, 1997

Gehlert S, Chang CH, Hartlage S: Symptom patterns of premenstrual dysphoric disorder as defined in the Diagnostic and Statistical Manual of Mental Disorders-IV. J Womens Health 8:75–85, 1999

Girdler SS, Pedersen CA, Straneva PA, et al: Dysregulation of cardiovascular and neuroendocrine responses to stress in premenstrual dysphoric disorder. Psychiatry Res 81:163–178, 1998

Graham CA, Sherwin BB: A prospective treatment study of premenstrual symptoms using a triphasic oral contraceptive. J Psychosom Res 36:257–266, 1992

Graze KK, Nee J, Endicott J: Premenstrual depression predicts future major depressive disorder. Acta Psychiatr Scand 81:201–206, 1990

Greene R, Dalton K: The premenstrual syndrome. BMJ I:1007–1014, 1953

Gurguis GN, Yonkers KA, Phan SP, et al: Adrenergic receptors in premenstrual dysphoric disorder, I: platelet alpha 2 receptors: Gi protein coupling, phase of menstrual cycle, and prediction of luteal phase symptom severity. Biol Psychiatry 44:600–609, 1998

Hahn PM, VanVugt DA, Reid RL: A randomized, placebo-controlled crossover trial of danazol for the treatment of premenstrual syndrome. Psychoneuroendocrinology 20:193–209, 1995

Halbreich U: Premenstrual dysphoric disorders: a diversified cluster of vulnerability traits to depression. Acta Psychiatr Scand 95:169–176, 1997

Halbreich U, Endicott J: Relationship of dysphoric premenstrual changes to depressive disorders. Acta Psychiatr Scand 71:331–338, 1985

Halbreich U, Smoller JW: Intermittent luteal phase sertraline treatment of dysphoric premenstrual syndrome. J Clin Psychiatry 58:399–402, 1997

Halbreich U, Tworek H: Altered serotonergic activity in women with dysphoric premenstrual syndromes. Int J Psychiatry Med 23:1–27, 1993

Halbreich U, Petty F, Yonkers K, et al: Low plasma gamma-aminobutyric acid levels during the late luteal phase of women with premenstrual dysphoric disorder. Am J Psychiatry 153:718–720, 1996

Hammarback S, Bäckström T: Induced anovulation as treatment of premenstrual tension syndrome. Acta Obstet Gynecol Scand 67:159–166, 1988

Hammarback S, Backstrom T, Holst J, et al: Cyclical mood changes as in the premenstrual tension syndrome during sequential estrogen-progestogen postmenopausal replacement therapy. Acta Obstet Gynecol Scand 64:393–397, 1985

Hargrove JT, Abraham GE: The incidence of premenstrual tension in a gynecologic clinic. J Reprod Med 27:721–724, 1982

Harrison WM, Endicott J, Nee J, et al: Characteristics of women seeking treatment for premenstrual syndrome. Psychosomatics 30:405–411, 1989

Harrison WM, Endicott J, Nee J: Treatment of premenstrual dysphoria with alprazolam: a controlled study. Arch Gen Psychiatry 47:270–275, 1990

Haskett RF, DeLongis A, Kessler RC: Premenstrual dysphoria: a community survey. Paper presented at the annual meeting of the American Psychiatric Association, Chicago, IL, May 1987

Hendrick V, Altshuler LL: Recurrent mood shifts of premenstrual dysphoric disorder can be mistaken for rapid-cycling bipolar II disorder. J Clin Psychiatry 59:479–480, 1998

Jermain DM, Preece CK, Sykes RL, et al: Luteal phase sertraline treatment for premenstrual dysphoric disorder: results of a double-blind, placebo-controlled, crossover study. Arch Fam Med 9:328–332, 1999

Johnson SR: The epidemiology and social impact of premenstrual symptoms. Clin Obstet Gynecol 30:367–376, 1987

Johnson SR, McChesney C, Bean JA: Epidemiology of premenstrual symptoms in a nonclinical sample, I: prevalence, natural history and help-seeking behaviour. J Reprod Med 33:340–346, 1988

Johnson TM: Premenstrual syndrome as a Western culture-specific disorder. Cult Med Psychiatry 11:337–356, 1987

Kaspi SP, Otto MW, Pollack MH, et al: Premenstrual exacerbation of symptoms in women with panic disorder. J Anxiety Disord 8:131–138, 1994

Kendler KS, Silberg JL, Neale MC, et al: Genetic and environmental factors in the aetiology of menstrual, premenstrual and neurotic symptoms: a population-based twin study. Psychol Med 22:85–100, 1992

Kendler KS, Karkowski LM, Corey LA, et al: Longitudinal population-based twin study of retrospectively reported premenstrual symptoms and lifetime major depression. Am J Psychiatry 155:1234–1240, 1998

Korzekwa MI, Lamont JA, Steiner M: Late luteal phase dysphoric disorder and the thyroid axis revisited. J Clin Endocrinol Metab 81:2280–2284, 1996

Kouri EM, Halbreich U: State and trait serotonergic abnormalities in women with dysphoric premenstrual syndromes. Psychopharmacol Bull 33:767–770, 1997

Kraemer GR, Kraemer RR: Premenstrual syndrome: diagnosis and treatment experiences. J Womens Health 7:893–907, 1998

Ladisich W: Influence of progesterone on serotonin metabolism: a possible causal factor for mood changes. Psychoneuroendocrinology 2:257–266, 1977

Lam RW, Carter D, Misri S, et al: A controlled study of light therapy in women with late luteal phase dysphoric disorder. Psychiatry Res 86:185–192, 1999

Landén M, Eriksson O, Sundblad C, et al: Compounds with affinity for serotonergic receptors in the treatment of premenstrual dysphoria: a comparison of buspirone, nefazodone and placebo. Psychopharmacology 155:292–298, 2001

Leather AT, Studd JW, Watson NR, et al: The treatment of severe premenstrual syndrome with goserelin with and without "add-back" estrogen therapy: a placebo-controlled study. Gynecol Endocrinol 13:48–55, 1999

Leibenluft E, Fiero PL, Rubinow DR: Effects of the menstrual cycle on dependent variables in mood disorders research. Arch Gen Psychiatry 51:761–781, 1994

Macmillan I, Young A: Bipolar II disorder vs premenstrual dysphoric disorder. J Clin Psychiatry 60:409–410, 1999

Marvan ML, Escobedo C: Premenstrual symptomatology: role of prior knowledge about premenstrual syndrome. Psychosom Med 61:163–167, 1999

Maskall DD, Lam RW, Misri S, et al: Seasonality of symptoms in women with late luteal phase dysphoric disorder. Am J Psychiatry 154:1436–1441, 1997

McLeod DR, Hoehn-Saric R, Foster GV, et al: The influence of premenstrual syndrome on ratings of anxiety in women with generalized anxiety disorder. Acta Psychiatr Scand 88:248–251, 1993

Meltzer H: Serotonergic dysfunction in depression. Br J Psychiatry 155(suppl 8):25–31, 1989

Menkes DB, Coates DC, Fawcett JP: Acute tryptophan depletion aggravates premenstrual syndrome. J Affect Disord 32:37–44, 1994

Merikangas KR, Foeldenyi M, Angst J: The Zurich Study, XIX: patterns of menstrual disturbances in the community: results of the Zurich Cohort Study. Eur Arch Psychiatry Clin Neurosci 243:23–32, 1993

Mezrow G, Shoupe D, Spicer D, et al: Depot leuprolide acetate with estrogen and progestin add-back for long-term treatment of premenstrual syndrome. Fertil Steril 62:932–937, 1994

Monteleone P, Luisi S, Tonetti A, et al: Allopregnanolone concentrations and premenstrual syndrome. Eur J Endocrinol 142:269–273, 2000

Morse CA, Dennerstein L, Farrell E, et al: A comparison of hormone therapy, coping skills training, and relaxation for the relief of premenstrual syndrome. J Behav Med 14:469–489, 1991

Morse G: Positively reframing perceptions of the menstrual cycle among women with premenstrual syndrome. J Obstet Gynecol Neonatal Nurs 28:165–174, 1999

Mortola JF: Premenstrual syndrome. Trends in Endocrinology and Metabolism 7:184–189, 1996

Mortola JF, Girton L, Beck L, et al: Diagnosis of premenstrual syndrome by a simple, prospective, and reliable instrument: the Calendar of Premenstrual Experiences. Obstet Gynecol 76:302–307, 1990

Muneyvirci-Delale O, Nacharaju VL, Altura BM, et al: Sex steroid hormones modulate serum ionized magnesium and calcium levels throughout the menstrual cycle in women. Fertil Steril 69:958–962, 1998

Nakayama K, Nakagawa T, Hiyama T, et al: Circadian changes in body temperature during the menstrual cycle of healthy adult females and patients suffering from premenstrual syndrome. Int J Clin Pharmacol Res 17:155–164, 1997

Nikolai TF, Mulligan GM, Gribble RK, et al: Thyroid function and treatment in premenstrual syndrome. J Clin Endocrinol Metab 70:1108–1113, 1990

O'Brien PM, Abukhalil IE: Randomized controlled trial of the management of premenstrual syndrome and premenstrual mastalgia using luteal phase–only danazol. Am J Obstet Gynecol 180 (1 pt 1):18–23, 1999

O'Brien PM, Abukhalil IE, Henshaw C: Premenstrual syndrome. Curr Opin Obstet Gynecol 5:30–37, 1995

Odber J, Cawood EH, Bancroft J: Salivary cortisol in women with and without perimenstrual mood changes. J Psychosom Res 45:557–568, 1998

Paddison PL, Gise LH, Lebovits A, et al: Sexual abuse and premenstrual syndrome: comparison between a lower and higher socioeconomic group. Psychosomatics 31:265–272, 1990

Parry BL: Mood disorders linked to reproductive cycle in women, in Psychopharmacology: The Fourth Generation of Progress. Edited by Bloom FE, Kupfer DJ. New York, Raven, 1995, pp 1029–1042

Parry BL: Light therapy of premenstrual depression, in Seasonal Affective Disorder and Beyond. Edited by Lam RW. Washington, DC, American Psychiatric Press, 1998, pp 173–191

Parry BL, Newton RP: Chronological basis of female-specific mood disorders. Neuropsychopharmacology 25:S102–S108, 2001

Parry BL, Mahan AM, Mostofi M, et al: Light therapy of late luteal phase dysphoric disorder: an extended study. Am J Psychiatry 150:1417–1419, 1993

Parry BL, Mostofi N, LeVeau B, et al: Sleep EEG studies during early and late partial sleep deprivation in premenstrual dysphoric disorder and normal control subjects. Psychiatry Res 85:127–143, 1999

Pearlstein T, Steiner M: Non-antidepressant treatment of premenstrual syndrome. J Clin Psychiatry 61(suppl):22–27, 2000

Pearlstein TB, Frank E, Rivera-Tovar A, et al: Prevalence of Axis I and Axis II disorders in women with late luteal phase dysphoric disorder. J Affect Disord 20:129–134, 1990

Pearlstein TB, Stone AB, Lund S, et al: Comparison of fluoxetine, bupropion, and placebo in the treatment of premenstrual dysphoric disorder. J Clin Psychopharmacol 17:261–266, 1997

Ramacharan S, Love EJ, Fick GH, et al: The epidemiology of premenstrual symptoms in a population based sample of 2650 urban women. J Clin Epidemiol 45:377–382, 1992

Rapkin AJ: The role of serotonin in premenstrual syndrome. Clin Obstet Gynecol 35:629–636, 1992

Rapkin AJ, Edelmuth E, Chang LC, et al: Whole blood serotonin in premenstrual syndrome. Obstet Gynecol 70:533–537, 1987

Rapkin AJ, Shoupe D, Reading A, et al: Decreased central opioid activity in premenstrual syndrome: luteinizing hormone response to naloxone. J Soc Gynecol Invest 3:93–98, 1996

Rapkin AJ, Morgan M, Goldman L, et al: Progesterone metabolite allopregnanolone in women with premenstrual syndrome. Obstet Gynecol 90:709–714, 1997

Rapkin AJ, Cedars M, Morgan M, et al: Insulin-like growth factor-1 and insulin-like growth factor-binding protein-3 in women with premenstrual syndrome. Fertil Steril 70:1077–1080, 1998

Reid RL: Premenstrual syndrome. Current Problems in Obstetrics, Gynecology, and Fertility 8:1–57, 1985

Rickels K, Freeman E, Sondheimer S: Buspirone in treatment of premenstrual syndrome (letter). Lancet 1:777, 1989

Rivera-Tovar AD, Frank E: Late luteal phase dysphoric disorder in young women. Am J Psychiatry 147:1634–1636, 1990

Roca CA, Schmidt PJ, Bloch M, et al: Implications of endocrine studies of premenstrual syndrome. Psychiatr Ann 26:576–580, 1996

Rojansky N, Halbreich U, Zander K, et al: Imipramine receptor binding and serotonin uptake in platelets of women with premenstrual changes. Gynecol Obstet Invest 31:146–152, 1991

Rubinow DR, Schmidt PJ: The treatment of premenstrual syndrome: forward into the past. N Engl J Med 332:1574–1575, 1995

Sarno AP, Miller EJ Jr, Lundblad EG: Premenstrual syndrome: beneficial effects of periodic low-dose danazol. Obstet Gynecol 70:33–36, 1987

Schmidt PJ, Grover GN, Roy-Byrne PP, et al: Thyroid function in women with premenstrual syndrome. J Clin Endocrinol Metab 76:671–674, 1993

Schmidt PJ, Purdy RH, Moore PH Jr, et al: Circulating levels of anxiolytic steroids in the luteal phase in women with premenstrual syndrome and in control subjects. J Clin Endocrinol Metab 79:1256–1260, 1994

Schmidt PJ, Nieman LK, Danaceau MA, et al: Differential behavioral effects of gonadal steroids in women with and in those without premenstrual syndrome. N Engl J Med 338:209–216, 1998

Seideman RY: Effects of a premenstrual syndrome education program on premenstrual symptomatology. Health Care for Women International 11:491–501, 1990

Smith RN, Studd JW, Zamblera D, et al: A randomised comparison over 8 months of 100 micrograms and 200 micrograms twice weekly doses of transdermal oestradiol in the treatment of severe premenstrual syndrome. Br J Obstet Gynaecol 102:475–484, 1995

Smith S, Rinehart JS, Ruddock VE, et al: Treatment of premenstrual syndrome with alprazolam: results of a double-blind, placebo-controlled, randomized crossover clinical trial. Obstet Gynecol 70:37–43, 1987

Steege JF, Stout AL, Knight DL, et al: Reduced platelet tritium-labeled imipramine binding sites in women with premenstrual syndrome. Am J Obstet Gynecol 167:168–172, 1992

Steinberg S, Annable L, Young SN, et al: A placebo-controlled clinical trial of L-tryptophan in premenstrual dysphoria. Biol Psychiatry 45:313–320, 1999

Steiner M: Female-specific mood disorders. Clin Obstet Gynecol 35:599–611, 1992

Steiner M, Wilkins A: Diagnosis and assessment of premenstrual dysphoria. Psychiatr Ann 26:571–575, 1996

Steiner M, Yonkers K: Depression in Women (pocketbook). London, England, Martin Dunitz, 1998, pp 7–12

Steiner M, Haskett RF, Carroll BJ: Premenstrual tension syndrome: the development of research diagnostic criteria and new rating scales. Acta Psychiatr Scand 62:177–190, 1980

Steiner M, Steinberg S, Stewart D, et al: Fluoxetine in the treatment of premenstrual dysphoria. N Engl J Med 332:1529–1534, 1995

Steiner M, Korzekwa M, Lamont J, et al: Intermittent fluoxetine dosing in the treatment of women with premenstrual dysphoria. Psychopharmacol Bull 33:771–774, 1997a

Steiner M, LePage P, Dunn E: Serotonin and gender specific psychiatric disorders. International Journal of Psychiatry in Clinical Practice 1:3–13, 1997b

Steiner M, Judge R, Kumar R: Serotonin re-uptake inhibitors in the treatment of premenstrual dysphoria: current state of knowledge. International Journal of Psychiatry in Clinical Practice 1:241–247, 1997c

Steiner M, Streiner DL, Steinberg S, et al: The measurement of premenstrual mood symptoms. J Affect Disord 53:269–273, 1999a

Steiner M, Yatham LN, Coote M, et al: Serotonergic dysfunction in women with pure premenstrual dysphoric disorder: is the fenfluramine challenge test still relevant? Psychiatry Res 87:107–115, 1999b

Stevinson C, Ernst E: Complementary/alternative therapies for premenstrual syndrome: a systematic review of randomized controlled trials. Am J Obstet Gynecol 185:227–235, 2001

Su TP, Schmidt PJ, Danaceau M, et al: Effect of menstrual cycle phase on neuroendocrine and behavioral responses to the serotonin agonist *m*-chlorophenylpiperazine in women with premenstrual syndrome and controls. J Clin Endocrinol Metab 82:1220–1228, 1997

Sundblad C, Modigh K, Andersch B, et al: Clomipramine effectively reduces premenstrual irritability and dysphoria: a placebo controlled trial. Acta Psychiatr Scand 85:39–47, 1992

Sundblad C, Hedberg MA, Eriksson E: Clomipramine administered during the luteal phase reduces the symptoms of premenstrual syndrome: a placebo controlled trial. Neuropsychopharmacology 9:133–145, 1993

Sundblad C, Wikander I, Andersch B, et al: A naturalistic study of paroxetine in premenstrual syndrome: efficacy and side-effects during ten cycles of treatment. Eur Neuropsychopharmacol 7:201–206, 1997

Sundström I, Andersson A, Nyberg S, et al: Patients with premenstrual syndrome have a different sensitivity to a neuroactive steroid during the menstrual cycle compared to control subjects. Neuroendocrinology 67:126–138, 1998

Sundström I, Nyberg S, Bixo M, et al: Treatment of premenstrual syndrome with gonadotropin-releasing hormone agonist in a low-dose regimen. Acta Obstet Gynecol Scand 79:891–899, 1999

Sveindóttir H: Prospective assessment of menstrual and premenstrual experiences of Icelandic women. Health Care for Women International 19:71–82, 1998

Sveindóttir H, Bäckström T: Prevalence of menstrual cycle symptom cyclicity and premenstrual dysphoric disorder in a random sample of women using and not using oral contraceptives. Acta Obstet Gynecol Scand 79:405–413, 2000

Taylor D: Effectiveness of professional-peer group treatment: symptom management for women with PMS. Res Nurs Health 22:496–511, 1999

Taylor DL, Mathew RH, Ho BT, et al: Serotonin levels and platelet uptake during premenstrual tension. Neuropsychobiology 12:16–18, 1984

Thys-Jacobs S, Alvir MJ: Calcium-regulating hormones across the menstrual cycle: evidence of a secondary hyperparathyroidism in women with PMS. J Clin Endocrinol Metab 80:2227–2232, 1995

Thys-Jacobs S, Starkey P, Bernstein D, et al: Calcium carbonate and the premenstrual syndrome: effects on premenstrual and menstrual symptoms. Premenstrual Syndrome Study Group. Am J Obstet Gynecol 179:444–452, 1998

Tuiten A, Panhuysen G, Koppeschaar H, et al: Stress, serotonergic function, and mood in users of oral contraceptives. Psychoneuroendocrinology 20:323–334, 1995

van den Akker OB, Stein GS, Neale MC, et al: Genetic and environmental variation in menstrual cycle: histories of two British twin samples. Acta Geneticoe et Gemellologiae (Roma) 36:541–548, 1987

Walker AF, De Souza MC, Vickers MF, et al: Magnesium supplementation alleviates premenstrual symptoms of fluid retention. J Womens Health 7:1157–1165, 1998

Walton J, Youngkin E: The effect of a support group on self-esteem of women with premenstrual syndrome. J Obstet Gynecol Neonatal Nurs 16:174–178, 1987

Wang M, Seippel L, Purdy RH, et al: Relationship between symptom severity and steroid variation in women with premenstrual syndrome: study on serum pregnenolone, pregnenolone sulfate, 5 α-pregnane-3,20-dione and 3 α-hydroxy-5-alpha-pregnan-20-one. J Clin Endocrinol Metab 81:1076–1082, 1996

Watson NR, Studd JW, Savvas M, et al: Treatment of severe premenstrual syndrome with oestradiol patches and cyclical oral noresthisterone. Lancet 2:730–732, 1989

West CP, Hillier H: Ovarian suppression with the gonadotrophin-releasing hormone agonist goserelin (Zoladex) in management of the premenstrual tension syndrome. Hum Reprod 9:1058–1063, 1994

Wikander I, Sundblad C, Andersch B, et al: Citalopram in premenstrual dysphoria: is intermittent treatment during luteal phases more effective than continuous medication throughout the menstrual cycle? J Clin Psychopharmacol 18:390–398, 1998

Woods NF, Lentz MJ, Mitchell ES, et al: Perceived stress, physiologic stress arousal, and premenstrual symptoms: group differences and intra-individual patterns. Res Nurs Health 21:511–523, 1998

World Health Organization: International Statistical Classification of Diseases and Related Health Problems, 10th Revision, Clinical Modification. Geneva, Switzerland, World Health Organization, 1996, p 717

Wurtman JJ: Depression and weight gain: the serotonin connection. J Affect Disord 29:183–192, 1993

Wyatt KM, Dimmock PW, Jones PW, et al: Efficacy of vitamin B-6 in the treatment of premenstrual syndrome: systematic review. BMJ 318:1375–1381, 1999

Wyatt K, Dimmock P, Jones P, et al: Efficacy of progesterone and progestogens in management of premenstrual syndrome: systematic review. BMJ 323:776–780, 2001

Yatham LN: Is 5-HT$_{1A}$ receptor subsensitivity a trait marker for late luteal phase dysphoric disorder? A pilot study. Can J Psychiatry 38:662–664, 1993

Yonkers KA: Anxiety symptoms and anxiety disorders: how are they related to premenstrual disorders. J Clin Psychiatry 58(suppl 3):62–67, 1997a

Yonkers KA: The association between premenstrual dysphoric disorder and other mood disorders. J Clin Psychiatry 58(suppl 15):19–25, 1997b

Yonkers KA, Halbreich U, Freeman E, et al: Symptomatic improvement of premenstrual dysphoric disorder with sertraline treatment: a randomized controlled trial. JAMA 278:983–988, 1997

Young SA, Hurt PH, Benedek DM, et al: Treatment of premenstrual dysphoric disorder with sertraline during the luteal phase: a randomized, double-blind, placebo-controlled crossover trial. J Clin Psychiatry 59:76–80, 1998

Yu M, Zhu X, Li J, et al: Perimenstrual symptoms among Chinese women in an urban area of China. Health Care for Women International 17:161–72, 1996

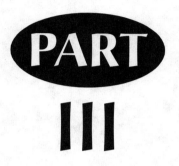

PART III

Schizophrenia and Related Disorders

Introduction

Schizophrenia is one of the most emotionally immobilizing diseases known to humans. It affects 1% of the adult world population, including 2 million Americans. The incidence of this illness is similar for men and women; however, men tend to show an earlier onset of illness, with symptoms such as distorted perceptions of reality, hallucinations, delusions, distorted thinking, dull emotional expressions, social isolation, withdrawal, unclear speech, and disorganized or catatonic behavior. Women have a later age at onset and less premorbid dysfunction. In this part, the authors concentrate on the different facets of sex differences in disease expression and response to treatment.

Within the first three chapters of this part, sex differences in the origin and progression of schizophrenia are explored. Chapter 8 begins by including observations about the etiological origins, premorbid course, and onset of the disease. Chapter 9 contains a review of 10 studies published in the past decade focusing on the sex effects of neurocognition and symptom expression. The central role of gonadal hormones in male and female differences in manifestation of schizophrenia is also included within this discussion. Finally, Chapter 10 features menopause with respect to the symptoms of schizophrenia. Mechanistically, estrogen may be exerting potential protective effects in schizophrenia through an antidopaminergic pathway. Preliminary clinical and epidemiological observations that females with schizophrenia have fewer psychotic symptoms at times of high estrogen levels and that menopause may aggravate the symptoms of schizophrenia support this hypothesis. However, it is clear that the role of estrogen in schizophrenia remains hypothetical.

The next two chapters in this part focus on drug effects on schizophrenia. Antipsychotic medication remains the cornerstone treatment for schizophrenia. The efficacy and side effect profile of conventional and atypical neuroleptics are considered with an emphasis on the clinical consequences (for women) of neuroleptic-induced hyperprolactinemia.

Finally, the last three chapters discuss specific women's issues in regard to this psychosis. Chapter 13 explores the effects of estrogens on schizophrenia, including an examination of the four separate lines of evidence that were originally proposed by Riecher-Rossler and Hafner. An overview of issues concerning women in the diagnosis and treatment of schizophrenia, as well as quality of life considerations and systems of care, is found in Chapter 14. Finally, the effect of schizophrenia on the family in this age of postinstitutionalization services and intervention is examined in Chapter 15.

Sex Differences in the Origins and Premorbid Development of Schizophrenia

Elaine F. Walker, Ph.D.
Deborah J. Walder, M.D.
Richard Lewine, Ph.D.
Rachel Loewy, B.A.

Numerous studies have documented sex differences in the clinical manifestation and course of schizophrenia, and these findings suggest that sex may have implications for prognosis and treatment (Lewine and Seeman 1995; Seeman 1995). More recently, as the empirical literature has accumulated, it has become apparent that sex differences also exist in the precursors of the illness. In this chapter, we examine the empirical literature dealing with differences between males and females in the putative origins and premorbid characteristics of schizophrenia.

With respect to the origins of the disorder, we first consider the evidence for sex differences in the contributions of both genetic factors and

This work was supported in part by a Research Scientist Development Award (MH00876) to Dr. Walker from the National Institute of Mental Health.

obstetrical complications. We then examine research findings on premorbid behavior, with an emphasis on childhood behavior problems that distinguish male and female patients. Finally, given the association between premorbid function and age at onset (Hafner and an der Heiden 1997), the evidence for sex differences in age at onset of illness is addressed.

As this overview of the literature illustrates, the sexes differ in the nature and course of premorbid impairment. They also may differ in the origins of their vulnerability to schizophrenia. A primary goal of our discussion is to explore the implications of these findings for understanding the epigenesis of sex differences.

BACKGROUND

Differences between males and females in the manifestation and rate of occurrence of illness are ubiquitous. They have been documented in neurological, cardiovascular, and respiratory conditions as well as in several psychiatric disorders. Two general classes of factors have been evoked to explain sex differences in illness: socialization experiences and biological processes. For example, it is assumed that sex differences in risk for cardiovascular disorders are a function of differences in both the rate of occurrence of risk behaviors and the influence of sex hormones. Similarly, sex differences in schizophrenia have been attributed to sex-role socialization and hormonal factors, particularly the influence of estrogen (Lewine and Seeman 1995).

One of the central questions debated in this literature is whether sex 1) influences the expression of a single illness or 2) is associated with differential risk for etiological subtypes of schizophrenia (Lewine 1981). Explanations of sex differences based on socialization and hormonal factors typically imply that sex is acting to moderate the clinical expression of a single illness. Of course, socialization and hormonal factors also could influence vulnerabilities to illness subtypes. Some in the field have proposed that the observed sex differences in schizophrenia are a consequence of differences between males and females in vulnerability to discrete etiological subtypes. Notable in this regard is a hypothesis offered by Murray and his colleagues (Castle et al. 1995; Murray et al. 1992b). These authors proposed that males predominate in a "neurodevelopmental" subtype of schizophrenia that has its origins in perturbations of fetal central nervous system (CNS) development. Thus, it is assumed that sex moderates vulnerability to subtypes of schizophrenia that involve different neuropathogenic mechanisms. Our review of the literature considers the relative merits of these alternative hypotheses.

In discussing the topic of sex differences in schizophrenia, it is important to keep two caveats in mind. First, as already noted, it is certainly plausible that the syndrome is not homogeneous with respect to etiology. Therefore, although we use the singular term *schizophrenia* for convenience, we do not assume a single etiology. Second, the validity of current diagnostic distinctions among the psychotic disorders has not been established. This is key to our interpretation of sex differences because changing diagnostic criteria have produced changes in the sex ratios within diagnostic categories (Burbach et al. 1984). Specifically, with the revised diagnostic criteria introduced in DSM-III (American Psychiatric Association 1980), pronounced affective symptoms became an exclusion criterion for schizophrenia, and this was associated with a significant decrease in the proportion of females meeting criteria for the disorder. The decrease appears to be a result of the fact that affective symptoms, although common in both male and female schizophrenia patients (Siris 1995), are more prevalent in psychotic women (Bardenstein and McGlashan 1990). This is reflective of the general trend for depressive disorders to be more common in women.

Whether contemporary diagnostic distinctions more accurately reflect the natural etiological boundaries of psychotic disorders remains to be established. In the interim, our interpretations of the findings on sex differences in schizophrenia must take these shifting boundaries into consideration. This note of caution is particularly relevant to the issue of sex differences in the genetic origins of schizophrenia.

GENETIC CONTRIBUTION

A genetic component in the etiology of schizophrenia has been well established (Gottesman 1991; Kendler et al. 1985), but the question of sex differences in the heritability of the disorder continues to be debated. The answer to this question has obvious implications for our understanding of possible sex differences in vulnerability to subtypes of schizophrenia.

Some early reports indicated that risk rates for schizophrenia were higher in the first-degree relatives of female probands than in the relatives of males. However, more recent studies have yielded inconsistent results, with some showing no sex difference. Changing diagnostic criteria and other methodological factors have made it difficult to judge the validity of the findings. Because an article by Goldstein (1995a) contains excellent overviews of this area of research, we do not present a comprehensive review here. Instead, we highlight the key issues and the general conclusions that can be drawn at this point.

Several of the first twin studies of schizophrenia reported higher concordance rates among female monozygotic and dizygotic twins than among male monozygotic or dizygotic pairs (Rosenthal 1962; Slater 1958). However, as pointed out by several authors (Gottesman 1991; Samuels 1978), these investigations were based on residents of mental institutions, which at the time were more highly populated by women with chronic disorders. This may have increased concordance rates for females because severity of symptoms is associated with a greater genetic component to the illness. Furthermore, the diagnostic criteria used at the time included syndromes that would currently be classified as mood disorders. As noted earlier, females have a much higher rate of depressive disorders than do males, and strong evidence indicates that these disorders are more heritable than schizophrenia (Gottesman 1991; Walker et al. 1991). Moreover, twin studies also indicate higher heritability for mood disorder in females than in males (Kendler et al. 1993).

Subsequent twin studies have generally failed to yield evidence of a sex difference in concordance rates for schizophrenia (Fischer 1973; Gottesman 1991; Kringlen 1968). It is noteworthy, however, that the Fischer (1973) and Kringlen (1968) studies showed higher female concordance for narrower definitions of schizophrenia but higher male concordance for broader definitions of schizophrenia. Stromgren (1987) reported similar findings.

Like the twin studies, investigations of the familial incidence of psychopathology have yielded inconsistent results. One of the earliest family history studies found a higher risk for psychosis in relatives of male probands, but the authors did not statistically compare the risk rates in families of male and female probands (Pollock et al. 1939). Several subsequent investigations systematically examined sex differences and found a higher rate of schizophrenia or spectrum disorders in relatives of female patients (Bellodi et al. 1986; Shimizu et al. 1987; Wolyniec et al. 1992). In contrast, some reports suggested no sex difference in familial risk (Murphy et al. 1997; Sturt and Shur 1985). In fact, Sham et al. (1994) used more stringent diagnostic criteria than those used in the early studies and found no difference in the risk for schizophrenia among relatives of male and female probands; however, they did find a higher rate of manic-depressive psychosis among relatives of females. In contrast, Wolyniec et al. (1992) found that the first-degree relatives of females had higher risk rates of nonaffective psychosis than did the first-degree relatives of males.

In an excellent critical review of the research in this area, Goldstein (1996) explored the effect that changing diagnostic criteria and methods would have on the results of twin and family studies of schizophrenia. If the diagnostic criteria used for probands were broad, and thus included more female patients with affective symptoms, then the relatives of the females would be expected to have an elevated rate of mood disorders. Moreover, if the diagnostic criteria applied to the relatives were also broad, then some relatives with mood disorder may have been given diagnoses of schizophrenia, thus further elevating the rate of affected relatives among the female probands. Clearly, the research findings on sex differences in the genetic liability for schizophrenia do not provide a firm basis for any specific conclusions about etiology, but they do suggest a critical point: namely, that sex differences in clinical presentation, particularly affective symptoms, may have significant implications for our understanding of schizophrenia. We return to this point later in the chapter.

OBSTETRICAL FACTORS

Numerous studies have shown that complications of pregnancy and delivery are associated with a higher rate of schizophrenia in the offspring. A subgroup of these investigations examined sex differences in the strength of this relation, and the results suggested that males may be more likely to manifest the behavioral sequelae of obstetrical complications.

A study by Foerster et al. (1991a) of consecutively admitted patients showed that male patients with schizophrenia were exposed to a higher rate of obstetrical complications than were female patients. Similar findings were reported by O'Callaghan et al. (1992) based on an investigation of a British cohort. The Danish study of high-risk offspring of schizophrenic mothers also found more obstetrical complications in the histories of male patients (Mednick et al. 1978). Taken together, the findings suggest that males may be more vulnerable to fetal insults to CNS development. Extending their research beyond fetal development, Nasrallah and Wilcox (1989) examined the medical histories of a large sample of patients with chronic schizophrenia and found that males were more likely to have a history of childhood brain injury.

In contrast to the above studies, one of the most comprehensive investigations to date found no sex differences in exposure to obstetrical complications (Verdoux et al. 1997). Verdoux et al. (1997) combined data on obstetrical factors for 854 patients with schizophrenia from several research groups. Although greater obstetrical complications were linked with earlier age at onset, no significant sex difference in the rate of complications was seen. Given the methodological strength of this study, the absence of significant sex differences is noteworthy.

A substantive body of literature now shows a relation between prenatal maternal viral infection and schizophrenia in offspring. Contrary to the research on other obstetrical complications, it has been reported that this association is more pronounced for females (Murray et al. 1992a, 1992b).

Although the evidence for sex differences in exposure to obstetrical complications is not compelling, it is nonetheless possible that males are uniquely sensitive to obstetrical complications. Casar et al. (1997) found that the strength of the association between history of obstetrical complications and adult neuropsychological deficits was stronger for male than for female patients with schizophrenia. Along these same lines, it has been reported that a stronger relation exists between obstetrical complications and neurological soft signs in male patients with schizophrenia (Lane et al. 1996), but this sex difference appears to be a general phenomenon rather than a unique characteristic of schizophrenia. Follow-up studies of community samples of children exposed to obstetrical complications have yielded similar results; males had more soft neurological signs (Hadders-Algra et al. 1988a) and greater behavioral deficits (Hadders-Algra et al. 1988b).

PREMORBID BEHAVIOR

The premorbid period has been of intense interest to researchers seeking to identify the earliest signs of vulnerability to schizophrenia. Over the past three decades, we have witnessed the accumulation of an extensive body of literature documenting behavioral dysfunction before the onset of the clinical syndrome labeled *schizophrenia*. Much of this research has focused on the adult years immediately preceding diagnosis (Mueser et al. 1990). Recent reviews of these findings concluded that males have more behavioral deficits, including impairment in occupational and interpersonal functioning, during this period (Haas and Garratt 1998; Tamminga 1997). Other research has examined the childhood and adolescent development of individuals who later develop schizophrenia. The present discussion focuses on this literature, with the goal of clarifying the nature and earliest age at onset of sex differences.

Research on premorbid childhood behavior in schizophrenia has relied on four methodological approaches: 1) follow-up studies of the adult psychiatric outcomes of large samples evaluated during childhood, 2) retrospective studies that obtain childhood archival data on diagnosed patients, 3) retrospective studies that rely on informants' descriptions of patients' premorbid behavior, and 4) prospective studies that assess subjects at risk for the disorder, typically offspring of schizophrenic patients (Walker et al. 1995b). The last approach is distinguished from the first three with respect to the representativeness of the patient samples. Specifically, prospective studies typically focus on the biological offspring of schizophrenic parents. Although this strategy has proved to be very fruitful, the fact that most patients with schizophrenia do not have a parent with the disorder may limit the generalizability of the findings. This may be particularly true of premorbid behavior. Some high-risk offspring are reared by their mentally ill parents, whereas others are placed in alternative settings, such as foster homes or institutions. In either case, many of these children experience nonoptimal caregiving, which may contribute to behavioral dysfunction, independent of risk for schizophrenia. Aside from this methodological limitation, prospective high-risk studies have a unique advantage with respect to systematically documenting the premorbid development of individuals at risk for schizophrenia.

Studies of premorbid behavior also vary in the nature of the measures used. Retrospective studies typically use scales that involve ratings of the quality of the patient's functioning in multiple domains. The most commonly used scale is the Cannon-Spoor Scale, which rates the patient on global adjustment during childhood and adolescence (Cannon-Spoor et al. 1982). In contrast, the sources of data typically used in retrospective and follow-up studies (e.g., school records, medical records, or childhood movies) contain less systematic information but often address more specific behavioral characteristics.

In summary, diverse measures and methodologies add to the complexity of this body of research. However, methodological diversity also confers an advantage with respect to the strength of the inferences that can be drawn. When the same pattern of findings is yielded by investigations that used different sampling procedures and data sources, it is less likely to be attributable to methodological artifact. Thus, the optimal approach to drawing inferences about sex differences in premorbid behavior is to identify commonalities in the findings across methodologies.

To our knowledge, the first comprehensive review of the literature on behavioral antecedents of schizophrenia was published in 1969. In this paper, Offord and Cross (1969) came to the following conclusions: 1) premorbid behavior among patients is diverse, with a subgroup showing significant adjustment problems and others manifesting a "normal" developmental course; 2) the behavior problems that precede schizophrenia include both disruptive, aggressive behavior and withdrawn, dependent tendencies; and 3) premorbid behavioral dysfunction is linked to poor prognosis.

Notably absent in this early review was a discussion of sex differences in premorbid behavior. In large part, this is because most of the studies published up to that time focused on populations (e.g., child guidance clinic referrals, military recruits) that contained few or no females. In the following overview, we limit our discussion to studies that examined sex differences in the premorbid adjustment of subjects for whom psychiatric outcome data are available. Thus, our discussion does not include reports on the behavior of high-risk children whose psychiatric outcomes are not yet known.

Among the earliest investigations that explored sex differences in premorbid childhood behavior was Watt's follow-back study of patients' school records (Watt 1972; Watt and Lubensky 1976; Watt et al. 1970). Teachers' annual reports from school records (elementary and high school) were systematically coded, and analyses showed significant sex differences. Among the preschizophrenic children, boys were more likely to be described as moody, unmotivated, abrasive, and noncompliant. Girls were described as overly inhibited, sensitive, and conforming. For both sexes, the preschizophrenic children's behavior problems increased over time, with a marked rise in adolescence (Watt 1972), but the pattern of longitudinal change differed for males and females. Before seventh grade, the primary factor distinguishing both male and female preschizophrenic children from same-sex control subjects was "emotional instability," with the preschizophrenic children seen as less emotionally mature, cheerful, and secure. In grades 7 through 12, the girls in the preschizophrenic group became increasingly introverted, whereas the boys became more disagreeable and noncompliant. Watt and his colleagues (Watt 1978; Watt and Lubensky 1976) replicated these results in an expanded sample, again finding preschizophrenic boys to be more abrasive and antisocial and preschizophrenic girls to be more introverted and emotionally unstable than their same-sex peers.

The validity of Watt's findings on sex differences in premorbid behavior is supported by the results of a prospective study of Danish offspring of schizophrenic parents. John et al. (1982) obtained teachers' comments from the school records of high-risk children. When compared with high-risk boys with healthy adult outcomes, the preschizophrenic boys were described as being noncompliant, inappropriate, and anxious, whereas the preschizophrenic girls were described as anhedonic and withdrawn. Both sexes were isolated from peers.

In a follow-up paradigm, Done et al. (1994) obtained psychiatric outcome data on a 1958 British birth cohort that was part of a national study of child development. Teachers completed behavior rating scales on the children during the elementary school years when they were ages 7 and 11 years. The behavior ratings of the preschizophrenic children were compared with those of same-sex subjects who had healthy adult outcomes. Analyses showed significant sex differences, with preschizophrenic boys showing more "overreaction" (i.e., cruel, hostile behavior) than did boys with healthy adult outcomes and preschizophrenic girls showing heightened overreaction and "underreaction" (i.e., social withdrawal, depression) when compared with other girls. For both sexes, the preschizophrenic subjects showed a pattern of escalating adjustment problems with age; however, the pattern differed for males and females. With increasing age, the preschizophrenic males became more overreactive, whereas the females became more underreactive, a pattern similar to that documented by the previous investigations.

Jones et al. (1995) conducted a similar follow-up study of a 1946 British birth cohort that was repeatedly evaluated between birth and age 16 years. Thirty patients with schizophrenia (10 female) were identified in this cohort, and they were compared with 4,716 subjects with no evidence of psychiatric illness. Analyses of teacher evaluations indicated that the preschizophrenic subjects were more anxious, solitary, and gloomy than the comparison group. However, these authors detected no significant sex differences, with the exception of higher ratings for girls on anxiety at age 13 years. In contrast to other studies, these authors failed to find an increase in disruptive or antisocial behavior in the preschizophrenic children.

Taken together, the above studies suggest two conclusions: 1) significant sex differences are seen in premorbid childhood behavior, and 2) the sex differences show an age-related increase in magnitude, with males becoming more disruptive and females becoming more withdrawn. The fact that similar findings emerged from studies that used very different methodologies lends support to their validity. Specifically, the above studies used prospective high-risk, follow-back, follow-up, and retrospective paradigms and converged on the same general pattern.

All of the above studies relied on archival sources of information (i.e., school records), and this has both advantages and disadvantages. The major advantage is that potential influences of rating biases due to knowledge of the individual's psychiatric outcome are eliminated. The primary limitation is that archival data are often nonsystematic and incomplete. Prospective studies overcome the latter obstacle.

In a prospective study of high-risk children in Israel, investigators obtained data on childhood behavior from interviews with parents, teachers, and the children themselves (Hans et al. 1992). These evaluations were conducted when the children were between ages 7 and 14 years. Fourteen years later, the subjects were reassessed to determine their psychiatric status. Of those located for follow-up, nine subjects (four female), all offspring of schizophrenic parents, met diagnostic criteria for schizophrenia spectrum disorder (i.e., schizophrenia or a Cluster A personality disorder). The researchers compared these children with those who showed no evidence of psychiatric symptoms at follow-up. Of the nine with spectrum outcomes, four had extreme social isolation and aggressive behavior in childhood, and all of these were males. In contrast, the females were perceived as shy and withdrawn, but not problematic, in childhood. Interestingly, self-reports obtained during childhood indicated that the females were more likely to express feelings of insecurity and social rejection.

Retrospective data on childhood and adolescent functioning also have identified sex differences. Foerster et al. (1991b) used a modified version of the Cannon-Spoor Scale and a measure of premorbid schizotypal signs and found that male patients with schizophrenia showed more premorbid spectrum symptoms and a higher rate of adjustment problems in middle and late childhood when compared with female patients. In a study conducted by Fennig et al. (1995), the authors found a significant increase in adjustment problems for both sexes during adolescence but a more pronounced increase in behavioral deficits among preschizophrenic males. Similarly, Larsen et al. (1996) used the Cannon-Spoor Scale and found striking sex differences in developmental trajectories, with male patients showing poorer adjustment and deteriorating more rapidly during adolescence than females.

To obtain a more detailed picture of the premorbid developmental trajectory in schizophrenia, we obtained detailed retrospective parental ratings of childhood behavior (Walker et al. 1995a, 1995b). Parents of young adult patients with schizophrenia were asked to rate the childhood behavior of all their offspring at four age periods: birth to 4 years, 4–8 years, 8–12 years, and 12–16 years. The rating scale included more than 100 items that described specific behavior problems that yielded multiple factors. Preschizophrenic subjects were compared with their same-sex healthy siblings. Across all but the first age period, preschizophrenic males showed significantly higher rates of externalized behavior problems (a factor defined by aggressive and delinquent behavior items) when compared with their same-sex siblings with healthy adult outcomes. The preschizophrenic boys also showed significantly more internalized behavior (a factor defined by social withdrawal, anxiety or depression, and somatic concerns), beginning in the 4–8 age period. In contrast, preschizophrenic females did not differ from their same-sex siblings in externalized behavior, but they did manifest more internalized problems, beginning in the 8–12 age period. The preschizophrenic females also exceeded the preschizophrenic males in the rate of internalized problems. Analyses of the behavior dimensions comprising the internalized factor indicated that the depression score differentiated the male and female preschizophrenic patients more than the other behavior ratings. Specifically, across age periods, preschizophrenic females showed higher rates of depression than did both their same-sex siblings and preschizophrenic males. Furthermore, the preschizophrenic females showed a more dramatic increase in depression ratings during adolescence when compared with the other groups. Studies of community samples also report an increase in depressive symptoms among adolescent girls (Gjerde and

Block 1996), so the developmental trend observed in preschizophrenic females by Walker et al. (1995a) suggests that these "normative" sex differences in depressive symptoms are more pronounced in preschizophrenic subjects.

In our research on the precursors of schizophrenia, we also obtained childhood home movies of these patients and their siblings (Walker et al. 1993). This allowed us to directly observe facial affect in naturalistic settings. We found that the preschizophrenic females manifested significantly less positive facial emotion than did their same-sex healthy siblings, preschizophrenic males, and nonschizophrenic males. These differences were apparent as early as infancy and became more pronounced in adolescence. Thus, direct observation yields results that converge with findings from studies of behavior ratings and suggests that preschizophrenic females are more dysphoric than males.

It is noteworthy that researchers have not reported sex differences in the earliest age at which premorbid behavioral dysfunction is detected. Thus, although the nature and course of precursors vary by sex, there is no difference in the point at which the trajectory deviates from that of same-sex comparison groups.

PREMORBID COGNITIVE FUNCTIONS

In 1984, we conducted a meta-analysis of the research findings on intelligence and schizophrenia (Aylward et al. 1984). Studies of both premorbid and postmorbid intellectual functioning were included. The former were primarily analyses of data from elementary- and high-school records. The results indicated that schizophrenia was associated with a significant intellectual deficit across the life span, including the premorbid period. When the effects of sex on the magnitude of the deficit were tested, preschizophrenic males showed significantly greater deficits relative to their same-sex peers and siblings than did preschizophrenic females. Although few studies of childhood intellectual functioning in schizophrenia have been done since the publication of this review, a study of early developmental problems found that preschizophrenic males were rated by their parents as showing more significant developmental delays (Goldstein et al. 1994).

AGE AT ONSET OF ILLNESS

It is well established that poor premorbid functioning is associated with an earlier age at onset of schizophrenia. The evidence of sex differences in premorbid functioning would therefore lead us to predict that females have a later age at onset than do males. This has, in fact, been documented in numerous reports since the beginning of the twentieth century. In the early 1900s, Kraepelin proposed that men develop schizophrenia at an earlier age than do women. This was replicated in many subsequent investigations, indicating an onset of illness 2–5 years earlier in males than in females.

However, concerns about methodological factors caused some to express doubt about the validity of the findings. It was suggested that reported sex differences in age at onset might be an artifact of sex differences in hospitalization rates (e.g., a reluctance to hospitalize females), marriage rates (e.g., female patients are more likely to have spousal caregivers), or other uncontrolled extraneous variables. However, more recent well-controlled studies indicated that these factors do not account for the findings. Several comprehensive reviews of the literature on sex differences in age at onset provide a more detailed discussion of the findings (Angermeyer and Kuhn 1988; Goldstein 1995b; Lewine 1978, 1981). In this overview, we focus on some contemporary investigations that address the methodological limitations of earlier studies.

To explore the effects of criteria used for designating clinical onset, Loranger (1984) used multiple indicators of onset age. He found that the mean age at onset of the male patients ($n = 100$) was approximately 5 years earlier than that of the female patients ($n = 100$), according to all of the following three criteria: 1) first treatment, 2) first hospitalization, and 3) immediate family's first awareness of psychotic symptoms. A meta-analysis of the literature by Angermeyer and Kuhn (1988) also showed that the sex difference in age at onset holds across onset criteria. Furthermore, Hafner et al. (1989) found that the higher mean age at first hospitalization among females was not attributable to diagnostic procedures, sex differences in help-seeking behavior, or occupational status. Studies that used international data found cross-cultural consistency in the sex difference in age at onset (Hambrecht et al. 1992; Jablensky and Cole 1997). Several other investigations have replicated the finding of earlier onset in males (Faraone et al. 1994; Folnegovic-Smalc et al. 1990; Gureje 1991; Hafner et al. 1992; Ohaeri 1992; Szymanski et al. 1995). It should be mentioned, however, that some researchers have not found a sex difference in age at onset (Beiser et al. 1993; Kendler and Walsh 1995; Kirov et al. 1996).

Evidence indicates that obstetrical complications and genetic factors moderate the relations between sex and age at onset. Kirov et al. (1996) found a mean age at onset 2.6 years earlier among patients with a history of at least one definite obstetrical complication when compared with patients with no history of obstetrical complications. This effect was entirely due to the male patients with histories of obstetrical complications who had, on average, an onset 3.5 years earlier. In contrast, no sex differences in age at onset among schizophrenic patients without a history of obstetrical complications were found. Gorwood et al. (1995) found no sex difference in age at onset among patients with schizophrenia and a positive family history of the illness, but the female onset age was later for patients without a family history. Albus and Maier (1995) also found an earlier age at onset in patients with a family history of schizophrenia as well as an absence of sex differences in age at onset among patients with a family history. Albus et al. (1994) suggested that the absence of sex differences in age at onset in familial cases indicates that genetic factors override the protective effect of estrogens. In other words, the penetrance of the genotype is not reduced by the antidopaminergic action of estrogen.

Other findings suggest that sex differences in age at onset may vary among subtypes of schizophrenia. Beratis et al. (1994) found that the onset for men was earlier than for women in the paranoid subtype of schizophrenia, but the disorder occurred earlier in women in the disorganized subtype. No significant sex difference was seen in the undifferentiated and the residual subtypes. Further research is needed to explore the relation of symptom profiles to age at onset in males and females.

Several hypotheses have been posited to account for sex differences in age at onset of schizophrenia. First, as noted earlier in this chapter, some investigators have suggested that schizophrenia has heterogeneous etiologies and that subtype(s) characterized by an early onset may be overrepresented in men (Angermeyer and Kuhn 1988; Castle et al. 1995). Studies showing that the sex difference in age at onset is greater for nonfamilial cases and those with evidence of obstetrical complications support this hypothesis. Second, it has been suggested that hormonal differences account for the findings, specifically that estrogen may confer protective effects and delay illness onset (Lewine 1988; Loranger 1984; Seeman 1985; Seeman and Lang 1990). Androgens, in contrast, may have a triggering effect that leads to an earlier clinical expression in males. Third, it has been proposed that cultural and social factors lead to stressful psychosocial experiences earlier for men than for women and that these trigger psychotic episodes (Loranger 1984). Among the alternative explanations offered to date, the psychosocial stress hypothesis seems least plausible, in that sex differences in age at onset have been shown across diverse cultures.

Finally, we must consider the possibility that the sexes do not differ in onset age but rather in age at illness detection. Angermeyer and Kuhn (1988) pointed out that the illness produces different symptoms in men and women. Males with the disorder tend to have more aggressive and criminal behavior as well as more frequent substance abuse than do female patients and thus may be noticed earlier. Furthermore, the more frequent occurrence of atypical schizophrenic syndromes in women may result in an initial diagnosis other than schizophrenia and only later in a diagnosis of schizophrenia. In other words, women may escape detection for a longer time after the first appearance of symptoms associated with schizophrenia.

Extending this line of thinking, our conceptualization of schizophrenia as having a discrete onset may lack validity. As our review has shown, many patients have significant abnormalities in behavior before diagnosis. Some preschizophrenic females may reach a clinical level of depression before exceeding the clinical threshold for psychotic symptoms. If schizophrenia is reconceptualized as a "process," the critical difference between males and females may lie in the nature of the developmental trajectory.

GENERAL DISCUSSION

Examination of the factors that distinguish the sexes in the premorbid period suggests an amplification of sex differences that characterize nonschizophrenic populations. The significance of sex differences in schizophrenia may be brought into clearer focus if we interpret the findings in light of the cognitive and socioemotional differences that have been shown to distinguish males and females.

For example, studies of community samples show that males are more likely than females to have cognitive deficits. Furthermore, cognitive impairment is associated with a broad range of behavior problems, including conduct disorder and attention-deficit disorder (Moffitt 1990) as well as schizophrenia. It may be, then, that the more pronounced premorbid cognitive performance deficits associated with schizophrenia in males reflect this generalized trend.

Similarly, disruptive behavior has been shown to be more common in healthy males than in females, and this sex difference is amplified in clinical samples (Ollendick and Herson 1998). For females, the counterpart is depression; in randomly selected samples, females are more likely to show depression than are males (Paradisio and Robinson 1998), and this sex difference becomes more pronounced in the preadolescent and adolescent period (Angold et al. 1998). As noted earlier, studies of adult patients with schizophrenia also have documented higher rates of depressive symptoms in female than in male patients (Bardenstein and McGlashan 1990; Lewine 1988).

The presence of affective symptoms, particularly depression, is linked to a better prognosis for schizophrenia and psychotic disorders in general (Grossman et al. 1991; Kay and Murrill 1990; Tsuang and Coryell 1993). This link is consistent with the findings of a more favorable prognosis for women with schizophrenia (Lewine 1988). At the same time, it appears that depressive symptoms in schizophrenia are at least partially genetically determined. Subotnik et al. (1997) found that depressive symptoms in first-episode schizophrenia patients were predicted by the rate of affective disorder in biological relatives. They concluded that a genetic liability to mood disorder, when present, modifies the expression of the schizophrenic syndrome. Although the authors did not address sex differences, their speculation has relevance to the data on sex differences in the family history of schizophrenia. If, as evidence suggests, females are generally more likely than males to express the genetic liability for depression, then women with schizophrenia would be expected to manifest affective symptoms as well as a family history of mood disorder. This again suggests the possibility that family history of affective illness contributes to the apparent elevation in family history of schizophrenia among female patients.

The origins of sex differences in vulnerability to depression are still debated, although biological explanations have gained increasing support as research has provided evidence for the persistence of the phenomenon across cohorts and cultures (see Seeman 1995 for reviews). Whatever the origins, it is well established that depression is linked to certain cognitive propensities. These include a tendency toward rumination that is characterized by heightened self-monitoring and inhibition (Broderick 1998). It has been proposed that the greater propensity to rumination among females contributes to their higher rate of depression, although it also may be that depression increases ruminative cognitions.

Research has documented other normative sex differences in cognitive style. Females engage in more self-monitoring and exercise greater self-control over impulse expression than males do (Gjerde and Block 1996). Research also has shown a normative tendency for males to show more overconfidence in their judgments than females do (Pulford and Colman 1997). In particular, males are more likely than females to express high confidence in their erroneous judgments.

These normative differences in cognitive style offer another vantage point on sex differences in schizophrenia. They may play a mediating role in the relation between sex and illness expression. We have found that women with psychotic disorders are more likely than their male counterparts to label themselves mentally ill and to acknowledge that their behavior and ideations are sometimes abnormal (Walker and Rossitor 1989). Furthermore, Walker and Rossitor found that significantly more female inpatients report that they are aware in advance when they are about to have "strange or illogical" thoughts and that they use cognitive strategies in an effort to prevent them. The first step in censuring the expression of bizarre ideations is to label them as such. Thus, the female tendency toward greater self-monitoring may increase self-censoring of bizarre ideations, thereby reducing overt symptom expression.

It is intriguing to consider how these differences in cognitive style might contribute to the well-documented sex differences in the course of schizophrenia. The positive symptoms of schizophrenia, particularly hallucinations and delusions, are key criteria in contemporary diagnostic taxonomies, and clinicians often rely solely on patients' self-reports to assess the presence of these symptoms. Given that males are less behaviorally inhibited and ruminative, they may be less reticent than females to report abnormal perceptual experiences and ideations with conviction and less likely to act on them. In other words, females may have a higher threshold for expressing confidence in the accuracy of atypical perceptual experiences and ideations. This could contribute to a later age at detection of symptoms, as well as a more favorable prognosis.

The idea that the clinical expression of schizophrenia is influenced by the patient's premorbid personality and cognitive characteristics is long-standing (Amminger et al. 1994; Zigler and Levine 1981). As the study of normative sex differences in human behavior has progressed, it has become apparent that males and females differ in their socioemotional and cognitive characteristics and that these differences are, in part, a consequence of biological factors that distinguish the sexes. Thus, positing a role for cognitive style factors in determining sex differences in schizophrenia does not negate the role of hormones or other biological factors.

CONCLUSION

We have reviewed the literature pertaining to the etiological origins, premorbid course, and onset of schizophrenia. Although the research has yielded ample evidence of sex differences, the studies had limitations that may compromise the generalizability of the findings. For example, some of the sample sizes were very small, and only a few investigations explored sex differences in the longitudinal course of the illness. Furthermore, the findings suggested potentially complex moderating effects of other factors on the relation between sex and the course of the disorder.

It is obvious that many important questions remain to be addressed in research on sex differences in schizophrenia. For example, taken together, the findings from studies of family history do suggest a higher rate of psychopathology in the biological relatives of female patients with schizophrenia. What is not clear, however, is whether this sex difference is due to a specific genetic liability for schizophrenia, for affective disorder, or for both. Further research in the area may shed light on broader issues of genetic determinants to schizophrenia and the manner in which its expression is moderated by other vulnerabilities. At the psychological level of analysis, the limited available data indicate that there are sex differences in the way patients with schizophrenia conceptualize and attempt to control their symptoms. More systematic research in this area, including studies of sex differences in self-monitoring, could help to elucidate the determinants of sex differences in illness onset and course. Finally, investigations aimed at elucidating neurohormonal contributions to sex differences in schizophrenia are greatly needed. By clarifying the effect of gonadal hormones on illness expression, we may gain insight into the neurotransmitters and brain regions involved in the disorder.

REFERENCES

Albus M, Maier W: Lack of gender differences in age at onset in familial schizophrenia. Schizophr Res 18:51–57, 1995

Albus M, Scherer J, Hueber S, et al: The impact of familial loading on gender differences in age at onset of schizophrenia. Acta Psychiatr Scand 89:132–134, 1994

American Psychiatric Association: Diagnostic and Statistical Manual of Mental Disorders, 3rd Edition. Washington, DC, American Psychiatric Association, 1980

Amminger GP, Mutschlechner R, Resch F: Social competence and adolescent psychosis. Br J Psychiatry 165:273, 1994

Angermeyer MC, Kuhn L: Gender differences in age at onset of schizophrenia: an overview. European Archives of Psychiatry and Neurological Sciences 237:351–364, 1988

Angold A, Costello EJ, Worthman CM: Puberty and depression: the roles of age, pubertal status and pubertal timing. Psychol Med 28:51–61, 1998

Aylward E, Walker E, Bettes B: Intelligence in schizophrenia: meta-analysis of the research. Schizophr Bull 10:430–459, 1984

Bardenstein KK, McGlashan TH: Gender differences in affective, schizoaffective and schizophrenic disorders: a review. Schizophr Res 3:159–172, 1990

Beiser M, Erickson D, Fleming JAE, et al: Establishing the onset of psychotic illness. Am J Psychiatry 150:1349–1354, 1993

Bellodi L, Bussoleni C, Scorza-Smeraldi R, et al: Family study of schizophrenia: exploratory analysis for relevant factors. Schizophr Bull 12:120–128, 1986

Beratis S, Gabriel J, Hoidas S: Age at onset in subtypes of schizophrenic disorders. Schizophr Bull 20:287–296, 1994

Broderick P: Early adolescent gender differences in the use of ruminative and distracting coping strategies. Journal of Early Adolescence 18:173–191, 1998

Burbach DJ, Lewine R, Meltzer HY: Diagnostic concordance for schizophrenia as a function of sex. J Consult Clin Psychol 52:478–479, 1984

Cannon-Spoor HE, Potkin SG, Wyatt RJ: Measurement of premorbid adjustment in chronic schizophrenia. Schizophr Bull 8:471–484, 1982

Casar C, Artamendi M, Gutierrez M, et al: Neuropsychological deficits, obstetric complications and premorbid adjustment in patients with the first psychotic episode. Actas Luso Esp Neurol Psiquiatr Cienc Afines 25:303–307, 1997

Castle DJ, Abel K, Takei N, et al: Gender differences in schizophrenia: hormonal effect or subtypes? Schizophr Bull 21:1–12, 1995

Done JD, Crow T, Johnstone E, et al: Childhood antecedents of schizophrenia and affective illness: social adjustment at ages 7 and 11. BMJ 309:699–703, 1994

Faraone SV, Chen WJ, Goldstein JM, et al: Gender differences in age at onset of schizophrenia. Br J Psychiatry 164:625–629, 1994

Fennig S, Putnam K, Bromet EJ, et al: Gender, premorbid characteristics and negative symptoms in schizophrenia. Acta Psychiatr Scand 92:173–177, 1995

Fischer M: Genetic and environmental factors in schizophrenia. Acta Psychiatr Scand 238(suppl):61–72, 1973

Foerster A, Lewis S, Owen M, et al: Low birth weight and family history of schizophrenia predict poor premorbid functioning in psychosis. Schizophr Res 5:13–20, 1991a

Foerster A, Lewis S, Owen M, et al: Pre-morbid adjustment and personality in psychoses: effects of sex and diagnosis. Br J Psychiatry 158:171–176, 1991b

Folnegovic-Smalc V, Folnegovic Z, Kulcar Z: Age of disease onset in Croatia's hospitalized schizophrenics. Br J Psychiatry 156:368–372, 1990

Gjerde PF, Block J: A developmental perspective on depressive symptoms in adolescence: gender difference in autocentric-allocentric modes of impulse regulation, in Adolescence: Opportunities and Challenges. Edited by Cicchetti D, Toth S. Rochester, NY, University of Rochester Press, 1996, pp 167–197

Goldstein J: Gender and the familial transmission of schizophrenia, in Gender and Psychopathology. Edited by Seeman MV. Washington, DC, American Psychiatric Press, 1995a, pp 201–226

Goldstein J: The impact of gender on understanding the epidemiology of schizophrenia, in Gender and Psychophathology. Edited by Seeman MV. Washington, DC, American Psychiatric Press, 1995b, pp 159–199

Goldstein J: Sex and brain abnormalities in schizophrenia: fact or fiction? Harv Rev Psychiatry 4:110–115, 1996

Goldstein JM, Seidman LJ, Santangelo S, et al: Are schizophrenic men at higher risk for developmental deficits than schizophrenic women? Implications for adult neuropsychological functions. J Psychiatr Res 28:483–498, 1994

Gorwood P, Leboyer M, Jay M, et al: Gender and age at onset in schizophrenia: impact of family history. Am J Psychiatry 152:208–212, 1995

Gottesman I: Schizophrenia Genesis: The Origins of Madness. New York, WH Freeman, 1991

Grossman LS, Harrow M, Goldberg JF, et al: Outcome of schizoaffective disorder at two long-term follow-ups: comparisons with outcome of schizophrenia and affective disorders. Am J Psychiatry 148:1359–1365, 1991

Gureje O: Gender and schizophrenia: age at onset and sociodemographic attributes. Acta Psychiatr Scand 83:402–405, 1991

Haas GS, Garratt LS: Gender differences in social functioning, in Handbook of Social Functioning in Schizophrenia. Edited by Mueser K, Tarrier N. Boston, MA, Allyn & Bacon, 1998, pp 149–180

Hadders-Algra M, Huisjes HJ, Touwen BC: Perinatal correlates of major and minor neurological dysfunction at school age: a multivariate analysis. Dev Med Child Neurol 30:472–481, 1988a

Hadders-Algra M, Huisjes HJ, Touwen BC: Perinatal risk factors and minor neurological dysfunction: significance for behaviour and school achievement at nine years. Dev Med Child Neurol 30:482–491, 1988b

Hafner H, an der Heiden W: Epidemiology of schizophrenia: tutorial. Can J Psychiatry 42:139–151, 1997

Hafner H, Riecher A, Maurer K, et al: How does gender influence age at first hospitalization for schizophrenia? A transnational case register study. Psychol Med 19:903–918, 1989

Hafner H, Riecher-Rossler A, Maurer K, et al: First onset and early symptomatology of schizophrenia: a chapter of epidemiological and neurobiological research into age and sex differences. Eur Arch Psychiatry Clin Neurosci 242:109–118, 1992

Hambrecht M, Maurer K, Hafner H, et al: Transnational stability of gender differences in schizophrenia? An analysis based on the WHO study on determinants of outcome of severe mental disorders. Eur Arch Psychiatry Clin Neurosci 242:6–12, 1992

Hans S, Marcus J, Hensen L, et al: Interpersonal behavior of children at risk for schizophrenia. Psychiatry 55:314–335, 1992

Jablensky A, Cole S: Is the earlier age at onset of schizophrenia in males a confounded finding? Results from a cross-cultural investigation. Br J Psychiatry 170:234–240, 1997

John RS, Mednick SA, Schulsinger F: Teacher reports as a predictor of a schizophrenia and borderline schizophrenia: a Bayesian decision analysis. J Abnorm Psychol 91:399–413, 1982

Jones P, Murray R, Rodger B: Childhood risk factors for adult schizophrenia in a general population birth cohort at age 43 years, in Neural Development and Schizophrenia. Edited by Mednick SA, Hollister JM. New York, Plenum, 1995, pp 151–176

Kay SR, Murrill LM: Predicting outcome of schizophrenia: significance of symptom profiles and outcome dimensions. Compr Psychiatry 31:91–102, 1990

Kendler KS, Walsh D: Gender and schizophrenia: results from an epidemiologically based family study. Br J Psychiatry 167:184–192, 1995

Kendler KS, Gruenberg AM, Tsuang MT: Psychiatric illnesses in first-degree relatives of schizophrenic and surgical control patients: a family study using DSM-III criteria. Arch Gen Psychiatry 42:770–779, 1985

Kendler KS, Pedersen N, Johnson L, et al: A pilot Swedish twin study of affective illness, including hospital- and population-ascertained subsamples. Arch Gen Psychiatry 50:699–706, 1993

Kirov G, Jones PB, Harvey I, et al: Do obstetric complications cause the earlier age at onset in male than female schizophrenics? Schizophr Res 20:117–124, 1996

Kringlen E: An epidemiological-clinical twin study on schizophrenia, in The Transmission of Schizophrenia. Edited by Rosenthal D, Kety S. Oxford, England, Pergamon, 1968, pp 49–63

Lane A, Colgan K, Moynihan F, et al: Schizophrenia and neurological soft signs: gender differences in clinical correlates and antecedent factors. Psychiatry Res 64:105–114, 1996

Larsen TK, McGlashan TH, Johannesen JO, et al: First episode schizophrenia, II: premorbid patterns by gender. Schizophr Bull 22:257–269, 1996

Lewine RR: Response complexity and social interaction in the psychophysical testing of chronic and paranoid schizophrenics. Psychol Bull 85:284–294, 1978

Lewine R: Sex differences in schizophrenia: timing or subtypes? Psychol Bull 90:432–444, 1981

Lewine RRJ: Gender and schizophrenia, in Handbook of Schizophrenia. Edited by Tsuang MT, Simpson JC. Amsterdam, The Netherlands, Elsevier Science, 1988, pp 379–397

Lewine RJ, Seeman MV: Gender, brain and schizophrenia: anatomy of differences/differences of anatomy, in Gender and Psychopathology. Edited by Seeman MV. Washington, DC, American Psychiatric Press, 1995, pp 131–158

Loranger AW: Sex difference in age at onset of schizophrenia. Arch Gen Psychiatry 41:157–161, 1984

Mednick SA, Schulsinger F, Teasdale TW, et al: Schizophrenia in high-risk children: sex differences in predisposing factors, in Cognitive Defects in the Development of Mental Illness. Edited by Serbin G. New York, Brunner/Mazel, 1978, pp 169–197

Moffitt T: Juvenile delinquency and attention deficit disorder: boys' developmental trajectories from age 3 to age 15. Child Dev 61:893–910, 1990

Mueser KT, Bellack AS, Morrison RL, et al: Social competence in schizophrenia: premorbid adjustment, social skill and domains of functioning. J Psychiatr Res 24:51–63, 1990

Murphy BM, Burke JG, Bray JC, et al: Lack of gender differences in familial schizophrenia. Irish Journal of Psychological Medicine 14:128–131, 1997

Murray RJ, O'Callaghan E, Takai N: Genes, viruses and neurodevelopmental schizophrenia. J Psychiatr Res 26:225–235, 1992a

Murray R, O'Callaghan E, Castle DJ, et al: A neurodevelopmental approach to the classification of schizophrenia. Schizophr Bull 18:319–332, 1992b

Nasrallah HA, Wilcox JA: Gender differences in the etiology and symptoms of schizophrenia: genetic versus brain injury factors. Ann Clin Psychiatry 1:51–53, 1989

O'Callaghan E, Gibson T, Colohan HA, et al: Risk of schizophrenia in adults born after obstetric complications and their association with early onset of illness: a controlled study. BMJ 305:1256–1259, 1992

Offord DR, Cross LA: Behavioral antecedents of adult schizophrenia: a review. Arch Gen Psychiatry 21:267–283, 1969

Ohaeri JU: Age at onset in a cohort of schizophrenics in Nigeria. Acta Psychiatr Scand 86:332–334, 1992

Ollendick T, Herson M: Handbook of Child Psychopathology, 3rd Edition. New York, Plenum, 1998

Paradisio S, Robinson RG: Gender differences in poststroke depression. J Neuropsychiatry Clin Neurosci 10:41–47, 1998

Pollock HM, Malzberg B, Fuller RG: Hereditary and Environmental Factors in the Causation of Manic-Depressive Psychoses and Dementia Praecox. Utica, NY, State Hospitals Press, 1939

Pulford BD, Colman AM: Overconfidence: feedback and item difficulty effects. Personality and Individual Differences 23:125–133, 1997

Rosenthal D: Familial concordance by sex with respect to schizophrenia. Psychol Bull 59:401–421, 1962

Samuels L: Sex differences in concordance rates for schizophrenia: finding or artifact? Schizophr Bull 4:14–15, 1978

Seeman MV: Interaction of sex, age, and neuroleptic dose. Compr Psychiatry 24:124–128, 1985

Seeman MV: Gender and Psychopathology. Washington, DC, American Psychiatric Press, 1995

Seeman MV, Lang M: The role of estrogens in schizophrenia gender differences. Schizophr Bull 16:185–194, 1990

Sham PC, Gottesman II, MacLean CJ, et al: Schizophrenia: sex and familial morbidity. Psychiatry Res 52:125–134, 1994

Shimizu A, Kurachi M, Yamaguchi N, et al: Morbidity risk of schizophrenia to parents and siblings of schizophrenic patients. Japanese Journal of Psychiatry and Neurology 41:65–70, 1987

Siris S: Depression in schizophrenia, in Contemporary Issues in the Treatment of Schizophrenia. Edited by Shrique C, Nasrallah HA. Washington, DC, American Psychiatric Press, 1995, pp 155–166

Slater E: The monogenic theory of schizophrenia. Acta Genetica et Statistica Medica 8:50–56, 1958

Stromgren E: Changes in the incidence of schizophrenia? Br J Psychiatry 150:1–7, 1987

Sturt E, Shur E: Sex concordance for schizophrenia in proband-relative pairs. Br J Psychiatry 147:44–47, 1985

Subotnik KL, Nuechterlein KH, Asarnow RF, et al: Depressive symptoms in the early course of schizophrenia: relationship to familial psychiatric illness. Am J Psychiatry 154:1551–1556, 1997

Szymanski S, Lieberman JA, Alvir JM, et al: Gender differences in onset of illness, treatment response, course, and biologic indexes in first-episode schizophrenic patients. Am J Psychiatry 152:698–703, 1995

Tamminga C: Gender and schizophrenia. J Clin Psychiatry 58:33–37, 1997

Tsuang M, Coryell W: An 8-year follow-up of patients with DSM-III-R psychotic depression, schizoaffective disorder, and schizophrenia. Am J Psychiatry 150:1182–1188, 1993

Verdoux H, Geddes JR, Takei N, et al: Obstetric complications and age at onset in schizophrenia: an international collaborative meta-analysis of individual patient data. Am J Psychiatry 154:1220–1227, 1997

Walker E, Rossitor J: Schizophrenic patients' self-perceptions: legal and clinical implications. The Journal of Psychiatry and Law 17:55–73, 1989

Walker E, Downey G, Caspi A: Twin studies of psychopathology: why do the concordance rates vary? Schizophr Res 5:211–221, 1991

Walker E, Grimes K, Davis D, et al: Childhood precursors of schizophrenia; facial expressions of emotion. Am J Psychiatry 150:1654–1660, 1993

Walker E, Weinstein J, Baum K, et al: Antecedents of schizophrenia: moderating influences of age and biological sex, in Search for the Cause of Schizophrenia. Edited by Hafner H, Gattaz W. New York, Springer-Verlag, 1995a, pp 21–42

Walker E, Davis D, Weinstein J, et al: Modal developmental aspects of schizophrenia across the life-span, in The Behavioral High-Risk Paradigm in Psychopathology. Edited by Miller G. New York, Springer-Verlag, 1995b, pp 121–157

Watt NF: Longitudinal changes in the social behavior of children hospitalized for schizophrenia as adults. J Nerv Ment Dis 55:42–54, 1972

Watt NF: Patterns of childhood social development in adult schizophrenia. Arch Gen Psychiatry 35:160–165, 1978

Watt NF, Lubensky AW: Childhood roots of schizophrenia. J Consult Clin Psychol 44:363–375, 1976

Watt NF, Stolorow RD, Lubensky AW, et al: School adjustment and behavior of children hospitalized for schizophrenia as adults. Am J Orthopsychiatry 40:637–657, 1970

Wolyniec PS, Pulver AE, McGrath JA, et al: Schizophrenia: gender and familial risk. J Psychiatr Res 26:17–27, 1992

Zigler E, Levine J: Premorbid competence in schizophrenia: what is being measured? J Consult Clin Psychol 49:96–105, 1981

9

Sex Differences in Neurocognitive Function in Schizophrenia

Anne L. Hoff, Ph.D.
William S. Kremen, Ph.D.

*T*he purpose of this chapter is to describe the literature on cognitive sex differences in schizophrenia, the methodological issues regarding studies in this area, and directions for future research. As documented in a number of publications (Jensvold et al. 1996; Seeman 1995), there has been great interest in understanding the effects of sex differences on clinical presentation and outcome, cognitive function, and biological variables such as brain morphometry and neurotransmitters in psychiatric disorders. The notion is that an understanding of sex differences in schizophrenia may be important in developing 1) a better understanding of the pathophysiology of the disorder and 2) more optimum treatments for both sexes.

In the study of schizophrenia, the general consensus has been that male patients develop the illness at an earlier age than female patients (Angermeyer and Goldstein 1989). Men have more negative and fewer affective symptoms than women (Goldstein and Link 1988; Lewine 1985). Men have a worse outcome and more severe course of illness than women, at least until the age of menopause for women (Goldstein 1988; Jonsson and Nyman 1991). Recent evidence strongly suggests that cognitive function is a reasonably good predictor of functional (social and occupational functioning) outcome (Green 1996). Thus, if female patients with schizophrenia have better outcomes than males, it is reasonable to expect that they should have better cognitive function than male patients.

The literature is less consistent with regard to whether male patients have more evidence of structural brain abnormalities than female patients. Studies have found greater evidence of abnormalities in women (Hoff 1994; Nasrallah et al. 1986), greater evidence of abnormalities in men (Lewine and Seeman 1995; Nopoulos et al. 1997), or the same degree of abnormality in both (Lauriello et al. 1997). Evidence also indicates that sex differences may be important in the familial transmission of schizophrenia (Faraone and Chen 1990; Goldstein 1995). For example, some evidence indicates a greater prevalence of schizophrenia in the biological relatives of women with schizophrenia and a greater prevalence of schizotypal personality disorder in the relatives of men with schizophrenia (Goldstein et al. 1990).

A factor related to sex differences in cognition may be that males are more vulnerable to the effects of pre- or perinatal insult (Lyon et al. 1989) and are more likely to have developmental disorders such as learning disabilities and attention-deficit disorders than are females (American Psychiatric Association 1994). Boys at high risk for schizophrenia are more likely to manifest premorbid neuromotor, IQ, social, and attentional deficits (E. Aylward et al. 1984; Erlenmeyer-Kimling and Cornblatt 1984; Watt et al. 1982). Because males are more likely to have neurodevelopmental abnormalities, they may be more likely to have cognitive processing disorders as adults.

Another factor that has been postulated to be related to symptomatic and onset differences between male and female patients with schizophrenia is that of gonadal hormones. Later age at onset and less severe course of illness in females have been linked to the protective antidopaminergic properties of estrogen (Seeman and Lang 1990). Female patients with schizophrenia have been shown to have lower estrogen levels than women without schizophrenia (Kopala et al. 1995; Riecher-Rossler et al. 1994), although there are few studies in which neuroleptics are known to reduce estrogen production (Carter et al. 1982). Studies of testosterone levels in males with schizophrenia are even less common, although some evidence has shown relatively higher levels in male patients with schizophrenia compared with control subjects (Oades and Schepker 1994). The effects of hormonal fluctuations on symptoms are evident in premenstrual and postpartum exacerbations of illness (Gerada and Reveley 1988; Kendell et al. 1987), and studies have shown that schizophrenia symptoms are most severe during the cycle when estrogen levels are lowest (Riecher-Rossler et al. 1994). These findings parallel those in female control subjects who perform better on measures of verbal production and memory at the midluteal point in the menstrual cycle, one of the times when estrogen levels are highest (Hampson 1990). Whether these effects on cognition are the same or more or less pronounced in patients with schizophrenia has not been adequately studied.

For the purpose of this chapter, we have identified 10 studies published in the past decade that have specifically addressed the issue of cognitive sex differences in schizophrenia. These studies are listed chronologically in Table 9–1. We also discuss one study of cognitive sex differences in biological relatives of patients with schizophrenia. All of these studies, including our own, have numerous methodological limitations that affect the interpretation of results. Before describing each study, we discuss these limitations.

METHODOLOGICAL ISSUES

Many of the methodological issues have been thoughtfully considered by other researchers, with a focus on the issue of sex differences in schizophrenia (Goldstein 1993, 1996; Walker and Lewine 1993). Recommendations for appropriate methodology also have been made.

Failure to Address Severity, Age at Onset, and Other Clinical Differences Between Male and Female Patients

Given that male patients have greater severity of illness than females do, cognitive abilities may be more affected in males than in females with schizophrenia. However, severity of illness is a multifaceted concept that may not always be measured in the same way across studies. Age at onset may be a component of severity or at least a characteristic related to severity of illness. Age at onset of illness relates to cognitive function in patients with schizophrenia (i.e., earlier age at onset is associated with worse cognitive ability) (Hoff et al. 1996; Johnstone et al. 1989). By virtue of their earlier age at onset, male patients would be more cognitively impaired than would their female counterparts. Moreover, in some cases, the differentiation between early and late onset may be somewhat arbitrary. When age at onset is not treated as a continuous variable, differences in the choice of a cut point may change results across studies.

Clinical symptomatology is another index of severity, although it changes over time. Correlations between symptoms and cognition in schizophrenia are not always particularly strong, and cognitive deficits

TABLE 9–1.   Summary of neuropsychological studies

Study	Characteristics of sample	Patients M	Patients F	Control Subjects M	Control Subjects F	Measures	Findings
Perlick et al. 1992	Chronically ill inpatients	15	11			Mattis Dementia Rating Scale	Female patients worse than males on conceptualization; female inpatients worse than male inpatients on construction, but female outpatients better than males
	Chronically ill outpatients	13	13				
Goldstein et al. 1994	"Mid-range prognostic group of schizophrenic patients" (inpatient)	28	21			Large battery	2 of 25 cognitive variables were significantly different; males worse than females on Visual-Verbal Test and Manual Position Sequencing Test, nonpreferred hand
Andia et al. 1995	Stabilized outpatients	53	32			H-R Neuropsychological Test Battery, WAIS-R	No difference between males and females on summary measures
Goldberg et al. 1995	Chronically ill inpatients	89	39			H-R Neuropsychological Test Battery, WAIS-R	2 of 31 significant differences
							0 of 28 significant differences
	Chronically ill inpatients	41	22			Memory battery	2 of 15 significant differences
	Inpatients (private hospital)	30	27			Screening battery	1 of 23 significant differences
	Schizophrenic twins from discordant monozygotic pairs	11	9			Large battery	5 of 97 significant differences, males better than females
Lewine et al. 1996	Recruited from private and public facilities (mostly from outpatient and briefly hospitalized population)	113	43	40	59	Large battery	For patients, females more impaired than males on measures of verbal and spatial memory and visual processing; for control subjects, males better than females on verbal IQ, grip strength, motor speed, and visual processing

TABLE 9–1.   Summary of neuropsychological studies *(continued)*

Study	Characteristics of sample	Patients M	Patients F	Control Subjects M	Control Subjects F	Measures	Findings
Lewine et al. 1997	71% inpatients 29% outpatients	130	61			Large battery	Early-onset males and late-onset females more impaired than late-onset males and early-onset females
Albus et al. 1997	First-episode inpatients	37	29	20	20	Large battery	No difference between male and female patients
Seidman et al. 1997	Stable outpatients	24	16	15	17	WCST UPSIT	Male patients more impaired than female patients on WCST
Goldstein et al. 1998 (subsample of Seidman et al. 1997)	Stable outpatients	17	14	13	14	Large battery	Group by sex interaction significant for executive function (male patients worse than female patients); effect sizes larger for male–male comparisons than female–female comparisons
Hoff et al. 1998	First-episode inpatients Chronically ill inpatients	41 56	17 18	56	18	Large battery	No difference between male and female patients after controlling for age at onset and symptoms

Note.   H–R=Halstead-Reitan;   UPSIT=University   of   Pennsylvania   Smell   Identification   Test;   WAIS-R=Wechsler   Adult   Intelligence   Scale—Revised; WCST=Wisconsin Card Sorting Test.

often persist even after relative remission of symptoms (Gold and Harvey 1993; Seidman et al. 1992). When cognition–symptom correlations are significant, they tend to be stronger for negative or disorganization symptoms than for delusions or hallucinations (Basso et al. 1998). Men with schizophrenia have more negative and fewer paranoid symptoms than women with schizophrenia (Goldstein and Link 1988); thus, men may manifest more cognitive impairment as well. Measures of social or occupational functioning are also indices of severity of illness. Goldstein (1996) recommended that only patients in remission be tested because sex differences may be blurred by the predominance of state-related effects when testing acutely ill patients. Although symptomatic differences still may be present, this strategy seeks to minimize possible effects of symptomatic differences on cognitive abilities between the sexes.

Sampling Biases

Goldstein (1996) pointed out that female patients with better outcomes are underrepresented in studies comparing chronically ill males with chronically ill females, thereby attenuating the differences that normally would be seen. By extension, sex differences should be relatively greater in younger, less chronically ill patients. Consequently, one might predict an age by sex interaction in which cognitive differences would be greater in younger than in older patients with schizophrenia. In a similar vein, Walker and Lewine (1993) argued that the threshold for involuntary treatment is lower for males than for females. As a result, involuntarily committed females in places such as state hospitals will have a higher severity of illness than their male counterparts. Following this line of reasoning, the prediction would be that in voluntary populations, which are less severely ill, male patients would show more impairment; among involuntary populations, female patients should show more impairment by virtue of their relatively greater severity of illness. Neither of these predictions has been adequately tested to date.

Heterogeneity of Patient Samples

Some studies have combined inpatients and outpatients, placing patients in different phases or acuity of illness together. Inconsistencies across different studies may be created by different distributions of newly admitted patients and relatively stable inpatients or outpatients between the sex groups. Given the considerations noted in the previous two subsections, these kinds of heterogeneity could easily obscure or create inconsistencies in sex difference findings.

Lack of a Control Group

Many studies have not included control subjects. Because sex differences exist in cognitive processes between males and females without schizophrenia (Collaer and Hines 1995; Halpern 1992), finding sex differences in patients with schizophrenia may reflect, in part, normally occurring variation between the sexes.

Poorly Matched Control Subjects

Inclusion of a control group is important, but it is equally important that patients and control subjects be appropriately matched on relevant demographic characteristics. Goldstein (1996) argued that control subjects must be matched to patients based on premorbid ability and that matching should occur *within* sex. Some studies have indicated that patients and control subjects were matched overall, but the lack of specific matching within sex made it difficult to properly interpret sex difference results. Ideally, patients and control subjects should be matched on (premorbid) intellectual capacity, race/ethnicity, and handedness. Current IQ or education should not be used as a matching variable because these are usually attenuated as a consequence of schizophrenic illness (Meehl 1970). Reasonable estimates of premorbid intellectual functioning include parental education or parental socioeconomic status and oral word recognition tests, such as the reading subtest of the Wide Range Achievement Test (WRAT-R or WRAT-III) or the National Adult Reading Test (Kremen et al. 1996).

Lack of Appropriate Statistics

Because of normally occurring sex differences, the true test of whether there are meaningful sex differences in the cognitive processes of patients with schizophrenia should be a significant group by sex interaction, in which it can be shown that sex differences in patients with schizophrenia are different from sex differences in control subjects. This interaction cannot be interpreted properly if, as indicated by Goldstein (1996), the subgroups composing it are not demographically matched within sex.

Small Sample Sizes

Effect sizes between male and female control subjects vary depending on the function being measured (e.g., verbal, spatial, analytic) and on the test used to measure it. Cognitive differences tend to be small in the general population, accounting for only about 4%–5% of the variance (Halpern

1992). Cohen's (1988) convention for small effect sizes was 0.20 or less. Hyde and Linn (1988), in their meta-analysis of verbal abilities, found effect sizes ranging from 0.02 in vocabulary to 0.33 in speech production; the average effect size was 0.11 across all verbal tasks, with females performing better than males. Effect sizes for visual-spatial abilities ranged from 0.13 on measures of spatial visualization to 0.91 for mental rotation tests, with males performing better than females (Linn and Petersen 1986). In general, females are superior to males on measures of verbal ability, particularly speech production or fluency, whereas males excel on measures that require visual-spatial processing, particularly if an element of mental rotation is involved. The lack of consistency in studies of cognitive sex differences in schizophrenia suggests that effect sizes for schizophrenia may be relatively small as well. If effect sizes on many cognitive tests are relatively small, larger samples are required to detect statistical significance between the sexes in both patient and control groups. Thus, some studies may lack adequate statistical power and may increase the risk of type II error (failure to detect presence of statistically significant differences) (Cohen 1988).

REVIEW OF STUDIES WITHOUT CONTROL GROUPS

Studies without control groups were generally the first to be conducted to determine sex differences in cognition in schizophrenia. Although these studies lacked an important component, they have given the field a start in addressing this issue. Perlick et al. (1992) studied 26 continuously hospitalized inpatients (>18 months) and 26 clinically stable outpatients (>3 years in the community without hospitalization) with chronic schizophrenia from an urban state hospital setting. Their measure of cognitive function was the Mattis Dementia Rating Scale, which provides measures of attention, memory, initiation and perseveration, conceptualization, and construction. Use of group (inpatient, outpatient) by sex analyses of covariance (ANCOVAs) with age, total Brief Psychiatric Rating Scale (BPRS) score, and age at onset as covariates showed that female patients were more impaired than male patients on the conceptualization scale (main effect for sex). Females also were more impaired than males on the construction scale in the inpatient sample but better than the males in the outpatient sample. This was the only significant interaction. Effect sizes on most of the scales between the sexes were much greater in the inpatient sample (>0.73) than in the outpatient sample (<0.26). These effect sizes suggest little difference in the outpatient sample. The strengths of this study were that the authors compared two homogeneous and well-characterized samples and also controlled for variables in their statistical analyses that could affect neuropsychological performance; however, the sample sizes were small, and there were ceiling effects on subtests of the Mattis Dementia Rating Scale. In addition, the Mattis Dementia Rating Scale may not be an appropriate test for patients with schizophrenia because it was designed for a different population and does not include a wide variety of cognitive measures.

Goldstein et al. (1994) studied 28 male and 21 female patients with schizophrenia recruited from the inpatient services of three teaching hospitals. These patients had been part of other studies that required them to be moderately treatment responsive (must have functioned well without antipsychotic medications for 4 consecutive months during the preceding 2 years and had no more than 6 months of continuous hospitalization). A neuropsychological battery consisting of 25 variables derived from 17 tests was administered. Male patients were significantly more impaired than females on two measures: the Visual-Verbal Test (a measure of abstract thinking) and the nonpreferred hand performance of the Manual Position Sequencing Test. Latent class analysis was used to identify possible subtypes; two classes of patients were detected. Class 1 was more likely to consist of patients who were male (100%) and who had developmental learning problems and negative symptoms. Class 2 was less likely to have learning difficulties and negative symptoms and more likely to be female (63%). In comparing the neuropsychological performances of these groups, Class 1 showed greater neuropsychological impairment than Class 2, particularly on measures of verbal intellectual functioning, fluency, and verbal memory.

The authors concluded that patients with schizophrenia and histories of early developmental problems had more neuropsychological dysfunction as adults and were more likely to be men. Developmental learning problems, which tend to be associated with verbal deficits, are more common in males in general. Nevertheless, these results still point to a cluster of characteristics that may be associated with sex differences and are likely to be relevant to treatment or outcome in schizophrenia. Unlike most other studies, the goal of this study was to simultaneously examine particular configurations of patient characteristics rather than to specifically study cognitive sex differences in schizophrenia. In terms of neurocognitive function specifically, few sex differences were seen; only 2 of 25 cognitive variables were significant.

Andia et al. (1995) studied 85 stable outpatients with schizophrenia referred from a university-affiliated outpatient service with the Wechsler Adult Intelligence Scale—Revised (WAIS-R) and summary measures of the Halstead-Reitan Neuropsychological Test Battery. Although clinical differences were found between male and female patients (women were more likely to have paranoid or disorganized subtypes, were taking less medication, and were more likely to be better educated, married, living independently, and employed than were men), no significant differences were seen between the sexes on the intellectual measures and summary measures of the Halstead-Reitan Battery. On the basis of demographic characteristics, female patients in the study appeared to be higher functioning than their male counterparts yet did not manifest any cognitive advantages. However, examination of only summary measures may have obscured differences in particular domains of function.

Goldberg et al. (1995) analyzed neuropsychological data from four separate cohorts of patients: two groups of patients with chronic schizophrenia from a tertiary care facility, a group of patients with schizophrenia from a private psychiatric hospital, and twins with schizophrenia from discordant monozygotic twin pairs. After computing 97 t tests from these four samples, they found that 5 of 97 were statistically significant, all in the direction of males performing better than females. Significant differences were not observed in any one sample more than the others.

REVIEW OF STUDIES WITH CONTROL GROUPS

Lewine et al. (1996) studied 156 patients with schizophrenia, 39 patients with schizoaffective disorder, and 99 control subjects, using a comprehensive neuropsychological test battery measuring language, executive function, verbal memory, spatial memory, visual processing, concentration, and motor function. Patients were recruited from both public and private facilities through the Clinical Research Program and Schizophrenic Disorders Program at the Emory University School of Medicine. The exact breakdown by facility or inpatient and outpatient status was not given. Data were analyzed separately for patient and control groups with one-way between-groups (male, female) analyses of variance on summary scores of the cognitive domains plus composite measures of left- and right-hemisphere functioning and individual test variables.

For the control subjects, males performed significantly better than females on the WAIS-R Verbal IQ, on measures of grip strength and motor speed (bilaterally), and on Judgment of Line Orientation, a measure of visual-perceptual ability. For the patients, males outperformed females on measures of verbal memory, spatial memory, visual processing, and putative right-hemisphere domains. The authors concluded that schizophrenia in women may be due to right-hemisphere dysfunction, although verbal memory also was one of the functions on which male patients performed better than female patients. Even though female patients in this study had a later age at onset, they were still more significantly impaired than males on neurocognitive measures. Symptoms as measured by the Scale for the

Assessment of Positive Symptoms were similar between the sexes. Group by sex interactions were not examined.

In a subsequent article based on a similar population and the same neuropsychological measures, Lewine et al. (1997) broke down male and female patient groups into early- and late-onset groups, defining early onset as 25 years or younger and late onset as older than 25 years at first psychiatric hospitalization. Several statistically significant sex by onset interactions were found: early-onset men and late-onset women were more significantly impaired than late-onset men and early-onset women. Although the authors had predicted that early-onset patients would be more cognitively impaired than later-onset patients, worse performance by late-onset women was not expected.

Albus et al. (1997) studied 66 patients in their first episode of schizophrenia consecutively recruited from acutely admitted inpatients at a state hospital in Germany with a battery of neuropsychological tests. Forty control subjects (20 males and 20 females) were matched to 40 of the first-episode patients on age, sex, and education. Raw test scores were converted to z scores and grouped into the following cognitive domains: verbal intelligence and language; spatial organization; verbal memory and learning; visual memory; short-term memory; visual-motor processing and attention; information processing and attention; and abstraction-flexibility. There were statistically significant main effects for the group, with patients performing worse than control subjects, and main effects for sex (females better than males on verbal intelligence and language, and males better than females on spatial organization). No statistically significant group by sex interactions were found, suggesting that sex did not modify cognitive dysfunction in these patients with schizophrenia.

Seidman et al. (1997) studied 40 clinically stable outpatients with chronic schizophrenia and compared them with 32 control subjects matched on age, sex, handedness, parental socioeconomic status, ethnicity, and premorbid intellectual ability estimated by the reading subtest of the WRAT-R. Neuropsychological tests included the Wisconsin Card Sorting Test (WCST), University of Pennsylvania Smell Identification Test, and auditory and visual versions of the Continuous Performance Test. There were statistically significant group effects for all of the tests (patients with schizophrenia worse than control subjects), main effects for sex on the WCST variables (females better than males), and group by sex interactions on the WCST variables (males with schizophrenia performing worse than females with schizophrenia).

Goldstein et al. (1998) studied 17 male and 14 female stable chronically ill outpatients with schizophrenia who were demographically matched, *within* sex, to control subjects. Age at onset also was similar in male and female patients. Subjects in this study were largely a subset of those in the study by Seidman et al. (1997). Their comprehensive neuropsychological test battery included the following functions: attention; language; verbal memory; nonverbal memory; and executive, visual-spatial, and motor function. Male patients were significantly worse than male control subjects on all functions; female patients were significantly worse than female control subjects on attention, executive, visual memory, and motor functions. Male patients performed worse than female patients on attention, executive, and verbal memory functions. The only significant group by sex interaction was for executive function, but power to detect interactions was low with the small sample sizes. Effect sizes for male–male comparisons were larger than effect sizes for female–female comparisons by 0.80 standard deviation for executive function, 0.60 standard deviation for language, and 0.74 standard deviation for visual-spatial ability, indicating that male patients had significantly greater degrees of cognitive impairment than did female patients relative to their respective control counterparts. Note that these differences in effect sizes were the same when looking at male versus female patients with schizophrenia compared with male versus female control subjects. It is not known how psychiatric symptoms may have related to cognitive impairment in these patients.

Hoff et al. (1998) evaluated two groups of patients with schizophrenia—a first-episode group ($n=58$) and a chronically institutionalized group ($n=74$)—and a group of normal control subjects ($n=74$), using a comprehensive battery of neuropsychological tests that measured the following domains: language, executive function, verbal memory, spatial memory, concentration/speed, and sensory-perceptual function. Because the groups were mismatched on age and premorbid intellectual ability (WRAT-R), the authors performed multivariate ANCOVAs on the groups of individual tests constituting each domain with age and WRAT-R scores as covariates. On the basis of previous work in which they found age at onset to be positively correlated with cognitive performance in patients with schizophrenia (Hoff et al. 1996), these investigators predicted that male patients would be more impaired than female patients by virtue of their earlier age at onset but that differences between the sexes would be eliminated after considering onset age as a covariate. Statistically significant main effects were observed for group (patients with schizophrenia more impaired than control subjects) and sex (males performed better than females on executive, spatial memory, and concentration/speed; females were better than males on verbal memory). There were significant group by sex interactions in the spatial memory and sensory-perceptual domains, with the post hoc comparison indicating that only chronically ill males were more impaired than chronically ill females. After including age at onset as an additional covariate, these group by sex interactions remained statistically significant.

Post hoc comparisons on individual tests indicated that chronically ill males were more impaired than chronically ill females on the Benton Visual Retention Test, whereas no significant differences were observed on other individual tests. Because chronically ill males had higher scores on the positive symptom scale of the BPRS and because both the positive and the negative symptom scales were associated with spatial memory variables (higher symptom scores associated with worse performance), positive and negative symptom scales were added as covariates in these analyses. Differences between chronically ill male and female patients were eliminated after accounting for variance due to symptomatic differences. It was concluded that cognitive sex differences in schizophrenia were not robust findings and were likely associated with symptomatic and age at onset differences between sexes. That is, it appears that severity of illness accounts for much more of the variance in neurocognitive performance than do sex differences.

The lack of sex differences in cognitive function in the first-episode patients could have been because this consecutive admission sample was tested a relatively brief time after admission (2–4 weeks). Thus, the influence of state-related factors may have obscured sex differences in cognition in this young, non–chronically ill sample. Compared with functioning closer to the time of admission, neurocognitive performance in schizophrenia tends to improve when patients are ready for discharge and may even improve further up to a year after discharge (Sweeney et al. 1991).

The Hoff et al. (1998) data in chronically ill patients, however, do not support the notion that an overrepresentation of severely ill females in involuntary settings would either attenuate differences between sexes or result in females having greater cognitive impairment than males. Chronically ill males were more impaired than chronically ill females on measures of spatial memory, although after symptomatology (male symptoms worse than female symptoms) was additionally controlled, these differences were eliminated.

NEUROCOGNITIVE FUNCTION IN THE RELATIVES OF PATIENTS WITH SCHIZOPHRENIA

As noted in the introduction to this chapter, some evidence suggests that sex differences may be important in the familial transmission of schizophrenia (Faraone and Chen 1990; Goldstein 1995). Several studies also have found neuropsychological deficits in nonpsychotic biological relatives of patients with schizophrenia compared with demographically matched nonschizophrenic control subjects (Cannon et al. 1994; Faraone et al. 1995;

Keefe et al. 1994; Mirsky et al. 1992), and it has been suggested that such deficits may reflect risk indicators for schizophrenia (Kremen et al. 1994). Consequently, Kremen et al. (1997) examined sex differences in neuropsychological function in 54 nonpsychotic relatives of patients with schizophrenia and 72 healthy control subjects. Relatives and control subjects were matched within sex on age, parental education, estimated intellectual ability (WRAT-R), and handedness. There were significant group by sex interactions for verbal memory and motor function and trends ($P<0.10$) toward significant interactions for auditory attention and mental control-encoding. With the exception of motor function, the female relatives accounted for most of the impairment. The results could not be accounted for by psychopathology in the relatives. These group by sex interactions remained for measures that were included in a 4-year follow-up study of this sample (Faraone et al. 1999).

A speculative explanation for the findings is that women may have a higher threshold than men for developing schizophrenia. Differing thresholds would imply a sex difference in the population prevalence of schizophrenia. Although controversial, some studies have indeed suggested higher rates of schizophrenia in men (Castle et al. 1994; Iacono and Beiser 1992a; Kendler and Walsh 1995). If women did have a higher threshold for developing the illness, then female relatives might be able to withstand greater impairments than men before developing psychotic symptoms. Consequently, in a sample that was limited to nonpsychotic relatives—as in the study by Kremen et al. (1994)—both less impaired men and more impaired women could be overrepresented.

Alternatively, these group by sex interactions might be explained, in part, by differences in estrogen levels between female relatives and female control subjects. Estrogen data were not available for these women. However, some data suggest that women with schizophrenia have lower-than-normal estrogen levels (Riecher-Rossler and Hafner 1993), and recent work by Hoff et al. (2001) indicated that estrogen levels are very strongly positively correlated with cognitive performance in women with chronic schizophrenia. Thus, certain hormonal abnormalities in women could reflect genetically mediated liability for schizophrenic cognitive impairment.

SUMMARY OF FINDINGS

We have reviewed 10 studies conducted in the past decade that examined a total of 698 male patients with schizophrenia and 372 female patients with schizophrenia on a variety of neuropsychological measures. Unfortunately, we were unable to perform a meta-analysis of these studies because 1) there was not enough overlap of the same neuropsychological measures, and 2) raw individual test data broken down by sex were frequently not reported. Based on our review of studies performed on this topic over the past decade, we believe that firm conclusions regarding cognitive sex differences in schizophrenia are not yet possible given the inconsistency of findings.

In direct comparisons of male and female patients on cognitive measures, 5 of the 10 studies found essentially no differences between the two groups. However, combining these studies presents problems because of the differences in patient sample and methodology. Two studies of first-episode inpatients (Albus et al. 1997; Hoff et al. 1998) did not find evidence of sex differences, although an argument could be made that because these patients were tested close to the time of admission, clinical state effects may have predominated over more traitlike cognitive differences. Studies of chronically ill inpatients showed a mixed pattern, with females worse than males (Perlick et al. 1992) or little evidence of sex differences (Goldberg et al. 1995; Goldstein et al. 1994; Hoff et al. 1998). Studies of more stable chronically ill outpatients showed a mixed pattern as well. Male patients were more impaired than females in one sample (Goldstein et al. 1998; Seidman et al. 1997) but showed essentially no cognitive differences in two other outpatient samples (Andia et al. 1995; Perlick et al. 1992). Lewine et al. (1996) found more cognitive impairment in females than in males, but their study included a mixture of inpatients and outpatients.

Factors that might account for the inconsistencies in these results are not readily apparent. Age at onset in these studies was either very similar for men and women or controlled for statistically. Other possible indicators of severity of illness such as symptom ratings, marital status, employment status, and living status also were similar or slightly better in female patients. Although these results did not suggest that sex differences in cognition varied as a function of inpatient versus outpatient status, a more careful examination of the outpatient samples is still relevant because arguments put forth by Goldstein (1996) and by Walker and Lewine (1993) suggested that sex differences in cognitive function should be more readily apparent in outpatients. In addition, these authors argued that sex differences would be attenuated in chronically ill samples because women with poor outcome would be overrepresented. Because all of the outpatient studies examined chronically ill patients, the studies conducted to date do not constitute an adequate test of these ideas.

In the outpatient sample studied by Perlick et al. (1992), female patients were nonsignificantly better than male patients on three of five scales, but the effect sizes were small (0.12–0.26). The largest effect size (0.41) was on the conceptualization scale, in which males performed better than females.

The effect size for the total Mattis Dementia Rating Scale score among these outpatients was 0.33, with females showing more overall impairment than males. Male and female outpatients in this study had similar age at onset, duration of illness, and BPRS symptom ratings.

In the study by Andia et al. (1995), female patients were significantly more likely to be paranoid subtype, employed, married, or living independently than were male patients. They also were significantly more educated than the men but did not differ in age at onset or symptoms rated according to the Scale for the Assessment of Negative Symptoms and Scale for the Assessment of Positive Symptoms. As already indicated, particular neuropsychological differences could have been overlooked because the authors examined only summary IQ and neuropsychological measures. Although the groups did not differ cognitively, one might have expected the female patients to have performed better than the males. That is, given the significantly higher education in the women and other clinical and demographic differences, one might expect better rather than equal performance, even on the global measures that were used. The literature suggests that recovered or less disabled patients who would not be part of these chronic samples are more likely to be women; however, based on several typical indices, the female patients who were in the Andia et al. sample were, in fact, less disabled and had better outcomes than the male patients but still had similar or worse cognitive function (given their educational differences).

The results of Seidman et al. (1997) and Goldstein et al. (1998) indicated that male outpatients were significantly worse than female outpatients on several neuropsychological functions. Effect sizes were moderate to large. Male and female patients had similar age at onset, duration of illness, and parental socioeconomic status. Although premorbid intellectual ability (WRAT-R) and education were not significantly different in male and female patients, IQ was significantly lower in male than in female patients. Thus, the pattern in this sample was in the opposite direction of the Andia et al. (1993) findings.

Based largely on likely selection bias, the argument made by Goldstein (1996) and by Walker and Lewine (1993) that sex differences will be attenuated in chronically ill samples is a compelling one. However, it does not appear to be sufficient to account for the varying results in these outpatient samples. Selection bias leading to a reduction in the presumed cognitive advantage of female over male patients with schizophrenia might explain a lack of differences; however, it cannot explain findings that go in opposing directions as noted. Thus, some other factor(s), in addition to selection bias, must be affecting the results.

The patient groups in these different studies were matched on demographic and clinical characteristics, or in the case of Andia et al. (1995),

common in males than in females. This issue remains unresolved, but some studies do suggest that the prevalence of schizophrenia is increased in males, even in first-episode patients (Castle et al. 1994; Iacono and Beiser 1992a, 1992b; Kendler and Walsh 1995). As we have already explained, the findings of group by sex interactions indicating the most impairment among nonpsychotic female relatives of patients with schizophrenia are consistent with an increased prevalence of schizophrenia among males (Kremen et al. 1997).

In addition to being more vulnerable to neurodevelopmental problems, males do not have the advantage that estrogen may confer on both cognition and symptoms in female patients. We believe that gonadal hormones may have an important role as a modulatory influence on cognition and symptoms in schizophrenia. In our own work, we have found very strong positive correlations (r_s of Global scale with estrogen=0.86) between average estrogen level (drawn weekly over 4 consecutive weeks) and neuropsychological performance in chronically hospitalized female patients with schizophrenia (Hoff et al. 2001). In male patients, testosterone levels were negatively correlated with neuropsychological performance but much less strongly than with estrogen. These findings suggest that gonadal hormones (particularly estrogen) are strongly associated with cognitive performance in schizophrenia. Thus, differences in hormone levels may be one factor accounting for some of the inconsistencies across studies.

Additional studies relating hormones to cognition and symptoms in schizophrenia are necessary to establish their role in this disorder. The greater neuropsychological impairment in nonpsychotic female relatives of schizophrenic patients also might be a function of reduced levels of estrogen. These findings in biological relatives suggest that neurocognitive impairment and/or reduced levels of estrogen also may be related to genetic influences in schizophrenia. Our data relating hormones to cognition (Hoff et al. 2001) also may have implications for the role of hormone replacement in the treatment of schizophrenia, parallel to the relatively recent use of estrogen therapies in patients with Alzheimer's disease (Henderson 1995).

In conclusion, we believe that sex differences are best viewed as a modulating influence on both cognitive function and symptom expression in this disorder. Two of the more likely pathways of these influences are differences in 1) vulnerability to neurodevelopmental abnormalities and 2) levels of gonadal hormones. As such, researchers should examine the possible influence of sex differences in studies of schizophrenia.

REFERENCES

Albus M, Hubmann W, Mohr F, et al: Are there gender differences in neuropsychological performance in patients with first-episode schizophrenia? Schizophr Res 28:39–50, 1997

American Psychiatric Association: Diagnostic and Statistical Manual of Mental Disorders, 3rd Edition, Revised. Washington, DC, American Psychiatric Association, 1987

American Psychiatric Association: Diagnostic and Statistical Manual of Mental Disorders, 4th Edition. Washington, DC, American Psychiatric Association, 1994

American Psychiatric Association: Diagnostic and Statistical Manual of Mental Disorders, 4th Edition, Text Revision. Washington, DC, American Psychiatric Association, 2000

Andia A, Zisook S, Heaton R, et al: Gender differences in schizophrenia. J Nerv Ment Dis 183:522–528, 1995

Angermeyer MC, Goldstein JM: Gender differences in schizophrenia: rehospitalization and community survival. Psychol Med 19:365–382, 1989

Aylward E, Walker E, Bettes B: Intelligence in schizophrenia: meta-analysis of the research. Schizophr Bull 10:430–459, 1984

Aylward GP, Pfeiffer SI, Wright A, et al: Outcome studies of low birth weight infants published in the last decade: a metaanalysis. J Pediatr 115:515–520, 1989

Basso MR, Nasrallah HA, Olson SC, et al: Neuropsychological correlates of negative, disorganized and psychotic symptoms in schizophrenia. Schizophr Res 31:99–111, 1998

Buka SL, Lipsett LP, Tsuang MT: Emotional and behavioral development of low-birthweight infants, in Advances in Applied Developmental Psychology. Edited by Friedman SL, Sigman MD. Norwood, NJ, Ablex, 1992, pp 21–36

Cannon TD, Zorrilla LE, Shtasel D, et al: Neuropsychological functioning in siblings discordant for schizophrenia and healthy volunteers. Arch Gen Psychiatry 51:651–661, 1994

Carter DA, McGarrick GM, Norton KR, et al: The effect of chronic neuroleptic treatment on gonadotropin release. Psychoneuroendocrinology 7:201–207, 1982

Castle DJ, Sham PC, Wessely S, et al: The subtyping of schizophrenia in men and women: a latent class analysis. Psychol Med 24:41–51, 1994

Cohen J: Statistical Power Analysis for the Behavioral Sciences, 2nd Edition. Hillsdale, NJ, Lawrence Erlbaum, 1988

Collaer M, Hines M: Human behavioral sex differences: a role for gonadal hormones during early development? Psychol Bull 118:55–107, 1995

Erlenmeyer-Kimling L, Cornblatt B: Biobehavioral risk factors in children of schizophrenic parents. J Autism Dev Disord 14:357–373, 1984

Faraone S, Chen W: Sex differences in the familiar transmission of schizophrenia. Br J Psychiatry 156:819–826, 1990

Faraone SV, Seidman LJ, Kremen WS, et al: Neuropsychological functioning among the nonpsychotic relatives of schizophrenic patients: a diagnostic efficiency analysis. J Abnorm Psychol 104:286–304, 1995

Faraone SV, Seidman LJ, Kremen WS, et al: Neuropsychological functioning among the nonpsychotic relatives of schizophrenic patients: a 4-year follow-up study. J Abnorm Psychol 108:176–181, 1999

Feinberg I: Schizophrenia: caused by a fault in programmed synaptic elimination during adolescence? J Psychiatr Res 4:319–334, 1982

Gerada C, Reveley A: Schizophreniform psychosis associated with the menstrual cycle. Journal of Preventative Psychiatry 1:5–15, 1988

Gold JM, Harvey PD: Cognitive deficits in schizophrenia. Psychiatr Clin North Am 16:295–312, 1993

Goldberg TE, Gold JM, Torrey EF, et al: Lack of sex differences in the neuropsychological performance of patients with schizophrenia. Am J Psychiatry 152:883–888, 1995

Goldstein J: Gender differences in the course of schizophrenia. Am J Psychiatry 145:684–689, 1988

Goldstein J: Sampling biases in studies on gender and schizophrenia: a reply. Schizophr Bull 19:9–14, 1993

Goldstein JM: Gender and the familial transmission of schizophrenia, in Gender and Psychopathology. Edited by Seeman MV. Washington, DC, American Psychiatric Press, 1995, pp 201–226

Goldstein JM: Sex and brain abnormalities in schizophrenia: fact or fiction? Harv Rev Psychiatry 4:110–115, 1996

Goldstein JM, Link BG: Gender and the expression of schizophrenia. J Psychiatr Res 22:141–155, 1988

Goldstein J, Faraone S, Chen W, et al: Sex differences in the familial transmission of schizophrenia. Br J Psychiatry 156:819–826, 1990

Goldstein JM, Seidman LJ, Santangelo S, et al: Are schizophrenic men at higher risk for developmental deficits than schizophrenic women? Implications for adult neuropsychological functions. J Psychiatr Res 28:483–498, 1994

Goldstein JM, Seidman LJ, Goodman JM, et al: Are there sex differences in neuropsychological functions among patients with schizophrenia? Am J Psychiatry 155:1358–1364, 1998

Green MF: What are the functional consequences of neurocognitive deficits in schizophrenia? Am J Psychiatry 153:321–330, 1996

Halpern DF: Sex Differences in Cognitive Abilities, 2nd Edition. Hillsdale, NJ, Lawrence Erlbaum, 1992

Hampson E: Variations in sex-related cognitive abilities across the menstrual cycle. Brain Cogn 14:26–43, 1990

Henderson VW: Alzheimer's disease in women: is there a role for estrogen replacement therapy? Menopause Management 4:10–13, 1995

Hoff AL: Gender differences in corpus callosum size in first-episode schizophrenics. Biol Psychiatry 35:913–919, 1994

Hoff AL, Harris D, Faustman WO, et al: A neuropsychological study of early onset schizophrenia. Schizophr Res 20:21–28, 1996

Hoff AL, Kremen WS, Wieneke M, et al: Association of estrogen levels with neuropsychological performance in women with schizophrenia. Am J Psychiatry 158:1134–1139, 2001

Hoff AL, Wieneke M, Horon R, et al: Sex differences in neuropsychological functioning of first episode and chronically ill schizophrenic patients. Am J Psychiatry 155:1437–1439, 1998

Hyde JS, Linn MC: Gender differences in verbal ability: a meta-analysis. Psychol Bull 104:53–69, 1988

Iacono W, Beiser M: Are males more likely than females to develop schizophrenia? Am J Psychiatry 149:1070–1074, 1992a

Iacono WG, Beiser M: Where are the women in first-episode studies of schizophrenia? Schizophr Bull 18:471–480, 1992b

Jensvold MF, Halbreich U, Hamilton JA: Psychopharmacology and Women: Sex, Gender, and Hormones. Washington, DC, American Psychiatric Press, 1996

Johnstone EC, Owens DG, Bydder GM, et al: The spectrum of structural brain changes in schizophrenia: age of onset as a predictor of cognitive and clinical impairments and their cerebral correlates. Psychol Med 19:91–103, 1989

Jonsson H, Nyman AK: Predicting long-term outcome in schizophrenia. Acta Psychiatr Scand 83:342–346, 1991

Keefe RS, Silverman JM, Roitman SE, et al: Performance of nonpsychotic relatives of schizophrenic patients on cognitive test. Psychiatry Res 53:1–12, 1994

Kendell RE, Chalmers JC, Platz C: Epidemiology and puerperal psychoses. Br J Psychiatry 150:662–673, 1987

Kendler KS, Walsh D: Gender and schizophrenia: results of an epidemiologically based family study. Br J Psychiatry 167:184–192, 1995

Kopala L, Good K, Honer W: Olfactory identification ability in pre- and postmenopausal women with schizophrenia. Biol Psychiatry 38:57–63, 1995

Kremen WS, Seidman LJ, Pepple JR, et al: Neuropsychological risk indicators for schizophrenia: a review of family studies. Schizophr Bull 20:103–119, 1994

Kremen WS, Seidman LF, Faraone SV, et al: The "3 Rs" and neuropsychological function in schizophrenia: an empirical test of the matching fallacy. Neuropsychology 10:22–31, 1996

Kremen WS, Goldstein JM, Seidman LJ, et al: Sex differences in neuropsychological function in non-psychotic relatives of schizophrenic probands. Psychiatry Res 66:131–144, 1997

Lauriello J, Hoff AL, Wieneke MH, et al: Similar extent of brain dysmorphology in severely ill women and men with schizophrenia. Am J Psychiatry 154:819–825, 1997

Lewine R: Schizophrenia: an amotivational syndrome in men. Can J Psychiatry 30:316–318, 1985

Lewine RR, Seeman MV: Gender, brain, and schizophrenia, in Gender and Psychopathology. Edited by Seeman MV. Washington, DC, American Psychiatric Press, 1995, pp 131–158

Lewine RR, Walker EF, Shurett R, et al: Sex differences in neuropsychological functioning among schizophrenic patients. Am J Psychiatry 153:1178–1184, 1996

Lewine RR, Haden C, Caudle J, et al: Sex-onset effects on neuropsychological function in schizophrenia. Schizophr Bull 25:51–61, 1997

Linn MC, Petersen AC: A meta-analysis of gender differences in spatial ability: implications for mathematics and science achievement, in The Psychology of Gender: Advances Through Meta-Analysis. Edited by Hyde JS, Linn MC. Baltimore, MD, Johns Hopkins University Press, 1986, pp 67–101

Lyon M, Barr CE, Cannon TD, et al: Fetal neural development and schizophrenia (clinical conference). Schizophr Bull 15:149–161, 1989

Meehl PE: Nuisance variables and the ex post facto design, in Minnesota Studies in the Philosophy of Science. Edited by Radner M, Winokur S. Minneapolis, University of Minnesota Press, 1970, pp 373–402

Mirsky AF, Lochhead SJ, Jones BP, et al: On familial factors in the attentional deficit in schizophrenia: a review and report of two new subject samples. J Psychiatr Res 26:383–403, 1992

Nasrallah HA, Andreason NC, Coffman J, et al: A controlled magnetic resonance imaging study of corpus callosum thickness in schizophrenia. Biol Psychiatry 21:274–282, 1986

Nopoulos P, Flaum M, Andreasen NC: Sex differences in brain morphology in schizophrenia. Am J Psychiatry 154:1648–1654, 1997

Oades RD, Schepker R: Serum gonadal steroid hormones in young schizophrenic patients. Psychoneuroendocrinology 19:373–385, 1994

Perlick D, Mattis S, Stastny P, et al: Gender differences in cognition in schizophrenia. Schizophr Res 8:69–73, 1992

Riecher-Rossler A, Hafner H: Schizophrenia and oestrogens: is there an association? Eur Arch Psychiatry Clin Neurosci 242:323–328, 1993

Riecher-Rossler A, Hafner H, Stumbaum M, et al: Can estradiol modulate schizophrenia symptomatology? Schizophr Bull 20:203–214, 1994

Seeman MV: Gender and Psychopathology. Washington, DC, American Psychiatric Press, 1995

Seeman MV, Lang M: The role of estrogens in schizophrenia gender differences. Schizophr Bull 16:185–194, 1990

Seidman LJ, Cassens GP, Kremen WS, et al: The neuropsychology of schizophrenia, in Clinical Syndromes in Adult Neuropsychology: The Practitioner Handbook. Edited by White RF. Amsterdam, The Netherlands, Elsevier Science, 1992, pp 381–449

Seidman LJ, Goldstein JM, Goodman JM, et al: Sex differences in olfactory identification and Wisconsin Card Sorting performance in schizophrenia: relation to attention and verbal ability. Biol Psychiatry 42:104–115, 1997

Sweeney JA, Haas GL, Keilp JG, et al: Evaluation of the stability of neuropsychological functioning after acute episodes of schizophrenia: one-year follow-up study. Psychiatry Res 38:63–76, 1991

Walker E, Lewine RR: Sampling biases in studies of gender and schizophrenia. Schizophr Bull 19:1–7, 1993

Watt NF, Grubb TW, Erlenmeyer-Kimling L: Social, emotional, and intellectual behavior at school among children at high risk for schizophrenia. J Consult Clin Psychol 50:171–181, 1982

Weinberger DR: Implications of normal brain development for the pathogenesis of schizophrenia. Arch Gen Psychiatry 44:660–669, 1987

10

Does Menopause Intensify Symptoms in Schizophrenia?

Mary V. Seeman, M.D.C.M., F.R.C.P.C., F.A.C.P.

*M*enopause constitutes an important psychological turning point in a woman's life, the point at which she ceases to be fertile. Many women hail this stage of life as liberation; some mourn it as loss (Avis and McKinlay 1991; Wilbur et al. 1995). The loss is literal in the sense that pituitary hormone levels gradually decline until ovarian follicles are no longer stimulated, secretion of estrogen and progesterone stops, and menstruation ceases. The potential for childbearing is over. More important, menopause, for many women, is a metaphor for growing old. The status and role of postmenopausal women vary, depending on culture and caste, but in most of the world today, status (power, respect, financial means) is lost at this stage of a woman's life. Menopause takes place at an average age of 50. Via built-in genetic mechanisms, menopause comes earliest to those women whose menarche, or menstruation onset, came latest. Given that women in developed countries are now living into their 80s, many women spend more than one-third of their lives in the postmenopausal state. The effect of menopause is, thus, important for all women but may be of special significance for those with a vulnerability to psychiatric disease (Hunter et al. 1986; Neri et al. 1997; Nijs 1998).

EFFECTS OF MENOPAUSE

The cessation of ovarian estrogen production causes several immediately experienced physical and emotional symptoms. More than 85% of postmenopausal women have intermittent hot flushes that usually last for 1–2 years but may, in one-quarter to one-half of postmenopausal women, continue for more than 5 years. Ten percent may continue to experience vasomotor symptoms as long as 15 years after the onset of menopause (Berg et al. 1988). Hot flushes are experienced as waves of unpredictable heat and perspiration that are socially embarrassing and that interrupt sleep and result in daytime fatigue because they so often occur at night. Urogenital atrophy leads to vaginal dryness, burning, and itching; painful intercourse; vaginal discharge or bleeding; vaginal narrowing; urethral inflammation with pain on voiding; urinary urgency and frequency; and occasional incontinence. These symptoms seriously interfere with personal and intimate life. They undermine feelings of self-worth and complicate sexual and interpersonal relationships.

For ill-understood hormonal reasons, many women gain weight at this time that they cannot lose, despite determined dieting and exercise. Breasts sag; skin loses its elasticity and becomes mottled; and hair dries, turns gray, and falls out. Women feel less and less attractive, especially when media fashions and men's desires favor the young. An immediate central nervous effect occurs as well. The ability to think and to remember wanes, and many women become increasingly irritable and anxious. This is accompanied by an anticipation of worse to come.

Although some of these effects may be social and cultural rather than biological (Holte and Mikkelsen 1991b), reports of vasomotor and urinary or vaginal symptoms, as well as fatigue and nervousness, come from Puerto Rico, Tanzania, Norway, Denmark, The Netherlands, Sweden, and Japan as well as North America (Holte and Mikkelsen 1991a; Koster and Davidsen 1993; Lock et al. 1988; Moore and Kombe 1991; Morales Pereira 1990; Oldenhave et al. 1993).

Eventually, the bone loss that begins at menopause brings with it chronic pain and a 50% risk of at least one bone fracture after menopause. Fifteen percent of postmenopausal women can anticipate a life-threatening hip fracture. This is the beginning of the stage of life when women, no longer protected by estrogens, become candidates for coronary heart disease. Both cardiovascular disease and osteoporosis bring pain, fear, decreased activity, and increasing isolation. Although there may be an evolutionary advantage to ending human female fertility at a relatively early age (even today, the risk of death in childbirth for a 40-year-old woman is seven times that for a 20-year-old woman) (Diamond 1996), for the individual woman, menopause can be considered a risk factor for psychosocial distress. An analogous syndrome can be experienced in men but is less well understood. Symptoms in men include impotence, weakness, and memory loss (Tan and Philip 1999).

Cawood and Bancroft (1996) studied the effect of menopause on the well-being of women and found the expected correlation with depression. The presence of depression, however, was not statistically correlated with any specific hormone deficiency but rather with lowered socioeconomics, poorer body image, and fatigue.

Individual differences in *rate* of change may be the reason that it has proven impossible to correlate mood states with any specific hormone level. When hormone changes are slow and gradual, equilibrium and accommodation are potentially achievable. Perhaps only the dramatic changes are reflected in mood shifts. On average, postmenopausal plasma estradiol decreases to less than 10% of the premenopausal values. How rapidly it declines in any one individual may be the determining factor behind clinical manifestations.

SCHIZOPHRENIA

There are several reported sex differences in schizophrenia. Women, relative to men, have a later age at onset of schizophrenia. They require lower neuroleptic doses to recover from an acute episode of psychosis, and they attain remission faster than men do. Maintenance doses of antipsychotic medication, at least in the premenopausal years, tend to be lower than those needed for men. Women show a tendency toward premenstrual and postpartum exacerbation of symptoms and have relatively few episodes of illness during pregnancy (Apfel and Handel 1992; Seeman and Lang 1990). These observations, sometimes supported and sometimes not, have led to the hypothesis that estrogens are "psychotoprotective" (Di Paolo 1994; Gattaz et al. 1994; Hafner et al. 1991; Magharious et al. 1998; Riecher-Rossler and Hafner 1993; Riecher-Rossler et al. 1994a, 1994b; Seeman 1995, 1996). One strong line of evidence supporting this hypothesis is that epidemiological studies show a second peak of onset of schizophrenia in women (but not men) around the time of menopause (Castle et al. 1995; Hafner and an der Heiden 1997). In addition, longitudinal outcomes, which are superior for women over men for the first 15 years of illness (Angermeyer et al. 1990; Davidson and McGlashan 1997; Harrison et al. 1996; Jonsson and Nyman 1984, 1991; Mason et al. 1995; Ram et al. 1992), gradually even out (Bleuler 1974; Ciompi 1980; Harding et al. 1987; Huber et al. 1975; Nyman and Jonsson 1983; Opjordsmoen 1991; Steinmeyer et al. 1989), suggesting that, at a time point approximating menopause, women's comparative advantage with respect to schizophrenia outcome wanes.

MENOPAUSE AND SCHIZOPHRENIA STUDY

Given the above findings and what we know about the effects of menopause on women in general, one would expect the severity of schizophrenia symptoms to increase in affected women as they approach menopause. To study this issue, I undertook a random chart review of 20 women first admitted for schizophrenia at the Clarke Institute of Psychiatry, Toronto, Ontario, Canada, between 1967 and 1975. To qualify for recruitment into this study, the women needed to still be attending outpatient services at the institute in 1995. In addition to reviewing the clinical records, I interviewed each of these women personally. All of the women interviewed at that stage reported either irregular menstrual cycles or no cycling at all. None were receiving hormone replacement therapy.

The working hypothesis of the study was that the chart review would show an increasing severity of psychotic symptoms and resultant disability beginning after age 40, at the time when estrogen levels usually begin to decrease. In the interview, I asked the women whether and when they experienced a downturn in the course of their illness and whether they could attribute this to a specific life event or a treatment change.

RESULTS

Thirteen of the 20 patients reported a decline in their functioning first apparent in their 40s. What distinguished these 13 from the other 7? No difference in premorbid competence, no difference in mean onset age of first psychotic symptom, and no overall difference in initial severity of the illness were found. Marriage did not distinguish the two groups. Two of the 7 who did not deteriorate after age 40 were married, compared with 4 of the 13 who did.

Perhaps the only difference that stood out is that 4 of the 13 who deteriorated had had a child, an only child, whom they had given up for adoption. A fifth had given custody of her only son to her husband, although she continued to stay in touch with the boy. In the other group, only 1 woman had had children (2 sons), and this woman had been able to keep her family together with the help of an especially supportive husband.

One can speculate that the advent of menopause for a woman whose only child was given away signals the end of the possibility of reparation, a meaning for the event that is qualitatively different from its significance to a woman who has been a parent or for whom this was never a choice.

Four of the seven who did not experience a downturn in their illness had worked all their adult lives, despite their symptoms and despite their repeated hospitalizations. I include in this group the woman with the two children who had stayed home and looked after her family. In the other group, most also had tried to work, although only two had been able to do so for the better part of their adult lives. This suggests that their illness had followed a relatively severe course even before their experience of a downturn. An alternative explanation is that the daily routine of working itself provides protection.

At the 1995 evaluation, 14 of the 20 women were being supported by government subsidies. Four were receiving a pension from work. One lived on a parental inheritance. The remaining woman was financially supported by her husband. At interview, 1 woman reported that, through her work, she was financially providing for both herself and her husband. Essentially, all of the 20 women lived at or near the poverty line. These women had always been poor—when finances had recently decreased, it was because of work loss or loss of a financially supportive relative or partner. In general, financial reverses did not seem to correlate with symptom exacerbation.

The history of substance abuse was frequent and contributed to the severity of current symptoms. Five of the 13 women who deteriorated abused alcohol or drugs, compared with only 1 who did so in the other group of 7.

One of the women in this study took her life by jumping from her apartment building window 1 year after the study interview. This woman heavily used substances and had been especially symptomatic since she lost her court battle over regaining custody of the child she lost to Children's Aid. Part of her story has been reported previously. She was called "Jane" in a book chapter, written shortly after she gave birth, which was intended to illustrate sex differences in treatment response in schizophrenia (Seeman 1995). At the time of the interview in 1995, this woman was clearly doing very poorly; she had multiple and frequent hospital admissions in the previous year, chaotic relationships, and severe cognitive pathology. No psychological precipitant was found to account for her suicide; it occurred in the context of cocaine abuse.

Four women, including the patient who had jumped to her death, had experienced long periods of homelessness. All these women were in the deteriorating group, and the periods of homelessness invariably occurred relatively late in the illness when parents and other close family members were either not alive or deliberately alienated. The phenomenon of family members refusing to have anything to do with their ill relative was unique to the deteriorating group.

In the 13 women who experienced a worsening of symptoms, 4 attributed it to the recent death of a parent. All of the women had reached the age when parental death was not uncommon. Two of those whose symptoms had not worsened also were interviewed during a period of recent mourning. In retrospect, for both groups, the effect of parental loss on symptom severity seemed to be delayed by several years.

In accordance with the initial hypothesis, most of the women in this small sample (but not all) showed a course of illness that is not typical in men: a relatively late onset of illness (after age 25), a relatively mild first decade of illness, and increasing age-related severity. In the 13 who had evidence of increased severity after age 40, the event of menstrual cessation sometimes, but far from always, coincided with a memorable downturn. In other words, if estrogen withdrawal plays a part in increasing symptom severity, its effect on the brain may not synchronize with its effect on the hypothalamic-pituitary-ovarian axis. Social deterioration at this late age was most closely correlated with three (perhaps interdependent) factors: substance abuse, loss of supports, and a family history of schizophrenia. Four of the 13 had a first-degree relative with schizophrenia; 1 was adopted and did not know her biological family history. In the other group, however, 2 of the 7 also reported a first-degree relative with schizophrenia.

DISCUSSION

If the menopausal period contributes to the risk of deterioration in schizophrenia, how does it do this? Can a declining level of gonadal hormones release a previously suppressed genetic influence? Can declining hormone levels sensitize women to the psychological stress of loneliness, abandonment, and poverty or to the cumulative stress of alcohol and drugs?

Of the various hormones, most is known about the effects of estrogens and their absence. Estrogen withdrawal in specific brain cells may release a cascade of events that, over time, might increase the severity of psychotic and cognitive symptoms. Rationales for such effects are based on what we know about estrogenic effects on neurotransmitter pathways, cognitive pathways, stress induction pathways, and, more directly, neuronal growth and atrophy.

Estrogens and Neurotransmitter Systems

Estrogenic influences on neurotransmitter levels probably operate through direct membrane effects on the electrical firing rate of neurotransmitter-secreting cells (Schumacher 1990). Whereas genomic effects of gonadal steroids are slow (minutes to hours), membrane effects are rapid, with a latency of microseconds to minutes. Estrogen effects have been reported in acetylcholine, serotonin, and dopamine pathways. Estrogen also enhances the progesterone-induced anxiolytic effect mediated through a potentiation of γ-aminobutyric acid (Smith 1994). Estrogens also potentiate excitatory amino acids such as glutamate and aspartate (Smith 1994).

Estrogens and Cognitive Pathways

Several case-control studies (Henderson et al. 1994; Paganini-Hill and Henderson 1996) suggested that women who use estrogen replacement therapy are less likely to develop Alzheimer's disease than are women who do not. More recent prospective studies also have observed a protective effect of estrogen on cognition (Kawas et al. 1997).

Until the recent discovery of a new estrogen receptor (ER-β) (Kuiper et al. 1996) and its localization in brain regions associated with learning, memory, and emotion (Shugrue et al. 1997), it was difficult to understand how estrogen replacement therapy could improve cognitive functions because ER-α is sparsely distributed in key cognitive regions such as neocortex, hippocampus, and basal forebrain nuclei. It is now thought that estrogens work through both of these receptors and that the two receptors coexist within the same cell.

Estrogens and Genes

Among the many genes suspected to be under the direct influence of estrogen are genes responsible for neuronal development, migration, growth, survival, dendritic spine formation and density, antioxidant activity, synaptic plasticity, neurodegeneration, and apoptosis secondary to glucose deprivation or to toxins (Birge 1997). Decreased estrogen levels at the time of menopause may activate or suppress these genes, leading to disrupted neuronal circuits and ensuing psychosis.

Selective Estrogen Receptor Modulators

Newly synthesized molecules, selective estrogen receptor modulators, act both as tissue-specific estrogen agonists and as antagonists in the sense that, to various extents and by a variety of intermediary means, they can either inhibit or enhance estrogen-induced activation of estrogen response element–containing genes (Kauffman and Bryant 1995). Raloxifene, one of the new selective estrogen receptor modulators, forms a raloxifene response element that does not itself bind directly to the DNA domain of the gene but activates it via an intermediate molecule. Other estrogen agonists may similarly take estrogen's place in turning on target genes.

CONCLUSION

Much evidence indicates that menopause may produce a variety of physical and psychosocial symptoms and that the symptoms of schizophrenia may be aggravated at this time. This could be an indirect and late effect of estrogen withdrawal. Addressing both hormonal and psychosocial issues may prove preventive (Graziottin 1999; Ritsher et al. 1997; Ryan et al. 1999; Shaver 1994). The advent of selective estrogen receptor modulators may, in the near future, make estrogen replacement a safe and effective option for women as they age.

REFERENCES

Angermeyer M, Kuhn L, Goldstein JM: Gender and the course of schizophrenia differences in treated outcomes. Schizophr Bull 16:293–307, 1990

Apfel RJ, Handel MH: Madness and Loss of Motherhood: Sexuality, Reproduction, and Long-Term Mental Illness. Washington, DC, American Psychiatric Press, 1992

Avis NE, McKinlay SM: A longitudinal analysis of women's attitudes toward the menopause: results from the Massachusetts Women's Health Study. Maturitas 13:65–79, 1991

Berg G, Gottwall T, Hammar M, et al: Climacteric symptoms among women aged 60–62 in Linköping, Sweden, in 1986. Maturitas 10:193–199, 1988

Birge SJ: The role of estrogen in the treatment of Alzheimer's disease. Neurology 48(suppl 7):S36–S41, 1997

Bleuler M: The long-term course of the schizophrenic psychoses. Psychol Med 4:244–254, 1974

Castle DJ, Abel K, Takei N, et al: Gender differences in schizophrenia: hormonal effect or subtypes? Schizophr Bull 21:1–12, 1995

Cawood EH, Bancroft J: Steroid hormones, the menopause, sexuality and well-being of women. Psychol Med 26:925–936, 1996

Ciompi L: The natural history of schizophrenia in the long term. Br J Psychiatry 136:413–420, 1980

Davidson L, McGlashan TH: The varied outcomes of schizophrenia. Can J Psychiatry 42:34–43, 1997

Diamond J: Why women change. Discover July:131–137, 1996

Di Paolo T: Modulation of brain dopamine transmission by sex steroids. Rev Neurosci 5:27–42, 1994

Gattaz WF, Vogel P, Riecher-Rossler A, et al: Influence of the menstrual cycle phase on the therapeutic response in schizophrenia. Biol Psychiatry 36:137–139, 1994

Graziottin A: Strategies for effectively addressing women's concerns about the menopause and HRT. Maturitas 33(suppl 1):S15–S23, 1999

Hafner H, an der Heiden W: Epidemiology of schizophrenia. Can J Psychiatry 42:139–151, 1997

Hafner H, Behrens S, De Vry J, et al: Oestradiol enhances the vulnerability threshold for schizophrenia in women by an early effect on dopaminergic transmission. Eur Arch Psychiatry Clin Neurosci 241:65–68, 1991

Harding CM, Brooks GW, Ashikaga T, et al: The Vermont longitudinal study of persons with severe mental illness, I: methodology, study sample and overall status 32 years later. Am J Psychiatry 144:718–726, 1987

Harrison G, Croudace T, Mason P, et al: Predicting the long-term outcome of schizophrenia. Psychol Med 26:697–705, 1996

Henderson VW, Paganini-Hill A, Emanuel CK, et al: Estrogen replacement therapy in older women. Arch Neurol 51:896–900, 1994

Holte A, Mikkelsen A: The menopausal syndrome: a factor analytic replication. Maturitas 13:193–203, 1991a

Holte A, Mikkelsen A: Psychosocial determinants of climacteric complaints. Maturitas 13:205–215, 1991b

Huber G, Gross G, Schüttler R: A long-term follow-up study of schizophrenia: psychiatric course of illness and prognosis. Acta Psychiatr Scand 52:49–57, 1975

Hunter M, Battersby R, Whitehead M: Relationships between psychological symptoms, somatic complaints and menopausal status. Maturitas 8:217–228, 1986

Jonsson H, Nyman K: Prediction of outcome in schizophrenia. Acta Psychiatr Scand 69:274–291, 1984

Jonsson H, Nyman AK: Predicting long-term outcome in schizophrenia. Acta Psychiatr Scand 83:342–346, 1991

Kauffman RF, Bryant HU: Selective estrogen receptor modulators. Drug Line 8:9, 1995

Kawas C, Resnick S, Morrison A, et al: A prospective study of estrogen replacement therapy and the risk of developing Alzheimer's disease. Neurology 48:1517–1521, 1997

Koster A, Davidsen M: Climacteric complaints and their relation to menopausal development—a retrospective analysis. Maturitas 17:155–166, 1993

Kuiper GG, Enmark E, Pelto-Huikko M, et al: Cloning of a novel estrogen receptor in rat prostate and ovary. Proc Natl Acad Sci U S A 93:5925–5930, 1996

Lock M, Kaufert P, Gilbert P: Cultural construction of the menopausal syndrome: the Japanese case. Maturitas 10:317–332, 1988

Magharious W, Goff DC, Amico E: Relationship of gender and menstrual status to symptoms and medication side effects in patients with schizophrenia. Psychiatry Res 77:159–166, 1998

Mason P, Harrison G, Glazebrook G, et al: The characteristics of outcome in schizophrenia at 13 years. Br J Psychiatry 167:596–603, 1995

Moore B, Kombe H: Climacteric symptoms in a Tanzanian community. Maturitas 13:229–234, 1991

Morales Pereira A: Climacteric and menopause: medical point of view. P R Health Sci J 9:85–87, 1990

Neri I, Demyttenaere K, Facchinetti F: Coping style and climacteric symptoms in a clinical sample of postmenopausal women. J Psychosom Obstet Gynaecol 18:229–233, 1997

Nijs P: Counselling of the climacteric woman: diagnostic difficulties and therapeutic possibilities. Eur J Obstet Gynecol Reprod Biol 81:273–276, 1998

Nyman AK, Jonsson H: Differential evaluation of outcome in schizophrenia. Acta Psychiatr Scand 68:458–475, 1983

Oldenhave A, Jaszmann LJ, Haspels AA, et al: Impact of climacteric on well-being: a survey based on 5213 women 39–60 years old. Am J Obstet Gynecol 168:772–780, 1993

Opjordsmoen S: Long-term clinical outcome of schizophrenia with special reference to gender differences. Acta Psychiatr Scand 83:307–313, 1991

Paganini-Hill A, Henderson VW: Estrogen replacement therapy and risk of Alzheimer's disease. Arch Intern Med 156:2213–2217, 1996

Ram R, Bromet EJ, Eaton WW, et al: The natural course of schizophrenia: a review of first admission studies. Schizophr Bull 18:185–207, 1992

Riecher-Rossler A, Hafner H: Schizophrenia and oestrogens: is there an association? Eur Arch Psychiatry Clin Neurosci 242:323–328, 1993

Riecher-Rossler A, Hafner H, Stumbaum M, et al: Can oestradiol modulate schizophrenic symptomatology? Schizophr Bull 2:203–214, 1994a

Riecher-Rossler A, Hafner H, Dütsch-Strobel A, et al: Further evidence for a specific role of estradiol in schizophrenia? Biol Psychiatry 36:492–495, 1994b

Ritsher JE, Coursey RD, Farrell EW: A survey on issues in the lives of women with severe mental illness. Psychiatr Serv 48:1273–1282, 1997

Ryan CA, Ghali WA, Boss RD, et al: Care during menopause: comparison of a women's health practice and traditional care. Journal of Women's Health and Gender Based Medicine 8:1295–1302, 1999

Schumacher M: Rapid membrane effects of steroid hormones: an emerging concept in neuroendocrinology. Trends Neurosci 13:359–362, 1990

Seeman MV (ed): Gender differences in treatment response to schizophrenia, in Gender and Psychopathology. Washington, DC, American Psychiatric Press, 1995, pp 227–251

Seeman MV: The role of estrogen in schizophrenia. J Psychiatry Neurosci 21:123–127, 1996

Seeman MV, Lang M: The role of estrogens in schizophrenia gender differences. Schizophr Bull 16:185–194, 1990

Shaver JL: Beyond hormonal therapies in menopause. Exp Gerontol 29:469–476, 1994

Shughrue PJ, Lane MV, Merchenthaler I: Comparative distribution of estrogen receptor-alpha and -beta mRNA in the rat central nervous system. J Comp Neurol 388:507–527, 1997

Smith SS: Female sex steroid hormones: from receptors to networks to performance: actions on the sensorimotor system. Prog Neurobiol 44:55–86, 1994

Steinmeyer EM, Marneros A, Deister A, et al: Long-term outcome of schizoaffective and schizophrenic disorders: a comparative study, II: causal-analytical investigations. Eur Arch Psychiatry Clin Neurosci 238:126–134, 1989

Tan RS, Philip PS: Perceptions of and risk factors for andropause. Arch Androl 43:97–103, 1999

Wilbur J, Miller A, Montgomery A: The influence of demographic characteristics, menopausal status, and symptoms on women's attitudes toward menopause. Womens Health 23:19–39, 1995

11

Sex-Related Differences in Antipsychotic-Induced Movement Abnormalities

Laurie A. Lindamer, Ph.D.
Jonathan P. Lacro, Pharm.D.
Dilip V. Jeste, M.D.

*T*he most effective symptomatic treatment for psychosis involves the use of neuroleptic or antipsychotic medications, but these are also associated with neurological side effects, including extrapyramidal symptoms (EPS) and tardive dyskinesia (TD). Acute EPS include acute dystonia, akathisia, and parkinsonism (rigidity, bradykinesia, and tremor). TD has been described as nonrhythmic, involuntary, choreiform movements. These motor abnormalities have been related to decreased quality of life, noncompliance with medication, violent behavior, and suicide attempts (Jeste and Caligiuri 1993). Consequently, identifying risk factors for the development of EPS and TD in patients with psychosis has been an active area of research.

This work was supported, in part, by National Institute of Mental Health Grants MH43693, MH51459, MH45131, MH49671, MH56398, and MH01580; the National Alliance for Research on Schizophrenia and Depression; and the Department of Veterans Affairs.

Sex differences in many aspects of schizophrenia, such as age at onset, clinical presentation, and response to treatment, have been well described (Andia and Zisook 1991; Tamminga 1997). The understanding of sex differences in side effect profiles of antipsychotic medication, particularly motor abnormalities, is less well studied. In this chapter, we provide an overview of data from selected studies that describe sex-related differences with respect to antipsychotic-induced movement abnormalities and discuss possible mechanisms underlying these existing differences. Last, we highlight methodological difficulties in conducting research in this area and describe the necessary areas that warrant further investigation.

SEX AND EXTRAPYRAMIDAL SYMPTOMS

Studies of EPS (antipsychotic-induced dystonia, akathisia, and parkinsonism) report prevalences varying from 2% to 90% in patients who are prescribed typical neuroleptic medication (Casey 1991). Little consensus exists regarding the risk factors for the development of antipsychotic-induced EPS, and the predictors seem to vary with the type of movement disorder. For example, severity of psychopathology and neuroleptic dosage have been reported to be important predictors of dystonia or akathisia (Aguilar et al. 1994; Chakos et al. 1992; Sachdev 1995), but psychopathology did not predict antipsychotic-induced parkinsonism (Caligiuri et al. 1997). Some studies (Caligiuri et al. 1997), but not all (Chakos et al. 1992; Chatterjee et al. 1995; Hoffman et al. 1987), identified age as a risk factor for parkinsonism.

The data are also inconsistent with regard to the role sex that plays in the development of EPS. In an early study of 3,775 patients (aged 4–89 years) taking various neuroleptic medications, more women (48%) than men (30%) developed EPS (Ayd 1961). Nearly twice as many women had parkinsonism and akathisia than did men; however, nearly twice as many men had dyskinesia (Ayd 1961). Some methodological limitations of this study, such as no characterization of patients with respect to diagnosis and the lack of objective measurement of EPS, make interpretation of these results difficult.

In a more recent study, Chakos et al. (1992) investigated the prevalence of risk factors for EPS in a sample of younger (16–40 years), treatment-naïve patients with schizophrenia who received fluphenazine. The researchers used the Simpson-Angus Extrapyramidal Rating Scale (Simpson and Angus 1970) and a modified version of the Simpson Dyskinesia Rating Scale (Simpson et al. 1979) and found that 36% of the treatment-naïve patients developed dystonia, 18% had akathisia, and 34% had parkinsonism. They also discovered that more females than males developed dystonia (50% vs. 25%); however, they found no sex differences in the prevalence of parkinsonism or akathisia, which is inconsistent with the findings of Ayd (1961). Szymanski et al. (1995) reported similar results. In their study, they observed a first-episode, neuroleptic-naïve group of patients with schizophrenia who were between the ages of 16 and 40 years and who were receiving fluphenazine. These authors found no sex differences for antipsychotic-related akathisia or parkinsonism as measured by the Simpson-Angus Extrapyramidal Rating Scale; however, they did find a sex-related difference in risk for acute dystonic episodes (48% women and 22% men), which is similar to the results of Chakos et al. (1992). In addition, no sex differences were found in a sample of newly treated middle-aged (mean age, 46 years) patients with schizophrenia using both clinical and instrumental ratings of parkinsonism (Caligiuri et al. 1997).

In summary, the role of sex in the development of antipsychotic-induced EPS seems to vary according to the type of motor abnormality. The prevalence of dystonia has been reported to be greater in women with schizophrenia than in men, whereas no sex differences were observed in akathisia or parkinsonism.

ESTROGEN AND EXTRAPYRAMIDAL SYMPTOMS

Some data are available on the effects of estrogen treatment of EPS but are limited to case studies or small open studies and focus mostly on parkinsonian symptoms. In both men and women, estrogen treatment seems to worsen symptoms of parkinsonism, both idiopathic and neuroleptic induced.

In a case study of a postmenopausal 64-year-old woman with Parkinson's disease, treatment with conjugated estrogens (0.625 mg) worsened her rigidity and bradykinesia but improved her symptoms of dyskinesia (Villeneuve et al. 1978, 1980). The authors also administered conjugated estrogens to three men with Parkinson's disease and found a worsening of parkinsonian symptoms in two of the men (Bedard et al. 1979).

In a small open study of male psychiatric patients, no changes were seen in neuroleptic-induced parkinsonian symptoms with the administration of estrogen (Villeneuve et al. 1980). Furthermore, Glazer et al. (1984) found no significant difference in neuroleptic-induced parkinsonian symptoms between a postmenopausal group of women who received estrogen and those who received placebo.

Some data on the estrogen treatment of parkinsonism suggest that estrogens have an antidopaminergic effect, worsening symptoms of rigidity and bradykinesia, whereas other data are consistent with the studies finding no sex differences in parkinsonian symptoms.

SEX AND TARDIVE DYSKINESIA

In review of the literature on sex and TD, some, but not all, studies have identified being female as a risk factor in the development of TD. Jeste and Caligiuri (1993) reported in a review article that increased age, female gender, mood disorders, organic brain dysfunction, and the presence of early EPS were risk factors for TD in some studies. Another group of researchers found that older age and female gender, respectively, appear to be the first and second most prominent risk factors for TD (Kane and Smith 1982; Kane et al. 1988). In a review, Yassa and Jeste (1992) found that the prevalence of TD was significantly greater for women than for men (26.6% vs. 21.6%). However, in another study, Jeste et al. (1995) found no sex difference in TD. In addition, Saltz et al. (1991) found a similar result in a longitudinal study of a large sample of older patients with diagnoses including organic mental disorders and psychosis. Because most of these patients were women (72%), sex differences may have been obscured.

These inconsistencies have led other researchers to investigate the effects of sex and age on TD (Yassa and Jeste 1988, 1997). These results showed that TD prevalence increases with age for women but not for men. TD appears to be equally distributed between the sexes in younger patients (younger than 50 years), but after age 70, many more women develop TD than do men. This finding suggests that the interaction between age and sex may better account for the differences in prevalence of TD than age or sex alone. Other researchers (Sandyk et al. 1993) found that postmenopausal women had more oral-facial TD than did premenopausal women. This age by sex interaction suggests a role for the reproductive hormone estrogen in the emergence of TD because postmenopausal estrogen levels are very low relative to premenopausal levels.

ESTROGEN AND TARDIVE DYSKINESIA

More direct evidence that estrogen plays a role in the development of TD comes from case reports. Some small studies have shown an improvement of symptoms with estrogen treatment in women (Bedard et al. 1977, 1979; Villeneuve et al. 1978) and also in men (Villeneuve et al. 1980). Bedard et al. (1977) reported a case study of a perimenopausal 51-year-old woman whose neuroleptic-induced TD (buccolinguomasticatory) improved with the cessation of menstruation. After 4 months of amenorrhea, the patient's menstrual cycles resumed and her TD subsequently worsened. The subsequent administration of conjugated estrogens (0.625 mg) decreased her TD. In another case study (Glazer and Nasrallah 1988), a 69-year-old woman had been treated with neuroleptics for paranoid symptoms and developed severe TD (Abnormal Involuntary Movement Scale [AIMS] score of 22). The patient's TD did not respond to common treatments, such as L-dopa, but did respond to conjugated estrogens (1.25 mg). Her AIMS score decreased to 14 in 2 months and to 9 in 4 months of treatment with estrogen.

Improvement of TD also has been reported in an open-label study of estrogen supplementation in neuroleptic-treated men with chronic schizophrenia (Villeneuve et al. 1980). In a crossover design, Koller et al. (1982) administered 2.5 mg of conjugated estrogens or placebo to a group of patients with various diagnoses, including Huntington's disease, levodopa-induced chorea, and TD. These authors concluded that estrogen may have only limited use in the treatment of chorea. Of the 10 patients with TD, however, 4 showed an improvement of symptoms, and the difference between the placebo and the treatment groups was nearly significant ($P=0.09$).

In a small double-blind trial, Glazer et al. (1984) administered conjugated estrogens (1.25 mg) to postmenopausal women with TD, most of whom had the diagnosis of schizophrenia or schizoaffective disorder. The AIMS score decreased by 38% in the estrogen group and 9% in the placebo group, which nearly reached statistical significance ($P=0.09$). After completion of the study and discontinuation of estrogen, the AIMS scores returned to near baseline levels. The authors cautioned that the estrogen group had less neuroleptic exposure and shorter duration of TD than did the placebo group, which may have influenced their response to estrogen treatment. In a different study, Glazer et al. (1983) examined the relation between levels of estradiol and severity of TD in postmenopausal women (44–67 years) and men (27–67 years), most of whom had a diagnosis of schizophrenia. They concluded that there was no association between these factors but noted that this study was limited to hypogonadal women; thus, the restriction of range of levels of estradiol could have produced low correlation coefficients.

ATYPICAL ANTIPSYCHOTIC MEDICATIONS AND MOTOR ABNORMALITIES

All of the information described earlier in this chapter involved the use of typical antipsychotics. The introduction of atypical agents represented a significant advancement in antipsychotic treatment. Experience with atypical agents such as clozapine, risperidone, olanzapine, and quetiapine has shown that the risk of EPS and TD is significantly lower relative to typical agents in younger (Casey 1996; Miller et al. 1998) and older patients (Jeste et al. 1999).

POSSIBLE BIOLOGICAL MECHANISMS FOR SEX-RELATED DIFFERENCES IN TARDIVE DYSKINESIA

Although other neurotransmitter systems may be involved, the dopamine system of the basal ganglia is most likely to play a role in the development of antipsychotic-induced TD and parkinsonism, although the exact mechanism is not yet known. Evidence from preclinical studies suggests that there are sex differences in dopamine transmission in the basal ganglia, which may underlie some of the sex differences seen in TD and parkinsonism. Furthermore, estrogen modulation of dopamine-mediated behavior and biochemistry has been documented. Data from these animal studies are inconsistent; some have found that estrogen enhances dopamine transmission, whereas others have found that it has an inhibiting effect. Here, we present selected studies that indicate a role for estrogen in the development and treatment of antipsychotic-induced motor abnormalities (Van Hartesveldt and Joyce 1986).

Sex differences have been noted in dopamine-mediated motor behavior and dopamine biochemistry in rats. For example, the removal of ovaries, but not testes, reduced dopamine-induced rotational behavior (Becker and Ramirez 1980), and differences in basal extracellular dopamine due to release, synthesis, and metabolism have been seen in the basal ganglia between ovariectomized and castrated rats (Becker 1990; Castner et al. 1993). These sex differences suggest that a reproductive hormone, such as estrogen, may be involved in the differential response of dopamine-mediated behavior and biochemistry of the rat striatum.

More direct evidence that estrogen influences dopamine biochemistry in the basal ganglia of rats comes from studies of estrogen treatment. Estrogens have been shown to reduce dopamine concentrations in the striatum and other subcortical areas (Van Hartesveldt and Joyce 1986). Treatment with estradiol in intact males and ovariectomized females increased the density of striatal dopamine D_2 receptors (Bazzett and Becker 1994; Di Paolo et al. 1981; Hruska and Silbergeld 1980). This result is independent of preparation of estradiol, independent of dosing (single vs. chronic), not related to prolactin, and specific to estradiol (Van Hartesveldt and Joyce 1986).

Estrogen administration has been used to study dopamine-mediated behavior in animals that model antipsychotic-induced motor abnormalities, such as TD and parkinsonism. For example, chronic treatment with a dopamine antagonist leads to the development of stereotyped behaviors in rats that can be compared to the involuntary movements of TD. As in TD, withdrawal of the dopamine antagonist results in an increase in dyskinesia. In rats, the administration of estrogens can produce withdrawal sensitivity similar to that seen with haloperidol (Gordon and Diamond 1981). Female adult rats treated chronically with haloperidol or estradiol benzoate showed increased stereotyped behavior on challenges with dopamine agonists. Gordon et al. (1980) reported a biphasic response to estrogen administration. Initially, doses of estradiol benzoate reduced the intensity and duration of stereotyped behavior in rats, but stereotyped behavior was enhanced more than 48 hours after hormone administration. The continued treatment with estradiol benzoate prevented an increase in stereotyped behavior (Gordon et al. 1980). A similar result was observed in male rats: estrogen administration produced an increase in stereotypy on challenge with a dopamine agonist.

Another animal model of TD is the monkey model of lingual dyskinesia (Bedard and Boucher 1986; Bedard et al. 1983). A lesion of the midbrain, including the substantia nigra, produces tongue rolling and protrusion, similar to what is seen in humans with TD, which worsens with the administration of dopamine agonists. In these animals, estradiol had a biphasic effect similar to that of haloperidol—an initial inhibition of dopamine-mediated behavior (tongue protrusion) followed by a facilitation. These preclinical studies suggest that one effect of estrogen is similar to that of neuroleptic medication. Dopamine antagonism by estrogen also was found with a model of neuroleptic-induced catalepsy. Treatment with haloperidol in male and female adult rats resulted in catalepsy that was potentiated by the administration of estradiol (Di Paolo et al. 1981).

RESEARCH LIMITATIONS AND AREAS FOR FUTURE RESEARCH

The influence of sex and more specifically the utility of estrogen treatment for motor abnormalities cannot yet be decided because these studies are small and vary considerably in methodology (e.g., age differences in samples; heterogeneity of diagnosis; type of estrogen treatment; and type, severity, and duration of motor abnormality). The role of sex in the development of motor abnormalities in patients taking atypical antipsychotic medication warrants further investigation.

REFERENCES

Aguilar EJ, Keshavan MS, Martinez-Quiles MD, et al: Predictors of acute dystonia in first-episode psychotic patients. Am J Psychiatry 151:1819–1821, 1994

Andia AM, Zisook S: Gender differences in schizophrenia: a literature review. Ann Clin Psychiatry 3:333–340, 1991

Ayd FJ: A survey of drug-induced extrapyramidal reactions. JAMA 175:1054–1060, 1961

Bazzett TJ, Becker JB: Sex differences in the rapid and acute effects of estrogen on striatal D2 dopamine receptor binding. Brain Res 637:163–172, 1994

Becker JB: Direct effect of 17 beta-estradiol on striatum: sex differences in dopamine release. Synapse 5:157–164, 1990

Becker JB, Ramirez VD: Sex differences in the amphetamine stimulated release of catecholamines from rat striatal tissue in vitro. Brain Res 204:361–372, 1980

Bedard PJ, Boucher R: Estradiol can suppress haloperidol-induced supersensitivity in dyskinetic monkeys. Neurosci Lett 64:206–210, 1986

Bedard P, Langelier P, Villeneuve A: Oestrogens and extrapyramidal system. Lancet 2:1367–1368, 1977

Bedard PJ, Langelier P, Dankova J, et al: Estrogens, progesterone, and the extrapyramidal system, in Advances in Neurology. Edited by Poirier LJ, Sourkes TLA, Bedard PJ. New York, Raven, 1979, pp 411–422

Bedard P, Boucher R, Di Paolo T, et al: Biphasic effect of estradiol and domperidone on lingual dyskinesia in monkeys. Exp Neurol 82:172–182, 1983

Caligiuri MP, Lacro JP, Rockwell E, et al: Incidence and risk factors for severe tardive dyskinesia in older patients. Br J Psychiatry 171:148–153, 1997

Casey DE: Neuroleptic drug-induced extrapyramidal syndromes and tardive dyskinesia. Schizophr Res 4:109–120, 1991

Casey DE: Side effect profiles of new antipsychotic agents. J Clin Psychiatry 57:40–45, 1996

Castner SA, Xiao L, Becker JB: Sex differences in striatal dopamine: in vivo microdialysis and behavioral studies. Brain Res 610:127–134, 1993

Chakos MH, Mayerhoff DI, Loebel AD, et al: Incidence and correlates of acute extrapyramidal symptoms in first episode of schizophrenia. Psychopharmacol Bull 28:81–86, 1992

Chatterjee A, Chakos M, Koreen A, et al: Prevalence and clinical correlates of extrapyramidal signs and spontaneous dyskinesia in never-medicated schizophrenic patients. Am J Psychiatry 152:1724–1729, 1995

Di Paolo TD, Poyet P, Labrie F: Effect of chronic estradiol and haloperidol treatment on striatal dopamine receptors. Eur J Pharmacol 73:105–106, 1981

Glazer WM, Nasrallah HA: Neuroendocrine aspects of tardive dyskinesia: the role of estrogen, prolactin, and dopamine, in Tardive Dyskinesia: Biological Mechanisms and Clinical Aspects. Edited by Wolf ME, Mosnaim AD. Washington, DC, American Psychiatric Press, 1988, pp 181–196

Glazer WM, Naftolin F, Moore DC, et al: The relationship of circulating estradiol to tardive dyskinesia in men and postmenopausal women. Psychoneuroendocrinology 8:429–434, 1983

Glazer WM, Naftolin F, Morgenstern H, et al: Estrogen placement and tardive dyskinesia. Psychoneuroendocrinology 10:345–350, 1984

Gordon JH, Diamond BI: Antagonism of dopamine supersensitivity by estrogen: neurochemical studies in an animal model of tardive dyskinesia. Biol Psychiatry 16:365–371, 1981

Gordon JH, Borison RL, Diamond BI: Estrogen in experimental tardive dyskinesia. Neurology 30:551–554, 1980

Hoffman WF, Labs SM, Casey DE: Neuroleptic-induced parkinsonism in older schizophrenics. Biol Psychiatry 22:427–439, 1987

Hruska RE, Silbergeld EK: Increased dopamine receptor sensitivity after estrogen treatment using the rat rotation model. Science 208:1466–1468, 1980

Jeste DV, Caligiuri MP: Tardive dyskinesia. Schizophr Bull 19:303–315, 1993

Jeste DV, Caligiuri MP, Paulsen JS, et al: Risk of tardive dyskinesia in older patients: a prospective longitudinal study of 266 patients. Arch Gen Psychiatry 52:756–765, 1995

Jeste DV, Lacro JP, Bailey A, et al: Lower incidence of tardive dyskinesia with risperidone compared with haloperidol in older patients. J Am Geriatr Soc 47:716–719, 1999

Kane JM, Smith JM: Tardive dyskinesia: prevalence and risk factors, 1959 to 1979. Arch Gen Psychiatry 39:473–481, 1982

Kane JM, Woerner M, Lieberman J: Tardive dyskinesia: prevalence, incidence, and risk factors. J Clin Psychopharmacol 8:52S–56S, 1988

Koller WC, Barr A, Biary N: Estrogen treatment of dyskinetic disorders. Neurology 32:547–549, 1982

Miller CH, Mohr F, Umbricht D, et al: The prevalence of acute extrapyramidal signs and symptoms in patients treated with clozapine, risperidone, and conventional antipsychotics. J Clin Psychiatry 59:69–75, 1998

Sachdev P: The epidemiology of drug-induced akathisia, part II: chronic, tardive, and withdrawal akathisias. Schizophr Bull 21:451–461, 1995

Saltz BL, Woerner MG, Kane JM, et al: Prospective study of tardive dyskinesia incidence in the elderly. JAMA 266:2402–2406, 1991

Sandyk R, Kay SR, Awerbuch GI: Subjective awareness of abnormal involuntary movements in schizophrenia. Int J Neurosci 69:1–20, 1993

Simpson GM, Angus JW: A rating scale for extrapyramidal side effects. Acta Psychiatr Scand Suppl 212:11–19, 1970

Simpson GM, Lee JH, Zoubok B, et al: A rating scale for tardive dyskinesia. Psychopharmacology 64:171–179, 1979

Szymanski S, Lieberman JA, Alvir JM, et al: Gender differences in onset of illness, treatment response, course, and biologic indexes in first-episode schizophrenic patients. Am J Psychiatry 152:698–703, 1995

Tamminga CA: Gender and schizophrenia. J Clin Psychiatry 58:33–37, 1997

Van Hartesveldt C, Joyce JN: Effects of estrogen on the basal ganglia. Neurosci Biobehav Rev 10:1–14, 1986

Villeneuve A, Langelier P, Bedard P: Estrogens, dopamine and dyskinesias. Can Psychiatr Assoc J 23:68–70, 1978

Villeneuve A, Cazejust T, Cote M: Estrogens in tardive dyskinesia in male psychiatric patients. Neuropsychobiology 6:145–151, 1980

Yassa R, Jeste DV: Gender differences in tardive dyskinesia: a critical review of the literature. Schizophr Bull 18:701–715, 1992

Yassa R, Jeste DV: Tardive dyskinesia 1988: thirty-one years later. J Clin Psychopharmacol 8:1S, 1988

Yassa R, Jeste DV: Gender as a factor in the development of tardive dyskinesia in neuroleptic-induced movement disorders, in Neuroleptic-Induced Movement Disorders. Edited by Yassa R, Vasquan Nair NP, Jeste DV. New York, Cambridge University Press, 1997, pp 26–40

12

Women and Antipsychotic Drugs

Focus on Neuroleptic-Induced Hyperprolactinemia

Ruth A. Dickson, M.D., F.R.C.P.C.
William M. Glazer, M.D.

*A*ntipsychotic drugs are the foundation of treatment for schizophrenia. These medications, first introduced in the 1950s, provide symptomatic treatment, not a cure, for schizophrenia and often must be taken chronically, throughout the human life cycle, from the onset of illness in adolescence or early adult years to old age. Sixty percent of the antipsychotics prescribed are to women, and approximately 30% of all antipsychotics are prescribed to women ages 20–50, the childbearing years (IMS America November 1996–April 1997). Only limited research has focused on the effects of these medications on hormonal systems. Because these drugs are prescribed as the treatments of choice for schizophrenia and schizoaffective disorder and often for other conditions such as mood disorders and severe personality disturbances that occur commonly in women, understanding the effect of antipsychotics on the endocrine system is imperative for optimal clinical management of these women.

Antipsychotic drugs are now broadly defined as being either old, typical, first-generation drugs (e.g., phenothiazines and butyrophenones) or new, atypical, second-generation drugs. The latter group of currently marketed drugs (e.g., clozapine, risperidone, olanzapine, and quetiapine), to a variable degree, 1) improve efficacy against positive and negative symptoms of schizophrenia; 2) treat comorbid syndromes such as depression; 3) cause less negative effect on or improve cognitive functioning; and 4) reduce side effects, primarily acute and chronic neurological movement disorders, compared with the older drugs (Arvanitis and Miller 1997; Green 1998; Kane and Freeman 1994; Marder et al. 1997; Tollefson et al. 1997).

The new antipsychotics also have variable propensities to induce hyperprolactinemia. Clozapine (Meltzer et al. 1979), olanzapine (Beasley et al. 1996; Crawford et al. 1997), and quetiapine (Arvanitis and Miller 1997) cause limited mild, or no clinically significant, prolactin elevation and collectively can be considered to be "prolactin-sparing" antipsychotics. In contrast, risperidone is comparable with typical neuroleptics in its propensity to raise serum prolactin levels (American Psychiatric Association 1997; Peuskins 1995). As clinical experience with the drugs has accumulated, the differential effect on prolactin secretion has been increasingly recognized as relevant to women's health (Canadian Clinical Practice Guidelines 1998; Canuso et al. 1998a; Currier and Simpson 1998a, 1998b).

Conceptualizing neuroleptic-induced hyperprolactinemia as a potentially serious adverse event requires a change in mind-set by psychiatrists. Historically, schizophrenia researchers have been intrigued by prolactin as an indirect measure of dopamine blockade, with limited interest in hyperprolactinemia as a medical side effect. Clinicians, until the 1990s and the introduction of the prolactin-sparing antipsychotics, had to accept neuroleptic-induced hyperprolactinemia as a part of antipsychotic therapy because efficacy was coupled with prolactin elevation just as it was with neurological motor abnormalities. The fact that clozapine, olanzapine, and quetiapine are efficacious antipsychotic drugs with minimal induction of movement disorders or hyperprolactinemia has reinforced that these are unwanted side effects of drug therapy that can be prevented and treated without sacrificing effective antipsychotic therapy.

In this chapter, we examine the consequences of high prolactin levels secondary to antipsychotic treatment in women and the benefits of avoiding or resolving this side effect when women are given prolactin-sparing antipsychotics. We recently completed a review of neuroleptic-induced hyperprolactinemia in both men and women (Dickson and Glazer 1999b); this chapter focuses on issues in women and updates available information.

WOMEN, CLINICAL TRIALS, AND ENDOCRINE SIDE EFFECTS OF ANTIPSYCHOTIC DRUGS

Less information is available on the side effects of the new drugs in women, particularly in those of childbearing age, than in men. Most subjects included in research protocols of the new antipsychotics were chronically ill men with schizophrenia (Beasley et al. 1996; Chouinard et al. 1993; Kane et al. 1988; Marder and Meibach 1994; Tollefson et al. 1997). This reflects research practices, access to study patients, and legal requirements at the time these trials were planned and initiated.

Adverse events data collected during premarketing trials of the new antipsychotic drugs likely underestimated the incidence and severity of female-specific endocrine side effects such as menstrual disturbances. Premenopausal women often were required to accept oral contraceptives or be incapable of conceiving as a condition of trial enrollment. Limited documentation of menstrual history and menopausal status pretrial increases the difficulty in estimating the percentage of the sample who are capable of experiencing menstrual side effects. Menstrual disturbances (or normalization of menses) may not become apparent in short-term (i.e., 8 weeks) trials; in fact, a common definition of amenorrhea is absence of menses for 6 months. In addition, no analysis was done of the effect of hormone replacement therapy or oral contraceptives on genitourinary side effects such as vaginal dryness or dyspareunia; this is a problem because supplemental estrogen in oral contraceptives may treat these symptoms, which, again, increases the likelihood that these side effects will be underestimated during clinical trials. Unfortunately, no scientifically rigorous, placebo-controlled, large-sample, longitudinal studies of rates of sexual and menstrual disturbances are available to show either induction or resolution of these endocrine-related side effects with the new antipsychotic drugs.

The failure to consider hormonal status of women during these trials not only influences accurate assessment of the prevalence and severity of reproductive endocrine side effects but also may confound interpretation of changes in psychopathology and cognition. For example, if a patient who is hypoestrogenized because of amenorrhea caused by neuroleptic-induced hyperprolactinemia enters a clinical trial and is prescribed an oral contraceptive as a condition of enrollment, this hormone replacement could affect her mental status (Lindamer et al. 1997; Seeman and Lang 1990). These changes then may be attributed to the test drug or may obscure the differences between placebo and active drug treatment. There is now no doubt that estrogen effects changes in multiple domains of mental functioning (Fink et al. 1996; McEwen 1997). Design of future clinical trials of new antipsychotic medications should include a sex-specific data analysis and consider the effect of supplemental sex steroids and menopausal status on endocrine function, schizophrenia symptoms, and comorbid syndromes such as depression.

PROLACTIN AND ANTIPSYCHOTIC DRUGS

Prolactin is an anterior pituitary peptide hormone whose major role in humans is in lactogenesis. Control of prolactin release is complex, with many physiological and neuroendocrine factors involved, but the neurotransmitter dopamine plays a primary role in regulation, acting as the principal prolactin inhibitory factor of prolactin synthesis and secretion by the pituitary lactotrope cells (Melmed 1995; Yazigi et al. 1997). Traditional neuroleptics elevate prolactin by dopamine blockade (i.e., by interfering with the normal inhibition of prolactin release) (Rubin 1987).

In a positron-emission tomography study that used labeled raclopride, an experimental drug highly selective for dopamine D_2 receptors, plasma prolactin concentrations were increased in patients with a D_2 occupancy greater than 50% and correlated with antipsychotic response (Nordstrom and Farde 1998). However, the relation between D_2 occupancy, prolactin levels, and antipsychotic efficacy is likely to be convoluted because clozapine, olanzapine, and quetiapine, all drugs with proven antipsychotic efficacy, do not cause sustained prolactin elevations.

No significant sex differences in prolactin levels are found in unmedicated patients with schizophrenia (Kuruvilla et al. 1992). However, antipsychotic drugs may induce a greater prolactin response in treated women than in men possibly because of greater sensitivity of the tuberoinfundibulum to dopamine blockade (Rubin 1987). No convincing evidence indicates that prolactin regulation in patients with schizophrenia is abnormal despite conceptualizations of schizophrenia as a "dopamine disease" or that gross abnormalities of prolactin secretion are characteristic of any psychiatric disorder (Rubin 1987; Sobrinho 1991).

HYPOTHALAMIC–PITUITARY–OVARIAN AXIS

The hypothalamus secretes gonadotropin-releasing hormone (GnRH) in a pulsatile manner with a frequency and amplitude that is necessary for normal pituitary secretion of luteinizing hormone (LH) and follicle-stimulating hormone (FSH). These gonadotropins then stimulate an ovarian response with normal follicle growth, resulting in normal menstrual cycles and—barring other pathology—intact reproductive function. Excessive secretion of prolactin inhibits the normal pulsatile secretion of GnRH. When GnRH pulses are suboptimal, the menstrual cycle will be distorted; this distortion may be minimal (e.g., continued regular menses with impaired follicular growth). Greater disruption of normal pulsatile GnRH secretion may induce a greater distortion of menstrual function, causing problems such as menses that are too frequent, infrequent, or excessively heavy, so-called menstrual chaos. Yet, further impairment of pulsatile GnRH secretion causes insufficient secretion of LH and FSH to result in a proper ovarian response, thus leading to a hypoestrogenized amenorrheic cycle (Corenblum 1993, 1997; Vance 1997; Yazigi et al. 1997).

Thus, in understanding the side effects of hyperprolactinemia, one must consider the direct effects of elevated prolactin and the secondary effects if the woman becomes hypogonadal. Deficient estrogen secretion may have immediate symptoms such as dyspareunia secondary to effects on genital tissue and effects on mental functioning (Seeman 1997) and later complications resulting from the lack of protection afforded by estrogen against osteoporosis (Biller et al. 1992; Schlechte et al. 1992) and cardiovascular disease (Shaarawy et al. 1997).

PROLACTIN AND BEHAVIORAL EFFECTS

Increased anxiety, depression, and hostility attributed to nonphysiological hyperprolactinemia have been reported in nonpsychotic women independent of estrogen status (Buckman 1985; Fava et al. 1981). Studies of prolactin secretion also show that prolactin can increase as a response to stress, albeit in highly individual and contextually dependent ways (see Sobrinho 1991 for a review of the neuropsychiatry of prolactin).

Given that neuroleptic-induced hyperprolactinemia can induce a hypogonadal state and that ovarian steroids produce profound effects in the brain unrelated to reproduction (Stahl 1997), hyperprolactinemia potentially has multiple effects on mental functioning. Estrogen is thought to modulate dopamine and therefore may improve neuroleptic responsiveness in women. The purported neuromodulating properties of estrogen have been proposed as a possible explanation for 1) the lower doses of typical neuroleptics required by younger women; 2) the exacerbation of psychosis in menopausal women with schizophrenia secondary to the loss of estrogen's protective effect; and 3) the psychiatric symptoms that, in general, worsen when estrogen levels are low and improve when they are high (Gattaz et al. 1994; Riecher-Rossler et al. 1994; Seeman 1996, 1997). Also, schizophrenia symptoms have improved with the use of estrogen replacement therapy in case reports (Kulkarni et al. 1996; Lindamer et al. 1997).

Estrogen also has a role in improving and maintaining specific cognitive functions, verbal memory, and, possibly, visual memory in women (Sherwin 1997, 1998). An intriguing example is that estrogen treatment in young girls with Turner's syndrome, who lack ovarian estrogen production because of a chromosomal abnormality, has a positive effect on nonverbal processing speed and speeded motor performance (Ross et al. 1998). The latter has been hypothesized as secondary to estrogen stimulating release of dopamine in the nigrostriatal system (McDermott 1993). Estrogen levels of 22 women with chronic schizophrenia were reported to be more related to measures of cognition than to symptomatology, but this relevant abstract contained few details (Hoff et al. 1997). Cognition of patients with schizophrenia has recently been a focus of intense interest, but the interplay of antipsychotic-induced endocrine changes and cognitive consequences has not, to our knowledge, been explored; however, given the effect of cognition on functional outcome, this area is of importance.

In summary, when women with schizophrenia are prescribed antipsychotic drugs that increase prolactin and secondarily induce lowered levels of sex hormones (relative for the individual), the effects of these changes on psychiatric symptoms and cognition are poorly understood. Conversely, when previously high prolactin levels and low levels of estrogen are normalized by switching to a new prolactin-sparing antipsychotic, the contribution through neuroendocrine mechanisms to changes in psychiatric symptoms and cognition has not been studied.

ANTIPSYCHOTIC DRUGS AND MENSTRUAL FUNCTIONING

That antipsychotics disrupt the hypothalamic-pituitary-ovarian axis has been known for many years. Menstrual disturbances are commonly associated with traditional antipsychotic treatment, with estimates of prevalence of 15%–50% (Santoni and Saubadu 1995) or as high as 91% (Ghadirian et al. 1982). Risperidone has been reported to induce amenorrhea in premenopausal women coincident with increases in prolactin levels that exceeded those found in women who received standard antipsychotics (Dickson et al. 1995). In these five cases, the doses of risperidone ranged from 3 to 6 mg, with an average dose of 4.8 mg, in line with more recent recommendations for lower doses of risperidone by the manufacturer.

Resolution of hyperprolactinemia and its complications with clozapine treatment has been described in a case report of an adolescent female (Bunker et al. 1997). In two recent cases of women aged 45 and 26, switching to olanzapine reduced serum prolactin levels, improved menstrual function, and reduced galactorrhea (Canuso et al. 1998b). However, the incidence of menstrual disturbances, their relation to the duration and chemical class of antipsychotic drug, and patient risk factors for the development of amenorrhea and secondary functional hypoestrogenism during drug treatment have not been adequately studied at a population level.

An early small case series of phenothiazine-treated patients reported premenopausal women with absent menses whose genitalia were described as compatible with the "climacterium" and in whom injection of progesterone did not cause withdrawal bleeding. Although endocrinological laboratory measurements were less sophisticated at that time, abnormalities of the hypothalamic-pituitary axis, particularly abnormal gonadotropin secretion, were reported (Taubert et al. 1966). Another small case series of six antipsychotic-treated women with menstrual disturbances found that 50% had a negative progesterone challenge test result, again indicating a hypoestrogenic state developing in a subgroup of women (Smith 1992). Why some, but not all, women develop endocrine disturbances with antipsychotic treatment is not known, but several factors have been postulated to be important, including the dose of drug, combinations of antipsychotics, and biological differences contributing to an individual's susceptibility (Beumont et al. 1974a). It has been suggested that amenorrhea often develops at serum prolactin levels greater than 60–100 ng/mL (Marken et al. 1992), but in our experience, this is highly variable; some women maintain normal cycles for extended periods of time despite high prolactin levels, and others develop disturbances early in the course of treatment despite relatively mild hyperprolactinemia.

Neuroleptic-induced hyperprolactinemia cannot be considered to be the sole precipitant or etiological factor in menstrual disturbances in women with diagnosed schizophrenia. Before the introduction of neuroleptics, women with schizophrenia were found to have abnormal menstrual cycles (Gregory 1957). Whether hypoestrogenism in women with schizophrenia occurs secondary to antipsychotic treatment and/or to the disease itself also has been debated (Riecher-Rossler et al. 1994). In addition, other causes of secondary menstrual disturbances (i.e., those that occur after menses have been established) develop in women with schizophrenia, just as in women without this disease. However, women with schizophrenia may be especially vulnerable to drug-induced disruption of their menstrual cycles given their underlying brain disease and preexisting menstrual disturbances. Thus, clinicians must document a menstrual history before starting antipsychotics and must monitor for menstrual disturbances during drug treatment, especially if they are prescribing drugs known to cause hyperprolactinemia.

The psychological sequelae of drug-induced menstrual chaos or amenorrhea in women with schizophrenia have, in general, been neglected by researchers and clinicians. For example, the loss of her "monthly marker" indicating whether she is pregnant or not may be distressing to a sexually active woman regardless of whether she has a serious mental illness. In women with impaired reality testing, the combination of amenorrhea, galactorrhea, and weight gain, all common side effects of neuroleptic treatment, may promote false beliefs of pregnancy. In the authors' clinical experience, the resumption of regular menses that occurs in some women treated with prolactin-sparing antipsychotics does affect psychological health, albeit in highly individual ways, modified by variables such as her stage in the life cycle, her attitude toward fertility, and cultural factors.

GALACTORRHEA, ANTIPSYCHOTIC DRUGS, AND PROLACTIN

Like menstrual disturbances, galactorrhea, defined as nonpuerperal milk production, has long been recognized as a side effect of antipsychotic treatment (Beumont et al. 1974b, 1975; Taubert et al. 1966) and, like menstrual abnormalities, has been an undervalued side effect. The estimated incidence during neuroleptic therapy has been reported to range from 10% to 57% (Windgassen et al. 1996). Premenopausal women who have been pregnant are at higher risk for developing galactorrhea secondary to prolactin-elevating antipsychotics, but this side effect is not rare in nulliparous women (Beumont et al. 1974b).

Galactorrhea, with normal menses and prolactin levels, may occur in up to 20% of women (Eastman 1990). A recent community survey of 1,000 healthy Anatolian women of reproductive age found that the prevalence of galactorrhea was 10.2%, with 2.9% amenorrheic and 19.6% oligomenorrheic, 88.2% parous, and 9.8% infertile. The authors concluded that galactorrhea is a common finding among unselected healthy women. It was idiopathic in 47.3% of the subgroup of 74 patients who were investigated. Only 10.8% had hyperprolactinemia; other causes cited included being postpartum, other drugs, fibrocystic breast disease, and in 4%, hypothyroidism (Sahin et al. 1998).

In antipsychotic-treated women, galactorrhea does not directly correlate with the prolactin level, and, as discussed above, not all nonpuerperal milk production is drug related. In one study, only two-thirds of the women in whom galactorrhea occurred as a side effect of neuroleptic treatment had documented elevated prolactin levels (Windgassen et al. 1996). In postmenopausal women, galactorrhea secondary to neuroleptic-induced hyperprolactinemia is uncommon unless concurrent estrogen replacement therapy is given because lactation requires an estrogen-primed breast (Birkenfeld and Kase 1994; Corenblum 1990; Vance 1997).

Because women with psychotic disorders who develop galactorrhea may not spontaneously disclose the problem, this side effect is underdiagnosed. In Wesselman's series, only 8 of the 28 women spontaneously divulged this side effect (Wesselmann and Windgassen 1995). Given the numerous side effects of antipsychotic treatment, some clinicians may consider galactorrhea as merely a nuisance rather than an important adverse effect of treatment. Milk production is for many women part of feminine identity, and in women with disturbed reality testing, drug-induced galactorrhea can be misinterpreted as evidence of pregnancy and, in part because of this misinterpretation, as a positive event affirming their generative potential. Others may find it distressing and embarrassing (Wesselmann and Windgassen 1995).

In women requiring antipsychotic therapy during the postpartum period, there may be advantages to prescribing a prolactin-sparing antipsychotic because lactation is often not desired. One case report supports this, describing the use of clozapine in treating a patient with a postpartum psychosis and mastitis (Kornhuber and Weller 1991). However, clozapine use is restricted because of the hematological risk, so the newer prolactin-sparing agents olanzapine and quetiapine may be useful in a wider range of women who require antipsychotic therapy postpartum.

SEXUALITY, ANTIPSYCHOTIC DRUGS, AND PROLACTIN

It is well accepted that neuroleptics do cause sexual problems in both sexes, including diminished desire, disorders of arousal, vaginal lubrication problems, and orgasmic dysfunction. These problems can be a result of the drug's direct pharmacological actions on sexual function or can be indirect, secondary to other side effects (Aizenberg et al. 1995; Crenshaw and Goldberg 1996; Lingjaerde et al. 1987). An example of the latter in patients treated with antipsychotics is akathisia, which may produce agitation and motor restlessness, thus affecting the desire for sexual relations.

A sexual history often is not included as part of a psychiatric assessment despite physicians' awareness that psychiatric disease, psychotropic drugs, and psychological sequelae of sexual dysfunction all may affect quality of life (Singh and Beck 1997). In our experience, this may be particularly true in patients with psychotic disorders, summed up by a female patient's remark: "No one ever asks us about this (sex). There is the assumption that because I have schizophrenia, I shouldn't have a sex life."

Crenshaw and Goldberg (1996) suggested that prolactin levels greater than 40 mg/mL can directly cause sexual dysfunction and that levels between 25 and 50 mg/mL should alert the physician to monitor sexual functioning. Ghadirian et al. (1982) found a correlation between elevated prolactin concentrations and sexual dysfunction in men with schizophrenia but not in women. Sexual dysfunction in hyperprolactinemic women does not seem to correlate with estrogen status and is not as simple as hypoestrogenism causing dyspareunia (Sobrinho 1991). The menstrual chaos that can occur secondary to neuroleptic-induced hyperprolactinemia also may indirectly affect sexual relationships because unpredictable menses can interfere with the desire to engage in and with access to partner-related sexual activity.

This apparent lack of correlation between prolactin levels and sexual dysfunction can be partly understood by the pharmacology of the drugs; typical antipsychotics affect multiple central and peripheral neural systems while elevating prolactin levels and, in some individuals, lowering levels of sex hormones. The evaluation of the effects of antipsychotics on sexual function in patients with schizophrenia is further complicated by the effect of the disease itself; the variable pharmacology and doses of the antipsychotic drugs used to treat it; the adherence of the patient to treatment prescribed; and the complex biological, psychological, and social factors and value systems that influence each individual's sexuality (Barnes et al. 1979; Crenshaw and Goldberg 1996; Segraves 1982, 1989).

Women may be reluctant to reveal information about reproductive and sexual dysfunction (i.e., spontaneous reporting is inadequate to assess these side effects) and/or may be unaware that such dysfunction may be medication induced. Assessment of individual patients is further confused by the polypharmacy that often occurs in clinical practice. For example, selective serotonin reuptake inhibitors (SSRIs) used to treat depression in schizophrenia are now well known to cause sexual dysfunction (Balon et al. 1993). Of interest, SSRIs may, in some women, also increase prolactin levels (Amsterdam et al. 1997).

Although the prolactin-sparing drugs clozapine, olanzapine, and quetiapine may improve sexual desire, arousal, and orgasmic capacity, to date no case reports have shown improvement in women's sexual functioning with these drugs. Two case reports of male patients switched from risperidone to prolactin-sparing drugs suggested that resolution of hyperprolactinemia improved ability to function sexually (Dickson and Glazer 1999a; Shiwach and Carnody 1998). In medical patients with hyperprolactinemia, libido is decreased, and dopamine agonists such as bromocriptine are successful in treating some, but not all, patients (Sobrinho 1991, 1993; Yazigi et al. 1997).

With the reduction in symptoms of schizophrenia and fewer drug side effects that occur in some women taking the new antipsychotic drugs, there may be new or renewed interest in romantic and/or sexual relationships. Resumption of menses may make the woman aware that she is once again a "normal" female capable of conception (Dickson et al. 2000). In some clozapine-treated women, yearning for a child occurs (Barnas et al. 1994; Waldman and Safferman 1993), but a concomitant change in sexual desire has not been reported. The contribution of hormonal factors to these changes is not clear. Given the complex array of individual vascular, neurological, and psychosocial factors and partner-related variables that contribute to satisfactory sexual relationships, it is unrealistic to expect that normalization of prolactin with prolactin-sparing antipsychotics will improve sexual functioning in all female patients. However, because prolactin elevations may contribute to sexual dysfunction either directly or indirectly, this should be considered in evaluating sexual dysfunction in each antipsychotic-treated woman because this factor is treatable.

Further research is needed in this area of schizophrenia and sexuality, but at a minimum, clinicians should routinely obtain a sexual history, be aware of the potential for iatrogenic sexual side effects from antipsychotic medications, and provide an environment where patients with schizophrenia can openly discuss their concerns about their sexuality.

FERTILITY, ANTIPSYCHOTIC DRUGS, AND PROLACTIN

The study of schizophrenia, antipsychotic drugs, and fertility, like the study of sexual functioning, is complex, with a multitude of biological and psychosocial factors influencing reproductive rates. Neuroleptic-induced hyperprolactinemia can reduce an individual's fertility by affecting both reproductive and sexual functioning, but it is just one of many factors that may influence reproductive capability. Psychosocial factors affect the amount of time in the hospital and, in turn, influence reproductive rates; for example, fertility of women with schizophrenia increased with deinstitutionalization (Odegard 1980) despite the widespread use of antipsychotic medication. Reduced reproductive fitness may occur secondary to the illness itself (Bassett et al. 1996). Therefore, although these medications affect fertility, many other factors clearly affect pregnancy rates in mentally ill women (Miller 1997).

When a woman's normal hormonal cyclicity is interrupted and an anovulatory amenorrheic state develops, fertility is, of course, impaired relative to her chance of conceiving with monthly ovulation. Normal levels of circulating prolactin also may play a role in maintaining early pregnancy. Hyperprolactinemia is a possible etiological agent in early pregnancy loss in a subgroup of women with histories of recurrent miscarriages (Hirahara et al. 1998), but the validity of this finding has been questioned given the design of this study (Dlugi 1998). No evidence indicates that neuroleptic-induced hyperprolactinemia permanently affects fertility (i.e., this is a reversible side effect).

With resolution of neuroleptic-induced hyperprolactinemia whether secondary to dose reduction, to discontinuing medication, or to switching to a prolactin-sparing antipsychotic drug, more regular menstrual cycles and more consistent ovulation may ensue, and the chance of conception therefore increases. Case reports of female patients conceiving when switched from typical antipsychotics to clozapine suggest that the normalization of reproductive functioning secondary to the prolactin-sparing property of clozapine may have increased the chance of conception (Dickson and Hogg 1998; Kaplan et al. 1995; Waldman and Safferman 1993). The youngest woman described in the limited clozapine and pregnancy case literature is 28 years old; whether more pregnancies will occur as clozapine is prescribed to younger women earlier in the course of their illnesses and therefore at a time in their life cycle of relatively higher fertility seems possible but is currently unknown (Dickson and Hogg 1998). Switching to olanzapine or quetiapine, which like clozapine is prolactin sparing relative to haloperidol and risperidone (Crawford et al. 1997; Tran et al. 1997), also may increase an individual's chances of conceiving. One case report of a woman who became pregnant when switched from typical antipsychotic treatment to olanzapine (Dickson and Dawson 1998) is very similar to the report of an unwanted pregnancy in a clozapine-treated woman (Kaplan et al. 1995).

Fertility of male clozapine patients has been commented on in an anecdotal report of clozapine-treated patients producing more children than their non-clozapine-treated peers in a day hospital population (Dickson and Edwards 1997). Resolution of impaired reproductive functioning induced by hyperprolactinemia, concurrent with improved symptom control and increased social interaction secondary to atypical antipsychotic treatment, has the potential to improve both sexes' reproductive capability. Assortative mating, in which sexual coupling among psychiatric patients increases above statistical chance, may occur; thus, changes in male psychiatric patients' sexual and/or reproductive capability are of importance to female psychiatric patients. Case reports suggest that increased reproductive capability, particularly with clozapine treatment, has occurred, but definitive research on changes in fertility of the seriously mentally ill at a population level is required. In the interim, it is prudent for clinicians to be aware of antipsychotic drugs' variable effects on prolactin secretion; to regularly inquire in a nonjudgmental manner about menses, sexual activity, and desire to have children as part of a comprehensive care plan for patients with schizophrenia; and to implement sex education and family planning programs.

Women who have been amenorrheic or who have had irregular periods may become pregnant shortly after switching drugs and be unaware of the pregnancy, thus exposing the fetus to the antipsychotic agent. Of the new-generation drugs, the most clinical experience has accumulated with the use of clozapine during pregnancy. No published case reports describe the use of risperidone, olanzapine, or quetiapine throughout pregnancy. Although a review of antipsychotic drugs and pregnancy is beyond the scope of this chapter, this rapidly evolving topic is of great importance given the frequent prescription of atypical drugs to women of childbearing age. Until more is known, it may be safer to switch to an older agent. However, this requires an individual risk–benefit assessment, especially in pregnant women with full or partial treatment resistance, because switching to an older agent may risk recurrence of acute psychosis, which ultimately may be of more danger to the mother and fetus than continuation of an effective newer medication (Canadian Clinical Practice Guidelines 1998). Given the desire of many seriously mentally ill women to bear and raise children, and their poor prognosis in retaining care of their children, the potential benefits of the new generation of drugs in improving this outcome warrant more research.

OSTEOPOROSIS, CARDIOVASCULAR DISEASE, AND ANTIPSYCHOTIC DRUGS

Gonadal steroids have metabolic effects beyond the reproductive system. Hypoestrogenism is a risk factor for both osteoporosis and cardiovascular disease in women. Neuroleptic-induced hyperprolactinemia, by inducing a hypoestrogenic state in a subgroup of antipsychotic-treated women, may increase the risk of decreased bone mineral density and cardiovascular disease. With both osteoporosis and cardiovascular disease, multiple risk factors interact in complex ways; hypoestrogenism induced by hyperprolactinemia is only one of many risk factors that patients with schizophrenia may have. Other risk factors, including smoking, sedentary lifestyle, and poor nutrition, that often present in patients with schizophrenia suggest that they may be at high risk for development of comorbid medical conditions (Abraham et al. 1995).

Prospective studies of bone loss in hyperprolactinemic women suggest that a decrease in bone mineral density is related to attendant estrogen deficiency and not to elevated prolactin level per se (Biller et al. 1992; Schlechte et al. 1992). Decreased bone mineral density, the hallmark of osteoporosis, has been reported in psychiatric patients (Ataya et al. 1988; Halbreich and Palter 1996; Halbreich et al. 1995), but a deficit of information on the effect of antipsychotic medications on rates and severity of osteoporosis and fracture rates in patients with schizophrenia remains. A case report of a young neuroleptic-treated woman showed improvement in bone mineral density following successful treatment of hyperprolactinemia and hypoestrogenism with bromocriptine (Kartaginer et al. 1990). The availability of new drugs that do not cause neuroleptic-induced hyperprolactinemia potentially lowers the risk of osteoporosis, but no studies have been reported that confirm that this in fact occurs.

Estrogen is thought to be cardioprotective in women; the largest increase in heart disease in women occurs around age 50, approximately the time of menopause, when production of endogenous estrogen declines (Stampfer et al. 1990). Hyperprolactinemic women with amenorrhea and low serum estrogen, compared with a control group, had a decrease in nitric oxide levels (known to affect vascular endothelium) associated with elevated blood pressure (Shaarawy et al. 1997). In a 6-week study, treatment with bromocriptine, a dopamine agonist, restored menses and increased serum nitric oxide and estrogen levels to those of healthy control subjects. More research is needed, but the authors of this study advised that adverse effects of hypoestrogenism secondary to hyperprolactinemia extend to the cardiovascular system.

BREAST CANCER, ANTIPSYCHOTIC DRUGS, AND PROLACTIN

Product labeling of prolactin-elevating antipsychotics advises that hyperprolactinemia increases the risk of breast cancer in animals. However, a review of endogenous hormones and breast cancer risk concluded that the cohort, case-control, and cross-sectional studies of prolactin levels do not provide consistent support for the hypothesis that elevated prolactin is associated with an increased risk of human breast cancer (Bernstein and Ross 1993). Available studies on prolactin and breast cancer and on antipsychotic drugs and breast cancer do not support switching to prolactin-sparing drugs as a preventive measure in women requiring antipsychotic drug treatment. For women with breast cancer who are taking antipsychotic medication, treatment should be conducted in consultation with breast cancer experts, assessing the potential risks and benefits of their antipsychotic prescription.

In general, prior studies have not supported an association between antipsychotic drugs and the subsequent development of breast cancer (Katz et al. 1967; Mortensen 1989, 1994; Overall 1978; Wagner and Mantal 1978). One recent study that did show an increased incidence of breast cancer in a small sample of neuroleptic-treated patients has been controversial (Goodwin 1997; Halbreich et al. 1996; Mortensen 1997; Torrey 1997). The authors of a small case series describing the pathology of breast cancer in neuroleptic-treated patients (12 female and 1 male) suggested that additional studies are warranted to characterize the biology of these neoplasms (Tsubura et al. 1992).

Because the widespread use of neuroleptics for severe psychiatric disorders did not occur until the late 1950s, earlier studies would not have included women who had received antipsychotic treatment throughout their entire life cycle and who with advancing age had now moved into the higher-risk age groups for the development of breast cancer. Given the relevance of this issue for women's health, it is important to conduct studies of these older women with modern detection techniques. Clinicians should ensure that seriously mentally ill women, like all women, have access to education about breast self-examination, regular breast examinations, and age-appropriate routine screening mammography (Dickson and Glazer 1999b).

TREATMENT OF NEUROLEPTIC-INDUCED HYPERPROLACTINEMIA

Optimal drug therapy for schizophrenia is complex and challenging; avoidance and treatment of hyperprolactinemia must be considered in the context of comprehensive care, with evaluation of the costs of this side effect to individual patients. Measuring prolactin levels is an important part of assessment for endocrine side effects, but the clinical objectives are to screen for endocrine abnormalities before initiating treatment and to monitor for and intervene appropriately should adverse events, as described in this chapter, occur. There is individual variability in end-organ susceptibility to hyperprolactinemia and in the length of time for side effects to manifest; therefore, prolactin levels must always be correlated with clinical findings.

If prolactin-related side effects do occur and are considered to be secondary to drug treatment, reduction of the antipsychotic has been the treatment of choice. If that is not possible, then symptomatic treatment with amantadine or bromocriptine has been advised (American Psychiatric Association 1997; Marken et al. 1992). However, psychiatrists have been reluctant to use these drugs with dopamine agonist properties for fear of exacerbating psychiatric symptoms; the limited information available suggests that bromocriptine therapy is tolerated by most antipsychotic-treated women without exacerbating their underlying psychiatric disorder (Smith 1992). Whether agents such as amantadine and bromocriptine are suitable for long-term use in patients with neuroleptic-induced hyperprolactinemia is unknown. Clinicians should be cognizant that reversal of hyperprolactinemia with these agents will correct anovulatory infertility (Yazigi et al. 1997).

Hypogonadism can be treated with hormone replacement therapy, estrogen, and progesterone, either cyclically or continuously (Vance 1997). Premenopausal patients who require contraception may be treated with oral contraceptives and in that way receive estrogen supplementation. However, direct effects of hyperprolactinemia (e.g., galactorrhea and reduced libido) would not be treated with this latter approach.

With the introduction of prolactin-sparing agents, switching a patient's antipsychotic therapy to one of these drugs (clozapine, olanzapine, or quetiapine) is a new option for avoiding and treating neuroleptic-induced hyperprolactinemia. This simplifies drug regimens by 1) eliminating the need to add another drug (dopamine agonist) to treat a side effect, 2) minimizing the necessity of progesterone challenge tests to monitor for functional hypoestrogenism in antipsychotic-treated amenorrheic women, and 3) reducing the need for hormone replacement therapy to treat drug-induced hypoestrogenism.

CONCLUSION

Until recently, interest has been limited in the clinical consequences of neuroleptic-induced hyperprolactinemia. In light of advances in endocrinology and the appreciation that changes in gonadal hormones influence not only reproductive systems but also neural networks, the development of antipsychotic drugs with fewer neuroendocrine side effects is potentially a significant advance for women who must take these drugs chronically to control their persistent mental illnesses. Sufficient information from the endocrinological literature and psychiatric case reports warrants caution when prescribing drugs that elevate prolactin levels. However, systematic, methodologically sound, longitudinal research is urgently needed to elucidate both short-term and long-term sequelae of antipsychotic-induced hyperprolactinemia in psychiatric populations.

REFERENCES

Abraham G, Friedman RH, Verghese C, et al: Osteoporosis and schizophrenia: can we limit known risk factors? Biol Psychiatry 38:131–132, 1995

Aizenberg D, Zemishlany Z, Dorfman-Etrog P, et al: Sexual dysfunction in male schizophrenic patients. J Clin Psychiatry 56:137–141, 1995

American Psychiatric Association: Practice guideline for the treatment of patients with schizophrenia. Am J Psychiatry 154(suppl 4):1–63, 1997

Amsterdam JD, Garcia-Espana F, Goodman D, et al: Breast enlargement during chronic anti-depressant therapy. J Affect Disord 46:151–156, 1997

Arvanitis LA, Miller BG: Multiple fixed doses of "Seroquel" (quetiapine) in patients with acute exacerbation of schizophrenia: a comparison with haloperidol and placebo. The Seroquel Trial 13 Study Group. Biol Psychiatry 42:233–246, 1997

Ataya K, Mercado A, Kartaginer J, et al: Bone density and reproductive hormones in patients with neuroleptic-induced hyperprolactinemia. Fertil Steril 50:876–881, 1988

Balon R, Yeragani VK, Pohl R, et al: Sexual dysfunction during antidepressant treatment. J Clin Psychiatry 54:209–212, 1993

Barnas C, Bergant A, Hummer M, et al: Clozapine concentrations in maternal and fetal plasma, amniotic fluid and breast milk (letter). Am J Psychiatry 151:945, 1994

Barnes TR, Bamber RW, Watson JP: Psychotropic drugs and sexual behaviour. Br J Hosp Med 21:594–600, 1979

Bassett AS, Alison B, Hodgkinson KA, et al: Reproductive fitness in familial schizophrenia. Schizophr Res 21:151–160, 1996

Beasley CM Jr, Sanger T, Satterlee W, et al: Olanzapine versus placebo: results of a double blind, fixed dose olanzapine trial. Psychopharmacology (Berl) 124:159–167, 1996

Bernstein L, Ross RK: Endogenous hormones and breast cancer risk. Epidemiol Rev 15:48–65, 1993

Beumont PJV, Gelder MG, Friesen HG, et al: The effects of phenothiazines on endocrine function, I: patients with inappropriate lactation and amenorrhoea. Br J Psychiatry 124:413–419, 1974a

Beumont PJV, Corker CS, Friesen HG, et al: The effects of phenothiazines on endocrine function, II: effects in men and post-menopausal women. Br J Psychiatry 124:420–430, 1974b

Beumont P, Bruwer J, Pimstone, B, et al: Brom-ergocryptine in the treatment of phenothiazine-induced galactorrhoea. Br J Psychiatry 126:285–288, 1975

Biller BMK, Baum HBA, Rosenthal DI, et al: Progressive trabecular osteopenia in women with hyperprolactinemic amenorrhea. J Clin Endocrinol Metab 75:692–697, 1992

Birkenfeld A, Kase NG: Functional anatomy and physiology of the female breast. Obstet Gynecol Clin North Am 21:433–444, 1994

Buckman M: Psychological distress in hyperprolactinemic women, in Prolactin: Basic and Clinical Correlates. Edited by MacLeod RM, Thorner MO, Scapagnini U. Padova, Italy, Livana Press, 1985, pp 601–608

Bunker MT, Marken PA, Schneiderhan ME, et al: Attenuation of antipsychotic-induced hyperprolactinemia with clozapine. J Child Adolesc Psychopharmacol 7:65–69, 1997

Canadian Clinical Practice Guidelines for the Treatment of Schizophrenia. Can J Psychiatry 43(suppl 2 revised):25S–39S, November 1998

Canuso CM, Goldstein JM, Green AI: The evaluation of women with schizophrenia. Psychopharmacol Bull 34:271–277, 1998a

Canuso CM, Hanau M, Jhamb KK, et al: Olanzapine use in women with antipsychotic-induced hyperprolactinemia (letter). Am J Psychiatry 155:1458, 1998b

Chouinard G, Jones B, Remington B, et al: A Canadian multicentre placebo-controlled study of fixed doses of risperidone and haloperidol in the treatment of chronic schizophrenic patients. J Clin Psychopharmacol 13:25–40, 1993

Corenblum B: Galactorrhea and hyperprolactinemia. Med Clin North Am 13:1569–1579, 1990

Corenblum B: Disorders of prolactin secretion, in Textbook of Gynecology. Edited by Copeland LJ. Philadelphia, PA, WB Saunders, 1993, pp 447–467

Corenblum B: Rise above normal when treating hyperprolactinemia. Canadian Journal of Diagnosis 14:133–144, 1997

Crawford AMK, Beasley CM Jr, Tollefson GD: The acute and long-term effect of olanzapine compared with placebo and haloperidol on serum prolactin concentrations. Schizophr Res 28:224–267, 1997

Crenshaw TL, Goldberg JP: Sexual Pharmacology: Drugs That Affect Sexual Functioning. New York, WW Norton, 1996, pp 307–316

Currier GW, Simpson GM: Antipsychotic medications and fertility. Psychiatr Serv 49:175–176, 1998a

Currier GW, Simpson GM: Pregnancy and clozapine: taking issue (editorial). Psychiatr Serv 49:997, 1998b

Dickson RA, Dawson DT: Olanzapine and pregnancy (letter). Can J Psychiatry 43:2, 1998

Dickson RA, Edwards A: Clozapine and fertility (letter). Am J Psychiatry 154:582–583, 1997

Dickson RA, Glazer WM: Hyperprolactinemia and male sexual dysfunction (letter). J Clin Psychiatry 60:125, 1999a

Dickson RA, Glazer WM: Neuroleptic induced hyperprolactinemia. Schizophr Res 35:S75–S86, 1999b

Dickson RA, Hogg L: Pregnancy of a patient treated with clozapine. Psychiatr Serv 49:1081–1083, 1998

Dickson RA, Dalby JT, Williams R, et al: Risperidone-induced prolactin elevations in premenopausal women with schizophrenia (letter). Am J Psychiatry 152:1102–1103, 1995

Dickson RA, Seeman MV, Corenblum B: Hormonal side effects in women: typical versus atypical antipsychotic treatment. J Clin Psychiatry 61(suppl 3):10–15, 2000

Dlugi AM: Hyperprolactinemic recurrent spontaneous pregnancy loss: a true clinical entity or a spurious finding? Fertil Steril 70:253–255, 1998

Eastman RC: Acromegaly, hyperprolactinemia, gonadotropin-secreting tumors, and hypopituitarism, in Diagnostic Endocrinology. Edited by Moore WT, Eastman RC. Toronto, Ontario, Canada, Decker, 1990, pp 33–56

Fava GA, Fava M, Kellner R, et al: Depression, hostility and anxiety in hyperpro-lactinemic amenorrhea. Psychother Psychosom 36:122–128, 1981

Fink G, Sumner BE, Rosie R, et al: Estrogen control of central neurotransmission: effect on mood, mental state and memory. Cell Mol Neurobiol 16:325–344, 1996

Gattaz WF, Vogel P, Riecher-Rossler A, et al: Influence of the menstrual cycle phase on the therapeutic response in schizophrenia. Biol Psychiatry 36:137–139, 1994

Ghadirian AM, Chouinard G, Annable L: Sexual dysfunction and plasma prolactin levels in neuroleptic-treated schizophrenic outpatients. J Nerv Ment Dis 170:463–467, 1982

Goodwin PJ: Breast cancer risk in psychiatric patients (letter). Am J Psychiatry 154:588, 1997

Green MF: Medications and neurocognition, in Schizophrenia From a Neurocog-nitive Perspective Probing the Impenetrable Darkness. Boston, MA, Allyn & Bacon, 1998, pp 103–120

Gregory BAJC: The menstrual cycle and its disorders in psychiatric patients—II. J Psychosom Res 2:199–224, 1957

Halbreich U, Palter S: Accelerated osteoporosis in psychiatric patients: possible pathophysiological processes. Schizophr Bull 22:447–454, 1996

Halbreich U, Rojansky N, Palter S, et al: Decreased bone mineral density in med-icated psychiatric patients. Psychosom Med 57:485–491, 1995

Halbreich U, Shen J, Panaro V: Are chronic psychiatric patients at increased risk for developing breast cancer? Am J Psychiatry 153:559–560, 1996

Hirahara F, Andoh N, Sawai K, et al: Hyperprolactinemic recurrent miscarriage and results of randomized bromocriptine treatment trials. Fertil Steril 70:246–252, 1998

Hoff AL, Wieneke M, Horon R, et al: Estrogen levels relate to neuropsychological function in female schizophrenics. Schizophr Res 24:107–108, 1997

IMS America: National Disease Therapeutic Index. November 1996–April 1997

Kane JM, Freeman HL: Towards more effective antipsychotic treatment. Br J Psy-chiatry 165(suppl 25):22–31, 1994

Kane J, Honihfeld G, Singer J, et al: Clozapine for the treatment resistant schizo-phrenic: a double blind comparison with chlorpromazine. Arch Gen Psychia-try 45:789–796, 1988

Kaplan B, Modai I, Stoler M, et al: Clozapine treatment and risk of unplanned pregnancy. J Am Board Fam Pract 8:239–241, 1995

Kartaginer J, Ataya K, Mercado A, et al: Osteoporosis associated with neuroleptic treatment—a case report. J Reprod Med 35:198–202, 1990

Katz J, Kunofsky S, Patton RE, et al: Cancer mortality among patients in New York mental hospitals. Cancer 20:2194–2199, 1967

Kornhuber J, Weller M: Postpartum psychosis and mastitis: a new indication for clozapine? Am J Psychiatry 148:1751–1752, 1991

Kulkarni J, de Castella A, Smith D, et al: A clinical trial of the effects of estrogen in acutely psychotic women. Schizophr Res 20:247–252, 1996

Kuruvilla A, Peedicayil J, Srikrishna G, et al: A study of serum prolactin levels in schizophrenia: comparison of males and females. Clin Exp Pharmacol Physiol 19:603–606, 1992

Lindamer LA, Lohr JB, Harris MJ, et al: Gender, estrogen, and schizophrenia. Psychopharmacol Bull 33:221–228, 1997

Lingjaerde O, Ahlfors UG, Bech P, et al: The UKU Side Effect Rating Scale: a new comprehensive rating scale for psychotropic drugs and a cross-sectional study of side effects in neuroleptic-treated patients. Acta Psychiatr Scand 334:1–100, 1987

Marder SR, Meibach RC: Risperidone in the treatment of schizophrenia. Am J Psychiatry 151:825–835, 1994

Marder SR, Davis JM, Chouinard B: The effects of risperidone on the five dimensions of schizophrenia derived by factor analysis: combined results of the North American trials. J Clin Psychiatry 58:538–546, 1997

Marken PA, Haykal RF, Fisher JN: Management of psychotropic-induced hyperprolactinemia. Clin Pharm 11:851–856, 1992

McDermott JL: Effects of estrogen upon dopamine release from the corpus striatus of young and aged female rats. Brain Res 606:118–125, 1993

McEwen BS: Ovarian steroids and the brain: implications for cognition and aging. Neurology 48(suppl 7):S8–S15, 1997

Melmed S (ed): The Pituitary. Cambridge, MA, Blackwell Science, 1995, pp 149–162

Meltzer HY, Goode DJ, Schyve PM, et al: Effect of clozapine on human serum prolactin levels. Am J Psychiatry 136:1550–1555, 1979

Miller LJ: Sexuality, reproduction, and family planning in women with schizophrenia. Schizophr Bull 23:623–635, 1997

Mortensen PB: The incidence of cancer in schizophrenic patients. J Epidemiol Community Health 12:185–194, 1989

Mortensen PB: The occurrence of cancer in first admitted schizophrenia patients. Schizophr Res 12:185–194, 1994

Mortensen PB: Breast cancer risk in psychiatric patients (letter). Am J Psychiatry 154:589, 1997

Nordstrom A, Farde L: Plasma prolactin and central D2 receptor occupancy in antipsychotic drug-treated patients. J Clin Psychopharmacol 18:305–310, 1998

Odegard O: Fertility of psychiatric first admissions in Norway 1936–1975. Acta Psychiatr Scand 62:212–220, 1980

Overall JE: Prior psychiatric treatment and the development of breast cancer. Arch Gen Psychiatry 35:898–899, 1978

Peuskins J: Risperidone in the treatment of patients with chronic schizophrenia: a multi-nation, multi-centre, double-blind, parallel-group study vs haloperidol. Br J Psychiatry 166:712–716, 1995

Riecher-Rossler A, Hafner H, Stumbaum M, et al: Can estradiol modulate schizophrenic symptomatology? Schizophr Bull 20:203–214, 1994

Ross JL, Roeltgen D, Feuillan P, et al: Effects of estrogen on nonverbal processing speed and motor function in girls with Turner's syndrome. J Clin Endocrinol Metab 83:3198–3204, 1998

Rubin RT: Prolactin and schizophrenia, in Psychopharmacology: The Third Generation of Progress. Edited by Meltzer HY. New York, Raven, 1987, pp 803–808

Sahin Y, Turan R, Kelestimur F: Prevalence of galactorrhea in normal women in Central Anatolia, in Abstracts of the 14th Annual Meeting of the European Society of Human Reproduction and Embryology, Vol 13. Oxford, United Kingdom, Oxford University Press, 1998, pp 345–346

Santoni JPH, Saubadu S: Adverse events associated with neuroleptic drugs: focus on neuroendocrine reactions. Acta Therapeutica 21:193–204, 1995

Schlechte J, Walkner L, Kathol M: A longitudinal analysis of premenopausal bone loss in healthy women and women with hyperprolactinemia. J Clin Endocrinol Metab 75:698–703, 1992

Seeman MV: The role of estrogen in schizophrenia. J Psychiatry Neurosci 21:123–127, 1996

Seeman MV: Psychopathology in men and women: focus on female hormones. Am J Psychiatry 154:1641–1647, 1997

Seeman MV, Lang M: The role of estrogens in schizophrenia: gender differences. Schizophr Bull 16:185–194, 1990

Segraves RT: Male sexual dysfunction and psychoactive drug use: review of a common relationship. Postgrad Med 71:227–233, 1982

Segraves RT: Effects of psychotropic drugs on human erection and ejaculation. Arch Gen Psychiatry 46:275–284, 1989

Shaarawy M, Nafei S, Abul-Nasr A, et al: Circulating nitric oxide levels in galactorrheic, hyperprolactinemic, amenorrheic women. Fertil Steril 68:454–459, 1997

Sherwin BB: Estrogen effects on cognition in menopausal women. Neurology 48(suppl 7):S21–S26, 1997

Sherwin BB: Cognitive assessment for postmenopausal women and general assessment of their mental health. Psychopharmacol Bull 34:323–326, 1998

Shiwach RS, Carnody TJ: Prolactogenic effects of risperidone in male patients: a preliminary study. Acta Psychiatr Scand 98:81–83, 1998

Singh SP, Beck AJ: No sex please, we're British. Psychiatr Bull 21:99–101, 1997

Smith S: Neuroleptic-associated hyperprolactinemia: can it be treated with bromocriptine? J Reprod Med 37:737–740, 1992

Sobrinho LG: Neuropsychiatry of prolactin: causes and effects. Baillieres Clin Endocrinol Metab 5:119–141, 1991

Sobrinho L: The psychogenic effects of prolactin. Acta Endocrinologica 129(suppl 1):38–40, 1993

Stahl SM: Estrogen makes the brain a sex organ. J Clin Psychiatry 58:421–422, 1997

Stampfer MJ, Colditz GA, Willett WC: Menopause and heart disease: a review. Ann N Y Acad Sci 592:193–203, 1990

Taubert HD, Haskins AL, Moszkowski EF: The influence of thioridazine upon urinary gonadotropin excretion. South Med J 59:1301–1303, 1966

Tollefson GD, Beasley CM Jr, Tran PV, et al: Olanzapine versus haloperidol in the treatment of schizophrenia and schizoaffective and schizophreniform disorders: results of an international collaborative trial. Am J Psychiatry 154:457–465, 1997

Torrey EF: Breast cancer risk in psychiatric patients (letter). Am J Psychiatry 154:588–589, 1997

Tran PV, Hamilton SH, Kuntz AJ, et al: Double-blind comparison of olanzapine versus risperidone in the treatment of schizophrenia and other psychotic disorders. J Clin Psychopharmacol 17:407–418, 1997

Tsubura A, Hatano T, Murata A, et al: Breast carcinoma in patients receiving neuroleptic therapy: morphologic and clinicopathologic features of thirteen cases. Acta Pathologica Japonica 42:494–499, 1992

Vance ML: New directions in the treatment of hyperprolactinemia. The Endocrinologist 7:153–159, 1997

Wagner S, Mantal N: Breast cancer at a psychiatric hospital before and after the introduction of neuroleptic agents. Cancer Res 38:2703–2708, 1978

Waldman MD, Safferman A: Pregnancy and clozapine (letter). Am J Psychiatry 150:168–169, 1993

Wesselmann U, Windgassen K: Galactorrhea: subjective response by schizophrenic patients. Acta Psychiatr Scand 91:152–155, 1995

Windgassen K, Wesselmann U, Schulze Monking H: Galactorrhea and hyperprolactinemia in schizophrenic patients on neuroleptics: frequency and etiology. Neuropsychobiology 33:142–146, 1996

Yazigi RA, Quintero CH, Salameh WA: Prolactin disorders. Fertil Steril 67:215–225, 1997

13

Can Estrogens Account for Sex Differences in Schizophrenia?

Kathryn Abel, Ph.D., M.R.C.P., M.R.C.Psych., M.A.
David J. Castle, M.Sc., M.D., M.R.C.P.

*I*n the search for the causes of schizophrenia, attention has increasingly been focused on sex differences in the presentation, course, and outcome of the condition (Castle and Murray 1991; DeLisi et al. 1989; Flor-Henry 1990; Goldstein 1995; Lewine 1988; Seeman 1995). The characteristics of schizophrenic illness in men tend to include earlier age at onset, poorer premorbid functioning, less favorable response to medication, and more frequent relapse compared with their female counterparts (Bardenstein and McGlashan 1990; Castle et al. 1993; Goldstein et al. 1989). In contrast, women with schizophrenia are more likely to manifest a later-onset illness, with less premorbid dysfunction and more "atypical" and affective symptoms (Bardenstein and McGlashan 1990; Goldstein and Link 1988). Also, those patients with a very late onset of illness ("late paraphrenia") show a massive female preponderance (Castle and Howard 1992).

Professor Robin Murray and Drs. Veronica O'Keane, Jim Van Os, and Tony Davies provided useful comments on earlier drafts of the manuscript. We are most grateful to Dr. Mary Seeman for useful discussions on this topic.

It has been proposed that these sex differences can, at least in part, be explained in terms of some factor in women (e.g., estrogen) serving to delay the onset and ameliorate the course of the illness (Hafner et al. 1989; Seeman 1986). The estrogen hypothesis rests, among other things, on the interpretation of four separate lines of evidence (Riecher-Rossler and Hafner 1993):

1. Experimental evidence of the effects of main estrogen on central neurotransmission: antidopaminergic effects, serotonergic effects
2. Historical reports of abnormal functioning of sexual organs in association with schizophrenia
3. Clinical data associating schizophrenic onset or relapse in women with times of low estrogen levels
4. Epidemiological data of sex differences in age at onset in schizophrenia, particularly the concept that a "postmenopausal peak" in incidence occurs in women, which is consequent to the decline in estrogen levels at that age (Hafner et al. 1989).

We evaluate the estrogen hypothesis by considering each of these lines of evidence in turn and then outline the role estrogens might play in the determination of sex differences in schizophrenia.

EXPERIMENTAL DATA

Estrogens and Dopamine

Estrogens and other steroid hormones have been known to be intimately involved in neural transmission and neurochemical function since the mid-nineteenth century (Berthold 1849). More recently, it has been shown that the brain has the properties of a target organ for hormones, with a distribution of hormone receptors unique for every hormone class (McEwen 1985). Estrogen has both up- and downregulating effects on dopamine systems in rats, depending on the experimental conditions. However, in monkeys, estrogen has been shown to have an action similar to that of haloperidol (Bedard et al. 1983). Furthermore, it is clear that different brain regions show different specificities for estrogen action. Therefore, the outcome of estrogen administration probably will differ, depending on the type and site of cell (McEwen 1991). This could be a result of different dopamine receptors being linked to different postreceptor systems, as is seen in the adrenergic receptor (Wessler et al. 1990). Di Paolo (1994) suggested that estradiol could be used to modify both hyper- and hypodopaminergic states. Thus, the mechanisms behind the varying actions of estrogens on the brain are complex, but dopaminergic systems appear to be particularly influenced by estrogens.

Important animal studies, notably those of Hafner et al. (1991), have attempted to address the functional effects of estrogen's action on the brain. Hafner et al. (1991) and Gattaz et al. (1991) investigated the effects of estradiol administration in neonatal and adult rats. They found that estradiol antagonized the behavioral effects of both haloperidol (catalepsy) and apomorphine (oral stereotypies, grooming, sitting behavior) but that these effects were consistently significant in only the neonatally treated rats, whose estradiol levels were 15 times greater than those of the rats treated in adulthood. These authors proposed that estradiol acted by downregulating dopamine receptors, but the discrepancy between the effect in neonatal and adult rats could reflect estrogenic action on brain maturation rather than on modulation of brain function. Consonant with this latter hypothesis, Lipska et al. (1993) found, in rats, that certain dopamine-related behavioral consequences of early hippocampal lesions do not manifest until early adulthood, and it appears that the timing of onset of such behaviors reflects brain maturational rather than hormonal changes.

Estrogens and Serotonin

Short-term estrogen treatment has been shown to increase the number of postsynaptic serotonin type 2A (5-HT_{2A}) receptors in the cerebral cortex and nucleus accumbens of rats (Fink and Sumner 1996) and to increase the number of postsynaptic 5-HT_{2A} receptors in humans (Travis et al. 1999). Several studies that used neuroendocrine challenge with specific serotonin probes consistently found that estrogen appears to increase central serotonin tone in healthy women of varying ages (O'Keane et al. 1991; van Amelsvoort et al. 2001). Other groups (Best et al. 1992; Halbreich et al. 1995) reported that short-term estrogen treatment in postmenopausal women enhanced serotonin responsivity. However, their probes (*m*-chlorophenylpiperazine [m-CPP], L-tryptophan) were less serotonin specific, so the conclusions regarding serotonergic effects are more limited. We have used the specific serotonergic probe difenfluramine in healthy postmenopausal women and shown that long-term estrogen replacement can reverse the apparent downregulation of serotonergic neurtotransmission that occurs following estrogen withdrawal at menopause (van Amelsvoort et al. 2001).

EARLY CLINICAL STUDIES

A connection between functioning of the nervous system and hormones was formulated by Berthold as early as 1849, whereas Beach (1898) implicated overactivity of the sex glands in the causation of dementia praecox. Kraepelin (1913) also drew attention to hormonal processes in schizophrenia, commenting on the considerable number of cases beginning during pregnancy or the puerperium. More directly, Mott (1919) reported "regressive atrophy" in 22 of 100 postmortem testes from dementia praecox patients and proposed an etiological role for underactivity of the sex glands. Kretschmer (1921) described "masculinization" or "feminization" of body type in association with female and male schizophrenia, respectively, and described genital hypoplasia in "the majority of all female schizophrenes."

Because these early accounts of hypogonadism and psychosis were conducted in the preneuroleptic era, the potential confounding effects of medication were avoided. However, the studies all had methodological flaws that make them of limited value. These flaws include the following: 1) the "schizophrenia" referred to was not operationally defined, which may have particular implication for female subjects who are less likely than their male counterparts to meet stringent diagnostic criteria for schizophrenia (Castle et al. 1993; Lewine et al. 1984); 2) the data were exclusively observational; 3) most studies omitted comparison with control groups of other mentally ill or healthy subjects; and 4) when sex hormone levels were measured, the number of subjects was small, and the "assays" were unstandardized, biological, and cross-sectional; again, few such studies included control subjects.

A further difficulty in interpreting these early studies is the potential confounding effect of poor conditions of care and general living standards of the mentally ill at this time, along with chronic illnesses such as tuberculosis. Indeed, tuberculosis alone may cause hypogonadism. Also, untreated mental illness is likely to have an independent secondary effect on gonadal functioning. For example, studies have shown that both nonpsychotic and psychotic mental illness can affect gonadal function in similar ways and that the psychic disturbance associated with illness may cause secondary hypothalamic dysfunction (Suwa et al. 1962, 1966; Whalley et al. 1989). Furthermore, more recent studies measuring hormonal levels have not shown consistent differences between schizophrenia subjects and control subjects in terms of gonadal hormone or gonadotropin levels (Arato et al. 1979; Czernik and Kleesiek 1979; Johnstone et al. 1977; Kulkarni et al. 1996; Tourney and Hatfield 1972, 1973). These data are all complicated by the difficulty of measuring hormone and gonadotropin levels in cycling premenopausal women. Unless women are assessed longitudinally and compared on identical cycle phases, interpretation of data between treated and untreated or ill and control groups is not very meaningful. In the treatment study of Kulkarni et al. (1996), women with schizophrenia all had relatively low estrogen levels at baseline while taking neuroleptic medication.

Smith et al. (in press) found that neuroleptic treatment has profound sexual effects in both men and women with schizophrenia. These effects are consistent with blunting of the gonadotropin axis.

CLINICAL PERSPECTIVE

Variations in the rates of psychosis in women paramenstrually, during pregnancy, postpartum, and at menopause are the basis of the clinical evidence cited in favor of a neuroleptic effect of estrogen (Riecher-Rossler and Hafner 1993). We have detailed elsewhere (Castle et al. 1995) the inconsistencies in the literature on psychotic disorders and hormonal changes in women and the problems these raise for the estrogen hypothesis of schizophrenia. First, the admission rates for psychiatric illness increase in the paramenstruum, but this effect is not exclusive to schizophrenia; indeed, it is more consistently shown for mood disorders (Ascher-Svanum and Miller 1990). Second, the vulnerability to psychosis in the puerperium is also largely the result of mood disorders and not schizophrenia (Kendell et al. 1987). In one of the few studies to examine specifically females with schizophrenia and their vulnerability to postpartum psychotic breakdown, Davies et al. (1995) divided patients into those fulfilling stringent Feighner criteria for schizophrenia ("narrow" group) and those meeting ICD-10 (World Health Organization 1992) but not Feighner criteria ("broad" group). They found that 43% of the broad group experienced a psychotic episode postpartum but that none of the narrow group was so afflicted. The conclusion was that estrogen flux postpartum has the potential to precipitate psychosis in more benign forms of schizophrenia (possibly particularly in those women with affective disorder admixture) but appears to have little, if any, role in the precipitation of illness in those women with a more severe form of illness.

Third, pregnancy itself, a time of high serum estrogen levels, does not appear to be a time of particular mental well-being for women with schizophrenia (McNeil et al. 1984). Yarden et al. (1966) found no difference in course of illness between 67 pairs of childbearing women with schizophrenia over a 5-year period. Davies et al. (1995) found that most of the women experienced symptoms during pregnancy rather than improvement. Fourth, menopause, associated with an excess of mood disorder (Ballinger 1990), has not consistently been shown to be a particularly vulnerable time for schizophrenia. Although some investigators, as detailed later in this chapter (see "Epidemiological Perspective"), have suggested a postmenopausal peak of first onset of schizophrenia in women, these investigators have not ascertained blood estrogen levels at the time of first onset or shown a consistent association between timing of menopause and timing of illness onset. A more likely explanation, and one upheld by Seeman in Chapter 10 in this volume, is that psychosocial factors rather than biological factors determine menopause effects at this time.

Another approach to this issue is directly to ascertain levels of psychopathology in relation to gonadal hormonal levels. Such data are sparse, and generally studies have concentrated on patients with affective disturbance rather than schizophrenia. In general, no consistent correlation has been found between the onset of psychosis and any plasma gonadal hormone level measured (Kuevi et al. 1983; Wieck 1989). However, there has been a recent increase in interest in gonadal hormonal levels and psychopathology ratings specifically in women with schizophrenia. Thus, Riecher-Rossler et al. (1994) measured estrogen levels in 32 women with acute schizophrenic relapse and reported that psychotic symptoms worsened with declining estradiol levels. The association was very striking in several subjects, in whom self-report and observer report of symptomatology corresponded. Furthermore, depression scores were not affected, discounting possible confounding by mood effects of estrogens. Of interest, however, was that all patients in the study had abnormally low estradiol levels, even though they had a history of normal menstrual cycles. This suggests normal gonadal function being disturbed by acute illness and neuroleptic medication; indeed, half of the women had anovulatory cycles. Furthermore, there were no control patients, making the results difficult to interpret. This is consistent with more recent findings by Smith et al. (in press) referred to in the previous section ("Early Clinical Studies").

In a direct test of the hypothesis that estrogens might ameliorate psychotic symptoms, Kulkarni et al. (1996) added 0.02 mg estradiol to the neuroleptic treatment regimen of 11 women in acute psychotic relapse. Compared with control patients receiving no estradiol, the treatment group showed more rapid improvement in both positive and negative psychotic symptoms, but by the eighth week of treatment, no differences were discernible between the groups. The authors suggested that estradiol may act as an antipsychotic agent or as a "catalyst" for neuroleptic responsiveness. Lindamer et al. (1997) described a case report of symptomatic improvement with estrogen replacement therapy in a 47-year-old woman with a diagnosis of schizophrenia. These intriguing findings require independent replication with longitudinal, double-blind, crossover studies but are clearly of potential therapeutic importance and underline the influence estrogens might have on the clinical expression of schizophrenia in women. The fact that the Kulkarni et al. study followed up women over two menstrual phases is of interest. Exogenous estrogen treatment may have effects on mood improvement and may render women anovulatory, as with the oral contraceptive pill (to which the dose used in this study is equivalent). If some women are particularly sensitive to the effects of physiological fluctuations in estrogens, then they may be more likely to improve if exogenous estrogen dampens these changes. A recently completed randomized, controlled study of estrogen add-on in women with a history of postpartum illness has not found improved response in women treated with estrogen (Seneviratne et al., personal communication).

EPIDEMIOLOGICAL PERSPECTIVE

Schizophrenia, on average, manifests earlier in males than in females by approximately 5 years (Lewine 1988). This is a worldwide finding (Hambrecht et al. 1992), independent of the way in which onset of the illness (Riecher et al. 1989) or the illness itself (Loranger 1984; Shimuzu et al. 1988) is defined. Furthermore, the sex-specific age-at-onset curves are quite different, as shown in the ABC study by Hafner et al. (1991) and the pooled data from the World Health Organization Determinants of Outcome Study (Hambrecht et al. 1992).

Our own case-register data from a defined catchment area (Castle et al. 1993) showed a marked single, early-onset peak for males with schizophrenia; a far lesser midlife peak; and insidious decline thereafter. Conversely, females had a far more even distribution over the years. Indeed, subjection of these data to an admixture analysis (Castle et al. 1998) showed that the male distribution was best described by two peaks, with modal onsets at 21 and 39 years, whereas the female distribution was better described by three peaks, with modal onsets at 22, 36, and 62 years. In other words, most women first developed schizophrenia at an age identical to first episodes in young men. The greatest difference in rates of schizophrenia between men and women occurs in the very late age at onset greater than 75 years (see Chapter 10), and it is this excess of women over men that draws the mean age of onset for women to the right. In addition, recent data emerging from the SOCRATES first-episode intervention study suggests that the women and men in the group showing earliest onset of schizophrenia appear remarkably similar with respect to symptoms and age at onset (Abel et al. 2002).

Any discrepancy that does exist in age at onset between women and men is difficult to explain on the basis of estrogen alone. Hafner et al. (1991) drew attention to an excess of schizophrenia in women in their mid to late 40s and attributed the excess to a decline in estrogens at this time. Although intriguing, there were no data on confirmed menstrual status at the time of psychotic breakdown, and it is well established (Treolar 1981) that selecting women on the basis of age produces an endocrinologically heterogeneous group. Also, the data reviewed above suggest that a midlife peak is also found in males (albeit a far less emphatic one).

Furthermore, the massive preponderance of females among those individuals with first onset in very old age ("late paraphrenia") (Castle and Howard 1992) cannot readily be accounted for in terms of a further decline in estrogen levels, which remain relatively unchanged in late postmenopause (Molnar et al. 1988). Some have suggested that a decline in adrenal function that occurs in late menopause (65–75 years) causes a loss of adrenal-derived estrogen and that this may in part explain the greater rise in rates of schizophrenia in older women (see Chapter 10). Also, the estrogen hypothesis would predict an equal sex prevalence in prepubertal schizophrenia. Although onset of schizophrenia before puberty is rare, reports of such cases tend to show an excess of males (Gillberg 1986; Green et al. 1984; Kraepelin 1919).

Apart from age at onset, sex differences frequently have been described in the course and outcome of schizophrenia, as referenced above. However, most of these data have assessed large groups of patients with various ages at onset. One study (Navarro et al. 1996) assessed course and outcome in women with the same early age at onset as men and found that in those with young age at onset, course and outcome were no different from those in men. Our recent first-episode intervention study also seems to confirm these findings in the earliest onset group (Abel et al. 2002).

Finally, and perhaps most difficult to reconcile with the estrogen hypothesis, is the epidemiology of bipolar disorder. If the role of estrogen is generally antidopaminergic, then it should exert a comparable "protective" effect in bipolar disorder, also strongly associated with increased dopamine activity (Diehl and Gershon 1992; Post et al. 1980). However, lifetime risk of bipolar disorder in females is either similar to or greater than that in males (Odegard 1972; Rawnsley 1982), and the age at onset in some studies is as much as 10 years earlier in females (Saugstad 1989).

CONCLUSION

In conclusion, it is unlikely that the estrogen hypothesis can provide an adequate explanation for the diversity of sex differences in the epidemiology, presentation, and outcome of schizophrenia. However, the hypothesis is of undoubted heuristic value, making both researchers and clinicians more aware of the possible effects of endogenous hormones in the central nervous system.

What role could gonadal hormones play in the differing presentation of schizophrenia in men and women? One factor of importance is that estrogens and other steroid hormones affect the brain directly through organizational effects during critical periods of neurodevelopment, which influences subsequent sex differences in behavior and cognitive abilities (Ames 1991; Kimura 1992). Testosterone, acting mainly via estrogen receptors (Seeman 1989), tends to slow development of the male brain, expressly the left hemisphere, making males more vulnerable to environmental brain insult during early development (Taylor 1969). In line with the neurodevelopmental theory of schizophrenia, it has been suggested (Murray et al. 1992) that such factors render men more prone to an early-onset, severe "neurodevelopmental" form of schizophrenia. On a related theme, women in general tend to show less lateralization of brain function than do men (McGlone 1980), conceivably making them more able to compensate for early brain insult. The converse of this is that a subtype of schizophrenic illness that has links to mood disorders is more common in women (Castle and Murray 1991), at least partly as a manifestation of the differing maturational effects of gonadal hormones (DeLisi et al. 1989).

Another consideration is that steroid hormones have activational effects, which are generally reversible and "manifest themselves as changes in chemical properties of neural tissue during endocrine cycles" (McEwen 1991). The behavioral consequences of these activational effects are indirectly seen in the clinical setting. This could, in part at least, suggest why estrogens might modulate psychotic symptoms (Kulkarni et al. 1996; Lindamer et al. 1997; Riecher-Rossler et al. 1994; Seeman 1996). Indeed, Seeman (1996) suggested that physiological estrogen fluctuation may allow modification of neuroleptic dosing in women.

Corticosteroids also have a prominent effect on mood in individuals without psychiatric disorders (Schatzberg et al. 1985). The data on menopausal and postpartum psychiatric illness suggest that during acute changes in steroid hormone levels, mood is affected (Kumar and Brockington 1988; Sherwin 1988), although the pattern of the relation of endocrine events to clinical states is not consistent (Schmidt and Rubinow 1991; Wieck 1989). Women tend to have more affective symptoms in the manifestation of schizophrenic illnesses (Goldstein and Link 1988) and are much more prone to mood disorder overall (Weissman and Klerman 1977). Thus, estrogens could have a role in determining the "affective flavoring" of schizophrenia in women.

Similarly, it may be not only that the role of gonadal hormones is to regulate receptors, as discussed earlier, but also that the effects of steroid hormones are themselves dependent on the receptor state at the time. In support of this idea, Di Paolo (1994) reported a stimulatory effect of estradiol on dopamine receptors when administered alone but an inhibitory effect when the dopamine receptors had been rendered supersensitive following haloperidol administration. Also, striatal dopamine release fluctuates with diurnal and estrus cycle changes, which again may reflect differing estrogen–dopamine interactions dependent on receptor state. The concept of receptor-sensitivity modification was applied by Friedhoff and Miller (1983) in the treatment of dyskinesias and could be similarly considered in schizophrenia. Thus, in the presence of a possible hyperdopaminergic state in schizophrenia, a relatively high estrogen-to-androgen ratio, as seen in women, could promote the development of affective symptoms, either elevating or depressing mood. In fact, it is likely that the activational and organizational hormonal effects interact, such that the developmental influences of hormones actually may define the eventual activational effects that a particular hormone may have in females or males (McEwen 1991).

In conclusion, the preliminary clinical findings suggesting that women with schizophrenia have fewer psychotic symptoms at times of high estrogen levels and the intriguing data suggesting an amelioration of psychotic symptoms by estrogen indicate that we should investigate further the potential therapeutic effects of gonadal hormones. However, if we are to establish a central role for gonadal hormones in the expression, and perhaps pathogenesis, of mental illness, then the organizational and activational functions established for estrogens in the brain must be integrated into an ever more complex understanding of neurotransmitter systems and neuronal function.

REFERENCES

Abel KM, Drake R, Lewis S: Sex differences in women and men with first episode psychosis: longitudinal analyses of the SOCRATES intervention trial. Presentation for the International First Episode Psychosis meeting, Davos, Switzerland, February 2002

Ames FR: Sex and the brain. S Afr Med J 80:150–152, 1991

Arato H, Erdos A, Polgar M: Endocrinological changes in patients with sexual dysfunction under long-term neuroleptic treatment. Pharmakopsychiatrie Neuropsychopharmakoologie 12:426–431, 1979

Ascher-Svanum H, Miller MJ: Premenstrual changes and psychopathology among psychiatric inpatients. Hosp Community Psychiatry 41:87–89, 1990

Ballinger CB: Psychiatric aspects of the menopause. Br J Psychiatry 156:773–787, 1990

Bardenstein KK, McGlashan TH: Gender differences in affective, schizoaffective, and schizophrenic disorders: a review. Schizophr Res 3:159–172, 1990

Beach F: Insanity in children. Journal of Mental Science 44:459–463, 1898

Bedard P, Boucher R, Daiglé M, et al: Similar effect of estradiol and haloperidol on experimental tardive dyskinesia in monkeys. Psychoneuroendocrinology 9:375–379, 1983

Berthold AA: Transplantation der Hoden. Archives of Anatomy and Physiology 16:42–50, 1849

Best NR, Rees MP, Barlow DH, et al: Effect of oestradiol treatment on 5-HT and dopamine-mediated neuroendocrine responses. J Psychopharmacol 6:483–488, 1992

Castle DJ, Howard R: What do we know about the aetiology of late onset schizophrenia? European Psychiatry 7:99–108, 1992

Castle DJ, Murray RM: The neurodevelopmental basis of sex differences in schizophrenia. Psychol Med 21:565–575, 1991

Castle DJ, Wessely S, Murray RM: Sex and schizophrenia: effects of diagnostic stringency, and associations with premorbid variables. Br J Psychiatry 162:658–664, 1993

Castle DJ, Abel K, Takei N, et al: Gender differences in schizophrenia: hormonal effect or subtypes? Schizophr Bull 21:1–12, 1995

Castle DJ, Sham P, Murray RM: Differences in distribution of ages of onset in males and females with schizophrenia. Schizophr Res 33:179–183, 1998

Czernik A, Kleesiek K: Die Wirkung von Depotneuroleptika auf die Hormonsekretion des Hypophysen-Vorderlappens. Nervenarzt 50:527–533, 1979

Davies A, McIvor RJ, Kumar C: Impact of childbirth on a series of schizophrenic mothers: a comment on the possible influence of oestrogen on schizophrenia. Schizophr Res 16:25–31, 1995

DeLisi L, Dauphinais D, Hauser P: Gender differences in the brain: are they relevant to the pathogenesis of schizophrenia? Compr Psychiatry 30:197–208, 1989

Diehl DJ, Gershon S: The role of dopamine in mood disorders. Compr Psychiatry 33:115–120, 1992

Di Paolo T: Modulation of brain dopamine transmission by sex steroids. Rev Neurosci 5:27–42, 1994

Fink G, Sumner BEH: Oestrogen and mental state. Nature 383:306, 1996

Flor-Henry P: Influence of gender in schizophrenia as related to other psychological syndromes. Schizophr Bull 16:211–227, 1990

Friedhoff AJ, Miller JC: Clinical implications of receptor sensitivity modification. Annu Rev Neurosci 6:121–148, 1983

Gattaz WF, Behrens S, De Vry J, et al: Östradiol hemmt Dopamin-vermittelte Verhaltensweisen bei Ratten: ein Tiermodell zur Untersuchung der geschlechtsspezifischen Unterschiede bei der Schizophrenie. Fortschr Neurol Psychiatr 1:1–44, 1991

Gillberg C: Teenage psychoses: epidemiology, classification and reduced optimality in the pre-, peri-, and neonatal periods. J Child Psychol Psychiatry 27:87–98, 1986

Goldstein JM: The impact of gender on understanding the epidemiology of schizophrenia, in Gender and Psychopathology. Edited by Seeman MV. Washington, DC, American Psychiatric Press, 1995, pp 159–200

Goldstein JM, Link BG: Gender and the expression of schizophrenia. J Psychiatr Res 22:141–155, 1988

Goldstein JM, Tsuang MT, Faraone SV: Gender and schizophrenia: implications for understanding the heterogeneity of the illness. Psychiatry Res 28:243–253, 1989

Green WH, Campbell M, Hardesty AS, et al: A comparison of schizophrenic and autistic children. Journal of the American Academy of Child Psychiatry 23:399–409, 1984

Hafner H, Riecher A, Maurer K, et al: How does gender influence age at first hospitalisation for schizophrenia? Psychol Med 19:903–918, 1989

Hafner H, Behrens S, De Vry J, et al: An animal model for the effects of estradiol on dopamine-mediated behaviour: implications for sex differences in schizophrenia. Psychiatry Res 38:125–134, 1991

Halbreich U, Rojansky N, Palter S, et al: Estrogen augments serotonergic activity in postmenopausal women. Biol Psychiatry 37:434–441, 1995

Hambrecht M, Maurer K, Hafner H, et al: Transnational stability of gender differences in schizophrenia. European Archives of Psychiatry and Neurological Sciences 242:6–12, 1992

Johnstone EC, Crow TJ, Mashiter K: Anterior pituitary hormone secretion in chronic schizophrenia: an approach to neurohumoral mechanisms. Psychol Med 7:223–228, 1977

Kendell RE, Chalmers JC, Platz C: The epidemiology of puerperal psychoses. Br J Psychiatry 150:662–673, 1987

Kimura D: Sex differences in the brain. Sci Am 267:81–87, 1992

Kraepelin E: Lectures on Clinical Psychiatry, 3rd Edition. Edited by Johnstone T. London, England, Baillieve, Tindall, and Cassell, 1913, pp 131–135, 356–359

Kraepelin E: Dementia Praecox and Paraphrenia. Edited by Robertson GM. Edinburgh, Scotland, E & S Livingstone, 1919, pp 230–231, 242–243

Kretschmer E: Physique and Character: An Investigation of the Nature of Constitution and of the Theory of Temperament, 2nd Edition. Edited by Miller E. London, England, Kegan Paul, Trench, Trubner, 1921

Kuevi V, Carson R, Dixson AF: Plasma amine and hormone changes in post-partum blues. Clin Endocrinol 19:43–51, 1983

Kulkarni J, de Castella A, Smith D, et al: A clinical trial of the effects of oestrogen in acutely psychotic women. Schizophr Res 20:247–252, 1996

Kumar R, Brockington IF: Motherhood and Mental Illness: Causes and Consequences. London, England, Butterworth, 1988

Lewine RJ: Gender and schizophrenia, in Handbook of Schizophrenia, Vol 3. Edited by Nasrallah HA. Amsterdam, The Netherlands, Elsevier, 1988, pp 379–397

Lewine RJ, Burbach D, Meltzer HY: Effect of diagnostic criteria on the ratio of male to female schizophrenic patients. Am J Psychiatry 141:84–87, 1984

Lindamer LA, Lohr JB, Harris JM, et al: Gender, estrogen and schizophrenia. Psychopharmacol Bull 33:221–228, 1997

Lipska BK, Jaskiw GE, Weinberger DR: Postpubertal emergence of hyperresponsiveness to stress and to amphetamine after neonatal excitotoxic hippocampal damage: a potential animal model of schizophrenia. Neuropsychopharmacology 9:67–75, 1993

Loranger AW: Sex differences in age at onset of schizophrenia. Arch Gen Psychiatry 41:157–161, 1984

McEwen BS: Basic research perspective: ovarian hormone influence on brain neurochemical functions, in Contemporary Issues in Obstetrics and Gynaecology, Vol 2: The Premenstrual Syndromes. Edited by Gise LH. New York, Churchill Livingstone, 1985, pp 21–33

McEwen BS: Steroid hormones are multifunctional messengers to the brain. Trends in Endocrinology and Metabolism 2:62–67, 1991

McGlone J: Sex differences in human brain asymmetry: a critical survey. Behav Brain Sci 3:215–263, 1980

McNeil TF, Kaij L, Malmquist-Larsson A: Women with non-organic psychosis: mental disturbance during pregnancy. Acta Psychiatr Scand 70:127–139, 1984

Molnar G, Takacs I, Bazsane Z: Endocrine changes in endogenous psychoses of climacteric and involution. European Journal of Psychiatry 2:147–158, 1988

Mott FW: Normal and morbid conditions of the testes from birth to old age in one hundred asylum and hospital cases. BMJ 2:737–742, 1919

Murray RM, O'Callaghan E, Castle DJ, et al: A neurodevelopmental approach to the classification of schizophrenia. Schizophr Bull 18:319–332, 1992

Navarro F, van Os J, Jones P, et al: Explaining sex differences in course and outcome in the functional psychoses. Schizophr Res 21:161–170, 1996

Odegard O: Epidemiology of the psychoses, in Psychiat der Gegenwart. Edited by Kisler KP, Meyer JE, Muller C, et al. Heidelberg, Germany, Springer Verlag, 1972, pp 213–258

O'Keane V, O'Hanlon M, Webb M, et al: *d*-Fenfluramine/prolactin response throughout the menstrual cycle: evidence for an oestrogen-induced alteration. Clin Endocrinol (Oxf) 34:289–292, 1991

Post RM, Jimerson DC, Bunney WE, et al: Dopamine and mania: behavioural and biochemical effects of dopamine receptor blocker pimozide. Psychopharmacology 67:297–305, 1980

Rawnsley K: Epidemiology of Affective Psychosis. London, England, Cambridge University Press, 1982, pp 134–136

Riecher A, Maurer K, Loffler W, et al: Schizophrenia: a disease of young single males? European Archives of Psychiatry and the Neurological Sciences 239:210–212, 1989

Riecher-Rossler A, Hafner H: Schizophrenia and oestrogens: is there an association? Eur Arch Psychiatry Clin Neurosci 242:323–328, 1993

Riecher-Rossler A, Hafner H, Stumbaum M, et al: Can oestrogens modulate schizophrenic symptomatology? Schizophr Bull 20:203–214, 1994

Saugstad LF: Social class, marriage, and fertility in schizophrenia. Schizophr Bull 15:9–42, 1989

Schatzberg AF, Rothschild AJ, Langlais PJ, et al: A corticosteroid/dopamine hypothesis for psychotic depression and related states. J Psychiatr Res 19:57–64, 1985

Schmidt PJ, Rubinow DR: Menopause-related affective disorders: a justification for further study. Am J Psychiatry 148:844–852, 1991

Seeman MV: Current outcome in schizophrenia: women vs men. Acta Psychiatr Scand 73:609–617, 1986

Seeman MV: Prenatal gonadal hormones and schizophrenia in men and women. Psychiatric Journal of the University of Ottawa 14:473–475, 1989

Seeman MV: Gender differences in treatment response in schizophrenia, in Gender and Psychopathology. Edited by Seeman MV. Washington, DC, American Psychiatric Press, 1995, pp 227–252

Seeman MV: The role of estrogen in schizophrenia. J Psychiatry Neurosci 21:123–127, 1996

Sherwin BB: Affective changes with estrogen and androgen replacement therapy in surgically menopausal women. J Affect Disord 14:177–187, 1988

Shimuzu A, Kurachi M, Noda M, et al: Influence of sex on age-at-onset of schizophrenia. Japanese Journal of Psychiatry and Neurology 42:35–40, 1988

Smith S, Wheeler M, Murray RM, et al: The effects of antipsychotic-induced hyperprolactinemia on the hypogonadal axis in women. J Clin Psychopharmacol, in press

Suwa N, Yamashita I, Owada H, et al: Psychic state and adrenocortical function: a psychophysiologic study of emotion. J Nerv Ment Dis 134:268–276, 1962

Suwa N, Yamashita I, Kozo I, et al: Psychic state and gonadal function: a psychophysiological study of emotion. J Nerv Ment Dis 143:36–46, 1966

Taylor DC: Differential rates of cerebral maturation between the sexes and between the hemispheres. Lancet 2:140–142, 1969

Tourney G, Hatfield L: Plasma androgens in male schizophrenics. Arch Gen Psychiatry 27:753–755, 1972

Tourney G, Hatfield L: Androgen metabolism in schizophrenics, homosexuals, and normal controls. Biol Psychiatry 6:23–36, 1973

Travis M, Mulligan O, Mulligan RS, et al: Preliminary investigation of the effect of oestradiol treatment on $5-HT_{2A}$ receptor binding: a single photon emission tomography (SPET) study using ^{123}I-5-I-R91150 (abstract). Neuroimage 9:S672, 1999

Treolar AE: Menstrual cyclicity and the pre-menopause. Maturitas 3:249–264, 1981

van Amelsvoort T, Abel KM, Robertson DM, et al: Prolactin response to d-fenfluramine in postmenopausal women on and off ERT: comparison with young women. Psychoneuroendocrinology 6:493–502, 2001

Weissman M, Klerman GL: Sex differences and the epidemiology of depression. Arch Gen Psychiatry 34:98–111, 1977

Wessler I, Dooley DJ, Osswald H, et al: Differential blockade by nifedipine and w-conotoxin GVIA of alpha-1 and beta-1 adrenoceptor-controlled calcium channels on motor nerve terminals of the rat. Neurosci Lett 108:173–178, 1990

Whalley LJ, Christie JE, Blackwood DHR, et al: Disturbed endocrine function in the psychoses, I: disordered homeostasis or disease process? Br J Psychiatry 155:455–461, 1989

Wieck A: Endocrine aspects of postnatal mental disorders. Baillieres Clin Obstet Gynaecol 3:857–877, 1989

World Health Organization: International Statistical Classification of Diseases and Related Health Problems, 10th Revision. Geneva, Switzerland, World Health Organization, 1992

Yarden PE, Max DM, Eisenbach Z: The effect of childbirth on the prognosis of married schizophrenic women. Br J Psychiatry 112:491–499, 1966

14

Women's Issues in the Treatment of Schizophrenia

Nicholas A. Keks, Ph.D., M.B.B.S., F.R.A.N.Z.C.P.
Natalie Krapivensky, M.B.B.S., F.R.A.N.Z.C.P.
Judy Hope, M.B., B.S.
Amgad Tanaghow, F.R.C.Psych. (U.K.), F.R.A.N.Z.C.P.
Christine Culhane, B.Pharm.

Schizophrenia is a disorder characterized by heterogeneity in presentation, treatment response, course, and outcome (Carpenter and Buchanan 1994). The treatment of schizophrenia is similarly complex and multidimensional. A treatment plan cannot be formulated based on diagnosis alone. The phase of illness, the mix of symptomatic manifestations, and the characteristics of the individuals with this devastating disorder must be considered (American Psychiatric Association 1997).

Sex (along with age) is the most basic of individual characteristics, yet until recently, it has received little attention in the formulation of treatment. Schizophrenia has sweeping effects across neurobiological, psychological, family, and social domains of patients. Clinicians should therefore take a broad and multiaxial approach to optimizing treatment outcomes, attending not only to symptoms but also to illness correlates (such as substance abuse, violence, and suicide) and quality-of-life issues (Lehman et al. 1995c). In all these respects, specific problems and considerations pertaining to women with schizophrenia should influence comprehensive service provision.

In this chapter, we address issues concerning women in the diagnosis of schizophrenia, treatment-relevant neurobiology, pharmacokinetics, treatment efficacy with typical and atypical antipsychotics, quality-of-life considerations, and systems of care. The aim of this chapter is to increase awareness of sex-specific factors in treatment to promote sensitive clinical practice that attempts to meet the particular needs of women in biological, psychological, and social respects.

OVERVIEW OF SCHIZOPHRENIA TREATMENT

There is now broad agreement that treatment of schizophrenia requires flexible integration of pharmacological, psychological, family-oriented, social, and vocational interventions within the context of a comprehensive, flexible, and patient-centered treatment system (Carpenter and Buchanan 1994; Kane and McGlashan 1995; Lehman et al. 1995b). The phase of illness is a key consideration in treatment planning and is most conveniently divided into 1) recent-onset illness, 2) remission (no signs of illness)/prophylactic treatment, 3) acute relapse, 4) maintenance phase (signs of illness remain), and 5) treatment-resistant illness (ongoing positive, negative, and cognitive symptoms unresponsive to medication) (Keks et al. 1989). Management plans differ considerably depending on illness phase, but specific illness features, associated problems, and behaviors also must be kept in mind (Lehman et al. 1995c). Additionally, the age and sex of the patient, physical state, resources, and specific needs must be considered. Illness and related factors that may be relevant in formulating the treatment of schizophrenia are listed in Table 14–1.

The advantages of providing treatment for those with severe, ongoing forms of the illness within an integrated service framework are increasingly apparent (Rosen 1992; Stein and Test 1980). Characteristics of such services include 24-hour availability, integrated community and hospital treatment, active outreach and crisis intervention, case management, and rehabilitation services. The increasing emphasis on treatment of patients with schizophrenia in the community poses specific challenges to women with this disorder in terms of meeting many specific needs, particularly safety and adequate support. Some specific social needs of women with schizophrenia are listed in Table 14–2.

TABLE 14–1. Illness characteristics that are targets for specific treatment intervention in schizophrenia

---

Positive symptoms
Negative symptoms
Cognitive symptoms
Anxiety and panic
Lack of insight
Depression
Iatrogenic symptoms
Mania
Motor symptoms
Violence or aggression
Suicide
Alcohol or drug abuse
Disturbance of sleep or sexual drive

TABLE 14–2. Specific psychosocial issues for women in the treatment of schizophrenia

---

Privacy
Safe environment
Access to financial assistance
Relationship information/counseling
Contraception
Sexually transmitted diseases
Unwanted pregnancy
Lactation
Parenting skills
Access to child care
Periodic separation from children
Long-term separation from children or loss of custody
Financial burden of children
Violence against women
Domestic violence
Sexual harassment/assault/rape

SEX-RELATED NEUROBIOLOGICAL ISSUES RELEVANT TO TREATMENT

The delineation of both anatomical and functional brain abnormalities in schizophrenia has significance not only for understanding the etiology and pathophysiology but also, ultimately, for treatment of the illness. Brain structural differences may underlie the differences between men and women with schizophrenia in age at onset, prevalence of negative symptoms, response to antipsychotics, and psychosocial adaptation. The advent of an increasing number of ways to image the brain has enabled researchers to extend this field of inquiry, and the number of published reports of brain morphology is increasing exponentially.

Different brain regions have received different degrees of scientific interest. To date, the results seem to confirm findings from previous postmortem research. Generally, results from magnetic resonance imaging (MRI) studies have proven to be even more inconsistent and difficult to interpret than results from earlier computed tomography (CT) investigations that mostly examined ventricular size. Although MRI has superior resolution to CT scanning, the studies generally test small numbers and tend to measure many small structures, which makes the findings more difficult to interpret. The choice of control group may be crucial, as demonstrated by failure to replicate results when the control group was changed to mirror the educational background of the patient group in one study (Andreasen et al. 1990). Other confounding variables include sex, age, time from diagnosis of disease, race, socioeconomic background, and stature.

Various aspects of brain morphology appear to distinguish patients from control subjects. CT studies in the 1980s found that patients with schizophrenia have larger ventricle-to-brain ratios (VBRs) than do control subjects (Flaum et al. 1993). Attempts have been made to correlate higher VBRs with poor premorbid adjustment (Weinberger et al. 1980b), cognitive impairment (Johnstone et al. 1976), and poor response to therapy (Weinberger et al. 1980a), highlighting the relevance of understanding structural brain abnormalities for treatment. More recently, MRI studies have supported the occurrence of larger ventricular size in patients with schizophrenia (Andreasen et al. 1990; Flaum et al. 1990). Furthermore, larger ventricles have been found particularly in male patients compared with control subjects, but no such difference has been found in females (Flaum et al. 1990); also, no difference in VBR was found between male and female patients. Andreasen's group also reported that patients with prominent negative symptoms had significantly larger ventricles than did patients with other subtypes of illness.

Several studies have indicated a greater likelihood of abnormal brain morphology in male than in female patients with schizophrenia (Andreasen et al. 1990; Flaum et al. 1990). The largest published MRI study to date was conducted by Flaum et al. (1993). This study evaluated and compared volumes of various brain regions in patients with schizophrenia and control subjects without schizophrenia and analyzed these by sex. The results showed that, compared with women, men have larger cranial and cerebral volumes, superior temporal gyrus, and third ventricle volumes. Cowell et al. (1996) also reported differences between symptomatic correlates of higher frontal lobe volumes between men and women with schizophrenia.

The corpus callosum is one area of the brain that has received considerable attention because of observed differences in its size between sexes in individuals without psychiatric disorders. The corpus is one of the structures that contains interhemispheric nerve bundle connections. For individuals without psychiatric disorders, larger size of the corpus callosum is correlated with better memory, attention, and concentration; faster speed of information processing; and improved executive functions and sensory-perceptual function. It has been postulated that the dysfunction of the corpus callosum and the associated deficiency of neural information transfer are related to cognitive deficits in schizophrenia, but this has not to date been supported by studies. It does appear, however, that cognitive deficits may be predictive of outcome in schizophrenia and that cognitive impairment differs between men and women at different stages of the disease (Perlick et al. 1992).

In the nonpsychiatric population, Raine et al. (1990) reported larger corpus callosum and anterior commissure in women than in men. However, available information on the size and sex differences of the corpus callosum in patients with schizophrenia is conflicting. Hoff et al. (1994), in a study of 62 first-episode patients, reported that women with a first episode of schizophrenia had a smaller total corpus callosum area than did control subjects, with no difference noted for men. In control subjects without schizophrenia, a larger corpus callosum was associated with better cognitive function, but no such relation emerged in patients with schizophrenia. These results are consistent with similar findings by Hauser et al. (1989) and Lewine et al. (1991) but contradict previous data from Nasrallah et al. (1986) and Raine et al. (1990), who found thicker corpus callosum in women compared with men. This inconsistency may be attributed to the different patient groups being studied. Hoff et al. (1994) examined first-episode patients, whereas Nasrallah et al. (1986) examined a sample of patients with chronic illness. The measures of corpus callosum also varied (total area vs. thickness), which may contribute to the observed difference in results.

The significance of the apparently greater deviations in male schizophrenia brain structure is unclear. Critics point to lack of clinical correlates and contradictory evidence, casting doubt on the importance of sex differences in schizophrenic brain structure (Kulkarni 1997). However, others have argued that males have a more severe form of schizophrenia, with earlier onset, poor premorbid adjustment, more negative symptoms, and poorer outcome. They also are more likely than female patients to have a history of pre- and perinatal complications and to have structural brain abnormalities (Murray and Lewis 1987; Murray et al. 1988). Murray (1991) argued that the most plausible explanation to account for all of these differences is that more males than females have the form of disease due to neurodevelopmental abnormality. He suggested that a neurodevelopmental perspective not only provides a causal explanation for the early-onset, severe form in males but also takes into account recent evidence regarding structural brain abnormalities.

Furthermore, Murray noted that electroencephalographic, neurochemical, and auditory evoked potential studies have suggested that left temporal lobe function has a more important role in schizophrenia. This is supported by MRI and neuropathological postmortem studies. It is proposed that a lesion in the left hemisphere would result in overcompensation by the right hemisphere and development of "pathological left-handedness." This theory has had some further support from studies that have associated left-handedness in schizophrenic patients with early onset of illness (Piran et al. 1982), more negative symptoms (Andreasen et al. 1982), increased ventricular size, and poor performance on neuropsychological tests (Katsanis and Iacono 1989).

Studies have reported left-lateralized striatal dopamine D_2 receptor binding in male patients with schizophrenia. Pilowsky et al. (1994) described male-characterized left-lateral asymmetry of striatal D_2 receptor binding in neuroleptic-naïve patients with schizophrenia. This finding has been replicated by Schroder et al. (1997) and Acton et al. (1997). The observed asymmetry was prominent in the drug-naïve state but diminished after administration of the conventional neuroleptic benperidol. This suggests that sex-related clinical differences in schizophrenia, such as response to treatment, may be related to the left-hemisphere predominance of D_2 receptors in men because this asymmetry may affect the binding of conventional neuroleptics.

Other authors have investigated the regional cerebral blood flow or asymmetries of glucose metabolic rates. These small studies of 10, 8, and 18 patients, respectively (Buchsbaum et al. 1992; Early et al. 1987; Potkin et al. 1994), did not address potential sex differences and were composed of mostly male patients. Nevertheless, their findings were consistent with the greater left than right striatal D_2 receptor binding and confirmed the characteristic male malfunction of the right striatum in schizophrenia.

In addition, there appears to be a difference in dopamine receptor sensitivity between men and women, which may be one factor contributing to possible superior efficacy of neuroleptics in women. This difference in receptor sensitivity is thought to be largely due to modulation of dopamine systems by estrogen. The neuroleptic-like antidopaminergic effect of estrogen has been reported in both preclinical animal behavior studies (Di

Paolo and Falardeau 1985) and biochemical studies, although results of the latter are inconsistent.

The components of the menstrual cycle associated with the lowest estrogen concentrations, the perimenstrual and luteal, have been associated with exacerbation of psychosis (Kulkarni 1997). The components of adjunctive estradiol have been found to be clinically beneficial in acute psychosis (Kulkarni et al. 1996). The detailed relations between sex steroids, sex, and schizophrenia are addressed in Chapter 13.

SEX-RELATED ISSUES IN DIAGNOSIS OF SCHIZOPHRENIA

The age at onset of schizophrenia in women is on average more than 5 years later than that in men (Lewine 1981) irrespective of whether the measured index is when symptoms were first noted, first treatment, or first hospitalization (Loranger 1984). Premorbidly, men with schizophrenia are more likely to be schizoid (Wolff and Chide 1980), whereas women appear to have better premorbid social adjustment (Salokongas 1983), although they are still impaired in comparison with same-sex peers (Andia and Zisook 1991).

There are conflicting data as to whether men and women differ symptomatically. Paranoid and schneiderian first-rank symptoms have been reported to be more common in women (Andia et al. 1995; Marneros 1984). It has been reported that men are more likely to have negative symptoms (Goldstein et al. 1990; Lewine 1985), but another study found more negative symptoms in first-episode women (Szymanski et al. 1995). Seeman (1996) suggested that the high prevalence of negative symptoms in men may be secondary to prescribed antipsychotic medication.

McGlashan and Bardenstein (1990), in the Chestnut Lodge study, found that at presentation, women had more symptoms related to depression than did men. However, others observed no differences, including no differences between men and women in the prevalence of depression (Addington et al. 1996; Goldstein and Link 1988). In a large study of early schizophrenia, Hafner et al. (1994) failed to find any symptomatic differences related to sex.

However, it is intriguing that the diagnostic system used for schizophrenia influences the male-to-female ratio. Major discrepancies in the ratio of men to women have been found between "broad" and "narrow" diagnostic systems (Lewine et al. 1984). One of the key differences between the narrow (e.g., Research Diagnostic Criteria; Spitzer et al. 1978) and the broad (e.g., schneiderian criteria) criteria is that the former exclude patients who present with affective subsyndromes, which may be more prevalent in women with psychosis (Keks et al. 1990).

Arguably, it is more appropriate for diagnosis to commence from the starting point of all patients with psychotic symptoms, and most clinicians tend to proceed in this way (Keks 1996). If the presentation of women with psychoses is associated with more affective symptomatology, then assignment to a diagnosis of schizophrenia and possibly access to appropriate therapy may be significantly influenced by the diagnostic system used. In many health systems, the provision of innovative treatments (which are invariably more expensive than conventional therapy) is contingent on the presence of schizophrenia, thus denying access to "atypical" cases. Table 14–3 compares the salient features of commonly used diagnostic systems for schizophrenia, emphasizing the existence of differing definitions for the disorder.

SEX-RELATED ISSUES IN PHARMACOKINETICS

Sex differences in pharmacokinetics have been extensively reviewed by Yonkers et al. (1992) and Pollock (1997). The luteal phase of the menstrual cycle may delay gastric transit time (Wald et al. 1981), which may increase bioavailability. The comparatively greater adiposity of women results in a larger volume of distribution, which eventually prolongs half-life and results in higher serum concentrations of drugs.

Evidence concerning sex differences in hepatic drug metabolism is conflicting (Yonkers et al. 1992). Endogenous or exogenous estrogen inhibits cytochrome P450 metabolism and monoamine oxidase activity (Pollock 1997). Differences in drug metabolism could occur in relation to menopausal status and hormone replacement therapy. Pregnancy can lead to the need for increased doses of psychotropic medication because of the accompanying physiological and hormonal changes.

With antipsychotics specifically, women receiving the same doses as men manifest higher plasma concentrations of fluphenazine (Simpson et al. 1990), thiothixene (Ereshefsky et al. 1991), chlorpromazine (Pollock 1997), and clozapine (Haring et al. 1989). Dose requirements of olanzapine are lower for women than for men, but no sex differences are apparent in doses of risperidone (van Peer et al. 1996).

SEX DIFFERENCES IN DOSE EXPERIENCE

Several studies suggested that younger women require lower doses of antipsychotic medication than do men and postmenopausal women (Mar-

TABLE 14–3. Comparison of diagnostic criteria for five diagnostic systems of schizophrenia

Diagnostic system	Positive symptoms	Negative symptoms	Course	Affective symptoms	Other
DSM-IV	Delusions, hallucinations, thought disorder, and disorganized behavior	Diagnostic if associated with positive symptoms	Continuous signs of illness for more than 6 months; major dysfunction	Schizoaffective and mood disorders excluded if mood episodes are brief during psychosis	Not due to substance abuse or medical condition
DSM-III-R	Specified delusions and hallucinations, formal thought disorder with other symptoms	Residual symptoms	Continuous signs of illness for more than 6 months; deterioration	Manic or depressive syndrome included if relatively brief	Not due to organic factor
ICD-10	Essentially schneiderian symptoms, formal thought disorder, and catatonic behavior of secondary importance	Listed but of secondary importance	Essentially cross-sectional (requires 1 month of illness)	If affective symptoms are present, they must follow psychotic symptoms	Excludes organic factor and drugs
Research Diagnostic Criteria	Specified delusions and hallucinations, qualified formal thought disorder, and grossly disorganized behavior	Not considered	Cross-sectional (duration>2 weeks)	No prominent manic or depressive symptoms	
Schneiderian	Characteristic positive symptoms	Not considered	Cross-sectional	Not considered	Excludes coarse brain disease

Source.   Modified from Keks et al. 1990.

riott and Hiep 1978; Seeman 1983; Yonkers et al. 1992). However, other naturalistic studies found that men and women received similar doses of antipsychotics (Addington et al. 1996; Galletly and Tsourtos 1997; Kulkarni 1997) or that women have received even higher doses (Zito et al. 1987). These findings suggest that some women may be receiving excessive doses of neuroleptics (Kulkarni 1997). A recent audit of 106 patients taking clozapine, risperidone, and conventional antipsychotics did not detect sex differences in dosing (Miller et al. 1998).

SEX-RELATED ISSUES AND EFFICACY OF ANTIPSYCHOTIC MEDICATION

It has been concluded authoritatively that women respond substantially better to antipsychotic medication than do men (Tamminga 1997; Yonkers et al. 1992). In a study of first-episode patients, 87% of the women, but only 55% of the men, achieved symptom remission with fluphenazine hydrochloride (Szymanski et al. 1995). However, the notion of superior response to conventional antipsychotics in women has been challenged by Pinals et al. (1996). These researchers compared 24 men and 20 women who were well matched on drug-free symptomatology and weight-adjusted conventional neuroleptic dose under double-blind, placebo-controlled conditions. All symptoms significantly improved, but no differences were seen between men and women. Whether there are sex differences in response to atypical antipsychotics needs to be clarified.

The availability of atypical antipsychotic medication constitutes a substantial therapeutic advance in the treatment of schizophrenia. For both men and women, evidence has shown superior efficacy for clozapine, risperidone, and olanzapine (particularly for negative but also for positive symptoms) and a lower risk of extrapyramidal side effects (Kane et al. 1988; Marder et al. 1997; Tollefson et al. 1997). A clinical consensus is emerging that new-generation antipsychotic medication should be considered first-line therapy in all phases of schizophrenia in view of the advantages of these drugs in comparison to conventional medications.

There appear to be no sex differences in efficacy with either risperidone (Marder et al. 1997) or olanzapine (Tollefson et al. 1997). Differences in efficacy between men and women also were not apparent with quetiapine; however, these studies involved only small numbers of women (Arvanitis et al. 1997; Peuskens and Link 1997). However, the female patients who had treatment-refractory schizophrenia appeared to respond less well than the men, although the difference was not statistically significant (Lieberman et al. 1994).

Reproductive implications of antipsychotic use by women are extensive. Those concerned with menstrual dysfunction and sexual dysfunction are covered elsewhere in this book, as are additional considerations arising from the tendency of many antipsychotics to induce significant hyperprolactinemia (see Chapter 12). The use of antipsychotics during pregnancy and lactation needs to be considered.

All of the antipsychotics cross the placenta into the fetus (Gelenberg and Keith 1998). There is no persuasive evidence of teratogenicity from antipsychotics, but clearly, the safe use of antipsychotic drugs has not been established. Significant experience is available with haloperidol, flupenthixol, zuclopenthixol, sulpiride, chlorpromazine, and trifluoperazine, which has been summarized by Bazire (1997). At worst, the teratogenicity of these antipsychotics is likely to be low, given decades of experience.

There do not appear to be indications of teratogenicity with risperidone, olanzapine, or clozapine to date. Again, safety of these compounds in pregnancy has not been established. There have been reports of pregnant women taking clozapine and giving birth to healthy babies (Dickson and Hogg 1998).

Apart from teratogenicity, antipsychotics can affect the fetus in a variety of ways and can cause a withdrawal syndrome and behavioral disturbances in the neonate (Gelenberg and Keith 1998). The use of antipsychotics in pregnancy is therefore problematic in both the first and the third trimesters and best avoided if possible. Unfortunately, the occurrence of psychosis during pregnancy poses its own major risks for the woman and the fetus, including physical self-neglect, substance abuse, and suicide. Failing to adequately treat the psychosis for a prolonged period also may worsen long-term outcome (Wyatt 1991). Drug selection will depend on careful consideration of the consequences of side effects for patient and fetus; for instance, postural hypotension may be more problematic during pregnancy. Use of the minimum effective dose is critical. Antipsychotics can be used in pregnancy, but the benefits should clearly outweigh the risks.

Breast-feeding by mothers taking antipsychotic medication is very difficult. Both typical and atypical drugs are excreted in the breast milk and are therefore liable to cause problems in the infant.

Some of the issues relevant to women in prescribing antipsychotic medication are given in Table 14–4.

WOMEN AND ADJUNCTIVE THERAPIES

Because therapeutic responsiveness of many patients with schizophrenia to antipsychotic medications can be inadequate (Tamminga 1997), clini-

TABLE 14–4.   Issues for women prescribed antipsychotic medication

Most appropriate drug for women

Efficacy (positive, negative, cognitive, affective symptoms)

Side effects (especially amenorrhea, galactorrhea, sexual dysfunction, weight gain)

Possibly lower doses needed with some antipsychotics for women in childbearing years

Standard doses needed after menopause

Pregnancy problems: possible teratogenicity, effects on fetus and infant after birth, altered pharmacokinetics

Lactation: antipsychotics expressed in breast milk, and some can accumulate in infant

cians often use adjunctive therapies, particularly electroconvulsive therapy, lithium, sodium valproate, carbamazepine, and anticholinergics (Johns and Thompson 1995). Although benzodiazepines may augment the antipsychotic effect of neuroleptics (Lingjaerde 1991), clinicians use benzodiazepines mostly in patients with acute psychosis who require sedative or anxiolytic effects in addition to antipsychotic medication (Hyman et al. 1995). Antidepressant medication also is frequently used during the course of treatment for schizophrenia because depression is quite common (Siris 1993; Siris et al. 1994). Although most evidence relates to imipramine, the use of selective serotonin reuptake inhibitors (SSRIs) is probably more appropriate (American Psychiatric Association 1997) in view of more favorable side effect profiles, particularly lower toxicity in overdose. However, the potential for pharmacokinetic interactions between antipsychotics and SSRIs exists, and the patient should be carefully monitored.

Issues for women in the prescription of therapies adjunctive to antipsychotics also include consideration of sex differences in pharmacokinetics, as well as use during pregnancy and lactation. Lithium and other mood stabilizers are implicated in teratogenicity; lithium is linked to cardiac abnormalities, and valproate has been associated with neural tube defects (Altshuler et al. 1996).

There is no indication of sex differences in efficacy of adjunctive medications in schizophrenia. With respect to sex-relevant side effects, menstrual irregularities can occur with serotonergic antidepressants and sodium valproate (Isojarvi et al. 1993). The relative effects of antidepressants and mood stabilizers on weight (which tends to increase with tricyclics and mood stabilizers and to remain steady or decrease with SSRIs) is also a relevant consideration for women given the propensity of antipsychotics to cause weight gain (Wirshing et al. 1999).

SEX DIFFERENCES IN COURSE AND OUTCOME OF SCHIZOPHRENIA

A major factor influencing the course of schizophrenia but relatively rarely addressed is the experience of the postpartum period. The prevalence of psychosis at this time is increased by a factor of 15. Although most psychoses are affective, the risk of both new cases and relapses of schizophrenia also increases dramatically (Kendell et al. 1987). Women with puerperal schizophrenia appear to have more affective symptoms. As indicated earlier in this chapter (see section "Sex-Related Issues in Diagnosis of Schizophrenia"), whether a patient is given a diagnosis of schizophrenia depends on the diagnostic system, some of which are highly exclusive of affective states (e.g., Research Diagnostic Criteria; Spitzer et al. 1978).

With respect to longer-term outcome, it is necessary to recall that the age at onset of schizophrenia is later in women than in men and, therefore, will affect women who are further advanced developmentally in occupational and psychosocial terms (which may improve longer-term outcome) (Kulkarni 1997).

Studies suggest that long-term outcome is better for women than for men. A Finnish study found that after 8 years, women were more likely to fully recover and to be better socially adjusted than were men (Salokongas 1983). Walter and Keward (1985) found that, in the longer term, women with schizophrenia were more likely to have better social relationships than were men. Prudo and Blum (1987) found that at 5 years, women were likely to have fewer symptoms and better social and occupational outcomes than were men. However, Childers and Harding (1990) failed to find sex differences in outcome for 82 subjects followed up for an average of 32 years.

Test et al. (1990), in reporting progress findings from the Wisconsin Community Care Study, indicated that after 2 years, women were more likely to participate in heterosexual relationships and behaviors and to be parents. Men, on the contrary, were more often in jail and committed suicide more frequently. In a cross-sectional study (Andia et al. 1995), women were more often married, living independently, employed, and better educated.

Interestingly, two classic long-term follow-up studies from the pre-neuroleptic era failed to detect a difference in outcome based on sex (Ciompi 1980; Loyd et al. 1985). This suggests that the differences in outcome between women and men stem from the treated course of the disease rather than its natural history (Andia and Zisook 1991). An additional factor may be illness phase, with women experiencing better outcomes during middle age but with both sexes then experiencing improvement after age 50 (Angermeyer et al. 1990).

QUALITY OF LIFE: WOMEN'S ISSUES IN ASSESSMENT AND TREATMENT

Quality-of-life–related outcomes are increasingly recognized as particularly and independently important in the assessment of outcome in psychoses. Assessment of quality of life allows the incorporation of the unique perspective of the patient into the evaluation of health status and psychiatric services (Barry and Zissi 1997). As will become apparent below, evidence indicates that the advantages of women over men in outcome on narrow outcome criteria may be reversed when quality-of-life indices are taken into account.

Although the assessment of quality of life is hampered by definitional and methodological dilemmas, it is generally understood to encompass both subjective and objective domains. It can involve direct and indirect assessment and can be generic or health and disease specific (Stedman 1996). Quality-of-life measurement in psychiatry has tended to move away from health-specific quality of life in favor of multiple domain and satisfaction measures that reflect the complex nature of outcomes. The evaluation of quality of life in psychotic patients has been regarded as unreliable (Orley et al. 1998). Although active psychosis may limit the assessment of quality of life, most researchers now acknowledge that evaluation is essential despite the limitations (Barry et al. 1993; Sullivan et al. 1992).

Research on the effects of chronic psychoses on quality of life has addressed two key aspects: the influence of psychopathology and the contribution of demographic variables.

Depression is well known to lower reported quality of life in the general population. This effect also occurs in those with chronic medical illness and in those with chronic psychiatric illness (Pyne et al. 1997). Recently, the effect of depressive symptoms on lowering quality-of-life perceptions in individuals with psychosis has been found to be more important than the presence of positive or negative symptoms.

As suggested earlier, women may be more prone to experience depression in psychoses and schizophrenia (McGlashan et al. 1990; Seeman 1996). Although studies of quality of life and psychopathology in psychosis have not specifically addressed sex differences, women with depressive symptoms probably are more likely to be at risk for poorer subjective quality of life. The diagnosis and treatment of depression is therefore of particular importance in optimizing the subjective experience of women with schizophrenia.

In the general population, the quality of life of men tends to be most strongly associated with satisfaction and material domains, especially finances, daily activities, and safety (Bharadwaj and Wilkening 1977). Women's quality of life is heavily influenced by satisfaction with family life; social domains such as family, social relationships, and living situation have the strongest effects. The determinants of quality of life among psychiatrically unwell women differ substantially. Life satisfaction in unwell women is most strongly related to daily activities and financial adequacy rather than social domains (Lehman et al. 1995a).

As already stated, women appear to be less impaired on objective psychosocial outcome criteria than men are. However, the overall quality of life of women with psychoses appears poorer than that of men (Lehman et al. 1995a). Thus, any outcome advantages in capacity to develop and sustain social relationships do not appear to translate into superior reported life satisfaction.

Miller and Finnerty (1996) found that women with schizophrenia were more likely than control subjects to have been raped, to engage in sexual risk behavior, to have more unwanted pregnancies and abortions, and to be victims of violence during pregnancy. They also were more likely to be unable to meet their children's basic needs and to have lost custody of their children.

Lehman et al. (1995a) advised specific psychosocial interventions for women with psychosis to achieve the level of quality of life similar to that of men. In particular, assistance with financial management, work opportunities, and social skills training were recommended. Miller and Finnerty (1996) also recommended provision of family planning and parenting training.

PSYCHOSOCIAL TREATMENT

Although the amount of evidence concerning the efficacy of psychological therapies in schizophrenia is limited (Lehman et al. 1995c), it is at the level of appropriately structured psychotherapeutic intervention that the most sex-sensitive treatment can be given to patients. The task of understanding, supporting, and attempting to meet the needs of the woman as a unique individual rather than as "schizophrenic" can be addressed. However, the psychotherapy needs to be flexible and tailored to the individual's capacity, especially in patients with residual illness (Carpenter and Buchanan 1994). Family psychoeducational approaches have been shown to reduce relapse rates and are clearly indicated in appropriate circumstances (Falloon et al. 1982; Hogarty et al. 1986).

Psychosocial skills training and psychoeducational and cognitive therapies may be particularly appropriate for improvement of basic living skills and coping strategies in patients with ongoing schizophrenia (American Psychiatric Association 1997).

Rehabilitation of patients with chronic schizophrenia has changed in emphasis since it was recognized that interventions must be ongoing to be effective. Interventions are broad and include emphasis on social relationships and vocational rehabilitation (Rosen 1992).

In structuring psychosocial interventions, clinicians should be aware of the sex differences between men and women with chronic schizophrenia that may be relevant to interventions. Mueser et al. (1995) found an association between memory and social skills in schizophrenic women but not in men. Performance on information-processing tasks was related to indices of social skill in women with schizophrenia. These findings suggest that cognitive therapies may be more effective for women with schizophrenia than for men.

Inpatient family intervention has been found to be more effective in women than in men during follow-up (Spencer et al. 1988).

SEX-SENSITIVE PSYCHIATRIC SERVICES

Following deinstitutionalization, which was largely achieved through the use of antipsychotic medications, it has become generally expected that people with chronic schizophrenia are as entitled as anyone else to live in the community rather than be subjected to long-term custodial care (Keks and Sacks 1996). However, to avoid adverse outcomes such as homelessness, the placement of people living in the community with chronic psychosis must be accompanied by adequate support and availability of an integrated system of service organization (Rosen 1992). The functional deficits associated with chronic schizophrenia tend to militate against the ability of patients to use multiple and diverse sources of service provision (Carpenter and Buchanan 1994).

Perhaps the most frequently cited model of integrated service provision has been the program developed in Madison, Wisconsin (Stein and Test 1980). This program involves assertive outreach, psychoeducation, team case management, crisis intervention, and use of general hospital psychiatric beds when necessary. Test et al. (1990) underlined the need for services to focus on treating the individual rather than merely the illness, thereby attending to sex-relevant needs. Social relationships, pregnancy, childbirth, and parenting are considered the most important issues for women. These and other issues are listed in Table 14–2.

Assistance with appropriate housing, financial support, training in parenting skills, and emotionally supportive case management should be available in service programs.

Psychosocial interventions for women should include a focus on relationship skills, contraception, information about sexually transmitted diseases and unwanted pregnancy, and specific sensitive management of sexual assault and violence. Psychiatric service staff are likely to require specific training in sex-sensitive practice and interventions targeted to issues relevant to women (Women's Advisory Group 1997).

The provision of adequate contraception for women with schizophrenia can be a major challenge in patients with significant functional impairment, in whom contraceptive efficacy may be poor. In these circumstances, women with schizophrenia may need intensive case management (which may include daily or twice-daily home visits) to provide the level of support necessary.

Women who are hospitalized on mixed-sex wards may be vulnerable to physical and sexual assault. Thomas et al. (1995) reported that 32% of the female psychiatric inpatients had been sexually molested and 4% had been sexually assaulted. Services must be acutely aware of the need to provide a safe and nonthreatening environment with adequate privacy (Women's Advisory Group 1997).

CONCLUSION

The treatment of schizophrenia is determined by consideration of illness phase, treatment-relevant characteristics of illness, and factors pertaining to the patient, such as age, physical state, and sex. Treatment must be comprehensive; although antipsychotic medication remains the cornerstone, a range of interventions needs to be offered, including psychological therapies, family therapy, social skills training, and rehabilitation, with particular focus on social and occupational functioning. Service provision in schizophrenia is best carried out within an integrated service network that is available around the clock, comprehensive in its elements (including financial assistance and appropriate accommodation), and delivered through case management to assist people who otherwise would be unable to access needed services.

Female gender is a critical variable in formulating therapeutic interventions. Clinicians must be aware of a variety of issues important to women with schizophrenia. The knowledge and skills to address particular needs of women are very important, especially those associated with reproduction, parenting, safety, and privacy. Schizophrenia usually is a devastating and chronic illness, which substantially diminishes quality of life. Interventions for women with schizophrenia need to address not only the illness of schizophrenia but also the person's particular perception of illness and its consequences on her psychosocial context.

REFERENCES

Acton PD, Pilowsky LS, Costa DC, et al: Multivariate cluster analysis of dynamic iodine-123 iodobenzamide SPET dopamine D2 receptor images in schizophrenia. Eur J Nucl Med 24:111–118, 1997

Addington D, Addington J, Pattern S: Gender and affect in schizophrenia. Can J Psychiatry 41:265–268, 1996

Altshuler LL, Cohen L, Szuba MP, et al: Pharmacologic management of psychiatric illness in pregnancy: dilemmas and guidelines. Am J Psychiatry 153:592–606, 1996

American Psychiatric Association: Practice guidelines for the treatment of patients with schizophrenia. Am J Psychiatry 154(suppl 4), 1997

Andia AM, Zisook S: Gender differences in schizophrenia: a literature review. Ann Clin Psychiatry 3:333–340, 1991

Andia AM, Zisook S, Heaton RK, et al: Gender differences in schizophrenia. J Nerv Ment Dis 183:522–528, 1995

Andreasen NC, Dennert JW, Olsen SA, et al: Hemispheric asymmetries and schizophrenia. Am J Psychiatry 139:427–430, 1982

Andreasen NC, Ehrhardt JC, Swayze VW, et al: Magnetic resonance imaging of the brain in schizophrenia: the pathophysiological significance of structural abnormalities. Arch Gen Psychiatry 47:35–44, 1990

Angermeyer MC, Kuhn L, Goldstein JM: Gender and the course of schizophrenia: differences in treated outcomes. Schizophr Bull 16:293–307, 1990

Arvanitis LA, Miller BG, the Seroquel Trial 13 Study Group: Multiple fixed doses of "Seroquel" (quetiapine) in patients with acute exacerbation of schizophrenia: a comparison with haloperidol and placebo. Biol Psychiatry 42:233–246, 1997

Barry MM, Zissi A: Quality of life as an outcome measure in evaluating mental health services: a review of the empirical evidence. Soc Psychiatry Psychiatr Epidemiol 32:38–47, 1997

Barry MM, Crosby C, Bogg J: Methodological issues in evaluating the quality of life of long-stay psychiatric patients. Journal of Mental Health 2:43–56, 1993

Bazire S: Psychotropic Drug Directory: The Professionals' Pocket Handbook and Aide Memoire. Jesses Farm, Mark Allen Publishing, 1997

Bharadwaj L, Wilkening EA: The prediction of perceived well-being. Social Indicators Research 4:421–439, 1977

Buchsbaum MS, Potkin SG, Siegel BV, et al: Striatal metabolic rate and clinical response to neuroleptics in schizophrenia. Arch Gen Psychiatry 49:966–974, 1992

Carpenter WT Jr, Buchanan RW: Schizophrenia. N Engl J Med 330:681–690, 1994

Childers SE, Harding CM: Gender, premorbid social functioning, and long-term outcome in DSM-III schizophrenia. Schizophr Bull 16:309–318, 1990

Ciompi L: The natural history of schizophrenia in the long term. Br J Psychiatry 36:413–420, 1980

Cowell PE, Kostianovsky DJ, Gur RC, et al: Sex differences in neuroanatomical and clinical correlations in schizophrenia. Am J Psychiatry 153:799–805, 1996

Dickson RA, Hogg L: Pregnancy of a patient treated with clozapine. Psychiatr Serv 49:1081–1083, 1998

Di Paolo T, Falardeau P: Modulation of brain and pituitary dopamine receptors by estrogens and prolactin. Prog Neuropsychopharmacol Biol Psychiatry 9:473–480, 1985

Early TS, Reiman EM, Raichle ME, et al: Left globus pallidus abnormality in never medicated patients with schizophrenia. Proc Natl Acad Sci U S A 84:561–563, 1987

Ereshefsky I, Saklad SR, Wantanabe MD, et al: Thiothixene pharmacokinetic interactions: a study of hepatic enzyme inducers, clearance inhibitors, and demographic variables. J Clin Psychopharmacol 11:296–301, 1991

Falloon IR, Boyd JL, McGill CW, et al: Family management in the prevention of exacerbation of schizophrenia: a controlled study. N Engl J Med 306:1437–1440, 1982

Flaum M, Arndt S, Andreasen NC: The role of gender in studies of ventricle enlargement in schizophrenia: a predominantly male effect. Am J Psychiatry 147:1327–1332, 1990

Flaum M, Swayze VW, O'Leary D, et al: Effects of diagnosis, laterality and gender on brain morphology in schizophrenia. Am J Psychiatry 152:704–714, 1993

Galletly CA, Tsourtos G: Antipsychotic drug doses and adjunctive drugs in the outpatient treatment of schizophrenia. Ann Clin Psychiatry 9:77–80, 1997

Gelenberg AJ, Keith S: Psychoses, in The Practitioner's Guide to Psychoactive Drugs, 4th Edition. Edited by Gelenberg AJ, Bassuk EL. New York, Plenum, 1998, pp 153–212

Goldstein JM, Link BG: Gender differences in the clinical expression of schizophrenia. J Psychiatr Res 22:141–155, 1988

Goldstein JM, Santangelo SL, Simpson JC, et al: The role of gender in identifying subtypes of schizophrenia: a latent class analytic approach. Schizophr Bull 16:263–275, 1990

Hafner H, Maurer K, Loffler W, et al: The epidemiology of early schizophrenia: influence of age and gender on onset and early course. Br J Psychiatry 164(suppl):29–38, 1994

Haring C, Meise U, Humpel C, et al: Dose-related plasma levels of clozapine: influence of smoking behavior, sex and age. Psychopharmacology 99:S38–S40, 1989

Hauser P, Dauphinais D, Berrettini W, et al: Corpus callosum dimensions measured by magnetic resonance imaging in bipolar affective disorder and schizophrenia. Biol Psychiatry 26:659–668, 1989

Hoff AL, Neal C, Kushner M, et al: Gender differences in corpus callosum size in first episode schizophrenics. Biol Psychiatry 35:913–919, 1994

Hogarty GE, Anderson CM, Reiss DJ, et al: Family psychoeducation, social skills training, and maintenance chemotherapy in the aftercare treatment of schizophrenia, I: one-year effects of a controlled study on relapse and expressed emotion. Arch Gen Psychiatry 43:633–642, 1986

Hyman SE, George A, Rosenbaum JF: Antipsychotic drugs, in Handbook of Psychiatric Drug Therapy, 3rd Edition. Boston, MA, Little, Brown, 1995, pp 5–42

Isojarvi JIT, Laatikainen TJ, Pakarinen AJ, et al: Polycystic ovaries and hyperandrogenism in women taking valproate for epilepsy. N Engl J Med 329:1383–1388, 1993

Johns CA, Thompson JW: Adjunctive treatments in schizophrenia: pharmacotherapies and electroconvulsive therapy. Schizophr Bull 21:607–619, 1995

Johnstone EC, Crow TJ, Frith CD, et al: Cerebral ventricular size and cognitive impairment in chronic schizophrenia. Lancet 2:924–926, 1976

Kane JM, McGlashan TH: Treatment of schizophrenia. Lancet 346:820–825, 1995

Kane J, Honigfeld G, Singer J, et al: Clozapine for the treatment-resistant schizophrenic: a double-blind comparison with chlorpromazine. Arch Gen Psychiatry 45:789–796, 1988

Katsanis J, Iacono WG: Association of left-handedness with ventricle size and neuropsychological performance in schizophrenia. Am J Psychiatry 146:1056–1058, 1989

Keks N: Schizophrenia. Australian Journal of Hospital Pharmacy 26:93–96, 1996

Keks N, Sacks T: Schizophrenia and the community. Med J Aust 164:583–584, 1996

Keks NA, Kulkarni J, Copolov DL: Treatment of schizophrenia. Med J Aust 151:462–467, 1989

Keks NA, Copolov DL, Kulkarni J, et al: Basal and haloperidol-stimulated prolactin in neuroleptic-free men with schizophrenia defined by 11 diagnostic systems. Biol Psychiatry 27:1203–1215, 1990

Kendell R, Chalmers J, Platz C: Epidemiology of puerperal psychoses. Br J Psychiatry 150:662–673, 1987

Kulkarni J: Women and schizophrenia: a review. Aust N Z J Psychiatry 31:46–56, 1997

Kulkarni J, de Castella A, Smith D, et al: A clinical trial of estrogen in acutely psychotic women. Schizophr Res 20:247–252, 1996

Lehman AF, Rachuba LT, Postrado LT: Demographic influences on quality of life among persons with chronic mental illness: evaluation and program planning. Evaluation and Program Planning 18:155–164, 1995a

Lehman AF, Thompson JW, Dixon LB, et al: Schizophrenia: treatment outcomes research—editors' introduction. Schizophr Bull 21:561–566, 1995b

Lehman AF, Carpenter WT Jr, Goldman HH, et al: Treatment outcomes in schizophrenia: implications for practice, policy, and research. Schizophr Bull 21:669–675, 1995c

Lewine R: Sex differences in schizophrenia: timing or subtypes? Psychol Bull 90:432–444, 1981

Lewine R: Schizophrenia: an amotivational syndrome in men. Can J Psychiatry 30:316–318, 1985

Lewine R, Ruback P, Metzer HY: Effects of diagnostic criteria on the ratio of male to female schizophrenic patients. Am J Psychiatry 141:84–87, 1984

Lewine RR, Flashman L, Gulley L, et al: Sexual dimorphism in corpus callosum and schizophrenia. Schizophr Res 4:63–64, 1991

Lieberman JA, Safferman AZ, Pollack S, et al: Clinical effects of clozapine in chronic schizophrenia: response to treatment and predictors of outcome. Am J Psychiatry 151:1744–1752, 1994

Lingjaerde O: Benzodiazepines in the treatment of schizophrenia: an updated survey. Acta Psychiatr Scand 84:453–459, 1991

Loranger AW: Sex differences in age at onset of schizophrenia. Arch Gen Psychiatry 41:157–161, 1984

Loyd D, Simpson JC, Tsuang MT: Are there sex differences in the long term outcome of schizophrenia? Comparisons with mania, depression and surgical controls. J Nerv Ment Dis 173:643–649, 1985

Marder SR, Davis JM, Chouinard G: The effects of risperidone on the five dimensions of schizophrenia derived by factor analysis: combined results of the North American trials. J Clin Psychiatry 58:538–546, 1997

Marneros A: Frequency of occurrence of Schneider's first rank symptoms in schizophrenia. Eur Arch Psychiatry Clin Neurosci 234:78–82, 1984

Marriott P, Hiep A: Drug monitoring at an Australian depot phenothiazine clinic. J Clin Psychiatry 39:206–212, 1978

McGlashan TH, Bardenstein KK: Gender differences in affective, schizoaffective, and schizophrenic disorders. Schizophr Bull 16:319–329, 1990

Miller CH, Mohr F, Umbricht D, et al: The prevalence of acute extrapyramidal signs and symptoms in patients treated with clozapine, risperidone, and conventional antipsychotics. J Clin Psychiatry 59:69–75, 1998

Miller LJ, Finnerty M: Sexuality, pregnancy and childrearing among women with schizophrenia-spectrum disorders. Psychiatr Serv 47:502–506, 1996

Mueser KT, Blanchard JJ, Bellack AS: Memory and social skill in schizophrenia: the role of gender. Psychiatry Res 57:141–153, 1995

Murray RW: The neurodevelopmental basis of sex differences in schizophrenia. Psychol Med 21:565–575, 1991

Murray RW, Lewis SW: Is schizophrenia a neurodevelopmental disorder? BMJ 295:681–682, 1987

Murray RW, Reveley AM, Lewis SW: Family history, obstetric complications and cerebral abnormality in schizophrenia, in Handbook of Schizophrenia, Vol 3. Edited by Nasrallah HA. Amsterdam, The Netherlands, Elsevier, 1988, pp 563–577

Nasrallah HA, Andreasen NC, Coffman JA, et al: A controlled magnetic resonance imaging study of corpus callosum thickness in schizophrenia. Biol Psychiatry 21:274–282, 1986

Orley J, Sazena S, Herman H: Quality of life and mental illness. Br J Psychiatry 172:291–293, 1998

Perlick D, Mattis S, Stasny P, et al: Gender differences in cognition in schizophrenia. Schizophr Res 8:69–73, 1992

Peuskens J, Link CG: A comparison of quetiapine and chlorpromazine in the treatment of schizophrenia. Acta Psychiatr Scand 96:265–273, 1997

Pilowsky LS, Costa DC, Ell PJ, et al: D2 dopamine receptor binding in the basal ganglia of anti-psychotic free schizophrenic patients: an I123-IBZM single photon emission CT study. Br J Psychiatry 164:16–26, 1994

Pinals DA, Malhotra AK, Missar CD, et al: Lack of gender differences in neuroleptic response in patients with schizophrenia. Schizophr Res 22:215–222, 1996

Piran N, Bigler ED, Cohen D: Motoric laterality and eye dominance suggest unique pattern of cerebral organization in schizophrenia. Arch Gen Psychiatry 39:1006–1010, 1982

Pollock BG: Gender differences in psychotropic drug metabolism. Psychopharmacol Bull 33:235–242, 1997

Potkin SG, Buchsbaum MS, Jin Y, et al: Clozapine effects on glucose metabolic rate in striatum and frontal cortex. J Clin Psychiatry 55:63–66, 1994

Prudo R, Blum AM: Five year outcome and prognosis in schizophrenia: a report from the London Field Research Center of the International Pilot Study of Schizophrenia. Br J Psychiatry 150:345–354, 1987

Pyne JM, Patterson TL, Kaplan RM, et al: Assessment of the quality of life of patients with major depression. Psychiatr Serv 48:224–230, 1997

Raine A, Harrison GN, Reynolds GP, et al: Structural and functional characteristics of the corpus callosum in schizophrenics, psychiatric controls and normal controls. Arch Gen Psychiatry 47:1060–1065, 1990

Rosen A: Community psychiatry services: will they endure? Current Opinion in Psychiatry 5:257–265, 1992

Salokongas RK: Prognostic implications of the sex of schizophrenic patients. Br J Psychiatry 142:145–151, 1983

Schroder J, Bubeck B, Silvestri S, et al: Gender differences in D2 dopamine receptor binding in drug-naïve patients with schizophrenia: an I 123-IBZM single photon emission CT study. Psychiatry Res 75:115–123, 1997

Seeman MV: Interaction of sex, age, and neuroleptic dose. Compr Psychiatry 24:125–128, 1983

Seeman M: Schizophrenia, gender, and affect. Can J Psychiatry 41:263–264, 1996

Simpson GM, Yadalam KG, Levinson DF, et al: Single dose pharmacokinetics of fluphenazine after fluphenazine decanoate administration. J Clin Psychopharmacol 10:417–421, 1990

Siris SG: Adjunctive medication in the maintenance treatment of schizophrenia and its conceptual implications. Br J Psychiatry Suppl 22:66–78, 1993

Siris SG, Bermanzohn PC, Mason SE, et al: Maintenance imipramine therapy for secondary depression in schizophrenia: a controlled trial. Arch Gen Psychiatry 51:109–115, 1994

Spencer J, Glick I, Haas G, et al: A randomized clinical trial of inpatient family intervention, III: effects at 6-month and 18-month follow-ups. Am J Psychiatry 145:1115–1121, 1988

Spitzer R, Endicott J, Robins E: Research Diagnostic Criteria: Instrument Number 58. New York, New York Psychiatric Institute, 1978

Stedman T: Approaches to measuring quality of life and their relevance to mental health. Aust N Z J Psychiatry 30:731–740, 1996

Stein LJ, Test MA: An alternative to mental hospital treatment, I: conceptual model, treatment program, and clinical evaluation. Arch Gen Psychiatry 37:409–412, 1980

Sullivan G, Wells KB, Leake B: Clinical factors associated with better quality of life in a seriously mentally ill population. Hosp Community Psychiatry 43:794–798, 1992

Szymanski S, Lieberman JA, Alvir JM, et al: Gender differences in onset of illness, treatment response, course, and biologic indexes in first-episode schizophrenic patients. Am J Psychiatry 152:698–702, 1995

Tamminga CA: Gender and schizophrenia. J Clin Psychiatry 58(suppl 15):33–37, 1997

Test MA, Burke SS, Wallisch LS: Gender differences of young adults with schizophrenic disorders in community care. Schizophr Bull 16:331–344, 1990

Thomas C, Bartlett A, Mezey GC: The extent and effects of violence among psychiatric in-patients. Psychiatr Bull 19:600–604, 1995

Tollefson GD, Beasley CM, Tran PV, et al: Olanzapine versus haloperidol in the treatment of schizophrenia and schizoaffective and schizophreniform disorders: results of an international collaborative trial. Am J Psychiatry 154:457–465, 1997

Van Peer A, Meulderman W, Woestenborghs R, et al: Clinical pharmacokinetics of risperidone, in Serotonin in Antipsychotic Treatment. Edited by Kane J, Moëller HJ, Awouters F. New York, Marcel Dekker, 1996, pp 277–292

Wald A, Van Thiel DH, Hoechstetter L, et al: Gastrointestinal transit: the effect of the menstrual cycle. Gastroenterology 80:1497–1500, 1981

Walter BJ, Keward HB: Gender differences in living conditions found among male and female schizophrenic patients: a follow-up study. Int J Soc Psychiatry 31:205–261, 1985

Weinberger DR, Bigelow LB, Kleinman JE, et al: Cerebral ventricular enlargement in chronic schizophrenia: an association with poor response to therapy. Arch Gen Psychiatry 37:11–13, 1980a

Weinberger DR, Cannon-Spoor E, Potkin SG, et al: Poor premorbid adjustment and CT scan abnormalities in chronic schizophrenia. Am J Psychiatry 137:1410–1423, 1980b

Wirshing DA, Wirshing WC, Kysar L, et al: Novel antipsychotics: comparison of weight gain liabilities. J Clin Psychiatry 60:358–363, 1999

Wolff S, Chide J: Schizoid personality in childhood: a controlled follow-up study. Psychol Med 10:85–100, 1980

Women's Advisory Group: Tailoring Services to Meet the Needs of Women. Melbourne, Australia, Victorian Government Department of Human Services, 1997

Wyatt RJ: Neuroleptics and the natural course of schizophrenia. Schizophr Bull 17:325–351, 1991

Yonkers KA, Kando JC, Cole JO, et al: Gender differences in pharmacokinetics and pharmacodynamics of psychotropic medication. Am J Psychiatry 149:587–595, 1992

Zito JM, Craig TJ, Wanderling J, et al: Pharmacoepidemiology in 136 hospitalized schizophrenic patients. Am J Psychiatry 144:778–782, 1987

15

Role of the Severely Mentally Ill in the Family

William B. Lawson, M.D., Ph.D.
Charlotte Kennedy, Ph.D.

*P*olicy changes have increased the likelihood that the severely mentally ill will either live in the community with their families or start families themselves. Economic factors and societal bias facing these individuals contribute to the burden of the severely mentally ill in the community, especially if they are ethnic minorities. The family of the mentally ill person faces unique stresses. These stresses are even greater if the mother is mentally ill. Women with schizophrenia are especially likely to become parents, often with limited resources. Nevertheless, the resilience of mothers with schizophrenia, accompanied by new treatment approaches in both psychoeducation and pharmacotherapy, as well as the relative success of ethnic minorities, provides optimism for the future.

EFFECT OF POLICY, TREATMENT, AND DEMOGRAPHIC SHIFTS

Much has been said about the effect of displaced severely mentally ill patients on the community as a result of deinstitutionalization and shorter hospital stays. Policymakers and institutional providers have focused on partial hospitalization, supportive living facilities, correctional facilities, and homeless shelters as ways to address these concerns of the severely mentally ill but have seldom addressed family needs. However, the largest percentage of the chronically mentally ill live with their families (Goldman 1982). Unfortunately, the effect of policy and treatment venues on family members is seldom considered.

In fact, recent policy decisions, new treatment interventions, and demographic changes have directly affected the extent to which the severely mentally ill interact with the family (Camann 1996). One major consequence of recent policy decisions and treatment advances has been the increasing likelihood that the severely mentally ill will form their own families. A major policy shift has been the decision to provide care for the severely mentally ill in the community rather than in large inpatient facilities. Deinstitutionalization and a lesser restrictive environment are now the standard of care. In the past, the sexes were segregated in large inpatient facilities with little likelihood of interaction, but now many individuals with severe mental illness spend much of the time in the community and with the opposite sex. An unanticipated consequence is that the fertility rate of mothers with schizophrenia has increased from below that of the general population in the 1950s to that of the general population since deinstitutionalization (Burr et al. 1979; Erlenmeyer-Kimling et al. 1969). In addition, newer antipsychotic medications have improved the prognosis for many patients with schizophrenia (Kane et al. 1988; Marder and Meibach 1994). The most dramatic gain has been in negative symptoms (i.e., the ability to express affect, to socialize, and to interact). In the past, the illness itself in addition to physical separation limited the capacity of many patients to form meaningful relationships with either peers or offspring. Successful treatment of the negative symptoms of schizophrenia now means that individuals with severe mental illness will be more likely to form relationships and families, have children, and keep them because of better symptom control.

Demographic trends interact with these policy and treatment consequences. Trends show that more individuals with schizophrenia are also becoming parents (Burr et al. 1979; Erlenmeyer-Kimling et al. 1969). In the general population, female-headed single-parent families have become more common (Bryant 1992). More women with schizophrenia than men are becoming parents, perhaps because schizophrenia has a later onset and causes fewer negative symptoms in women (Caton et al. 1999; White et al. 1995). Consequently, women with severe mental illness are not only more likely to have children than in the past but also more likely to raise them, either as single parents or as part of family units (Miller and Finnerty 1996; Mowbray et al. 1995a, 1995b; White et al. 1995). Today, women with severe mental illness are as likely to have children as women in the general population (Mowbray et al. 1995a; White et al. 1995). Pregnancies are often unplanned (Miller and Finnerty 1996). In addition, females with mental illness are more likely to have been married but are also more likely to be divorced (White et al. 1995). As a result, many do not have partners at some point in the life of the child. Despite the increased likelihood of being single parents, they want to keep their children and are electing more than ever to raise them (White et al. 1995).

ECONOMIC BURDEN

Increasingly, there has been an appreciation of the family burden that mothers face when a family member has schizophrenia. Economic and emotional stresses are common (Goldman 1982). When the mother has schizophrenia, these stressors are multiplied. Only a minority of mothers are able to provide consistent nurturing of their children because of the chronic, relapsing nature of the disorder (White et al. 1995). Custody loss is very high (Miller and Finnerty 1996; Mowbray et al. 1995a). Those mothers who are able to maintain their mothering role face economic concerns. Having a family member with schizophrenia is expensive. The annual direct costs may exceed the median family income, especially if a hospitalization occurs (Lawson 1986; Muller and Caton 1983). In the general population, single-parent families have lower-than-average incomes, and families headed by a female overwhelmingly have incomes below the poverty line (Bryant 1992). The limited employability associated with schizophrenia further exacerbates the difficulty of finding employment when a child needs care. The economic demands make essentials difficult to attain and luxuries impossible to attain. The individual with schizophrenia depends heavily on relatives in times of stress, thus shifting the economic burden to other family members (Tolsdorf 1976). A hospitalization dramatically increases the financial demands because of the direct cost of care of the illness itself, the need for a caregiver if there is a dependent child, and other indirect costs from the unpredictable and disruptive nature of such an event (Lawson 1986).

Another trend is the increasing percentage of ethnic minorities in the population (Bryant 1992). Increasingly, a larger percentage of the population with schizophrenia will be minorities. African Americans with schizophrenia are more likely to be parents, to be female, and to have been married in the past (White et al. 1995). However, minorities face additional economic stressors. Minorities consistently have an income lower than that of Caucasians (Lawson 1986). Minorities may have less access to resources

for economic reasons. African Americans may have less access to health services in general and mental health services in particular, which further ac-
centuates family burden (Lawson 1986).

BURDEN FROM BIAS

The family with a schizophrenic member also faces an increasing burden
because of prejudicial beliefs about schizophrenia. The family of a well
mother but ill offspring faces the stigma of blame. Historically, the mother
was thought to be a precipitant of the schizophrenic process (Lawson
1986). Theorists emphasized the importance of the family in the emergence of schizophrenic symptoms. Family dynamics were considered a major etiological factor in the development of schizophrenia. The family's
communication style transmitted the disorder, particularly through the
mother. Therapy was directed toward "devictimizing" the schizophrenic
member; deviant behavior was considered a sick role to be deemphasized,
and disturbed speech and behavior were comments on the underlying family process. The overwhelming message, whether overt or covert, was that
schizophrenia was caused by personal experience with family members,
and the key family member was believed to be the mother (Terkelsen
1983).

This approach extended to explaining racial/ethnic differences as well.
Schizophrenia was thought to be more common among African Americans
(Adebimpe 1981). Because the African American family often did not fit the
traditional model of the nuclear family, it was considered pathological.
Moreover, the African American family often was stereotyped as matriar-
chal and therefore unstable. The family was thus considered a "tangle of
pathology." Consequently, female-headed households were thought to be
part of the blame for the perceived higher prevalence of psychopathology
among African Americans (Lawson 1986).

Subsequent studies have not confirmed either view. Twin and family
studies have consistently failed to show a significant role of rearing practices as a key etiological factor in schizophrenia (Lawson 1986). These
studies also have tended to fail to show any substantive role of the mother
in the etiology of schizophrenia. Rather, biological factors such as genetics
or various prenatal stresses, such as infectious agents, have been emphasized in current thinking about the etiology of schizophrenia. This view has
been fortified by consistent findings of biological abnormalities in the biochemistry of severely mentally ill patients, even if they are not useful as diagnostic markers (Lawson 1990). Moreover, structural and functional
abnormalities of the brain have been consistently reported with various

structural and functional imaging and neuropathological procedures. Nevertheless, the belief that the family or mother is somehow to be blamed remains strong among laypersons and some therapists not familiar with recent advances in biological psychiatry (Lawson 1986).

BURDEN OF AN ILL FAMILY MEMBER

More recently, the tendency has been to think of the family interaction not as an etiological agent but as a stressor that may lead to relapse. Emotional overinvolvement and high levels of criticism by family members were highly predictive of symptomatic relapse (Vaughn et al. 1984). Interventions such as psychoeducation have been advocated as a way of preventing such outcomes and helping family members. These interventions can help address the stresses that can cause a readmission and can provide support for other family members in the face of significant family burden (Lamb and Oliphant 1978). However, such interventions, although potentially valuable, are seldom provided to families with a schizophrenic mother and can easily be used punitively to perpetuate stereotypes about "schizophrenogenic families" (Doll 1976; Terkelsen 1983).

There is now widespread recognition that some of the perceived dysfunctionality seen in families with schizophrenic members may be a consequence of the family attempting to adapt to an ill member (Doll 1976). The presence of a family member with mental illness may be emotionally distressing to the rest of the family. Family members report difficulties in dealing with unexpected and irrational anger, unjustified suspicions, episodes of psychotic behavior, mood shifts, irregular sleep, binge eating, destruction of household objects, physical threats and attacks, and suicide attempts (Hatfield 1985). Many of the regressed features and maladaptive behavior in the patient, once attributed to "institutionalization," persisted despite briefer hospital stays and are now believed to be a core symptom of the illness (Johnstone et al. 1981). Families were exposed to new economic and emotional stresses that were minimized in the past by lengthy hospitalizations.

Newer treatments also can increase family stress. Newer medication has resulted in marked improvement for patients who had not responded to other treatment (Kane et al. 1988; Marder and Meibach 1994). This overtly positive result may present challenges to families who have adapted to the patient as an ill person who cannot behave differently and deserves sympathy. The family may become resentful when the patient becomes less ill and is in better control (Conley and Baker 1990). The mother, who previously had an apathetic, asocial offspring whom she considered lost, now might face a stressful undoing of the grief reaction. Family members have difficulty handling a rational individual whose arguments were once considered irrational or who is no longer predictably withdrawn but might show a full range of emotions, including anger (Conley and Baker 1990).

BURDEN AND THE ILL MOTHER

The mentally ill mother faces the additional burden of child rearing. Treatment, including medication, can be both helpful and a burden (Nicholson et al. 1998a). Although side effects are less of a problem with newer medication, many agents still cause sedation, which may leave the mother with few personal resources to keep up with an active child. Inadequately treated negative symptoms may have the same result. Moreover, participating in treatment programs may conflict with the time needed for child rearing. Conversely, mothers may put their children's needs first and fail to address their medical needs such as keeping appointments or taking medication.

Those with severe mental illness have to cope with not being able to distinguish the normal stress of child rearing from the symptoms of their illness (Nicholson et al. 1998a). They may blame themselves for the normal problems of childhood or adolescence. Conversely, raising a child can be motivation to recover. Custody loss is a common threat and, as noted above, occurs frequently (White et al. 1995). Psychotic mothers are especially highly likely to lose their child. The loss of a child is often considered painful if the child is relinquished voluntarily or through custody loss (Miller 1997).

Mothers with mental illness face additional concerns as a result of the illness itself. There is little doubt that major mental illness can compromise child-rearing ability because of either positive psychotic symptoms or the more insidious negative symptoms (Rogosch et al. 1992). Moreover, severe mental illness, especially paranoid schizophrenia, is a risk factor for violence (Tardiff 1988). Nevertheless, most mentally ill women raise their children safely (Nicholson et al. 1998a). However, there are reports of mentally ill mothers killing their children, and these negative instances may be more influential in the eyes of the public and misinformed family members because they are consistent with the stereotype of the dangerous mentally ill patient. Mothers with schizophrenia are universally believed never to be capable of safely raising future children. However, one report found otherwise, showing that women who killed their children were at low future risk for harming any other children (Jacobsen and Miller 1998).

Family and extrafamilial factors further complicate the life of the mentally ill mother. As noted earlier in this chapter, a partner is often not available because of an unplanned pregnancy or a divorce (Miller and Finnerty 1996; White et al. 1995). When a partner is present, he can be helpful in providing emotional and economic support, in being available in times of crisis, and by making the child-rearing process less demanding. However, the relationship with a partner is often less than ideal. Fewer than half of the women with severe mental illness have romantic or intimate relationships (Ritsher et al. 1997). Moreover, the partners may undermine the status of the mother or even undermine treatment (Nicholson et al. 1998b). They may have unrealistic expectations or may be frankly abusive. Women with psychotic symptoms are especially likely to be victimized (Ritsher et al. 1997). The mentally ill spouse is vulnerable to abuse because she is perceived as being the sick member of the partnership; because she may have too few resources to survive outside the marriage, especially with a child; and because she often has low self-esteem and may blame herself (Nicholson et al. 1998a, 1998b). Having a well spouse is a two-edged sword because he may be necessary for the woman to retain custody or to maintain family resources, but he also may be more likely to gain sole custody and to consider her superfluous (Nicholson et al. 1998b).

The ill mother may face stigmatization from the family. Family members who do not understand mental illness may blame the mother for any problems that arise (Nicholson et al. 1998b). Other family members also may undermine the mentally ill mother. They may reinforce a sick role (Conley and Baker 1990; Nicholson et al. 1998b). Grandparents and other members of extended families can be seen as helpful, especially among minorities (Lawson 1986). However, they may become so successful that the mother becomes jealous (Nicholson et al. 1998b). The grandparents may be resentful at having to raise another family, or they simply may not be physically capable of the child-rearing demands.

Outside agencies also can be a mixed blessing. As noted earlier, the mother is often stigmatized and frequently loses custody of her children (White et al. 1995). These mothers are often judged by social service agencies to be unable to care for their children (Nicholson et al. 1998a, 1998b). Mental health service agencies, while addressing the needs of the patient, may contribute to a disregard of the needs of child rearing (Nicholson et al. 1998b). Often, services such as backup care in case of hospitalization are simply not provided, and the needs of the patient as a mother are not addressed (Nicholson et al. 1998b). Although approaches such as psychoeducation can be extremely helpful both to the ill mother and to the family as a whole, such services usually are not provided (Dixon et al. 1999).

RACIAL/ETHNIC MINORITIES

As noted earlier in this chapter (see section "Economic Burden"), minority families face additional pressures. African Americans and Hispanics tend to have schizophrenia overdiagnosed and mood disorders overlooked (Adebimpe 1981). However, studies have not confirmed the finding of an excess risk of schizophrenia, suggesting that concerns about the pathological nature of the black family are overblown at best (Lawson 1986). African American and Hispanic families have differential and sometimes adverse experiences with the mental health system when they have access at all. African Americans are more likely to be hospitalized, to be involuntarily committed, and to be placed in seclusion or restraints than are European Americans (Flaherty and Meagher 1980; Lawson et al. 1994; Lindsey et al. 1989; Soloff and Turner 1982; Strakowski et al. 1995). Moreover, African Americans are more likely than Caucasians to receive as-needed medication and higher doses of antipsychotic medication (Chung et al. 1995; Flaherty and Meagher 1980; Strakowski et al. 1993). These suboptimal treatment approaches further reduce the likelihood of optimal outcome, a necessity for child-rearing mothers. Furthermore, they reduce the likelihood of follow-up treatment in the mental health system. In fact, many minorities either delay seeking treatment in the standard mental health system or seek treatment outside of the system (Neighbors 1984). Moreover, minorities are less likely to receive psychoeducation for the mentally ill mother or family members (Dixon et al. 1999).

RECOMMENDATIONS AND REASONS FOR OPTIMISM

Despite the concerns raised in this chapter, the outlook for families with mentally ill members and for mothers raising their own children is bright. Approaches such as psychoeducation have substantial effects on families with ill members (Conley and Baker 1990). Newer pharmacological treatments, including the atypical medications, significantly reduce the risk of hospitalization, which is a major economic stress for many families (Addington et al. 1993). Moreover, many of the disruptive behaviors are better controlled. For the mother with mental illness, the lower frequency of side effects, including sedation, and the reduced likelihood of depression and negative symptoms mean a greater likelihood of a positive relationship with a partner or the family and an increased likelihood of successful child rearing (Addington et al. 1993; Tollefson et al. 1997, 1998). As noted earlier, despite the many difficulties, these women are having families and keeping their children (White et al. 1995). They have a strong desire to develop normal lives for themselves and their children (Mowbray et al. 1995b).

Making family psychoeducation more available and addressing the financial burden that families face would greatly reduce family stress. Moreover, the limitations of families must be recognized (Conley and Baker 1990). Their resources, both emotional and financial, are not limitless. As noted, the family may be a source of distress for the mentally ill mother when resources are limited. Consequently, addressing the emotional issues of the extended family and partners can be as important as addressing the needs of the "sick" member (Nicholson et al. 1998b). Systems need to recognize the special needs of mentally ill mothers, including identifying resources when hospitalization is necessary, separating the stresses of "normal" child rearing from the difficulty of having an illness, and incorporating the needs of the child when the treatment plan for the mother is developed (Nicholson et al. 1998b).

Despite the financial limitations, minority families may have special advantages. African Americans often have more tolerance for deviant behavior and believe that a mentally ill member deserves sympathy rather than rejection (Hatfield 1985). They often have extended families that have a strong tradition of sharing resources and have adopted institutions such as informal adoptions, informal support for elderly members, and greater tolerance for the mentally ill (Griffith and Mathewson 1981; Griffith et al. 1980). They also have alternatives to the mental health center, including the church, which can play a major role for the "well" members of the family (Griffith and Mathewson 1981; Griffith et al. 1980). Additional research in the coping strategies of minority families may provide other solutions to addressing the needs of the severely mentally ill within the context of a family (Lawson 1986).

REFERENCES

Addington DE, Jones B, Bloom D, et al: Reduction of hospital days in chronic schizophrenia treated with risperidone: a retrospective study. Clin Ther 14:917–926, 1993

Adebimpe VR: Overview: white norms and psychiatric diagnosis of black patients. Am J Psychiatry 138:279–285, 1981

Bryant BE: United States population: the changing face of the United States, in the World Almanac and Book of Facts. New York, World Almanac, 1992

Burr WA, Falek A, Strauss LT, et al: Fertility in psychiatric outpatients. Hosp Community Psychiatry 30:527–531, 1979

Camann MA: Family focused mental health policy. Issues in Mental Health Nursing 17:479–486, 1996

Caton LM, Cournos F, Dominguez B: Parenting and adjustment in schizophrenia. Psychiatr Serv 50:239–243, 1999

Chung H, Mahler JC, Kakuna T: Racial differences in the treatment of psychiatric inpatient. Psychiatr Serv 46:586–591, 1995

Conley RR, Baker RW: Family response to improvement by a relative with schizophrenia. Hosp Community Psychiatry 41:898–901, 1990

Dixon L, Lyles A, Scott J, et al: Service to families of adults with schizophrenia: from treatment recommendations to dissemination. Psychiatr Serv 50:233–238, 1999

Doll W: Family coping with the mentally ill: an unanticipated problem of deinstitutionalization. Hosp Community Psychiatry 27:183–185, 1976

Erlenmeyer-Kimling L, Nichol S, Rainer JD, et al: Changes in fertility rates in schizophrenic patients in New York State. Am J Psychiatry 125:916–927, 1969

Flaherty JA, Meagher R: Measuring racial bias in inpatient treatment. Am J Psychiatry 137:679–682, 1980

Goldman HH: Mental illness and family burden: a public health perspective. Hosp Community Psychiatry 33:557–560, 1982

Griffith EE, Mathewson MA: Communitas and charisma in a black church service. J Natl Med Assoc 73:1023–1027, 1981

Griffith EE, English T, Mayfield V: Possession, prayer, and testimony: therapeutic aspects of the Wednesday night meeting in a black church. Psychiatry 43:120–128, 1980

Hatfield A: Psychological costs of schizophrenia to the family. Soc Work 23:355–359, 1978

Jacobsen T, Miller LJ: Mentally ill mothers who have killed: three cases addressing the issue of future parenting capability. Psychiatr Serv 49:650–657, 1998

Johnstone EC, Owens DG, Gold A, et al: Institutionalization and the defects of schizophrenia. Br J Psychiatry 139:195–203, 1981

Kane J, Honifield G, Singer J, et al: Clozapine for the treatment resistant schizophrenic: a double-blind comparison versus chlorpromazine. Arch Gen Psychiatry 45:789–796, 1988

Lamb H, Oliphant E: Schizophrenia, through the eyes of families. Hosp Community Psychiatry 29:803–806, 1978

Lawson WB: Chronic mental illness and the black family. American Journal of Social Psychology 5:57–61, 1986

Lawson WB: Biological markers in neuropsychiatric disorders: racial and ethnic factors, in Family, Culture, and Psychobiology. Edited by Sorel E. New York, Levas, 1990, pp 79–89

Lawson WB, Hebler N, Holladay J, et al: Race as a factor in inpatient and outpatient admissions and diagnosis. Hosp Community Psychiatry 45:72–74, 1994

Lindsey KP, Paul GL, Mariotto MJ: Urban psychiatric commitments: disability and dangerous behavior of black and white recent admissions. Hosp Community Psychiatry 40:286–294, 1989

Marder SR, Meibach RC: Risperidone in the treatment of schizophrenia. Am J Psychiatry 151:825–835, 1994

Miller LJ: Sexuality, reproduction, and family planning in women with schizophrenia. Schizophr Bull 23:623–635, 1997

Miller LJ, Finnerty M: Sexuality, pregnancy, and childrearing among women with schizophrenia-spectrum disorders. Psychiatr Serv 47:502–506, 1996

Mowbray CT, Oyserman D, Zemencuk JK, et al: Motherhood for women with serious mental illness: pregnancy, childbirth, and the postpartum period. Am J Orthopsychiatry 65:21–38, 1995a

Mowbray CT, Oyserman D, Ross S: Parenting and the significance of children for women with a serious mental illness. Journal of the Mental Health Association 22:189–200, 1995b

Muller CF, Caton CL: Economic costs of schizophrenia: a post discharge study. Med Care 21:92–104, 1983

Neighbors HW: The distribution of psychiatric morbidity in black Americans: a review and suggestion for research. Community Ment Health J 20:169–181, 1984

Nicholson J, Sweeney EM, Geller JL: Mothers with mental illness, I: the competing demands of parenting and living with mental illness. Psychiatr Serv 49:635–642, 1998a

Nicholson J, Sweeney EM, Geller JL: Mothers with mental illness, II: family relationships and the context of parenting. Psychiatr Serv 49:643–649, 1998b

Ritsher JE, Coursey RD, Farrell EW: A survey on issues in the lives of women with severe mental illness. Psychiatr Serv 48:1273–1282, 1997

Rogosch FA, Mowbray CT, Bogat A: Determinants of parenting attitudes in mothers with severe psychopathology. Dev Psychopathol 4:469–487, 1992

Soloff PA, Turner SM: Patterns of seclusion: a prospective study. J Nerv Ment Dis 169:37–44, 1982

Strakowski SM, Shelton RC, Kolbrener ML: The effects of race and comorbidity on clinical diagnosis in patients with psychosis. J Clin Psychiatry 54:96–102, 1993

Strakowski SM, Lonczak HS, Sax KW, et al: The effects of race on diagnosis and disposition from a psychiatric emergency service. J Clin Psychiatry 56:101–107, 1995

Tardiff K: Management of the violent patient in an emergency situation. Psychiatr Clin North Am 11:539–549, 1988

Terkelsen KG: Schizophrenia and the family, II: adverse effects of family therapy. Fam Process 22:191–200, 1983

Tollefson GD, Beasley CM Jr, Tran PV, et al: Olanzapine versus haloperidol in the treatment of schizophrenia and schizoaffective and schizophreniform disorders: results of an international collaborative trial. Am J Psychiatry 154:457–465, 1997

Tollefson GD, Sanger TM, Lu Y, et al: Depressive signs and symptoms in schizophrenia: a prospective blinded trial of olanzapine and haloperidol. Arch Gen Psychiatry 55:250–258, 1998

Tolsdorf CC: Social networks, support, and coping: an exploratory study. Fam Process 4:407–418, 1976

Vaughn CE, Snyder KS, Jones S, et al: Family factors in schizophrenic relapse: replication in California of British research on expressed emotion. Arch Gen Psychiatry 41:1169–1177, 1984

White CL, Nicholson J, Fisher WH, et al: Mothers with severe mental illness caring for children. J Nerv Ment Dis 183:398–403, 1995

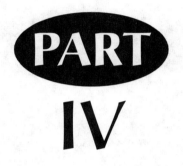

PART IV

Dementia and Related Disorders

Introduction

Alzheimer's disease (AD) is a fatal, progressive, neurodegenerative disorder that is characterized by a loss of cognitive ability and severe behavioral abnormalities. In America, this most common cause of dementia affects more than 4 million people; 5%–10% of all persons older than 65 and 50% of all persons older than 85 have this disease. It is the fourth leading cause of death in industrialized societies, preceded only by heart disease, cancer, and stroke.

Like mood disorders, AD has been reported to be more prevalent in women than in men, which may be explained by the longer life spans of women compared with men. On average, women live 7–8 years longer than men do, and age appears to be the single most important risk factor for AD. Most patients with AD are older than 80, the age at which women outnumber men by nearly two to one. However, it is implicit that other indefinable factors contribute to this finding because prevalence rates remain higher for women, even after adjusting for age.

Chapter 16 provides a comprehensive overview of the etiology, epidemiology, diagnosis, treatment, and management of AD as it relates to both men and women. An overview of the National Institute on Aging's mission and programs also is included. The subsequent chapters in this part are more sex specific.

In Chapters 17 and 18, the basic neurobiology defining estrogen's actions in the brain and the central role of gonadal steroids in the prevention and treatment of AD are explored. Recent experimental, epidemiological, and clinical trial studies have suggested that estrogen replacement therapy may afford some protective effect against the cognitive symptoms of AD. Furthermore, postmenopausal women receiving estrogen replacement therapy appear to have reduced risk of AD and a delay in the onset of the disease.

In Chapter 19, caring for the patient with AD and the challenges the caregiver faces are discussed. It has been said that AD can be more stressful for the caregiver than it is for the patient. AD not only directly affects a far greater proportion of women than men but also is a women's issue because the burden of informal community caregiving for those with AD usually is provided by women.

Overview of Alzheimer's Disease Research From the National Institute on Aging

Neil S. Buckholtz, Ph.D.

*A*lzheimer's disease (AD) is a progressive brain disorder that occurs gradually and results in memory loss, behavior and personality changes, and a decline in thinking abilities that cannot be reversed. These mental losses are related to the death of brain cells and the breakdown of the connections between them. The course of this disease varies from person to person, as does the rate of decline. On average, patients with AD live for 8–10 years after they receive the diagnosis; however, the disease can last for up to 20 years. The risk of developing AD increases with age, but AD and dementia symptoms are not a part of normal aging. AD and other dementing disorders in old age are caused by diseases. In the absence of a disease, the human brain often can function well into the tenth decade of life and beyond.

AD is the most common cause of dementia among people aged 65 and older and affects as many as 4 million Americans; slightly more than half of these people receive care at home, whereas the others are in many different health care institutions. The prevalence of AD doubles every 5 years

I wish to thank Drs. Creighton Phelps, Steven Snyder, and Marcelle Morrison-Bogorad for their helpful information and suggestions.

beyond age 65, and some studies indicate that nearly half of all persons aged 85 and older have symptoms of AD. In most industrialized countries, the 85 and older age group is the fastest growing segment of the population older than 65. The current number of Americans aged 85 and older is approximately 4 million and is expected to total nearly 8.5 million by the year 2030, according to the Bureau of the Census, and some experts who study population trends suggest that the number could be even greater. As more and more people live longer, the number of people affected by diseases of aging, including AD, grows.

AD places a heavy economic burden on caregivers and on society. A recent study estimated that the cost of caring at home or in a nursing home for one AD patient with severe cognitive impairments, not including indirect losses in productivity or wages, is more than $47,000 a year. For a disease that can span from 2 to 20 years, the overall cost of AD to families and to society is staggering. The annual economic toll of AD in the United States in terms of health care expenses and lost wages of both patients and their caregivers is estimated at $80–$100 billion. Thus, AD is a major health problem and expense for the United States. Until researchers find a way to cure or prevent AD, a large and growing number of people will be at risk. Providing and financing the care of this growing older population will increase the strain on our already burdened health care system.

The National Institute on Aging (NIA) is part of the federal government's National Institutes of Health (NIH). One of the NIA's main goals is to enhance the quality of life of older people by expanding knowledge about the aging brain and nervous system. The NIA has primary responsibility for conducting research aimed at finding ways to prevent, treat, and cure AD. The NIA's AD research support has important implications for public policy. Changes in the way the brain works are associated with many age-related losses that lead to institutional care. Changes in the brain that significantly affect the senses, movement, and the ability to think influence the quality of life of older people. For people with AD, a decline in these abilities limits independence, affects self-image, and influences the attitudes of others. Ultimately, these attitudes determine the nature and quality of health care services that patients with AD receive. The goal of research on AD is to identify early treatments that will change the disease's course or reduce its severity. Although no cure exists yet for AD, there is reason to be optimistic. Recent advances in understanding how this devastating illness affects the brain are suggesting new strategies for treating and preventing AD.

Research into the basic biology of the aging nervous system is critical to understanding what goes wrong in the brain of a person with AD. Understanding how nerve cells lose their ability to communicate with one another and why some nerve cells die in only certain areas of the brain is at the center of scientific efforts to discover what causes AD. Many researchers are working to slow AD's progression, delay its onset, or, eventually, prevent it altogether. In looking for better ways to diagnose AD, investigators strive to identify markers of dementia, develop and improve ways to test patients, determine causes and assess risk factors, and improve case-finding and sampling methods for population studies. Scientists also seek better ways to treat AD, improve a patient's ability to function, and support caregivers of patients with AD. The NIA provides support for all aspects of AD research, including basic etiology, epidemiology, diagnosis, treatment, and management, and the Alzheimer's Disease Centers program. In the following sections, I briefly discuss the focus of these areas and review some recent examples of the types of new findings that have provided insights into the pathophysiology of AD and its clinical manifestations, which will provide new targets for drug development and treatment.

ETIOLOGY OF ALZHEIMER'S DISEASE

Prominent cellular hallmarks of AD neuropathology include the loss of neurons and synapses from characteristically vulnerable areas of brain, the formation of neurofibrillary tangles, and the accumulation of amyloid β-peptide in senile plaques within the central nervous system (CNS) and cerebrovasculature. The etiology and pathogenesis of AD, whether sporadic or familial form, appears to be complex and multigenic. In addition to the amyloid cascade hypothesis, which posits that amyloid β-peptide 1-42 has direct and toxic effects on neurons with consequent development of dementia, other less directly linked factors may influence the etiology and pathogenesis of AD. Likely factors include 1) phosphorylation-dependent mechanisms that underlie cytoskeletal degeneration and neurofibrillary tangle formation; 2) the disruption of key trafficking and signaling proteins that might affect amyloid precursor protein (APP) metabolism or cell integrity; 3) the induction of apoptosis; 4) the generation of excitotoxins and disrupted ion homeostasis; 5) altered mitochondrial function; 6) oxidative stress and cytotoxic actions of free radical/reactive oxygen species; and 7) microglial, endothelial, and astroglial cell involvement in inflammatory responses, including the synthesis and release of toxic cytokines, acute-phase reactants, and complement proteins. The functional implications to the neuron of either the amyloid cascade hypothesis or one of the other nonamyloid mechanisms have not yet been fully explored and delineated. Several distinct or even overlapping mechanisms may lead to AD pathology through the formation of plaques and tangles and cell loss. The precise roles that any of these factors has in the development of AD are largely unknown.

Genetic research has identified a link between AD and genes on four chromosomes—1, 14, 19, and 21. The genes on chromosomes 1, 14, and 21 are associated with inherited early-onset cases, and the gene on chromosome 19 is associated with the late-onset or sporadic form of AD. With respect to the early-onset form, the first of these genes to be identified was the *APP* gene on chromosome 21. Two other genes for the presenilin proteins 1 and 2 on chromosomes 14 and 1, respectively, were identified in 1995. These genes were identified largely through linkage studies and account for approximately 50% of the inherited early-onset cases. However, they account for only a small fraction of all AD cases. In 1993, the *APOE* gene on chromosome 19 was associated with late-onset AD, and the ε4 isoform (*APOE* ε4) is considered to be a risk factor gene.

Transgenic and Knockout Models

Several transgenic and knockout models of AD have been developed, including several related to APP and amyloid β-peptide generation. These small animal models have been designed to overexpress either human APP or human APP–derived amyloid β-peptide fragments or the presenilins. With the emergence of transgenic animal models that recapitulate at least some of the features of AD, it can be argued that the genetic and neuropathological underpinnings of human AD derive from processing of the APP into amyloidogenic fragments—most notably, a fragment called amyloid β-peptide 1-42. There is a growing list of mouse models of AD developed with mutant forms of human APP and presenilin proteins, both of which, in humans, predispose to early-onset AD. The accumulation of amyloid β-peptide in these models, together with research (epidemiological, genetic, and experimental) on the influence of the naturally occurring *APOE* ε4, has added credence to the argument that posits amyloid β-peptide as a principal determinant in the development of AD. However, it is also possible to argue that amyloid β-peptide generation and deposition in plaque is but one factor among several other molecular and/or cellular changes that result in the development of this dementing illness.

Over the past several years, these transgenic models have provided insight into the pathogenesis of AD, but no mouse model yet exists that has all of the features seen in AD. Some of the features of AD have been successfully modeled, including region-specific deposition of plaques and learning and memory impairments, making this approach useful for the study of the mechanisms that underlie these facets of AD pathology. An example of a successful transgenic mouse model is the line developed by

Hsiao et al. (1996), in which amyloid β-peptide deposition occurs by age 11–13 months and behavioral deficits in Y- and water-mazes can be recognized by age 10 months.

Tauopathies and Tangles

The development of the hallmark neurofibrillary lesions in AD follows both a temporal and a spatial pattern with respect to brain region, cell layer, and cell type affected. In AD, the cytoskeleton of the neuron becomes deranged, and these cytoskeletal proteins are deposited as abnormal, paired helical filaments. The paired helical filaments in these neurofibrillary lesions are composed exclusively of abnormally phosphorylated forms of the tau protein. Tau, an abundant phosphoprotein in neurons, is found largely in axons, where it appears to stabilize microtubules of the cytoskeleton. In a normal human brain, six isoforms of tau are found. These vary in size from 352 to 441 amino acids and are derived from a single gene by alternative splicing of messenger RNA. Carboxyl-terminal, three or four tandem repeats of 31 or 32 amino acids each, is one key feature of the tau sequence. These tandem repeats constitute the microtubule binding domains. In AD brains, tau protein is 3–20 times more phosphorylated than normal and at sites different from those in normal brains. As a consequence, normal binding to microtubules is impeded, leading to loss of intracellular transport of macromolecules and tau aggregation into paired helical filaments. Several neurodegenerative diseases are characterized by tau aggregation into insoluble filaments. However, until recently, there has been no evidence from genetic studies that mutations in the *TAU* gene itself could be an initiating factor in any of these diseases.

Reports from three independent laboratories now describe the involvement of different *TAU* gene mutations on chromosome 17 in several large families with multisystem tauopathy and presenile dementia (Hutton et al. 1998; Poorkaj et al. 1998; Spillantini et al. 1998). In this complex of diseases, the presenting symptom usually is a personality change because the frontal cortex is primarily affected. The pathology is marked by the aggregation of tau protein in both neurons and glia, neuronal cell loss, neuronal and glial inclusions, and an overabundance of astroglial cells in both gray and white matter. The anatomical distribution and the biochemical characteristics of the tau deposits are different from the distributions and characteristics present in AD and other neurodegenerative diseases characterized by tau accumulation. No amyloid deposits are present. The examination of *TAU* gene dysfunction in neurodegenerative disorders such as AD, in which the accumulation of insoluble deposits of tau is a pathological feature, is now all the more important. In addition, a better understanding of the underlying pathogenic bases of abnormal protein folding and aggregation in these disorders may well provide clues to other age-dependent CNS diseases characterized by protein aggregation such as AD itself, Parkinson's disease, and Huntington's disease.

Amyloid β-Peptide Generation, Amyloid β-Peptide–Derived Diffusible Ligands, and Amyloid β-Peptide Fibril Breakers

Although the precise function of the APP, which gives rise, metabolically, to amyloid β-peptide, remains unknown, at least some of the consequences of that metabolism are becoming clearer. For example, amyloid β-peptide has both trophic and toxic effects on nearby neuronal processes and is an inducer of neuronal apoptosis. Furthermore, vascular amyloid deposition may compromise the function of the cerebrovasculature, which could lead to some of the characteristic pathognomonic changes seen in the amyloidoses.

Many researchers believe that aggregated, insoluble amyloid in plaques is the chief source of toxicity in AD, but some evidence indicates that more soluble amyloid β-peptide precursors also might be metabolically active. A recent article by Lambert et al. (1998) showed that with concentrations as low as 5 nmol/L, small, diffusible amyloid β-peptide 1-42 oligomers referred to as ADDLs (for amyloid β-peptide–derived diffusible ligands) could kill mature neurons in hippocampal slice cultures. It is believed that ADDLs form in the brain when certain inflammatory proteins such as apolipoprotein J or clusterin combine with amyloid β-peptide. It will be crucial to pinpoint toxicity related to different steps and branch points along the amyloid cascade and to determine precisely the cellular and subcellular sites at which the toxicity occurs. These results raise the question of the relative neurotoxicity of soluble and insoluble forms of amyloid β-peptide. ADDLs have not yet, however, been identified in human brain.

Increased amyloid β-peptide generation, fibril and aggregate formation, and the resulting neurotoxicity may lead to AD. One approach to developing drugs affecting the pathological cascade in AD is to investigate conditions under which fibril formation from amyloid β-peptide can be slowed or blocked. Recently, a 5–amino acid residue peptide was shown to inhibit amyloid β-peptide fibrillogenesis in vitro, to dissolve preformed fibrils in vivo, and to prevent fibril-induced death of neuroblastoma cells (Soto et al. 1998). The peptide, iAβ5, was modeled on amino acid residues in the central hydrophobic region of the N-terminal domain of amyloid β-peptide. Importantly, co-injection of a 20-fold molar excess of iAβ5 into the amygdala in a rat model of cerebral amyloid β-peptide deposition resulted

article by Tang et al. (1998) reported on a population-based longitudinal study of more than 1,000 Caucasians, Hispanics, and African Americans in a community in New York City that examined the risk of clinically diagnosed AD among people with and without an *APOE* ε4 allele. They found that the presence of an *APOE* ε4 allele was a determinant of risk for AD in Caucasians, but Hispanics and African Americans had an increased risk of AD regardless of *APOE* genotype, suggesting that other genes or environmental risk factors may contribute to the increased risk in Hispanics and African Americans.

In contrast, a prevalence and 3-year incidence study of more than 4,000 African American and Caucasian individuals in the Piedmont area of North Carolina by Fillenbaum et al. (1998) did not show a difference in AD prevalence or incidence between African Americans and Caucasians. This study examined all types of dementia, but there were no differences in type of dementia, and the majority (69%) was AD alone or together with another dementing disorder. Thus, these initial studies are not always consistent in their conclusions regarding the effect of *APOE* ε4 on the risk of AD, especially in African Americans, and further clarification is needed.

DIAGNOSIS OF ALZHEIMER'S DISEASE

The clinical diagnosis of AD has improved as the result of the work of many investigators. In specialized research facilities, clinical diagnosis by research neurologists now approaches 90% concordance with the subsequent neuropathological diagnosis. However, important questions and gaps in knowledge remain. Work must continue on the search for reliable, valid, and easily attainable biological markers that can identify cases very early in the course of disease when treatment may be most effective. Neuropsychological tests are needed that can pinpoint the sequence of deficits common to AD and separate people very early in the course of AD from people who are experiencing cognitive deficits from other causes.

Early and accurate diagnosis of AD has a major effect on the progress of research on dementia and is of extreme concern to patients and their families. The NIA's objective is to support research aimed at the development and evaluation of reliable and valid multidimensional diagnostic procedures and instruments for the identification of AD and other dementias of older individuals such as vascular dementias. The areas of research include

* Development of preclinical and antemortem diagnostic markers of dementias, including biochemical, imaging, or behavioral markers of early-stage AD

- Differential diagnosis of dementing diseases, including development and testing of screening batteries, neuropsychological tests, neuroimaging techniques, and clinical and neuropathological assessments
- Development and testing of instruments for screening for cognitive disorders, for inferring etiology, for assessing risk factors, and for determining family history
- Improvement of case-finding techniques, evaluation and refinement of diagnostic criteria, and further advances in epidemiological sampling and design

Improvement in the diagnosis of AD with a variety of procedures will provide a high correlation between clinical signs and neuropathology. One significant outcome is that it would allow patients and families to know what stage of the illness they are dealing with and to plan for the future. It also could provide for a significant improvement in the planning and design of drug trials because drugs would be more effective in altering the course of disease in patients with less severe illness, and these methods could provide means of identifying patients early in the course of the illness when they have had the smallest degree of cognitive loss. Thus, the earlier and more accurate the diagnosis, the greater will be the gain in slowing or eventually halting the clinical course of the illness, in determining its natural history, and in differentiating potential subtypes that could provide information about etiology and treatment. However, very early diagnosis has at least some potential negative consequences, such as increased anxiety about having a diagnosis with limited treatment options and questions about future insurability.

Mild Cognitive Impairment

One aspect of clinical diagnosis assuming a greater role is that of assessing questionable AD, also referred to as mild cognitive impairment—i.e., individuals who have a memory problem but do not meet the generally accepted criteria for AD, such as National Institute of Neurological and Communicative Disorders and Stroke–Alzheimer's Disease and Related Disorders Association or DSM-IV-TR (American Psychiatric Association 2000) criteria. This group is important because it is known that about 15%–20% of these individuals per year will progress to AD, which is much greater than the overall incidence rate for healthy age-matched individuals of about 1%–2% per year. Thus, if individuals with mild cognitive impairment could be identified reliably, treatments could be given that would delay or prevent the progression to diagnosed AD. This is the rationale for the Alzheimer's Disease Cooperative Study trial on vitamin E or donepezil for mild cognitive impairment discussed in the "Treatment and Management of Alzheimer's Disease" section later in this chapter.

The evaluation of mild cognitive impairment spans the boundary between normal aging and AD. One important focus in the mild cognitive impairment area is which criteria to use to identify people with mild cognitive impairment. One assessment instrument that is widely used to stage dementia is the Clinical Dementia Rating (CDR) Scale (Morris 1993). The CDR Scale is derived from an assessment of six categories of function (memory, orientation, judgment and problem solving, community affairs, home and hobbies, and personal care). Each category is rated on a scale of 0 to 3 (i.e., 0, 0.5, 1, 2, or 3). These individual category ratings are then used to generate an overall CDR score by a series of standardized rules that weigh some categories more heavily than others. A CDR score of 0 indicates normal cognition; 0.5 is questionable AD; and 1, 2, and 3 are mild, moderate, and severe AD, respectively. There seems to be general agreement on a CDR score of 0.5 as a necessary criterion for mild cognitive impairment, but questions remain about heterogeneity within the CDR 0.5 category (some scientists believe that individuals with dementia can be found within the 0.5 category) and what other neuropsychological measures to add—such as delayed recall, which has proved to be a sensitive measure of early memory change—to make the assessment more reliable in predicting who will progress to AD. The Alzheimer's Disease Cooperative Study will address some of these issues in the upcoming instrument development protocol for the mild cognitive impairment trial.

Early Diagnosis of Alzheimer's Disease Using Neuroimaging

Neuroimaging studies are attempting to assess whether aspects of brain function and/or structure can be measured to identify individuals at risk for AD before they develop the symptoms of the disease. Some groups now have data that suggest this may be possible. Convit et al. (1997) studied three groups of subjects with magnetic resonance imaging (MRI) in a cross-sectional analysis: 1) nonimpaired elderly persons, 2) individuals with minimal cognitive impairment who were at risk for AD, and 3) patients with AD. They found that hippocampal volume reductions separated the group at risk for AD from the nonimpaired group, correctly classifying 74%. The hippocampus was anatomically specific in that it and no other temporal lobe region separated nonimpaired from minimal cognitive impairment groups. In the contrast between individuals with minimal cognitive impairment and those with AD, the fusiform gyrus volume improved the ability of the hippocampal volume to separate these two groups, from

74% to 80%. Jack et al. (1997) also used MRI and reported a similar result, with total hippocampal volume measurement as the best discriminator of control subjects from at-risk (CDR score=0.5) individuals.

Johnson et al. (1998) published data from a study to determine whether single photon computed emission tomography (SPECT) measurements obtained when subjects were first seen could predict which individuals would subsequently progress to a diagnosis of AD. Four groups of subjects were followed up for a minimum of 2 years: 1) nonimpaired at baseline and nonimpaired at follow-up; 2) questionable at baseline (CDR score=0.5) and questionable at follow-up; 3) questionable at baseline and diagnosed with probable AD at follow-up (referred to as "convertors"); and 4) probable AD at baseline. The study found that four brain regions significantly differentiated the nonimpaired persons from the convertors as measured at baseline: bilateral regions of the anterior and posterior cingulate, the hippocampal formation, and the anterior thalamus. The subjects with AD also had decreased perfusion in the temporoparietal cortical regions. Thus, these results suggest that SPECT data can be successfully applied to the preclinical prediction of AD. Although the SPECT data were collected when the subjects were in the questionable stage, the data could identify more than 80% of the subjects who would progress to the point at which they met criteria for AD.

TREATMENT AND MANAGEMENT OF ALZHEIMER'S DISEASE

The objective of the NIA's AD treatment and management effort is to alter—by reducing, reversing, or slowing—the cognitive and behavioral manifestations of AD and eventually to delay the onset of AD and prevent it entirely. The primary manifestation of dementia is intellectual and cognitive deterioration. An effort has begun to test pharmacological agents for efficacy in modifying this aspect of AD; currently, four drugs are approved by the U.S. Food and Drug Administration for treatment of AD (tacrine, donepezil, rivastigmine, and galantamine), and several compounds are currently in clinical trials sponsored by pharmaceutical companies. Notwithstanding these efforts, however, no effective, generally useful treatment for AD is available (i.e., a treatment that works on large numbers of patients, maintains its effectiveness for a long period, works in both early and late stages of the disease, improves functioning of patients in activities of daily living as well as on sensitive neuropsychological measurements, and has no serious side effects). Also, both pharmacological and behavioral treatments for the behavior disorders associated with AD are needed. These behaviors include verbal and/or physical aggression, agitation, wandering, depression, sleep disturbances, and delusions, and they contribute significantly to institutionalization. Alleviation of these behaviors could thus contribute greatly to the prevention of institutionalization, to the maintenance of patients' dignity, to the reduction of stress on caregivers, and to reductions of cost to families and to the government.

Clinical Trials

The major AD clinical trials effort of the NIA is the Alzheimer's Disease Cooperative Study. This consortium of 42 sites was set up to perform clinical trials on compounds that large pharmaceutical companies generally would not be interested in. This would include drugs that are off patent or were patented and marketed for another use but might be useful for treatment of AD or novel compounds from individual investigators or from small companies without adequate resources for clinical trials. The types of drugs that could potentially ameliorate symptoms and modify the disease process are varied but include antioxidants, anti-inflammatories, and compounds affecting estrogenic, neurotrophic, and neurotransmitter processes.

During its initial grant period, the Alzheimer's Disease Cooperative Study initiated four drug studies and two studies of assessment instruments for AD clinical trials, one in English and the other in Spanish. The initial Alzheimer's Disease Cooperative Study of the antioxidants selegiline, vitamin E, or the combination over a 2-year period to assess any delay of progression has been published (Sano et al. 1997). Results showed that all three drug treatments versus placebo delayed the progression of AD in moderately impaired patients by about 6 months, as measured by time to reach one of four milestones (death, institutionalization, loss of activities of daily living, progression to severe AD), but did not affect cognitive measures. The English-language version of the instrument protocol has been published (Ferris and Mackell 1997), and these instruments are available to any group that wants to use them. Some have already been incorporated into pharmaceutical company trials. Results have been published from the agitation study (Teri et al. 2000), the prednisone study (Aisen et al. 2000), and the estrogen study (Mulnard et al. 2000). Results from the Spanish-language instrument protocol are being prepared for publication.

The Alzheimer's Disease Cooperative Study was funded in 1996 for an additional 5 years. It remains the major initiative for AD clinical trials in the federal government, addressing treatments for both cognitive and behavioral symptoms. This is part of the NIA's effort to facilitate the discovery, development, and testing of new drugs for the treatment of AD. For example, the Alzheimer's Disease Cooperative Study began a Phase I safety study of a compound, AIT-082, which the NIA supported through a small business grant and through preclinical toxicity testing in an NIA contract. This compound seems to stimulate the production of neurotrophins in the brain. A study of the usefulness of melatonin for sleep disturbances in patients with AD has been completed. Other studies that were initiated by the Alzheimer's Disease Cooperative Stufdy during this funding cycle include a study of whether vitamin E or donepezil can prevent the onset of AD in people with mild cognitive impairment, an anti-inflammatory treatment study of naproxen versus rofecoxib versus placebo, a study using divalproex sodium to modify agitation in nursing home patients, and an instrument development study for assessing mild cognitive impairment.

Management of Behavior Disorders of Alzheimer's Disease

Relatively little systematic research attention has been given to developing either pharmacological or behavioral interventions for the behavior disorders of AD such as wandering; disturbed sleep; pacing; agitation; feeding, bathing, and dressing difficulties; incontinence and toileting difficulties; screaming and other vocalizations; aggression and violence; and inappropriate sexual behavior. Research on the behavioral modification of these behavior disorders could be particularly important because it could indicate ways to avoid overmedication and multiple medications and could provide tools for families and other caregivers that replace physical and chemical restraints. The overarching goal is to reduce the severity and frequency of the disruptive behavior, to allow the patients to live in the least restrictive environment and manner, to maximize dignity and independence, to retain or reestablish self-care practices, and to alleviate caregiver burden.

Some interventions to ameliorate these symptoms are being systematically developed and tested, including the effects of exercise, sleep hygiene, and strategies for coping with activities of daily living on reducing agitation and other negative behaviors. Better control of these behaviors will improve care and delay institutionalization. Related research focuses on reducing the effects of caregiving on the health and well-being of the caregivers. As another part of this effort, family-relevant measures of patient function are being developed by the Caregiving, Health Services and Outcomes Research in Dementia (CHORD) project.

Behavioral intervention studies are often complex in design and labor and time intensive. Nevertheless, the potential significance of an effective treatment, either pharmacological or behavioral, that would ameliorate the behavioral symptoms would be enormous from many perspectives, including the increase in emotional and social well-being of the affected individual and his or her family and caregivers and the decreased economic costs to families and society. Research also is needed that addresses multimodal treatment approaches, such as combined pharmacological and behavioral interventions for managing behavior disorders.

Alzheimer's Disease Centers

The principal objectives of the Alzheimer's Disease Centers Program are to promote research, training, education, technology transfer, and multi-center and cooperative studies of the etiology, diagnosis, treatment, and clinical-neuropathological correlations. The national Alzheimer's Disease Centers were authorized by Congress (Public Health Service Act, Section 445) and funded by the NIA. The first 15 of these centers were conceived as comprehensive Research Centers (P50s). These centers all have an administrative core, a clinical core, a neuropathology core, and an education and information transfer core. Some centers include other optional cores, such as neuroimaging and data analysis cores. In addition to core facilities, the comprehensive centers have fully funded research projects. To diversify the centers geographically and to better distribute limited funds, only core support was provided to the second group of 13 Alzheimer's Disease Centers. These Alzheimer's Disease Core Centers (P30s) provide resources and expertise to investigators who obtain their primary research support from independent grants. The core centers provide the investigators with well-characterized patients, patient and family information, and tissue and biological specimens for use in research projects. There are currently 29 centers (17 P50s and 12 P30s).

Satellite Diagnostic and Treatment Clinics

A program to add Satellite Diagnostic and Treatment Clinics, linked to the existing Alzheimer's Disease Centers, was initiated in 1990. The goal of this initiative was to use the satellite clinics to target minority, rural, or other underserved populations to increase the heterogeneity of the research patient pool. It also permits special population groups to participate in research protocols and clinical drug trials associated with the parent center. The inclusion of patients with different characteristics allows investigators to answer questions about the appropriate diagnosis and treatment and management of AD that are more likely to be applicable to the broader United States population. Additionally, a more diverse patient pool facilitates investigations of the genetics of AD in minority groups, development of screening tests and neuropsychological examination procedures in minority group members and poorly educated patients, and studies of caregiving and family burden in rural and minority group cohorts. All satellites are designed to facilitate research and are organized to promote data gathering in the support of specific research questions.

Data Coordinating Center

In 1999, the NIA began support of the National Alzheimer's Coordinating Center to accomplish the following goals: 1) promote comparability among the Alzheimer's Disease Centers, 2) provide administrative information for management of the overall program, 3) index resources that are available at each center, and 4) promote the conduct of collaborative AD research.

As research on AD has progressed, it has become increasingly apparent that not only is AD genetically heterogeneous but also the dementias of aging are a family of diseases with a variety of overlapping phenotypes. Vascular dementia, Lewy body disease, hippocampal sclerosis, Parkinson's dementia, frontotemporal dementia, and other less common neurodegenerative diseases can, to a greater or lesser degree, mimic the symptoms and the pathology of AD. AD manifests in different genetic and physiological contexts, which may affect the clinical expression of the disease, including time of onset, symptoms, rate of progression, and response to treatment. For example, a significant percentage of AD coexists with vascular disease or Lewy body disease. At present, virtually no data on heterogeneity are available because of the limited numbers of patients seen at any one center. Access to larger data sets will allow characterization of the rarer and mixed phenotypes and genetic and ethnic differences that would not be possible with the smaller numbers of subjects in individual centers. By pooling patient information from many centers, it also will be possible to begin to identify potential biomarkers that will help to diagnose the different entities, permit characterization of disease course, and monitor response to treatment. Thus, opportunities for new and larger-scale, multisite collaborative studies on AD will be possible by combining resources, thereby increasing the power for symptom characterization, genetic analyses, neuroimaging profiles, and other studies. Moreover, with autopsy confirmation of many cases in a disease such as AD that has no specific diagnostic test for sporadic cases, these aggregate data are especially valuable. The first such example of a transcenter study is described in the following section.

Utility of *APOE* in Alzheimer's Disease Diagnosis

Although *APOE* ε4 is strongly associated with increased risk of AD, its value for diagnosing AD has not been clear. Investigators at 26 Alzheimer's

Meyer MR, Tschanz JT, Norton MC, et al: APOE genotype predicts when—not whether—one is predisposed to develop Alzheimer disease. Nat Genet 19:321–322, 1998

Morris JC: The Clinical Dementia Rating (CDR): current version and scoring rules. Neurology 43:2412–2414, 1993

Mulnard RA, Cotman CW, Kawas C, et al: Estrogen replacement therapy for treatment of mild to moderate Alzheimer disease. JAMA 283:1007–1015, 2000

Poorkaj P, Bird TD, Wijsman E, et al: Tau is a candidate gene for chromosome 17 frontotemporal dementia. Ann Neurol 43:815–825, 1998

Rogers J, Griffin WST: Inflammatory mechanisms of Alzheimer's disease: basic research, clinical studies and future directions, in Neuroinflammation: Mechanisms and Management. Edited by Wood P. Totowa, NJ, Humana Press, 1997, pp 177–193

Sano M, Ernesto C, Thomas R, et al: A controlled trial of selegiline, alpha-tocopherol, or both as treatment for Alzheimer's disease. N Engl J Med 336:1216–1222, 1997

Soto C, Sigurdsson EM, Morelli L, et al: Beta-sheet breaker peptides inhibit fibrillogenesis in a rat model of amyloidosis: implications for Alzheimer's therapy. Nat Med 4:822–826, 1998

Spillantini MG, Murrell JR, Goedert M, et al: Mutation in the tau gene in familial multiple system tauopathy with presenile dementia. Proc Natl Acad Sci U S A 95:7737–7741, 1998

Stewart WF, Kawas C, Corrada M, et al: Risk of Alzheimer's disease and duration of NSAID use. Neurology 48:626–632, 1997

Sze CI, Troncoso JC, Kawas C, et al: Loss of the presynaptic vesicle protein synaptophysin in hippocampus correlates with cognitive decline in Alzheimer disease. J Neuropathol Exp Neurol 56:933–944, 1997

Tang MX, Stern Y, Marder K, et al: The *APOE*-ε4 allele and the risk of Alzheimer's disease among African-Americans, whites, and Hispanics. JAMA 279:751–755, 1998

Teri L, Logsdon RG, Peskind E, et al: Treatment of agitation in AD: a randomized, placebo-controlled clinical trial. Neurology 55:1271–1278, 2000

West MJ, Coleman PD, Flood DG, et al: Differences in the pattern of hippocampal neuronal loss in normal ageing and Alzheimer's disease. Lancet 344:769–772, 1994

Xu H, Gouras GK, Greenfield JP, et al: Estrogen reduces neuronal generation of Alzheimer beta-amyloid peptides. Nat Med 4:447–451, 1998

17

Estrogen Replacement as a Prospective Treatment for Alzheimer's Disease

Rebecca M. Evans, M.D.
Martin R. Farlow, M.D.

*A*lzheimer's disease (AD) is the most common cause of dementia. AD is characterized by progressive deterioration of memory and other cognitive functions and impairment in activities of daily living. The prevalence of dementia in the United States is approximately 1%–2% at age 65 and doubles every 5 years thereafter to as much as 30%–50% of the population by age 85 (Evans et al. 1989; Jorm et al. 1987).

Most of those affected with AD are women. Why are more women than men affected with AD? An obvious answer might be that women live longer than men. When prevalence rates for AD are adjusted for age, however, women still have higher rates than men (Jorm et al. 1987; Rocca et al. 1991). Most studies of the incidence of AD also confirm higher rates in women (Katzman et al. 1989; Molsa et al. 1982; Payami et al. 1996; Rorsman et al. 1986). Another potential reason for higher rates of AD in women than in men may be the intrinsic biological differences between the sexes. Women have more estrogen, and men have more testosterone. Every woman undergoes menopause, in which the levels of estrogen produced by her body significantly and suddenly decline (Chakravarti et al. 1976). The average

age at menopause in developed countries is 51 years. The average life expectancy of women is 78 years, resulting in almost one-third of a woman's life spent in a hypoestrogenic state. In contrast, each man continues to produce testosterone throughout his life, with only a minimal and gradual decline in testosterone levels over time (Lund et al. 1999). The simple and intuitive observation that estrogen loss may be associated with the increased incidence of AD in women has led to the many basic scientific and clinical studies investigating the effects of estrogen on the brain.

Estrogen, of course, has long been known to have many diverse effects throughout the body. Estrogen replacement therapy (ERT) is often used short term to lessen uncomfortable side effects associated with menopause, such as hot flashes, vaginal dryness, and insomnia (Campbell and Whitehead 1977). Estrogen therapy also is often considered for long-term use in postmenopausal women to help prevent osteoporosis, reduce lipid levels, and prevent atherosclerosis (Palacios 1999). Until recently, it was presumed to reduce the risk of cardiac disease (Hulley et al. 1998). Most recently, ERT has been believed to have positive effects on cognitive function and has been thought to be useful in preventing the onset of Alzheimer's dementia and in treating AD.

In addition to the higher prevalence and incidence rates of AD in women, other factors have contributed to the consideration and study of estrogen as a therapeutic treatment for AD. Cell culture and animal models support a significant and varied role for estrogen within the brain, affecting not only the areas associated with reproduction but also other regions. Much of this research finds that estrogen is both neurotrophic and neuroprotective, actions relevant to the mechanisms associated with the pathological changes found in AD. Clinical studies of cognition in healthy postmenopausal women have found beneficial effects of estrogen. Epidemiological studies suggest that estrogen reduces the risk for AD. Although these clinical studies have many methodological issues, the overall impression has been that estrogen may be useful for prevention or treatment of AD.

This impression was contradicted by the negative results from three recent double-blind, placebo-controlled trials of ERT as a treatment for AD (Henderson et al. 2000; Mulnard et al. 2000; Wang et al. 2000). None of these studies found any beneficial effects for ERT in slowing the progression or treating the symptoms of AD. These results argue against a therapeutic role for ERT in AD but do not exclude the possibility of significant effects for ERT on prevention of AD. Two recent meta-analyses of epidemiological studies examining ERT and risk for AD concluded that the use of ERT in postmenopausal women was associated with a significant reduction in the risk for AD (Hogervorst et al. 2000; Yaffe et al. 1998).

In the following sections, the basic effects of estrogen that are relevant to the prevention and treatment of neurodegenerative disease are reviewed. Studies of the effects of estrogen on cognition in postmenopausal women without AD are only briefly discussed, with emphasis placed on discussion of the clinical studies that are particularly relevant to AD.

HORMONAL CHANGES IN WOMEN AND MEN WITH AGING

In premenopause, the ovaries produce estrogen predominantly in the form of estradiol. In the systemic circulation, about 25% of the estradiol is converted to estrone and the remainder metabolized to estriol. In the periphery and the brain, estradiol has a higher affinity for estrogen receptors than estrone. Estrone has low receptor affinity (O'Connell 1995). The ovaries begin to fail a few years before menopause (mean age=51), producing estradiol erratically (Judd 1987). At menopause, estradiol levels decrease dramatically to only 1% of average mid–menstrual cycle levels. Estrone is less affected, being present at 50% of premenopause levels. Following menopause, the primary source of estradiol is via androstenedione, which is metabolized to estrone and then to estradiol in the adipose tissue (O'Connell 1995).

In contrast to women, men do not have a sudden change in hormonal levels in midlife. Rather, testosterone levels decline by about 1% per year after age 40 (Lund et al. 1999). Elderly men maintain higher testosterone and estradiol levels than do postmenopausal women (Maas et al. 1997). Within the brain, testosterone is converted to estradiol by aromatase (Balthazart and Ball 1998; Naftolin 1994). Clinically significant testosterone deficiency is diagnosed in relatively few men, whereas all women experience estrogen deficiency as a normal biological function after menopause. Only recently have potential effects of androgen loss on cognition in men been explored. As with the studies of estrogen, studies of the effect of androgen levels on cognition in elderly men vary in findings, from no effect to a small decline on various neuropsychological tests (Alexander et al. 1998; Barrett-Conner et al. 1999; Janowsky et al. 1994; Lund et al. 1999).

NEUROBIOLOGICAL EFFECTS OF ESTROGEN

Estrogen produces its effects on the brain through several cellular and molecular mechanisms. We emphasize the neuroprotective and trophic actions that are relevant to the aging brain and to AD (Figure 17–1). More complete and detailed discussion of the neurobiological effects of estrogen

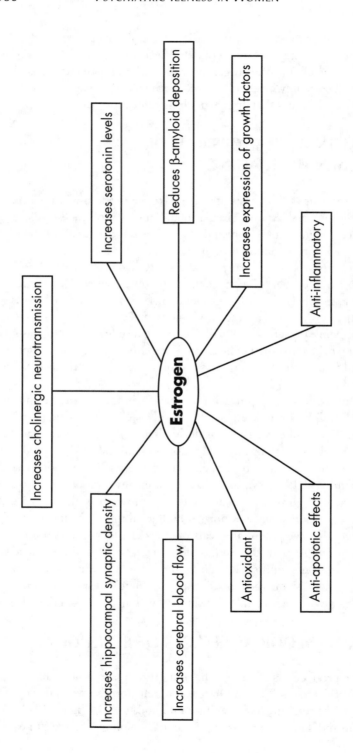

FIGURE 17–1.   The multiple trophic effects of estrogen in the brain that may influence the progression and onset of Alzheimer's disease.

can be found in several excellent recent reviews (Bicknell 1998; Garcia-Segura et al. 2001; McEwen and Alves 1999; Woolley 1999).

Genomic and Nongenomic Actions of Estrogen

Historically, estrogen's activities were thought to be genomic and mediated by classic intracellular estrogen receptors (McEwen and Alves 1999). Genomic effects are those that are delayed in onset and long in duration. Classic estrogen receptors were initially located only in the hypothalamus and pituitary gland, brain areas relevant to reproduction. More recently, estrogen receptors have been located throughout the brain in areas important in cognition, mood, and attention. Estrogen receptors are present in the hippocampus, cerebral cortex, caudate, putamen, basal forebrain cholinergic system, midbrain raphe and serotonergic system, dopaminergic system, and locus coeruleus and noradrenergic system (McEwen et al. 1997). Two types of classic estrogen receptors are known: $ER\alpha$, found primarily in brain areas that govern reproduction, and $ER\beta$, much more widely distributed throughout the brain, including the cortex and cerebellum (Shughrue et al. 1997). The interaction of estrogen with these estrogen receptors plays a role in apoptosis, axonal regeneration, and general trophic support of neurons.

Genetic polymorphisms in estrogen receptors might increase the risk for AD. A twofold increase in one estrogen receptor polymorphism was found in women with sporadic AD as compared with women without AD in an Italian population (Brandi et al. 1998). These estrogen receptor polymorphisms might alter receptor binding with estrogen, resulting in reduced neuroprotection and increased risk for AD.

Estrogen also has nongenomic actions. These actions protect or affect nerve cell activity but occur too rapidly to involve activation or repression of gene expression through known estrogen receptors. These nongenomic actions may modulate neurotransmitter function and antioxidant activities of estrogen (Garcia-Segura et al. 2001).

Both the genomic and the nongenomic actions of estrogen are mediated through various intracellular signaling cascades. Estrogen directly prevents free radical production via the structural form of one of its steroid rings (McEwen 1999). Estrogen upregulates antiapoptotic proteins (Garcia-Segura et al. 1998; Pike 1999), activates second messengers (Zhou et al. 1997), phosphorylates cyclic adenosine monophosphate (cAMP) response element binding (CREB) protein (Gu et al. 1996), activates mitogen-activated protein kinase (MAP) (Singh et al. 1999), directly excites neurons (Gu et al. 1999), and acts on calcium homeostasis (Joels and Karst 1995; Morley et al. 1992). The diversity of mechanisms and effects produced by estrogen have important therapeutic implications for the use of selective estrogen receptor modulators (SERMs) such as tamoxifen and raloxifene. SERMs are structurally different compounds from estrogen and have different agonist and antagonist properties (Garcia-Segura et al. 2001). Differences in action result in benefit for some aspects of drug action but also could result in undesirable effects in other areas.

Whether through genomic or nongenomic effects, estrogen acts to protect the brain from neurodegenerative processes in two primary ways. First, estrogen has a trophic influence on the structure and function of neurons in several areas, including the hippocampus, the basal forebrain, and the serotonergic, noradrenergic, and dopaminergic systems. Second, estrogen exerts a protective effect through its antioxidant and antiapoptotic properties (McEwen 1999). Estrogen also may protect against neurodegenerative diseases through its interactions with glial cells and its effects on blood vessels.

Neuronal Plasticity

In the early stages of AD, neuronal loss occurs predominantly in the hippocampus, especially in the CA1 region. The degree of neuronal loss correlates with the extent of memory impairment (Bobinski et al. 1998; Sass et al. 1990). The localization of estrogen receptors to the hippocampus suggests that estrogen may modulate learning and memory. This theory is supported by pathological studies and behavioral studies of aged rats and ovariectomized rats.

Estrogen is associated with synaptic density of the hippocampal CA1 pyramidal neurons in female rats but not in male rats. Intrinsic differences in spine density between the sexes may provide a biological basis as to why a sex difference exists in susceptibility to AD. In female rats, synaptic density of the pyramidal neurons fluctuates with phases of the estrous cycle, with synaptic density increasing with increasing estrogen levels and decreasing between the days of proestrus and estrus (when progesterone levels increase and estrogen levels decrease) (Galea et al. 1997; Gould et al. 1990; Lewis et al. 1995; McEwen and Woolley 1994; McEwen et al. 1997).

In ovariectomized adult female rats, the number and density of CA1 pyramidal cell spines and synapses decrease. If estradiol is replaced, the decrease can be prevented or reversed (Gould et al. 1990; Washburn et al. 1997; Woolley and McEwen 1992). These estrogen-induced structural changes appear to correlate with differences found on behavioral tests of hippocampal function between ovariectomized rats that have and have not been treated with estrogen. In rats, paradigms that test spatial memory are the best indicator of hippocampal function, whereas in humans, hippocampal function is best assessed by tests of verbal memory. Aged female rats with low estrogen levels perform significantly worse than rats with high estrogen levels in a Morris water maze, a spatial memory test (Juraska and Warren 1996). Ovariectomized rats that are treated with estrogen show improvements in speed and accuracy on other spatial memory tests, including the radial maze task and reinforced T-maze alternation tasks (Daniel et al. 1997; Fader et al. 1996; Luine et al. 1998). Performance on a measure of working memory, the two-choice water escape task, deteriorated in ovariectomized rats but did not change in rats maintained on long-term ERT (O'Neil et al. 1996). Ovariectomy also results in deterioration on tests of active avoidance behavior (Singh et al. 1994). When estrogen is replaced, performance improves relative to the untreated group. These behavioral experiments suggest that improved learning and working memory in rats may be associated with greater synaptic density in the hippocampus, which appears to be promoted by higher levels of estrogen (Singh et al. 1994).

Estrogen may stimulate dendritic sprouting in several ways. Hippocampal immunocytochemistry and cell culture studies suggest that estrogen interacts with ERα on inhibitory γ-aminobutyric acid (GABA) interneurons, transiently suppressing GABAergic function (McEwen 1999; Woolley and McEwen 1994; Woolley et al. 1997). This disinhibits CA1 neurons, resulting in upregulation of N-methyl-D-aspartate (NMDA) receptors and new synaptic formation. When NMDA receptors are blocked, estrogen is unable to induce synapse formation.

Estrogen also may affect synaptic growth through interactions with neurotrophins. Estrogen decreases the expression of brain-derived neurotrophic factor (BDNF) in the GABA interneurons in the hippocampus, inducing dendritic spine growth in pyramidal neurons (Murphy et al. 1998). Another neurotrophin, insulinlike growth factor-1 (IGF-1), stimulates the differentiation and survival of neuronal populations at least partly via an interactive and synergistic action with estrogen (Fernandez-Galaz et al. 1999; Toran-Allerand et al. 1988). IGF-1 and estradiol also have mutually dependent effects in protecting hippocampal neurons from kainic acid–induced degeneration (Azcoitia et al. 1999). The increased vulnerability of neurons to damage with aging may be explained in part by the decline in both IGF-1 production and estrogen with age (Lamberts et al. 1997). Estrogen's actions through neurotrophin receptors and genes may be one of the primary pathways by which it improves neuronal survival and dendritic growth, increases synaptic density, and maintains neuronal arborization in the hippocampus.

Estrogen and the Cholinergic System

The cholinergic neurotransmitter system consists of the nucleus basalis of Meynert and the septal nucleus in the basal forebrain and the neuronal projections to the amygdala, hippocampus, and cortical regions. The primary neurotransmitter in the cholinergic system is acetylcholine. Cholinergic neurotransmission plays a vital role in attention and memory. In AD, the brain undergoes the loss of cholinergic neurons and corresponding loss of acetylcholine (Bartus et al. 1982; Coyle et al. 1983). One marker for cholinergic activity is the level of choline acetyltransferase (ChAT), the rate-limiting enzyme for acetylcholine synthesis. In patients with AD, loss of ChAT correlates with loss of cognitive function (Baskin et al. 1999). Rodents are one of the primary animal models used to study AD, and analogous to what happens in men or women affected with AD, aged rats lose cholinergic neurons and manifest impaired spatial memory. Infusions of nerve growth factor (NGF) into the brain stop cholinergic neuronal loss and improve spatial memory deficits (Fischer et al. 1987). ChAT levels in the frontal cortex and hippocampus decline after ovariectomy in female rats, and high-affinity choline uptake also decreases (O'Malley et al. 1987; Singh et al. 1993, 1994). ERT after ovariectomy increases activity of ChAT in the basal forebrain, increases potassium-stimulated acetylcholine release, and prolongs survival of cholinergic neurons (Gibbs et al. 1997; Honjo et al. 1992; Luine 1985; O'Malley et al. 1987). The increased cholinergic activity correlates with better performance on behavioral memory tasks in the ovariectomized rats that are given ERT as compared with untreated rats. Estrogen also reverses short-term cognitive deficits in ovariectomized rats that have been induced by scopolamine, an anticholinergic agent (Dohanich et al. 1994).

Estrogen promotes survival of cholinergic neurons through a variety of mechanisms. Estrogen interacts directly with ERα on the cholinergic neurons and acts indirectly through effects on NGF and BDNF. Estrogen stimulates the promotor regions of genes for NGF and BDNF, which are synthesized in the hippocampus and transported retrogradely to the basal forebrain (Fischer et al. 1987; Singh et al. 1993, 1995; Toran-Allerand et al. 1992). NGF and BDNF bind with low-affinity NGF receptors that are colocalized with ERα. Ovariectomized rats lose messenger RNA (mRNA) for NGF and BDNF in the hippocampus, followed by a decline in cholinergic activity and deterioration on memory and learning task performance. ERT partially restores all of these deficits (Fischer et al. 1987; Singh et al. 1993).

Estrogen and Other Neurotransmitters

Although cholinergically innervated neurons are most affected in AD, brain regions innervated by other neurotransmitter systems also degenerate (Palmer and DeKosky 1993). The serotonergic, noradrenergic, and dopaminergic systems are all modulated by ovarian steroids.

The serotonergic system regulates mood and cognition. Abnormalities in serotonergic functioning are associated with depression, a mood disorder that frequently accompanies AD and that may, in fact, be the harbinger of memory loss (Meltzer et al. 1998). Higher concentrations of serotonin are present throughout the brain of female rats as compared with male rats (Carlsson and Carlsson 1988; Carlsson et al. 1985; Rosencrans 1970). Synthesis and turnover of 5-hydroxytryptamine (5-HT), a marker of serotonergic activity, are also increased in female rats. Estrogen replacement increases serotonin levels and affects serotonergic receptor density in ovariectomized rats (Biegon et al. 1983; Clarke and Maayani 1990; Cone et al. 1981; Di Paolo et al. 1983; Johnson and Crowley 1983; Summer and Fink 1995). Response to antidepressant drugs in animal models of depression and anxiety is facilitated by estrogen treatment (Kendall et al. 1982). Estrogen's actions on the serotonergic neurotransmitter system may partly explain the improved mood and affect that have been reported to occur in women receiving ERT (Barrett-Conner and Kritz-Silverstein 1993; Ditkoff et al. 1991; Klaiber et al. 1997; Sherwin 1988).

Estrogen also has trophic effects in the catecholaminergic system. When monkeys are ovariectomized, the number of cortical neurons declines markedly. ERT increases neuronal density, and ERT plus progesterone improves catecholaminergic innervation as assessed by increased tyrosine hydroxylase activity (Kritzer and Kohama 1998). Estrogen inhibits the activity of monoamine oxidase (MAO), a key enzyme responsible for metabolizing catecholamines (Luine et al. 1975). By inhibiting the actions of MAO, estrogen may indirectly increase levels of norepinephrine and dopamine. The studies discussed above found positive effects of ERT on the noradrenergic system, but other studies suggested that ERT may reduce noradrenergic tone in other brain regions (Tseng et al. 1997).

Pro- and antidopaminergic effects of estrogen are seen in the nigrostriatal and mesolimbic dopaminergic system of animals, depending on the dose and time course of ERT (Di Paolo et al. 1983; McEwen et al. 1994). In the aging brain, the number of dopaminergic neurons decreases (Morgan 1987). Studies in rats and humans suggest that high doses of estrogen have antidopaminergic effects (Barber et al. 1973; Hruska and Silbergeld 1980). (Because the dopaminergic system does not significantly contribute to AD symptoms, the reader is referred to the previously mentioned reviews for more information.)

NEUROPROTECTIVE PROPERTIES OF ESTROGEN

It has been known for many years that the addition of estrogen to neuronal cultures improves viability and survival of neurons (Garcia-Segura et al.

2001). Estrogen also has more specific properties that protect against cell death, including antioxidant and antiapoptotic activities. In primary cortical culture studies, estradiol prevents neuronal death induced by various stressors, including anoxia (Zaulyanov et al. 1999), AMPA toxicity (Zaulyanov et al. 1999), cytochrome oxidase inhibitor sodium azide, kainate, NMDA (Regan and Guo 1997), glutamate toxicity (Singer et al. 1996; Zaulyanov et al. 1999), iron (Vedder et al. 1999), and pro-oxidant hemoglobin (Regan and Guo 1997). Neuroprotective effects of estradiol also have been reported in studies that used cell lines derived from various types of neurons. Estrogen prevents hydrogen peroxide or glutamate-induced cell death in NT2 neurons, PC12 cells, and mouse neuroblastoma (Neuro 2a) cells (Bonnefont et al. 1998; Singer et al. 1998). Estradiol also prevents neuronal loss from serum deprivation in SK-N-SH human neuroblastoma cell cultures (Green et al. 1997) and from lipid peroxidation in hippocampal HT 22 cells (Vedder et al. 1999).

Hippocampal neurons are very sensitive to injury from glycopenia (Bishop and Simpkins 1995) or excessive amounts of corticosteroids. Preincubation with estrogen prevents glycopenia-induced neuronal damage in cell cultures (Bishop et al. 1994). Glucocorticoids produce atrophy of the apical dendrites of pyramidal neurons and neuronal loss in the CA3 hippocampal region of rats (Sapolsky et al. 1985; Woolley et al. 1990), and in cell cultures, glucocorticoids exacerbate injury from glutamate, β-amyloid, or glucose deficiency. The addition of estrogen to these cultures reduces injury from the combined excitotoxins and glucocorticoids (Goodman et al. 1996).

Estrogen's protective effect against oxidants appears to be mediated in part by the intrinsic structure of this steroid, the estrogen A ring steroid, because studies find that 17α-estradiol, 17β-estradiol, and estriol all reduce the generation of free radical estrogen receptors in the absence of living cells or cellular extracts, whereas other steroids are ineffective (Mooradian 1993). Other protective actions are mediated by binding with estrogen receptors or by direct effects on the neurons, as discussed previously in this chapter.

The neuroprotective effects of estrogen also may occur through the modulation by estrogen of the expression of specific proteins that regulate cell death (apoptosis) (Garcia-Segura et al. 1998). It upregulates the expression of Bcl-XL and Bcl-2, antiapoptotic proteins, and downregulates Nip-2 and Par-4, proapoptotic molecules (Chan et al. 1999; Guo et al. 1998; Pike 1999; Singer et al. 1998; Vegeto et al. 1999). Bcl-2 also promotes axonal growth and regeneration and decreases the production of reactive oxygen species (Bogdanov et al. 1999; Holm and Isacson 1999). Par-4, a proapoptotic protein, is upregulated in vulnerable neurons in AD brains. In hippocampal neuronal cultures, the expression of Par-4 and cell death from trophic factor deprivation is prevented by pretreatment with estradiol. The up- or downregulation of proteins involved in apoptosis may be one of the mechanisms through which estrogen manifests antioxidant actions.

In the cell culture studies described earlier in this chapter, in vitro antioxidant effects of estrogen have generally been observed at supraphysiological concentrations of the hormone. Lower dosages, dosages that are likely to be given clinically and that optimally induce estrogen receptor-medicated gene transcription, do not provide neuroprotection (Garcia-Segura et al. 2001). High doses of estradiol are known to be toxic to some neuronal populations, such as hypothalamic neurons (Desjardins et al. 1995), and may be toxic to other as-yet-unidentified or unstudied groups of neurons. Additionally, in most of these studies, estrogen prevented neuronal death and injury only when given before or at the same time as the toxin; it was ineffective when given after the oxidative insult (Garcia-Segura et al. 2001).

There is much less in vivo evidence (as opposed to much in vitro data) for neuroprotection by estrogen that applies to the theory that estrogen plays a significant role in protecting against the development of AD. Pretreatment with estrogen reduces neuronal loss in experimental animal studies of ischemia and anoxia. In rats, ERT given before middle cerebral artery occlusion reduces neuronal loss in ovariectomized females as compared with untreated rats (Simpkins et al. 1997). Estrogen also decreases the expression of the amyloid precursor protein (APP) after focal ischemia in ovariectomized rats (Shi et al. 1998).

In patients with AD, baseline cortisol levels have been elevated, suggesting excess glucocorticoid activity (Greenwald et al. 1986). Increasing cognitive impairment has been correlated with increasing cortisol levels (Heuser et al. 1988; Martignoni et al. 1992). ERT might help prevent or attenuate hippocampal neuronal injury resulting from elevated cortisol levels in women with AD, but to date, no studies have evaluated cortisol levels in patients with AD before and after ERT.

Effects of Estrogen on Cerebral Vasculature

The antiatherogenic lipid-lowering actions of estrogen are well known. Estrogen also has other effects on the cerebral vasculature, which may indirectly protect neuronal function. Platelet aggregation and leukocyte adhesion contribute to clot formation in cerebral ischemia. These processes are reduced by estrogen (Santizo and Pelligrino 1999). Estrogen induces vasodilatation (Hurn et al. 1995; Pelligrino et al. 1998) and decreases the response to injury of arterial smooth muscle (Applebaum-Bowden et al. 1989; Gangar et al. 1991; Polderman et al. 1993; Sullivan et al. 1995). Central nervous system vascular disease is increasingly recognized as contributing to the development and expression of AD. If ERT helps protect both large and small vessels from atherogenic changes, then the risk for AD may be reduced.

Estrogen and Glial Cells

Glial cells—astrocytes and microglia—support normal neuronal function in the brain. Estrogen receptors are present on glial cells (Azcoitia et al. 1999), and estrogen appears to regulate the morphology of glia (Garcia-Segura et al. 1996) and to downregulate the microglial proliferation and reactive gliosis seen with almost any type of neuronal injury (Garcia-Estrada et al. 1993). Glial cells may mediate actions of estrogen on neuronal plasticity and neuroprotection (Garcia-Segura et al. 1999). In astrocytes that have been exposed to β-amyloid or lipopolysaccharides, estrogen decreases the production of cytokines, such as nuclear factor kappa B (NF-κB) (Dodel et al. 1999). NF-κB activation initiates an inflammatory cascade that is thought to contribute to the formation of senile plaques found in AD. Another protein produced by glial cells, glial fibrillary acidic protein, increases with aging. Estrogen decreases these levels, opposing an effect of aging (Nichols et al. 1993).

Apolipoprotein E (apoE), a protein that is expressed by microglia and astrocytes, is important for normal membrane function and synaptic plasticity. Expression of apoE is increased in response to neuronal injury and results in increased synaptic sprouting. Studies of apoE knockout mice found that estrogen was unable to stimulate the synaptic sprouting that normally occurs in response to injury in the absence of apoE (Stone et al. 1998). When estrogen is present, apoE expression is upregulated, enhancing synaptic growth. This suggests another mechanism by which estrogen may modulate AD risk.

Effects of Estrogen on Amyloid and Tau

β-Amyloid is a neurotoxic peptide that is deposited in the senile plaques and vasculature of the brains of patients with AD. Only small quantities of β-amyloid are normally deposited in the brain with aging (Armstrong 1985). β-amyloid is derived from APP, a large transmembrane protein found in normal neurons. APP is released when neuronal injury occurs (Regland and Gotfries 1992) and can be broken down by either of two pathways. If APP is cleaved within the β-amyloid protein by α-secretase, a nonamyloidogenic amino-terminal fragment results, called soluble APP (sAPP). If β-secretase cleaves APP at the amino-terminus of the β-amyloid region, followed by further cleavage by γ-secretase, one of the β-amyloid proteins is formed (Sisodia et al. 1990). In vitro studies of mouse, rat, and human cortical neurons have found that physiological concentrations of β-estradiol increase the percentage of APP that is processed to sAPP and markedly decrease the production of β-amyloid (Xu et al. 1998). Cell culture experiments show that estrogen potentiates the neuroprotective effects of the cholinesterase inhibitors tacrine and donepezil and decreases the toxicity of β-amyloid (Svensson and Nordberg 1998). Estrogen induces the expression of Bcl-XL, an antiapoptotic protein, reducing the apoptosis caused by β-amyloid (Pike 1999). Whether the same neuroprotective effects occur in humans remains to be shown.

Neurofibrillary tangles are also a pathological hallmark of AD. These intracellular tangles are composed of abnormally phosphorylated tau, a component of microtubules. Microtubules support the structure of the axon and also function in axonal transport. Estradiol induces the neuronal expression of tau, potentially stabilizing the microtubules and maintaining neuronal viability (Ferreira and Caceres 1991; Lorenzo et al. 1992).

As discussed in the previous subsection, estrogen upregulates expression of apoE, stimulating hippocampal neuronal sprouting (Stone et al. 1998; Teter et al. 1999). However, estrogen administration in women increases the metabolism and decreases plasma levels of apoE (Applebaum-Bowden et al. 1989; Honjo et al. 1995). The effect of ERT on brain levels of apoE in women has not been studied.

Changes in the cerebral vasculature may help initiate or accelerate the pathogenic processes of AD. β-Amyloid is deposited in senile plaques as well as in cerebral blood vessels. When β-amyloid is given intravenously to rats, extensive damage to the peripheral mesenteric vessels occurs, similar to the inflammatory changes seen in AD (Rhodin et al. 1998). Conjugated estrogens given for 2 weeks before the β-amyloid infusions prevent the vascular damage (Rhodin et al. 1998). Similar effects from estrogen may protect the human brain.

The studies reviewed above present primarily positive effects of estrogen. Cell culture and animal data suggest that estrogen has a wide range of neuroprotective and trophic effects in the brain. Estrogen acts on the cholinergic and serotonergic neurotransmitter systems, influences synaptic density in the hippocampus, protects neurons against injury from a variety of oxidants, interacts with glial cells, and reduces damage to the cerebral vasculature. Specific actions of estrogen on APP metabolism and apoE are particularly relevant to AD. All of these diverse actions provide support for the hypothesis that estrogen helps protect against AD and positively affects cognitive performance.

However, as previously noted, not all effects of estrogen in the brain are protective or trophic. In rats, estrogen is toxic to neurons in some areas and promotes neuronal survival in others. In many of the rat studies, neuroprotective and antioxidant effects of estrogen were found only at supraphysiological levels, levels that would never be used clinically.

Most of these experimental studies support clinical research findings on estrogen's effects in the prevention of AD and have suggested that estrogen would be effective as an actual treatment for AD.

ESTROGEN REPLACEMENT THERAPY AND WOMEN WITH NORMAL COGNITION

Many of the clinical studies on estrogen replacement have focused on tests of cognition in healthy postmenopausal women. Because these women, by definition, have normal cognitive functioning, tests to detect change in cognition related to ERT must be very sensitive. For any given study, large batteries of neuropsychological tests were given. This, in itself, increased the statistical probability of finding one or two spurious significant differences between groups. A recent and extensive review of these studies by Hogervorst et al. (2000) concluded that ERT in healthy postmenopausal women had small, positive, but inconsistent effects on verbal memory, abstract reasoning, and information processing. Larger effects of ERT were found in epidemiological studies than in experimental studies. An analysis of whether the type of ERT used by women differentially affected cognitive function concluded that conjugated equine estrogens had the least effect as compared with oral or intramuscular estradiol preparations. Because women in these studies had completely normal cognition, it should be remembered that differences found in any specific test between treated and untreated women may be statistically significant, but the functional significance is likely to be minimal. Interested readers are referred to several review articles on the topic of ERT in women with normal cognition (Haskell et al. 1997; Hogervorst et al. 2000; Ottowitz and Halbreich 1995). We do not attempt to further discuss these studies but focus on studies that address the prevention of AD by ERT and the treatment of AD with ERT.

EPIDEMIOLOGICAL STUDIES OF ESTROGEN REPLACEMENT THERAPY AND THE RISK OF ALZHEIMER'S DISEASE

Several epidemiological case-control studies and two prospective cohort studies have investigated whether ERT in postmenopausal women alters the risk of developing AD (Table 17–1). More retrospective case-control studies than prospective studies have been conducted on ERT and AD risk because retrospective studies are easier to do, generally being shorter and less expensive. The odds ratios (ORs) found in the case-control studies varied, from finding of a trend for increased risk of AD with ERT use (Amaducci et al. 1986; Heyman et al. 1984), to no effect on risk (Brenner et al. 1994; Graves et al. 1990), to a trend for decreased risk of AD with ERT (Broe et al. 1990; Mortel and Meyer 1995; Paganini-Hill and Henderson 1994), and to significantly reduced risk (Baldereschi et al. 1998; Henderson et al. 1994; Lerner et al. 1997; Slooter et al. 1999; Waring et al. 1999). Both of the prospective cohort studies, the Manhattan study (Tang et al. 1996) and the Baltimore Longitudinal Study of Aging (Kawas et al. 1997), found reduced ORs for AD of approximately 50% in the women who were ever users of ERT.

The two earliest case-control studies (Amaducci et al. 1986; Heyman et al. 1984) found that postmenopausal ERT increased the risk for AD. Heyman et al. (1984) studied 28 women with AD matched by age and race to 56 control subjects who were interviewed by telephone. Information on ERT use was obtained from the spouse. ERT was used by only 7.5% of the control subjects and 15% of the patients with AD, for an OR of 2.4 (95% confidence interval [CI]=0.7–7.8). Amaducci et al. (1986) conducted a study of 116 patients with AD, of whom 75 were women, matched by age and sex to a total of 97 hospitalized outpatient control subjects. ERT was used by 12% of those with AD, 13% of the hospitalized control subjects, and 8% of the outpatient control subjects, based on the information given by proxies, with an OR for AD risk of 1.7 (95% CI=0.4–5.9). These studies had various methodological limitations, the most significant of which was that only a few control subjects in each trial used ERT. This limits the ability to detect whether ERT had an effect on AD risk. Information on ERT use was collected retrospectively, after dementia onset, from proxies. This could result in bias if control subjects and informants for patients with AD recalled past exposure differently.

The studies by Brenner et al. (1994) and Graves et al. (1990) found no effect of ERT on AD risk. Graves et al. (1990) compared 60 women with AD with 60 control subjects. Information on ERT by patients with AD was collected from a surrogate. ERT was used by 16% of the control subjects and by 18% of the patients with AD, with a resulting OR of 1.2 (95% CI=0.5–2.6).

In the Group Health Cooperative study, 107 women with probable AD were compared with 120 age- and sex-matched control subjects (Brenner et al. 1994). Computerized pharmacy records were used to ascertain and semiquantitate ERT use. ERT was classified as "ever use" or "never use"

TABLE 17–1. Epidemiological studies of risk for Alzheimer's disease (AD) with estrogen replacement therapy (ERT) use

Study	Design	N (women)	AD/Control subjects	ERT information	AD:Control subjects, ERT use, %	Risk	OR, 95% CI	Covariates	Type, dosage, and duration of ERT
Heyman et al. 1984	Case–control	120 (84)	28/56	Surrogate	15:7.5	×0.5	2.4 (0.7–7.8)	Age, sex, ethnicity, region	Use vs. no use
Amaducci et al. 1986	Case–control	213	116/97	Surrogate	12:8	×1.3	1.7 (0.4–5.9)	Age, sex, region	Use of ERT in menopause vs. no use (50% of AD and control subjects, no information)
Graves et al. 1990	Case–control	260 (120)	60/60	Surrogate	18:16	×1.1	1.2 (0.5–2.6)	Age, sex	Use vs. no use
Broe et al. 1990	Case–control	340 (212)	106/106	Surrogate	8:11	×1.4	0.8 (0.4–1.6)	Age, sex, region	>6 months of ERT vs. no use or <6 months of ERT
Brenner et al. 1994	Case–control	227	107/120	Pharmacy files	49:48	×1.0	1.1 (0.6–1.8)	Age, education, ethnicity, marriage, smoking, hysterectomy, progesterone	Ever vs. never use, also current vs. former, oral vs. vaginal and number of scripts written
Henderson et al. 1994	Case–control	235	143/92	Self/Surrogate	7:18	×2.7	0.3 (0.1–0.8)	Age, education	Current use vs. no current use

TABLE 17–1. Epidemiological studies of risk for Alzheimer's disease (AD) with estrogen replacement therapy (ERT) use *(continued)*

Study	Design	N (women)	AD/Control subjects	ERT information	AD:Control subjects, ERT use, %	Risk	OR, 95% CI	Covariates	Type, dosage, and duration of ERT
Paganini-Hill and Henderson 1994	Nested case-control	534	71/398/65 other dementia	Self	38:46	×1.2	0.7 (0.4–1.2)	Age, age at menarche and menopause, type of menopause, antihypertensive medication, stroke, weight	Duration and duration
Mortel and Meyer 1995	Case-control	306	93/148/65 vascular dementia	Self, surrogate, medical records	12:20	×1.8	0.6 (0.3–1.2)	Age	Use vs. no use
Tang et al. 1996	Prospective	1,124	167/957	Self	5:15	×3.0	0.4 (0.2–0.9)	Age, education, ethnicity	OR based on ever vs. never use, duration>1 year reduces risk, delays onset
Lerner et al. 1997	Case-control	246 (152)	74/78	Surrogate	25:45	×1.8	0.4; 0.6 adjusted for age; 0.9 (not significant) adjusted for education (0.3–0.9)	Age, education	Not studied

TABLE 17–1. Epidemiological studies of risk for Alzheimer's disease (AD) with estrogen replacement therapy (ERT) use *(continued)*

Study	Design	N (women)	AD/Control subjects	ERT information	AD:Control subjects, ERT use, %	Risk	OR, 95% CI	Covariates	Type, dosage, and duration of ERT
Kawas et al. 1997	Prospective	472	34/438	Self	27:46	×1.9	0.5 (0.2–1.0)	Age, age at menarche and menopause, education	Oral and transdermal effective; duration, no effect
Baldereschi et al. 1998	Observational/ cross-sectional	1,568	92/1,417/ 59 other dementia	Self	3:12	×4.0	0.2 (0.1–0.8)	Age, age at menarche and menopause, education, smoking, number of children, alcohol, weight	Ever used vs. never used
Slooter et al. 1999	Case-control from population-based study	228	109/119	Surrogate	10:20	×2.0	0.3 (0.1–0.9)	Age, education	Not studied
Waring et al. 1999	Case-control	444	222/222	Medical records	5:10	×2.0	0.4 (0.2–1.0)	Age, education, age at menopause	No dose effect; control subjects more likely to use ERT>6 months

Note. Sorted by year published. CI=confidence interval; OR=odds ratio.

and, for ever users, whether ERT use was current or past. Information on the numbers of prescriptions filled and on oral and vaginal ERT was collected. Approximately 50% of both patients with AD and control subjects had used ERT, with an OR of 1.1 (95% CI=0.6–1.8) for ever users versus never users. When the use of oral estrogen was analyzed alone for ever users versus never users, the OR was 0.7 (95% CI=0.4–1.5); the OR for vaginal use only was 1.3 (95% CI=0.7–2.3). The results suggested a trend (although not statistically significant) toward effectiveness of oral ERT for AD prevention.

Three case-control studies (Broe et al. 1990; Mortel and Meyer 1995; Paganini-Hill and Henderson 1994) found a trend toward decreased AD risk with ERT use. Broe et al. (1990) studied 170 patients with AD, of whom 106 were women who were matched by age and sex to an equal number of control subjects. Eight percent of the women with AD and 11% of the control subjects used ERT. The OR for greater than 6 months of ERT use was 0.8 (95% CI=0.4–1.6).

The Leisure World study used a nested case-control design, with each patient with AD matched by age to four control subjects (Paganini-Hill and Henderson 1994). Information on oral ERT use was collected prospectively by self-report when the 8,877 women initially enrolled in the study in 1981–1985, but AD cases were identified retrospectively by diagnosis on the death certificate. ERT was used by almost 50% of the cohort. Of the 2,529 women in the cohort who died before 1993, 138 cases of AD were identified. Each patient with AD was matched by birth and death date to five women who died without any mention of dementia on the death certificate. ERT users had a 30% lower risk of AD than did nonusers (OR=0.7), suggesting a trend, although not statistically significant. A more recent analysis of the cohort in 1996 identified 248 cases of AD based on death certificate diagnosis out of 3,760 deceased women (Paganini-Hill and Henderson 1996). The risk of AD was reduced by one-third for ERT users compared with nonusers (relative risk=0.65, 95% CI=0.49–0.88). In this study, the risk was reduced for users of either oral or nonoral forms of estrogen. The risk for AD was further decreased with increasing dosage and increasing duration of oral ERT, with the lowest risk found in those women who used conjugated estrogens long term and at high doses (OR=0.48; 95% CI=0.49–0.88). Because the information on ERT use was collected prospectively, the accuracy of these observations should be high. The use of death certificates for diagnosis has clear limitations. Often, only the proximate cause of death is listed, and a chronic disease such as AD might not be mentioned. Mild AD may not be diagnosed at the time of death. These factors would tend to underestimate the true numbers of AD cases, making estrogen look more protective than it actually is.

Mortel and Meyer (1995) conducted a retrospective case-control study with a postmenopausal clinic population in Texas. They identified 93 women with probable AD and 65 women with probable ischemic vascular disease and matched them with 148 control subjects. Only current estrogen use was investigated. Of the patients with AD, 11 (12%) were taking ERT, whereas 29 (20%) of the control group were taking ERT. The OR for AD risk for current oral ERT users as compared with nonusers was 0.6 (95% CI=0.3–1.2).

Waring et al. (1999) reported a case-control study comparing 222 patients with AD with 222 control subjects without AD. Information on estrogen use was obtained from medical records. Only those who had used ERT for greater than 6 months were considered to be exposed. The relative reduction in risk for AD in women using ERT was 0.4, which was statistically significant (95% CI=0.2–1.0, P=0.04). Lerner et al. (1997) found that 25% of the 74 patients with AD had used ERT compared with 45% of the 78 control subjects. The unadjusted OR was 0.4, but after adjusting for age and education, the OR was no longer significant at 0.9. When ERT use was combined with a history of smoking, the OR was significant at 0.4 (95% CI=0.0–0.7). Other studies have found a reduced risk for AD with smoking; thus, the significant OR may be primarily due to this effect.

A retrospective case-control study conducted in Los Angeles, California, by Henderson et al. (1994) identified 143 patients with AD and 92 control subjects. Of the patients with AD, 70 were confirmed by autopsy, and 73 had clinically diagnosed probable AD. Estrogen use was current in 10 (7%) of the patients with AD and in 17 (18%) of the control subjects as assessed by self or caregiver report. Age and educational status were not significantly different between the two groups. A statistically significant reduced risk for AD (OR=0.3, 95% CI=0.1–0.8) was found for current users as compared with noncurrent users. Also, those patients with AD who were taking estrogen had a significantly higher mean score on the Mini-Mental State Examination (MMSE, Folstein et al. 1975) than did patients with dementia not taking ERT (14.9 vs. 6.5).

A recent retrospective case-control study on AD and ERT use was conducted in Italy with a sample of 1,582 postmenopausal women (Baldereschi et al. 1998). Probable AD was diagnosed in 92 women in the sample. Of the 1,476 control women, 183 (12.4%) had ever used ERT; of those with AD, only 3 (3%) had ever used ERT. Women who had ever used ERT had a risk for AD that was 75% lower than those who had never used ERT (OR=0.2). The risk reduction remained essentially the same after adjusting for education, age, body weight, age at menarche, age at menopause, and number of children. The effect of ERT duration could not be evaluated because of the small number of patients with AD who had ever taken ERT.

The Rotterdam and Utrecht Aging Study (Slooter et al. 1999) identified 109 women with the onset of AD before age 65 who had been given diagnoses between 1980 and 1987 and matched them with 119 women of the same age and place of residence who were randomly selected from the municipal population register. Patients with AD had used ERT less frequently than control subjects (10% vs. 20%). A significantly reduced OR for AD risk in those who had ever used ERT was found after adjusting for age and education (OR=0.3, 95% CI=0.1–0.9). The mean age at onset was 58 for the AD group. This study differs from the other case-control studies in that it focused on early-onset AD. The frequency of the *APOE* ε4 allele is likely to be higher in early-onset AD groups than in groups with age at onset after 70 because *APOE* ε4 lowers the age at onset in Caucasians. No interaction was found, however, between estrogen use and cases with at least one ε4 allele.

Prospective epidemiological studies are the gold standard in observational research. A large population must be followed up to obtain an incidence of disease that will allow the analysis to reach statistical significance. These studies avoid the recall bias that can be a significant problem in case-control studies by gathering information on risk factors and disease occurrence at periodic intervals. Because these studies are resource intensive and expensive, only a limited number of studies are funded. Such studies, of course, do not prove causality but may find significant associations. Because these studies are not randomized, confounding factors, such as co-morbid disease; medication use and compliance; and ERT type, dosage, and duration, may not be evenly distributed among groups but may be adjusted for in the analysis. Of course, unknown confounders may remain.

In the Manhattan cohort, 1,124 older women were followed up prospectively in a community-based study (Tang et al. 1996). All participants were required to be cognitively normal, as assessed by a detailed psychometric assessment at the first interview. Information on estrogen use, duration, and type of preparation also was obtained at this time. Age, education, and ethnic group were adjusted for in the analysis. Over the 1–5-year follow-up period, 167 incident cases of AD were identified. Sixteen percent of the women who had never used ERT developed AD, whereas only 6% of those who had ever used ERT were diagnosed with AD. Women who had ever used ERT had a greater than 50% reduction in the risk of developing AD (relative risk=0.4, 95% CI=0.2–0.9). Of those ever users who did develop AD, the age at disease onset was significantly higher than in never users who developed dementia. Most of the women used conjugated estrogens. The primary drawback to this study was the limited number of years of follow-up. Information on duration of ERT is discussed in the next subsection.

The Baltimore Longitudinal Study of Aging (Kawas et al. 1997) followed up 472 post- or perimenopausal women prospectively for up to 16 years. Ever users were considered women who had used oral or transdermal estrogen at any time, based on self-report, with information obtained every 2 years. Thirty-four incident cases of AD were identified, of which 9 were ERT users. Age and educational status were not significantly different between the two groups. In the nondemented group, 230 were ever users (53%). The risk of developing AD in ever users of ERT was reduced by more than 50% (relative risk=0.5, 95% CI=0.2–1.0) as compared with never users. The major limitation of this study was the small number of incident cases of AD, which limited statistical power.

Epidemiological Studies and Estrogen Replacement Therapy Type, Dosage, Duration, and Mode of Delivery Data

In most of these epidemiological studies, information on ERT dosage, duration, route of administration, and formulation and whether progesterone was used was either not collected or very limited. The Leisure World study examined duration of use (Paganini-Hill and Henderson 1994, 1996). A trend toward declining ORs with increasing duration of conjugated equine estrogens use was found, with an OR of 0.8 for 3 years or less, OR of 0.5 for 4–14 years, and OR of 0.4 for 15 years or greater. The Manhattan study also assessed the relation between duration of ERT and reduction in AD risk (Tang et al. 1996). A significant linear trend for the effect of duration of ERT use on the risk for AD was found. Women in this study who used ERT for longer than 1 year (average duration=13.6 years) had an OR of 0.1 for the risk of AD as compared with women who used ERT for less than 1 year (average=4 months), for whom the OR was 0.5 (Tang et al. 1996). Waring et al. (1999) found that control subjects were more likely to have used ERT for more than 6 months. Brenner et al. (1994) found a lower OR for those who were currently using estrogen as compared with past users. Kawas et al. (1999) did not find any effect on the risk for AD related to duration of use, even though this study had the longest duration of follow-up.

Only two of the case-control studies examined in Table 17–1 studied dosage of ERT. Paganini-Hill and Henderson (1994) found that the OR for AD had a trend toward reduced risk with increasing dosage of conjugated estrogens. The OR was 0.8 for less than 0.625 mg/day of conjugated estrogens and 0.5 for greater than 1.25 mg/day of conjugated estrogens. Waring et al. (1999) did not find an effect for dosage. Only three studies evaluated the risk for AD with regard to route of ERT administration. Kawas et al. (1997)

reported protective effects for both oral and transdermal estrogen. Brenner et al. (1994) and Waring et al. (1999) found that oral ERT was more effective than transdermal or vaginal use. In the Manhattan study (Tang et al. 1996), the age at onset for AD was significantly later in women who had used ERT than in women who did not use ERT. In most of these studies, the majority of women used conjugated estrogens, which are composed primarily of estrone sulfate (Ditkoff et al. 1991). None of the studies had sufficient numbers of women using oral or intramuscular estradiol to be able to compare ORs for use of ERT with those for use of estrone or estradiol. Brain estrogen receptors are more sensitive to estradiol than to estrone (O'Connell 1995). Given the limited number of studies that have analyzed dose, duration, or method of administration, and the conflicting results of the studies that did evaluate these factors, no definite conclusions can be drawn about the influence of these parameters of ERT use on risk for AD.

Meta-Analyses of Studies of Estrogen Replacement Therapy and the Risk of Alzheimer's Disease

The studies just mentioned have been the subject of meta-analyses in two articles. Yaffe et al. (1998) found a summary OR of 0.7 (95% CI=0.5–1.0; P for heterogeneity=0.11) for AD for the eight case-control (Amaducci et al. 1986; Brenner et al. 1994; Broe et al. 1990; Graves et al. 1990; Henderson et al. 1994; Heyman et al. 1984; Mortel and Meyer 1995; Paganini-Hill and Henderson 1994) and the two prospective studies (Kawas et al. 1997; Tang et al. 1996) combined. Meta-analysis of only the eight case-control studies for AD found a summary OR of 0.8 (95% CI=0.6–1.2; P for heterogeneity=0.11). For the combined prospective studies, the summary OR was 0.5 (95% CI=0.3–0.8, P for heterogeneity=0.86).

Hogervorst et al. (2000) performed a meta-analysis of all of the studies listed in Table 17–1. The summary OR was 0.6 (95% CI=0.5–0.7; P for heterogeneity=0.03), consistent with a protective effect for ERT in reducing risk for AD, but significant heterogeneity was present among studies. The amount of heterogeneity declined significantly when the individual studies subjected to meta-analysis were restricted to those with sample sizes greater than 250. In these studies, the summary OR was even lower at 0.5 (95% CI=0.4–0.6; P for heterogeneity=0.36). The authors noted that when the sample size of the studies analyzed was less than 250, the OR was not significant (0.8, 95% CI=0.6–1.1), and the amount of heterogeneity was highly significant ($P<0.0001$). Additionally, meta-analysis of the studies conducted after 1994 found that the OR was lower at 0.5 (95% CI=0.5–0.7; $P=0.12$) than that of pre-1994 studies (OR=1.08, 95% CI=0.7–1.7; $P=0.02$), even though the later studies controlled more rigorously for potential confounding factors. In summary, these two meta-analyses support individual study findings of a reduced risk for AD with the use of estrogen postmenopausally.

Study Drawbacks and Confounders

In virtually all of these epidemiological studies, women used ERT for reasons other than prevention of dementia, so the outcomes were not likely to be biased by expectations of a protective effect of estrogen. Most of the case-control studies were not population based, which also may result in bias. Academic or tertiary medical centers are more likely to see patients with a higher educational level and potentially higher socioeconomic status than would be found in a population-based study. However, all of the retrospective studies that were population based (Baldereschi et al. 1998; Slooter et al. 1999; Waring et al. 1999) found significantly reduced ORs for risk of AD with ERT use. The two prospective population-based studies also found similarly reduced ORs.

Primarily two confounders may have significantly influenced the results of the above epidemiological studies. One potential bias is the accuracy of the history of ERT use. The second confounder is the effect of education and socioeconomic status.

ERT use in these studies was ascertained by questioning the subjects themselves or a surrogate (friend or relative) or by reviewing medical or pharmacy records. Subjects, especially those with AD, may not accurately recall use of ERT. Reduced reporting of ERT use by patients with AD would result in ERT appearing more protective than it actually is. Surrogates also may give inaccurate responses because they may not be fully aware of the subject's history of medication use. Surrogates are more likely to be unaware of ERT, to underestimate its use, and to be unable to provide information on type, dose, or duration of ERT. This would make ERT appear less protective for AD than it is in reality. Pharmacy or medical records might tend to be more complete but only if the subject consistently obtained medical care or prescriptions at places that are covered in these records. Prospective studies might avoid these problems if the subjects were initially enrolled at the time they may have been using ERT. However, this would require a longitudinal study that follows up participants over many years. ERT also may spuriously appear to prevent dementia if in fact physicians do not prescribe ERT to women who have prodromal AD or early dementia because of concerns over cost, compliance, undetected side effects, or usefulness of the therapy when significant cognitive problems are present. Physicians are more likely to give ERT to healthy women, especially to women who ask for this therapy.

Another significant confounder may be educational level. Although most of the studies adjusted for age, many did not adjust for educational level. Women using ERT tend to be younger, more highly educated, and in a higher socioeconomic group than nonusers (Barrett-Conner 1998). Higher levels of education and socioeconomic status are known to protect against AD (Tang et al. 1996). Postmenopausal women who use ERT also may be healthier before the onset of menopause than nonusers, as documented in one prospective study (Matthews et al. 1996). Blood pressure, cholesterol levels, plasma insulin, weight, alcohol use, and exercise were all better before menopause in the group that began using ERT postmenopause as compared with the group that did not use estrogen. Hence, the protective effect of ERT in AD may be due to the underlying health and lifestyles of ERT users rather than a direct result of ERT use.

In summary, the more recent large epidemiological studies generally have shown a reduction in the risk for AD associated with prior or current ERT use. Only very limited and contradictory data suggest that either higher dosages of ERT or longer duration of ERT further decreases the risk for AD. Whether women who use ERT have a later age at AD onset than those who do not use ERT is also unclear. Overall, however, these studies suggest that there may be a rationale for use of ERT in the prevention of AD in women who do not have contraindications to treatment and who are willing to accept the potential risks that also exist with ERT.

CLINICAL TRIALS OF ESTROGEN AS A TREATMENT FOR ALZHEIMER'S DISEASE

Several lines of evidence from clinical studies have suggested that ERT may be a useful treatment for AD. In addition to the epidemiological studies suggesting that ERT reduces the risk of developing AD, case-control studies have found that women with AD who were taking ERT had higher MMSE scores than did women with AD not taking ERT (Henderson et al. 1996; Henderson et al. 1994). In another study, the largest difference in performance between women with AD who used ERT and those who did not was on a naming task (Henderson et al. 1996). Hippocampal function is crucial for these semantic memory tasks, and these findings correlate with animal experiments that show that estrogen increases hippocampal neuronal density. If estrogen deficiency contributes to susceptibility to AD or to disease progression, then all women with AD should perform more poorly on cognitive tests than do men with AD. Clinically normal women tend to have higher scores on tests of naming ability than men do (Cohen and Wilkie 1979; Halpern 1992). Most cognitive domains are equally impaired in men and women with AD, except for naming tasks and other measures of semantic memory, which are likely to be impaired earlier and to a greater extent in women (Henderson and Buckwalter 1994; Ripich et al. 1995). A study of 1,648 patients with AD found that the 881 women not using ERT scored higher (worse) on the Alzheimer's Disease Assessment Scale, cognitive subscale (ADAS-cog; this neuropsychological test of cognition has been widely used in AD trials and is well validated as an outcome measure), than did men, controlling for age and educational level, whereas the 89 women taking ERT had lower (better) scores on the ADAS-cog than did the 676 men (Doraiswamy et al. 1997). The findings from these studies suggest that estrogen may be useful in maintaining cognition in women with AD.

UNCONTROLLED, UNBLINDED TRIALS OF ESTROGEN REPLACEMENT THERAPY IN ALZHEIMER'S DISEASE

Several experimental studies of ERT in women with AD have been reported. In this section, we focus briefly on the unblinded and uncontrolled trials (Fillet 1994; Fillet et al. 1986; Honjo et al. 1989; Ohkura et al. 1994a, 1994b, 1995b; Weiss 1987) followed by a more complete discussion of the blinded and controlled studies (see Table 17–2). All of the uncontrolled trials had small patient numbers and were brief, with the exception of one trial of 5 months' duration (Ohkura et al. 1995b). Only two of these uncontrolled trials found no improvement with ERT (Fillet 1994; Weiss 1987). The remainder found improvement on some of the tests of cognitive function for those patients taking ERT.

In an open-label, uncontrolled trial conducted by Fillet et al. (1986), seven women with AD were given 2 mg/day of estradiol over 6 weeks. Significant improvement was found on the MMSE and Randt Memory Test in three of the seven women; no change was found on the Global Deterioration Scale, Blessed Dementia Index, or Mattis Dementia Rating Scale. In the absence of a control group, a practice or learning effect could not be ruled out in this study. The women who improved cognitively also had significant improvement on the Hamilton Rating Scale for Depression.

In another uncontrolled, unblinded trial (Honjo et al. 1989), six of seven women with AD who received 1.25 mg/day of conjugated estrogens significantly improved on the New Screening Test for Dementia (Otsuka et al. 1987), and five of seven improved on the Hasegawa Dementia Scale (Hasegawa et al. 1974). The control group of seven women with AD did not receive any placebo tablets and had no change in test scores.

Ohkura et al. (1994a, 1994b, 1995a, 1995b) published four open-label trials of ERT in women with AD; two were of 6 weeks' duration, and two were of 5 months' duration. Improved cognition was reported in the treated groups in all studies. In one of the trials of 6 weeks' duration, the 15 patients with AD treated with ERT had improved scores on the MMSE, Hasegawa Dementia Scale, and Hamilton Rating Scale for Depression (Ohkura et al. 1994a). In this unblinded study, no changes occurred in the 15 control subjects with AD over the 6 weeks. In one of the trials of 5 months' duration, four of seven patients with AD taking 0.625 mg/day of conjugated estrogens plus progesterone had improvement in MMSE and Hasegawa Dementia Scale scores (Ohkura et al. 1995b). No control group was used. The other 5-month unblinded study by Ohkura et al. (1994b) found less decline in the MMSE scores in the 10 women with AD treated with 0.625 mg/day of conjugated estrogens as compared with the 10 patients with AD in the untreated group.

Both of the uncontrolled trials that had negative outcomes also were small and brief. Of the five women with AD treated with 1 mg of estradiol for at least 14 days in the uncontrolled, unblinded trial by Weiss (1987), three had no improvement at the end of 28 days on the MMSE, Global Deterioration Scale, Buschke Selective Reminding Test, and Word Fluency Test; one patient deteriorated, and one dropped out of the trial. A crossover study by Fillet (1994) randomized eight women with probable AD to treatment with a transdermal estradiol 0.05-mg patch twice a week or placebo. The study duration was 3 months. No significant changes were present in the MMSE, Paired Associates, or Bradburn Affect Balance Scale (mood) tests.

The MMSE often was used as an outcome measure in these trials, but it is usually regarded as being relatively insensitive to change in cognition, especially over brief time intervals, and is not used as a primary outcome measure in AD clinical drug trials. Many of these studies did not assess or exclude baseline depression, making it difficult to rule out a confounding effect of ERT on improvement in mood and affect causing improvement in cognition. The lack of blinding and absence of control groups renders these studies highly subject to investigator bias for positive outcomes with ERT. These trials also had inadequate power. Other limitations of the above interventional trials include short duration of treatment and cognitive screens that have not been widely validated and that often lack sensitivity.

DOUBLE-BLIND, PLACEBO-CONTROLLED TRIALS OF ESTROGEN REPLACEMENT THERAPY IN ALZHEIMER'S DISEASE

Seven randomized, double-blind, placebo-controlled trials of estrogen in AD have been published (Table 17–2). Honjo et al. (1993) enrolled 14

TABLE 17–2. Double-blind, placebo-controlled trials of estrogen replacement therapy (ERT) for Alzheimer's disease (AD)

Study	AD; treated: untreated, n	MMSE at enrollment	Dose of conjugated estrogens	Duration	Outcome measures	Results between drug and placebo group
Honjo et al. 1993	7:7	17/18	1.25 mg/day	3 weeks	MMSE, HSD, NSD	7/7 treated MMSE 18–22 (baseline to end); control subjects no change
Asthana et al. 1996	5:5	21	0.1 mg transdermal estradiol	8 weeks	Verbal memory (Buschke Delayed Free Recall test, Boston Naming, Visual Paired Associates)	Treated improved 1/3 tests from baseline; control subjects no change
Birge 1997	10:10	Mild, CDR<2	0.625 mg/day + medroxyprogesterone acetate	9 months	CIBIC, Blessed Dementia Index, Visual Paired Associates, Trail-Making tests	8/10 treated improved CIBIC, Blessed Dementia Index (baseline to end); control subjects 5/10 no change, 5/10 decline
Asthana et al. 1999	6:6	20	0.05 mg transdermal estradiol	8 weeks	Buschke Delayed Free Recall test, Revised Token Test, Wechsler Memory Scale, Visual Reproduction, Stroop Test, paragraph recall, MMSE, Blessed Dementia Index	Treated improved all but MMSE, Blessed Dementia Index, paragraph recall; control subjects no change
Henderson et al. 2000	42	10–26	1.25	16 weeks	ADAS-cog, CGIC, ADL/IADL, GDS, MADSR	All results NS
Mulnard et al. 2000	120	12–28	0.625 mg/day, 1.25 mg/day	12 months	CGIC, MMSE, CDR, ADAS-cog, Ham-D	All results NS
Wang et al. 2000	50	10–26	1.25 mg/day	12 weeks	CASI, CDR, CIBIC, BEHAVE-AD, Ham-D	All results NS

TABLE 17–2. Double-blind, placebo–controlled trials of estrogen replacement therapy (ERT) for Alzheimer's disease (AD) *(continued)*

Note. Sorted by year published.

ADAS-cog = Alzheimer's Disease Assessment Scale, cognitive subscale; ADL/IADL = activities of daily living/independent activities of daily living; BEHAVE-AD = Behavioral Pathology in Alzheimer's Disease; CASI = Cognitive Ability Screening Instrument; CDR = Clinical Dementia Rating Scale; CGIC = Clinical Global Impression of Change Scale; CIBIC = Clinician's Interview-Based Impression of Change; GDS = Geriatric Depression Scale; Ham-D = Hamilton Rating Scale for Depression; HSD = Hasegawa Dementia Scale; MADRS = Montgomery-Åsberg Depression Rating Scale; MMSE = Mini-Mental State Examination; NS = *P* between drug and placebo group was not significant; NSD = New Screening Test for Dementia.

women with probable AD (mean age=84) and gave conjugated estrogen 1.25 mg/day or placebo for 3 weeks. Significant improvement was found in the MMSE, Japanese New Screening Test for Dementia, and Hasegawa Dementia Scale scores in seven of the seven treated women. Because mood and affect were not assessed, these cognitive changes may have been caused by a positive effect of ERT on mood.

Asthana et al. (1996) reported a double-blind, placebo-controlled study of transdermal estradiol 0.1 mg given over 8 weeks to five women with probable AD compared with a control group of five women. The five treated women had significant improvement in verbal memory, as measured by the Buschke Delayed Free Recall test. A trend was found for improved naming on the Boston Naming Test and for improved visual memory on the Visual Paired Associates Test. In a similar study, 12 postmenopausal women with probable AD were randomized to a 0.05-mg transdermal estradiol patch or a placebo patch (Asthana et al. 1999) for 8 weeks. Memory and attention were significantly improved in the treated group relative to baseline; the control group had no change.

Preliminary results of a 9-month double-blind, placebo-controlled trial of ERT were reported by Birge (1997). Ten women with mild AD (Clinical Dementia Rating [CDR] Scale score<2) and without depression (Geriatric Depression Scale score<5) were randomized to treatment with conjugated equine estrogens 0.625 mg/day and medroxyprogesterone acetate 5 mg/day for 13 days every third month, and 10 women were randomized to placebo. Eight of the 10 ERT patients showed improvement on the Clinician's Interview-Based Impression of Change. Improvement relative to baseline in the ERT group was reported on tests of concentration and memory, including the Short Blessed Dementia Index, Trail-Making Test, and Paired Associates Learning test. Five of the 10 control subjects had no improvement, and 5 showed a decline on the Clinician's Interview-Based Impression of Change over the 9 months. Specific statistical data on these test results have not been published.

These studies had few patients and limited statistical power. The studies by Birge (1997) and Asthana et al. (1996) compared treated and untreated patients with their own baselines, a practice that is generally viewed as not being rigorous enough to suggest drug efficacy. The standard clinical trial practice is to compare treated and placebo groups to each other on outcome measures.

Rigorous double-blind, placebo-controlled studies on the use of ERT in AD had been lacking until recently. During 2000, the results of three large double-blind, placebo-controlled trials of conjugated estrogens in women with AD were reported (Henderson et al. 2000; Mulnard et al. 2000; Wang et al. 2000). None of the studies found beneficial effects for conjugated estrogens on the symptoms and course of AD. Henderson et al. (2000) conducted a 16-week double-blind, placebo-controlled treatment trial of conjugated estrogens in 42 women with mild to moderate AD. Half (21) of the participants received 1.25 mg/day of conjugated equine estrogens; the remainder were given placebo. Other antidementia drugs, such as cholinesterase inhibitors, were not allowed. The primary outcome measure was the ADAS-cog. In untreated patients with AD, ADAS-cog scores deteriorate by 7–10 points per year out of a total score of 70. Secondary outcome measures in the trial were the Alzheimer's Disease Cooperative Study Clinical Global Impression of Change (CGIC) Scale, a measure of overall functional status that assesses behavior, cognition, and ability to perform daily activities. Another secondary outcome measure used in more fully assessing the patient's functioning was an activities of daily living/independent activities of daily living (ADL/IADL) scale (Lawton and Brody 1969). Two of the women dropped out of the trial before the first evaluation. Completer analysis of the 40 women in the trial at 4 weeks and 36 women at 16 weeks found no significant differences between placebo and treated groups in ADAS-cog, CGIC, or ADL/IADL scale scores at 4 or 16 weeks. Post hoc analysis of subsections of the ADAS-cog found no significant differences between conjugated estrogens and placebo groups. This study had limited statistical power because of small sample size, but the 4-month duration is as long as that of cholinesterase inhibitor trials, in which a mean change of three to four points in favor of those taking cholinesterase inhibitors has been uniformly found at 4 months.

Another trial of estrogen in the treatment of AD enrolled 120 women with mild to moderate AD who had previously had hysterectomies (Mulnard et al. 2000). Women were randomized to one of three treatment groups: 0.625 mg/day of conjugated estrogens, 1.25 mg/day of conjugated estrogens, or placebo. Stable use of cholinesterase inhibitors was allowed. The duration of the trial was 12 months. The CGIC Scale was the primary outcome measure; secondary outcomes measures included the MMSE, the ADAS-cog, and the CDR Scale and specific tests for change in mood, motor function, activities of daily living, memory, attention, and language. Intent-to-treat analysis of the CGIC score found no significant difference between the estrogen-treated groups and the placebo group. The numerous neuropsychological tests that were secondary outcome measures showed no difference between estrogen and placebo groups. The CDR Scale score, a measure of global functioning, was significantly worse in the estrogen-treated groups than in the placebo group at 12 months ($P=0.01$), suggesting that the estrogen-treated groups actually did worse, even though higher percentages of estrogen-treated women were taking cholinesterase inhibitors than were those given placebo (24% for low-dosage conjugated estrogens and 23% for high-dosage conjugated estrogens vs. 13% for placebo).

The study by Wang et al. (2000) evaluated 1.25 mg/day of conjugated estrogens and placebo in 50 women aged 60 years and older with mild to moderate AD (MMSE score=10–26) in a 12-week treatment trial. Other antidementia medications were not allowed. The primary outcome measures were the Clinician's Interview-Based Impression of Change, the Cognitive Ability Screening Instrument (CASI), and the CDR Scale. Secondary outcome measures included the Hamilton Anxiety Scale and the Hamilton Rating Scale for Depression. No difference between treatment groups was found in any of the primary or secondary outcome measures in the intent-to-treat analysis of 6- and 12-week data. One death occurred in the placebo group; in the conjugated estrogens group, 11 of 25 (44%) had uterine bleeding, although only one woman withdrew from the trial because of this adverse drug effect.

The authors of these studies speculated that estrogen still may have some positive effects in AD, such as in use with cholinesterase inhibitors or in those with specific *APOE* genotypes. The neurotrophic and neuroprotective effects of estrogen on the cholinergic system found in preclinical studies suggest that estrogen might have synergistic actions when administered with cholinesterase inhibitor drugs. In a retrospective analysis of the effects of oral ERT on outcome measures in a 30-week pivotal tacrine trial (Knapp et al. 1994), women receiving tacrine and ERT had significantly better outcomes than did women receiving tacrine alone (Schneider et al. 1996). Of the 343 women assigned to treatment, 323 women had evaluable data, with 46 (14.2%) taking ERT. Of this group, 118 completed the trial, and 15 (12.7%) were taking ERT. The ERT consisted predominantly of oral conjugated estrogens, with a few patients taking estradiol or estrone sulfate, and 8 patients using concomitant medroxyprogesterone. The median duration of ERT use was 11 years. A significant improvement was found in ADAS-cog scores in the completer group receiving tacrine plus ERT as compared with the placebo group. Among completers, ERT use, although not duration of use, and nonuse of progesterone as well as increasing tacrine dose were independently associated with a better 30-week outcome on the ADAS-cog as analyzed by forward stepwise multiple linear regression. This publication was a retrospective subanalysis that was not planned for at trial inception; therefore, these results should be interpreted cautiously. One report found that the concomitant use of estrogen with tacrine raised plasma levels of the cholinesterase inhibitors, suggesting that positive drug interactions may not be from additional neuron-specific actions but may be related to drug metabolism (Laine et al. 1999). In contrast to the Schneider study, the trial by Mulnard et al. (2000) concluded that women taking ERT did worse, even though greater numbers of this group were taking cholinesterase inhibitors.

In summary, the small clinical studies of ERT use in AD suggested efficacy, but the three randomized, double-blind, placebo-controlled trials of sufficient power found no benefit for conjugated estrogens in the treatment of AD. The trial by Mulnard et al. suggested that conjugated estrogens may actually have adverse effects on cognition.

CONCLUSION

The experimental data on estrogen's effects in cell cultures and in animals suggest that estrogen has many important and vital effects on brain function, effects that may help prevent the onset of neurodegenerative disease. Many of these effects may specifically affect the pathogenetic processes that occur in AD.

Epidemiological studies suggest that estrogen use significantly decreases the risk for AD in women. Two different meta-analyses of the observational epidemiological studies found that the risk of dementia was decreased among those who used ERT (Hogervorst et al. 2000; Yaffe et al. 1998). Although the magnitude of this ERT effect was relatively modest, such a risk reduction would be of tremendous benefit in reducing the devastating social and economic costs associated with AD. However, the results of these epidemiological studies may have been confounded by selection and observation bias, so caution is needed in interpretation. Estrogen users tend to be better educated and healthier than nonusers and may differ in other demographic variables and lifestyle choices. The validity of the data is limited by the use of historical information that is subject to recall bias. Most important, a clear dose–response relation or effect for duration of use of estrogen on risk for AD has not been found.

With regard to the use of ERT for the treatment of AD, small observational trials of ERT in women with AD suggested some effectiveness, but three recent larger randomized, placebo-controlled trials in women with AD found no effect of ERT on cognition, function, or disease course. At present, the negative results from the three double-blind, randomized studies of ERT in AD appear reasonably definitive. ERT does not appear to be indicated for use in the treatment of AD. Some authors have speculated that estrogen may be useful in slowing the progression of mild cognitive impairment to AD, but given the unequivocally negative results of the AD trials, it seems unlikely that this would have a significant effect in mild cognitive impairment. Several hypotheses have been ventured as to why ERT may be effective in prevention of AD but not in treatment. One biologically plausible reason is that after the clinical appearance of AD, estrogen may have too weak of an effect to slow the momentum of the pathological and inflammatory changes already present.

The discrepancies between observational epidemiological studies and large randomized, double-blind trials are illustrated by the recent publication of the Heart and Estrogen/Progestin Replacement Study Research Group results (Hulley et al. 1998). Observational studies found lower rates of coronary heart disease in postmenopausal women who took ERT than in women who did not. In the Heart and Estrogen/Progestin Replacement Study, 2,763 postmenopausal women with coronary artery disease were treated with estrogen plus progesterone or placebo over an average 4.1-year follow-up period. The treated women did not have a reduction in the overall rate of coronary artery disease and experienced an increase in thromboembolic events and gallbladder disease.

Whether estrogen truly reduces the risk of developing AD is a question that remains to be answered. Several large prospective studies of estrogen use in healthy postmenopausal women are under way that should provide the answer to this question. One prospective study is the Women's Health Initiative Randomized Trial, an ongoing prospective trial of ERT compared with placebo (Shumaker et al. 1998). It will conclude in 2006. The Women's Health Initiative Memory Study is an associated ancillary trial to assess the effects of ERT on cognition and the risk of developing AD. Eight thousand postmenopausal women will be studied over 10 years. The second study is the Women's International Study of Long Duration Oestrogen After the Menopause (WISDOM) (Wren 1998), which will end in 2010.

Other questions about the use of ERT remain. It is not known what happens to estrogen receptors in postmenopausal women. Are receptors downregulated as a result of lack of estrogen exposure, and do they stay downregulated after an interval without sufficient estrogen? Is acute estrogen exposure sufficient to maintain receptor sensitivity? If the prospective studies find that ERT is protective for AD, what is the optimal dosage, time course, and route of administration for estrogen to produce desirable effects? Do short treatments of ERT provide neuroprotection? Are conjugated estrogens efficacious, or would estradiol be better? Are high or lower dosages more effective, and is exogenous estrogen as effective as endogenously formed estrogen (i.e., aromatized locally within the brain at the sites needed)? Future investigations of ERT in prevention of neurological disease should consider these questions.

Given the above findings from clinical trials, ERT cannot be recommended for use in women for the treatment of AD. The question of whether ERT is beneficial in the prevention of AD will be answered in several years. Currently, the results from the Heart and Estrogen/Progestin Replacement Study, the potential for adverse side effects, and the ongoing question of whether long-term ERT significantly increases the risk of breast and uterine cancer indicate that any potential benefits must be cautiously weighed against the known risks of ERT use for each individual woman.

REFERENCES

Alexander GM, Swerdloff RS, Wang C, et al: Androgen-behavior correlations in hypogonadal men and eugonadal men, II: cognitive abilities. Horm Behav 33:85–94, 1998

Amaducci LA, Fratiglioni L, Rocca WA, et al: Risk factors for clinically diagnosed Alzheimer's disease: a case-control study of an Italian population. Neurology 36:922–931, 1986

Applebaum-Bowden D, McLean P, Steinmetz A, et al: Lipoprotein, apolipoprotein, and lipolytic enzyme changes following estrogen administration in postmenopausal women. J Lipid Res 30:1895–1906, 1989

Armstrong RA: Beta-amyloid deposition in the medial temporal lobe in elderly non-demented brains and in Alzheimer's disease. Dementia 6:121–125, 1985

Asthana S, Craft S, Baker LD, et al: Transdermal estrogen improves memory in women with Alzheimer's disease (abstract). Society for Neuroscience Abstracts 22:200, 1996

Asthana S, Craft S, Baker LD, et al: Cognitive and neuroendocrine response to transdermal estrogen in postmenopausal women with AD: results of a placebo-controlled, double-blind pilot study. Psychoneuroendocrinology 24:657–677, 1999

Azcoitia I, Sierra A, Garcia-Segura LM: Neuroprotective effects of estradiol in the adult rat hippocampus: interaction with insulin-like growth factor-I signaling. J Neurosci Res 58:815–822, 1999

Baldereschi M, Di Carlo A, Lepore V, et al: Estrogen-replacement therapy and Alzheimer's disease in the Italian Longitudinal Study on Aging. Neurology 50:996–1002, 1998

Balthazart J, Ball CF: New insights into the regulation and function of brain estrogen synthase (aromatase). Trends Neurosci 21:2243–2249, 1998

Barber PV, Arnold AG, Evans G: Recurrent hormone dependent chorea: effects of oestrogens and progesterone. Clin Endocrinol (Oxf) 5:291–293, 1973

Barrett-Conner E: Rethinking estrogen and the brain. J Am Geriatr Soc 46:918–920, 1998

Barrett-Conner E, Kritz-Silverstein D: Estrogen replacement therapy and cognitive function in older women. JAMA 260:2637–2641, 1993

Barrett-Conner E, Goodman-Gruen D, Patay B: Endogenous sex hormones and cognitive function in older men. J Clin Endocrinol Metab 84:3681–3685, 1999

Bartus RT, Dean RL, Beer B, et al: The cholinergic hypothesis of geriatric memory dysfunction. Science 217:408–414, 1982

Baskin DS, Browning JL, Pirozzolo FJ, et al: Brain choline acetyltransferase and mental function in Alzheimer disease. Arch Neurol 56:1121–1123, 1999

Bicknell RJ: Sex-steroid actions on neurotransmission. Curr Opin Neurol 11:667–671, 1998

Biegon A, Reches A, Snyder L, et al: Serotonergic and noradrenergic receptors in the rat brain: modulation by chronic exposure to ovarian hormones. Life Sci 32:2015–2021, 1983

Birge SJ: The role of estrogen in the treatment of Alzheimer's disease. Neurology 48(suppl 7):S36–S41, 1997

Bishop J, Simpkins JW: Estradiol enhances brain glucose uptake in ovariectomized rats. Brain Res Bull 36:315–320, 1995

Bishop J, Singh M, Bodor ET, et al: Estradiol stimulates glucose uptake and has cytoprotective effects in rat C6 glioma cells (abstract). Society for Neuroscience Abstracts 20:694, 1994

Bobinski M, de Leon MJ, Tarnawski M, et al: Neuronal and volume loss in CA1 of the hippocampal formation uniquely predicts duration and severity of Alzheimer disease. Brain Res 805:267–269, 1998

Bogdanov MB, Ferrante RJ, Mueller G, et al: Oxidative stress is attenuated in mice overexpressing BLC-2. Neurosci Lett 262:33–36, 1999

Bonnefont AB, Munoz FJ, Inestrosa NC: Estrogen protects neuronal cells from the cytotoxicity induced by acetylcholinesterase-amyloid complexes. FEBS Lett 441:220–224, 1998

Brandi ML, Becherini L, Gennari L, et al: Estrogen receptor polymorphism in sporadic Alzheimer's disease. Neurobiol Aging 4(suppl):120, 1998

Brenner DE, Kukull WA, Stergachis A, et al: Postmenopausal estrogen replacement therapy and the risk of Alzheimer's disease: a population-based case-control study. Am J Epidemiol 140:262–267, 1994

Broe GA, Henderson AS, Creasey H, et al: A case-control study of Alzheimer's disease in Australia. Neurology 40:1698–1707, 1990

Campbell S, Whitehead M: Oestrogen therapy and the menopausal syndrome. Clin Obstet Gynecol 4:33–47, 1977

Carlsson M, Carlsson A: A regional study of sex differences in rat brain serotonin. Prog Neuropsychopharmacol Biol Psychiatry 12:53–61, 1988

Carlsson M, Svensson K, Eriksson E, et al: Rat brain serotonin: biochemical and functional evidence for a sex difference. J Neural Transm 63:297–313, 1985

Chakravarti D, Collins WP, Forecast JD, et al. Hormonal profiles after the menopause. BMJ 2:784–786, 1976

Chan SL, Tammariello SP, Estus S, et al: Prostate apoptosis response-4 mediates trophic factor withdrawal-induced apoptosis of hippocampal neurons: actions prior to mitochondrial dysfunction and caspase activation. J Neurochem 73:502–512, 1999

Clarke WP, Maayani S: Estrogen effects on 5-HT$_{1A}$ receptors in hippocampal membranes from ovariectomized rats: functional and binding studies. Brain Res 518:287–291, 1990

Cohen D, Wilkie F: Sex-related differences in cognition among the elderly, in Sex-Related Differences in Cognitive Functioning. Edited by Wittig MA, Petersen AC. New York, Academic Press, 1979, pp 147–157

Cone RI, Davis GA, Goy RW: Effects of ovarian steroids on serotonin metabolism within grossly dissected and microdissected brain regions of the ovariectomized rat. Brain Res Bull 7:639–644, 1981

Coyle JT, Price DL, DeLong MR: Alzheimer's disease: a disorder of cortical cholinergic innervation. Science 219:1184–1190, 1983

Daniel JM, Fader AJ, Spencer AL, et al: Estrogen enhances performance of female rats during acquisition of a radial arm maze. Horm Behav 32:217–225, 1997

Desjardins GC, Beaudet A, Meaney MJ, et al: Estrogen-induced hypothalamic β-endorphin neuron loss: a possible model of hypothalamic aging. Exp Gerontol 30:253–267, 1995

Di Paolo T, Daigle M, Picard V, et al: Effect of acute and chronic 17b-estradiol treatment on serotonin and 5-hydroxyindole acetic acid content of discrete brain nuclei of ovariectomized rat. Exp Brain Res 51:73–76, 1983

Ditkoff EC, Gary WG, Christo M, et al: Estrogen improves psychological function in asymptomatic postmenopausal women. Obstet Gynecol 78:991–995, 1991

Dodel RC, Du Y, Bales KR, et al: Sodium salicylate and 17β-estradiol attenuate nuclear transcription factor NF-κB translocation in cultured rat astroglial cultures following exposure to amyloid A β(1-40) and lipopolysaccharides. J Neurochem 73:1453–1460, 1999

Dohanich GP, Fader AJ, Javorsky DJ: Estrogen and estrogen-progesterone treatments counteract the effect of scopolamine on reinforced T-maze alternation in female rats. Behav Neurosci 108:988–992, 1994

Doraiswamy PM, Bieber F, Kaiser L, et al: The Alzheimer's Disease Assessment Scale: patterns and predictors of baseline cognitive performance in multicenter Alzheimer's disease trials. Neurology 48:1511–1517, 1997

Evans DA, Funkenstein H, Albert MS, et al: Prevalence of Alzheimer's disease in a community population of older persons: higher than previously reported. JAMA 262:2551–2556, 1989

Fader AJ, Hendricson AE, Dohanich GP: Effects of estrogen treatment on T-maze alternation in female and male rats (abstract 547.6). Society for Neuroscience Abstracts 22:1386, 1996

Fernandez-Galaz MC, Naftolin F, Garcia-Segura LM: Phasic synaptic remodeling in the rat arcuate nucleus during the estrous cycle depends on insulin-like growth factor-I receptor activation. J Neurosci Res 55:286–292, 1999

Ferreira A, Caceres A: Estrogen-enhanced neurite growth: evidence for a selective induction of tau and stable microtubules. J Neurosci 11:392–400, 1991

Fillet H: Estrogens in the pathogenesis and treatment of Alzheimer's disease in postmenopausal women. Ann N Y Acad Sci 743:233–238, 1994

Fillet H, Weinreb H, Cholst I, et al: Observations in a preliminary open trial of estradiol therapy for senile dementia-Alzheimer's type. Psychoneuroendocrinology 11:337–345, 1986

Fischer WI, Wictorin K, Bjorklund A, et al: Amelioration of cholinergic neuron atrophy and spatial memory impairment in aged rats by nerve growth factor. Nature 329:65–68, 1987

Folstein MF, Folstein SE, McHugh PR: Mini-mental state: a practical method for grading the cognitive state of patients for the clinician. J Psychiatr Res 12:189–198, 1975

Galea LAM, McEwen BS, Tanapat P, et al: Sex differences in dendritic atrophy of CA3 pyramidal neurons in response to chronic restraint stress. Neuroscience 81:689–697, 1997

Gangar KF, Vyas S, Whitehead M, et al: Pulsatility index in internal carotid artery in relation to transdermal oestradiol and time since menopause. Lancet 338:839–842, 1991

Garcia-Estrada J, del Rio JA, Luquin S, et al: Gonadal hormones down-regulate reactive gliosis and astrocyte proliferation after a penetrating brain injury. Brain Res 628:271–278, 1993

Garcia-Segura LM, Chowen JA, Naftolin F: Endocrine glia: role of glial cells in the brain actions of steroid and thyroid hormones and in the regulation of hormone secretion. Front Neuroendocrinol 17:180–211, 1996

Garcia-Segura LM, Cardona-Gomez P, Naftolin F, et al: Estradiol upregulates Bcl-2 expression in adult brain neurons. Neuroreport 9:593–597, 1998

Garcia-Segura LM, Naftolin F, Hutchison JB, et al: Role of astroglia in estrogen regulation of synaptic plasticity and brain repair. J Neurobiol 40:574–584, 1999

Garcia-Segura LM, Azcoitia I, DonCarlos LL: Neuroprotection by estradiol. Prog Neurobiol 63:29–60, 2001

Gibbs RB, Hashash A, Johnson DA: Effects of estrogen on potassium-stimulated acetylcholine release in the hippocampus and overlying cortex of adult rats. Brain Res 749:143–146, 1997

Goodman Y, Bruce AJ, Cheng B, et al: Estrogens attenuate and corticosterone exacerbates excitotoxicity, oxidative injury, and amyloid β-peptide toxicity in hippocampal neurons. J Neurochem 66:1836–1843, 1996

Gould E, Westlind-Danielsson A, Frankfurt M, et al: Sex differences and thyroid hormone sensitivity of hippocampal pyramidal cells. J Neurosci 10:996–1003, 1990

Graves AB, White E, Koepsell TD, et al: A case-control study of Alzheimer's disease. Ann Neurol 28:766–774, 1990

Green PS, Bishop J, Simplins JW. 17α-Estradiol exerts neuroprotective effects on SK-N-SH cells. J Neurosci 17:511–515, 1997

Greenwald BS, Mathe AA, Mohs RC, et al: Cortisol and Alzheimer's disease, II: dexamethasone suppression, dementia severity, and affective symptoms. Am J Psychiatry 143:442–446, 1986

Gu G, Rojo AA, Zee MC, et al: Hormonal regulation of CREB phosphorylation in the anteroventral periventricular nucleus. J Neurosci 16:3035–3044, 1996

Gu Q, Korach KS, Moss RL: Rapid action of 17β-estradiol on kainate-induced currents in hippocampal neurons lacking intracellular estrogen receptors. Endocrinology 140:660–666, 1999

Guo Q, Fu W, Xie J, et al: Par-4 is a mediator of neuronal degeneration associated with the pathogenesis of Alzheimer disease. Nat Med 4:957–962, 1998

Halpern DF: Sex Differences in Cognitive Abilities, 2nd Edition. Hilldale, NJ, Lawrence Erlbaum, 1992

Hasegawa K, Inoue K, Moriya K: An investigation of dementia rating scale for the elderly. Clin Psychiatry 16:965–969, 1974

Haskell S, Richardson ED, Horowitz RI: The effect of estrogen replacement therapy on cognitive function in women: a critical review of the literature. J Clin Epidemiol 50:1249–1264, 1997

Henderson VW, Buckwalter JG: Cognitive deficits of men and women with Alzheimer's disease. Neurology 44:90–96, 1994

Henderson VW, Paganini-Hill A, Emanuel CK, et al: Estrogen replacement therapy in older women: comparisons between Alzheimer's disease cases and non-demented control subjects. Arch Neurol 51:896–900, 1994

Henderson VW, Watt L, Buckwalter JG: Cognitive skills associated with estrogen replacement in women with Alzheimer's disease. Psychoneuroendocrinology 21:421–430, 1996

Henderson VW, Paganini-Hill A, Miller BL, et al: Estrogen for Alzheimer's disease in women: randomized, double-blind, placebo-controlled trial. Neurology 54:295–301, 2000

Heuser IJ, Litvan I, Juncos JL, et al: Cortisol baseline secretion and memory performance in patients with dementia of the Alzheimer type, in Senile Dementias: Second International Symposium. Edited by Agnoli A, Cahn J, Lassen N. Paris, France, John Libby Eurotext, 1988, pp 351–353

Heyman A, Wilkinson WE, Stafford JA, et al: Alzheimer's disease: a study of epidemiological aspects. Ann Neurol 15:335–341, 1984

Hogervorst E, Williams J, Burge M, et al: The nature of the effect of female gonadal hormone replacement therapy on cognitive function in post-menopausal women: a meta-analysis. Neuroscience 101:485–512, 2000

Holm K, Isacson O: Factors intrinsic to the neuron can induce and maintain its ability to promote axonal outgrowth: a role for Bcl-2? Trends Neurosci 22:269–273, 1999

Honjo H, Ogino Y, Naitoh K, et al: In vivo effects by estrone sulfate on the central nervous system-senile dementia (Alzheimer's type). Journal of Steroid Biochemistry 34:521–525, 1989

Honjo H, Tamura T, Matsumto Y, et al: Estrogen as a growth factor to central nervous cells: estrogen treatment promotes development of acetylcholinesterase-positive basal forebrain neurons transplanted in the anterior eye chamber. J Steroid Biochem Mol Biol 41:633–635, 1992

Honjo H, Ogino Y, Tanaka K, et al: An effect of conjugated estrogen on cognitive impairment in women with senile dementia: Alzheimer's type: a placebo-controlled, double-blind study. Journal of the Japan Menopause Society 1:167–171, 1993

Honjo H, Tanaka K, Kashiwagi T, et al: Senile dementia-Alzheimer's type and estrogen. Horm Metab Res 27:204–207, 1995

Hruska RE, Silbergeld EK: Estrogen treatment enhances dopamine receptor sensitivity in the rat striatum. Eur J Pharmacol 61:397–400, 1980

Hulley S, Grady D, Bush T, et al: Randomized trial of estrogen plus progestin for secondary prevention of coronary heart disease in postmenopausal women. Heart and Estrogen/Progestin Replacement Study (HERS) Research Group. JAMA 280:605–613, 1998

Hurn PD, Littleton-Kearney MT, Kirsch JR, et al: Postischemic cerebral blood flow recovery in the female: effect of 17β-estradiol. J Cereb Blood Flow Metab 15:666–672, 1995

Janowsky JS, Oviatt SK, Orwoll ES: Testosterone influences spatial cognition in older men. Behav Neurosci 108:325–332, 1994

Joels M, Karst H: Effects of estradiol and progesterone on voltage-gated calcium and potassium conductances in rat CA1 hippocampal neurons. J Neurosci 15:4289–4297, 1995

Johnson MD, Crowley WR: Acute effects of estradiol on circulation luteinizing hormone and prolactin concentrations and on serotonin turnover in individual brain nuclei. Endocrinology 113:1935–1941, 1983

Jorm AF, Korten AE, Henderson AS: The prevalence of dementia: a quantitative integration of the literature. Acta Psychiatr Scand 76:465–479, 1987

Judd HL: Oestrogen replacement therapy: physiological considerations and new applications. Baillieres Clin Endocrinol Metab 1:177–206, 1987

Juraska JM, Warren SG: Spatial memory decline in aged, non-cycling female rats varies with the phase of estropause (abstract 547.12). Society for Neuroscience Abstracts 22:1387, 1996

Katzman R, Aronson M, Fuld P, et al: Development of dementing illness in an 80-year-old volunteer cohort. Ann Neurol 25:317–324, 1989

Kawas C, Resnick S, Morrison A, et al: A prospective study of estrogen replacement therapy and the risk of developing Alzheimer's disease: the Baltimore Longitudinal Study of Aging. Neurology 48:1517–1521, 1997

Kendall DA, Stancel GM, Enna SJ: The influence of sex hormones on antidepressant-induced alterations in neurotransmitter receptor binding. J Neurosci 2:354–360, 1982

Klaiber EL, Broverman DM, Vogel W, et al: Relations of serum estradiol levels, menopausal duration, and mood during hormonal replacement therapy. Psychoneuroendrocrinology 22:549–558, 1997

Knapp MJ, Knopman DS, Solomon PR, et al, for the Tacrine Study Group: A 30-week randomized controlled trial of high-dose tacrine in patients with Alzheimer's disease. JAMA 271:985–991, 1994

Kritzer MF, Kohama SG: Ovarian hormones influence the morphology, distribution, and density of tyrosine hydroxylase immunoreactive axons in the dorsolateral prefrontal cortex of adult rhesus monkeys. J Comp Neurol 395:1–17, 1998

Laine K, Palovaara S, Tapanainen P, et al: Plasma tacrine concentrations are significantly increased by concomitant hormone replacement therapy. Clin Pharmacol Ther 66:602–608, 1999

Lamberts SW, van den Beld AE, van der Lely AJ: The endocrinology of aging. Science 278:419–424, 1997

Lawton MP, Brody EM: Assessment of older people: self-maintaining and instrumental activities of daily living. Gerontologist 9:179–186, 1969

Lerner A, Koss E, Debanne S, et al: Smoking and estrogen replacement therapy as protective factors against AD. Lancet 349:403–404, 1997

Lewis C, McEwen BS, Frankfurt M: Estrogen-induction of dendritic spines in ventromedial hypothalamus and hippocampus: effects of neonatal aromatase blockade and adult GDX. Brain Res Dev Brain Res 87:91–95, 1995

Lorenzo A, Diaz H, Carrer H, et al: Amygdala neurons in vitro: neurite growth and effects of estradiol. J Neurosci Res 33:418–435, 1992

Luine VN: Estradiol increases choline acetyltransferase activity in specific basal forebrain nuclei and projection areas of female rats. Exp Neurol 89:484–490, 1985

Luine VN, Khylchevskaya RI, McEwen BS: Effect of gonadal steroids on activities of monoamine oxidase and choline acetylase in rat brain. Brain Res 86:293–306, 1975

Luine VN, Richards ST, Wu VY, et al: Estradiol enhances learning and memory in a spatial memory task and effects levels of monoaminergic neurotransmitters. Horm Behav 34:149–162, 1998

Lund BC, Bever-Stille KA, Perry PJ: Testosterone and andropause: the feasibility of testosterone replacement therapy in elderly men. Pharmacotherapy 19:951–956, 1999

Maas D, Jochen A, Lalande B: Age-related changes in male gonadal function: implications for therapy. Drugs Aging 11:45–60, 1997

Martignoni E, Costa A, Sinforiani E, et al: The brain as a target for adrenocortical steroids: cognitive implications. Psychoneuroendocrinology 17:343–354, 1992

Matthews KA, Kuller LH, Wing RR, et al: Prior to the use of estrogen replacement therapy: are users healthier than nonusers? Am J Epidemiol 143:971–978, 1996

McEwen BS: The molecular and neuroanatomical basis for estrogen in the central nervous system. J Clin Endocrinol 84:1790–1797, 1999

McEwen BS, Alves SE: Estrogen actions in the central nervous system. Endocr Rev 20:279–307, 1999

McEwen BS, Woolley CS: Estradiol and progesterone regulate neuronal structure and synaptic connectivity in adult as well as developing brain. Exp Gerontol 29:431–436, 1994

McEwen BS, Chao H, Anjulo J: Glucocorticoid and estrogen effects on the nigrostriatal and mesolimbic dopaminergic systems, in Trophic Regulation of the Basal Ganglia. Edited by Fuxe K, Agnati L, Bjelke B, et al. London, England, Pergamon, 1994, pp 67–88

McEwen BS, Alves SE, Bulloch K, et al: Ovarian steroids and the brain: implications for cognition and aging. Neurology 48:S8–S15, 1997

Meltzer CC, Smith G, DeKosky ST, et al: Serotonin in aging, late-life depression, and Alzheimer's disease: the emerging role of functional neuroimaging. Neuropsychopharmacology 18:407–430, 1998

Molsa PK, Marttila RJ, Rinne UK: Epidemiology of dementia in a Finnish population. Acta Neurol Scand 65:541–552, 1982

Mooradian AD: Antioxidant properties of steroids. J Steroid Biochem Mol Biol 45:509–511, 1993

Morgan DG: The dopamine and serotonin systems during aging in human and rat brain: a brief review. Prog Neuropsychopharmacol Biol Psychiatry 11:153–157, 1987

Morley P, Whitfield JF, Vanderhyden BC, et al: A new, nongenomic estrogen action: the rapid release of intracellular calcium. Endocrinology 131:1305–1312, 1992

Mortel KF, Meyer JS: Lack of postmenopausal estrogen replacement therapy and the risk of dementia. J Neuropsychiatry Clin Neurosci 7:334–337, 1995

Mulnard RA, Cotman CW, Kawas C, et al: Estrogen replacement therapy for treatment of mild to moderate Alzheimer disease: a randomized controlled trial. JAMA 283:1007–1015, 2000

Murphy DD, Cole NB, Segal M: Brain-derived neurotrophic factor mediates estradiol-induced dendritic spine formation in hippocampal neurons. Proc Natl Acad Sci U S A 95:11412–11417, 1998

Naftolin F: Brain aromatization of androgens. J Reprod Med 39:257–261, 1994

Nichols NR, Day JR, Laping NJ, et al: GFAP mRNA increases with age in rat and human brain. Neurobiol Aging 14:421–429, 1993

O'Connell MB: Pharmacokinetic and pharmacologic variation between different estrogen products. J Clin Pharmacol 35:18S–24S, 1995

Ohkura T, Isse K, Akazawa K, et al: Evaluation of estrogen treatment in female patients with dementia of the Alzheimer type. Endocr J 41:361–371, 1994a

Ohkura T, Isse K, Akazawa K, et al: Low-dose estrogen replacement therapy for Alzheimer disease in women. Menopause 1:125–130, 1994b

Ohkura T, Teshima Y, Isse K, et al: Estrogen increases cerebral and cerebellar blood flows in postmenopausal women. Menopause 2:13–18, 1995a

Ohkura T, Isse K, Akazawa K, et al: Long-term estrogen replacement therapy in female patients with dementia of the Alzheimer type: 7 case reports. Dementia 6:99–107, 1995b

O'Malley CA, Hautamaki RD, Kelly M, et al: Effects of ovariectomy and estradiol benzoate on high affinity choline uptake, ACh synthesis, and release from rat cerebral cortical synaptosomes. Brain Res 403:389–392, 1987

O'Neil MF, Means LW, Poole MC, et al: Estrogen affects performance of ovariectomized rats in a two-choice water-escape working memory task. Psychoneuroendocrinology 21:51–65, 1996

Ottowitz WE, Halbreich U: Mood and cognitive change following estrogen replacement therapy in postmenopausal women. CNS Drugs 4:161–167, 1995

Otuska T, Shimonaka J, Kitamura T, et al: A new screening test for dementia. Clin Psychiatry 29:395–402, 1987

Paganini-Hill A, Henderson VW: Estrogen deficiency and risk of Alzheimer's disease in women. Am J Epidemiol 140:256–261, 1994

Paganini-Hill A, Henderson VW: Estrogen replacement therapy and risk of Alzheimer's disease. Arch Intern Med 156:2213–2217, 1996

Palacios S: Current perspectives on the benefits of HRT in menopausal women. Maturitas 33:S1–13, 1999

Palmer AM, DeKosky ST: Monoamine neurons in aging and Alzheimer's disease. J Neural Transm [Gen Sect] 91:135–159, 1993

Payami H, Zareparsi S, Montee KR, et al: Gender difference in apolipoprotein E-associated risk for familial Alzheimer disease: a possible clue to the higher incidence of Alzheimer disease in women. Am J Hum Genet 58:803–811, 1996

Pelligrino DA, Santizo R, Baughman VL, et al: Cerebral vasodilating capacity during forebrain ischemia: effects of chronic estrogen depletion and repletion and the role of neuronal nitric oxode synthase. Neuroreport 9:3285–3291, 1998

Pike CJ: Estrogen modulates neuronal Bcl-x$_L$ expression and β-amyloid-induced apoptosis: relevance to Alzheimer's disease. J Neurochem 72:1552–1563, 1999

Polderman KH, Coen D, Stehouwer A, et al: Influence of sex hormones on plasma endothelin levels. Ann Intern Med 118:429–432, 1993

Regan RF, Guo Y: Estrogens attenuate neuronal injury due to hemoglobin: chemical hypoxia, and excitatory amino acids in murine cortical cultures. Brain Res 764:133–140, 1997

Regland B, Gotfries CG: The role of amyloid β-protein in Alzheimer's disease. Lancet 340:467–469, 1992

Rhodin JAG, Thomas T, Sutton ET, et al: Protective action of estrogen against amyloid β-peptide induced vascular damage and inflammatory response (abstract). Neurobiol Aging 19(suppl 4S):1304, 1998

Ripich DN, Petrill SA, Whitehouse PJ, et al: Gender differences in language of AD patients: a longitudinal study. Neurology 45:299–302, 1995

Rocca WA, Hofman A, Brayne C, et al: Frequency and distribution of Alzheimer's disease in Europe: a collaborative study of 1980–1990 prevalence findings. Ann Neurol 30:381–390, 1991

Rorsman B, Hagnell O, Lanke J: Prevalence and incidence of senile and multi-infarct dementia in the Lundby Study: a comparison between the time periods 1947–1957 and 1957–1972. Neuropsychobiology 15:122–129, 1986

Rosencrans JA: Differences in brain area 5-hydroxytryptamine turnover and rearing behavior in rats and mice of both sexes. Eur J Pharmacol 9:379–382, 1970

Santizo R, Pelligrino DA: Estrogen leukocyte adhesion in the cerebral circulation of female rats. J Cereb Blood Flow Metab 19:1061–1065, 1999

Sapolsky RM, Krey LC, McEwen BS: Prolonged glucocorticoid exposure reduces hippocampal neuron number: implications for aging. J Neurosci 5:1222–1227, 1985

Sass KJ, Spencer DD, Kim JH, et al: Verbal memory impairment correlates with hippocampal pyramidal cell density. Neurology 40:1694–1697, 1990

Schneider LS, Farlow MR, Henderson VW, et al: Effects of estrogen replacement therapy on response to tacrine in patients with Alzheimer's disease. Neurology 46:1580–1584, 1996

Sherwin BB: Affective changes with estrogen and androgen replacement therapy in surgically postmenopausal women. J Affect Disord 14:177–187, 1988

Shi J, Panickar KS, Yang SH, et al: Estrogen attenuates over-expression of beta-amyloid precursor protein messenger RNA in an animal model of focal ischemia. Brain Res 810:87–92, 1998

Shughrue PJ, Lane MV, Merchenthaler I: Comparative distribution of estrogen receptor-α and -β mRNA in the rat central nervous system. J Comp Neurol 388:507–525, 1997

Shumaker SA, Reboussin BA, Espeland MA, et al: The Women's Health Initiative Memory Study (WHIMS): a trial of the effect of estrogen therapy in preventing and slowing the progression of dementia. Control Clin Trials 19:604–621, 1998

Simpkins JW, Rajakumar G, Zhang YQ, et al: Estrogens may reduce mortality and ischemic damage caused by middle cerebral artery occlusion in the female rat. J Neurosurg 87:724–730, 1997

Singer CA, Rogers KL, Strickland TM, et al: Estrogen protects primary cortical neurons from glutamate toxicity. Neurosci Lett 212:13–16, 1996

Singer CA, Rodgers KL, Dorsa DM: Modulation of Bcl-2 expression: a potential component of estrogen protection in NT2 neurons. Neuroreport 9:2565–2568, 1998

Singh M, Meyer EM, Simpkins JW: Ovariectomy reduces ChAT activity and NGF mRNA levels in the frontal cortex and hippocampus of female Sprague-Dawley rats. Neuroscience Abstracts 14:254, 1993

Singh M, Meyer EM, Millard WJ, et al: Ovarian steroid deprivation results in a reversible learning impairment and compromised cholinergic function in female Sprague-Dawley rats. Brain Res 644:305–312, 1994

Singh M, Meyer EM, Simpkins JW: The effect of ovariectomy and estradiol replacement on brain-derived neurotrophic factor messenger ribonucleic acid expression in cortical and hippocampal brain regions of female Sprague-Dawley rats. Endocrinology 136:2320–2324, 1995

Singh M, Setalo GJ, Guan X, et al: Estrogen-induced activation of mitogen-activated protein kinase in cerebral cortical explants: convergence of estrogen and neurotrophin signaling pathways. J Neurosci 19:1179–1188, 1999

Sisodia SS, Koo EH, Beyreuther K, et al: Evidence that β-amyloid protein in Alzheimer's disease is not derived by normal processing. Science 248:492–495, 1990

Slooter AJC, Bronzova J, Witteman JCM, et al: Estrogen use and early onset Alzheimer's disease: a population-based study. J Neurol Neurosurg Psychiatry 67:779–781, 1999

Stone DJ, Rozovsky I, Morgan TE, et al: Increased synaptic sprouting in response to estrogen via an apolipoprotein E-dependent mechanism: implications for Alzheimer's disease. J Neurosci 18:3180–3185, 1998

Sullivan TJ, Karas RH, Aronovitz M, et al: Estogen inhibits the response-to-injury in a mouse carotid artery model. J Clin Invest 96:2482–2488, 1995

Summer BE, Fink G: Estrogen increases the density of 5-hydroxytryptamine(2A) receptors in cerebral cortex and nucleus accumbens in the female rat. J Steroid Biochem Mol Biol 54:15–20, 1995

Svensson AL, Nordberg A: Estrogen, tacrine and donepezil attenuate β-amyloid induced toxicity in PC12 cells (abstract). Neurobiol Aging 19(suppl 4S):1087, 1998

Tang MX, Jacobs D, Stern Y, et al: Effect of oestrogen during menopause on risk and age at onset of Alzheimer's disease. Lancet 348:429–432, 1996

Teter B, Harris-White ME, Frautschy SA, et al: Role of apolipoprotein E and estrogen in mossy fiber sprouting in hippocampal slice culture. Neuroscience 91:1009–1016, 1999

Toran-Allerand CS, Ellis L, Pfenninger KH: Estrogen and insulin synergism in neurite growth enhancement in vitro: mediation of steroid effects by interactions with growth factors? Brain Res 469:87–100, 1988

Toran-Allerand CD, Miranda RC, Bentham WDL, et al: Estrogen receptors colocalize with low affinity nerve growth factor receptors in cholinergic neurons of the basal forebrain. Proc Natl Acad Sci U S A 89:4668–4672, 1992

Tseng JY, Kolb PE, Raskind MA, et al: Estrogen regulates galanin but not tyrosine hydroxylase gene expression in the rat locus coeruleus. Mol Brain Res 50:100–106, 1997

Vedder H, Anthes N, Stumm G, et al: Estrogen hormones reduce lipid peroxidation in cells and tissues of the central nervous system. J Neurochem 72:2531–2538, 1999

Vegeto E, Pollio G, Pellicciari C, et al: Estrogen and progesterone induction of survival of monoblastoid cells undergoing TNF-α-induced apoptosis. FASEB J 13:793–803, 1999

Wang PN, Liao SQ, Liu RS, et al: Effects of estrogen on cognition, mood, and cerebral blood flow in AD: a controlled study. Neurology 54:2061–2066, 2000

Waring SC, Rocca WA, Peterson RC, et al: Postmenopausal estrogen replacement therapy and risk of AD: a population-based study. Neurology 52:965–970, 1999

Washburn SA, Lewis CE, Johnson JE, et al: 17α dihydroequilenin increases hippocampal dendritic spine density of ovariectomized rats. Brain Res 758:241–244, 1997

Weiss BL: Failure of nalmefene and estrogen to improve memory in Alzheimer's disease. Am J Psychiatry 144:386–387, 1987

Woolley CS: Effects of estrogen in the CNS. Curr Opin Neurobiol 9:349–354, 1999

Woolley CS, McEwen BS: Estradiol mediates fluctuation in hippocampal synapse density during the estrous cycle in the adult rat. J Neurosci 12:2549–2554, 1992

Woolley C, McEwen BS: Estradiol regulates hippocampal dendritic spine density via an N-methyl-D-aspartate receptor dependent mechanism. J Neurosci 14:7680–7687, 1994

Woolley CS, Gould E, McEwen BS: Exposure to excess glucocorticoids alters dendritic morphology of adult hippocampal pyramidal neurons. Brain Res 531:225–231, 1990

Woolley C, Weiland NG, McEwen BS, et al: Estradiol increases the sensitivity of hippocampal CA1 pyramidal cells to NMDA receptor-medicated synaptic input: correlation with dendritic spine density. J Neurosci 17:1848–1859, 1997

Wren BG: Megatrials of hormonal replacement therapy. Drugs Aging 12:3433–3448, 1998

Xu H, Gouras GK, Greenfield JP, et al: Estrogen reduces neuronal generation of Alzheimer β-amyloid peptides. Nat Med 4:447–451, 1998

Yaffe K, Sawaya G, Lieberburg I, et al: Estrogen therapy in postmenopausal women: effects on cognitive function and dementia. JAMA 279:688–695, 1998

Zaulyanov LL, Green PS, Simpkins JW: Glutamate receptor requirement for neuronal cell death from anoxia-reoxygenation: an in vitro model for assessment of the neuroprotective effects of estrogens. Cell Mol Neurobiol 19:705–718, 1999

Zhou Y, Watters JJ, Dorsa DM: Estrogen rapidly induces the phosphorylation of the cAMP response element binding protein in rat brain. Endocrinology 137:2163–2166, 1997

18

Gonadal Steroid Influences on Adult Neuropsychological Function

Scott D. Moffat, Ph.D.
Susan M. Resnick, Ph.D.

OVERVIEW OF STEROID HORMONE EFFECTS

Accumulating evidence from both human and nonhuman species indicates that gonadal steroids may play an important role in the development and expression of behavior, both early in development and later in life. Traditionally, the actions of gonadal steroids have been classified as either *organizational* or *activational*, depending on the timing and duration of the effects (Phoenix et al. 1959). Although a strict dichotomy between these two modes of action has been challenged by numerous experimental findings (Arnold and Breedlove 1985), this classification scheme still serves as a useful framework for understanding the anatomical, physiological, and behavioral effects of steroids (Beatty 1992; Breedlove 1992a; Goy and McEwen 1980).

Organizational effects of gonadal steroids tend to occur early in life, typically in prenatal or early postnatal development. Organizational effects

We thank Dr. Pauline Maki for helpful comments on an earlier version of this chapter.

result in permanent structural changes in the brain or exert other long-term cellular and metabolic effects and are typically associated with a critical period (Arnold and Breedlove 1985). Once this critical period passes, the steroid loses its potential to exert an organizing effect on the brain and subsequent behavior (Whalen 1968).

The activational effects of steroids, which are the focus of this chapter, are not associated with a developmental critical period and result in relatively transient changes in behavior and neurophysiology that occur over periods of seconds, hours, or days. These effects occur only when the steroids are present, after which the behavioral and physiological effects diminish (Arnold and Breedlove 1985; Breedlove 1992b; McEwen 1981). Rather than permanent neuroanatomical changes, activational effects of steroids are thought to involve changes in receptor numbers (MacLusky and McEwen 1978), transient structural changes in neurons (Gould et al. 1990), temporary fluctuations in neurotransmitter levels or synthesis (Arnold and Breedlove 1985; McEwen 1981), or direct effects of steroids on the cell membrane that alter neurotransmission (McEwen 1991). It is noteworthy that activational effects of hormones are frequently dependent on earlier organizational effects of gonadal steroids (Breedlove 1992b).

In nonhuman species, several behavioral systems are responsive to the hormonal environment in both adult and developing animals. Although not always the case, gonadal steroids often exert maximal effects on behaviors that are differentially expressed in males and females. The diverse behavioral systems whose development and expression are sensitive to gonadal steroids include sexual and maternal behavior, overall activity levels, open field activity, aggression, juvenile play, feeding and taste preferences, avoidance learning, motor behavior, and song production in songbirds (Beatty 1992; Becker et al. 1992). Of particular interest to researchers investigating hormonal contributions to human abilities is the observation that gonadal steroids exert a marked influence on rodent spatial memory (Roof and Havens 1992; Stewart et al. 1975; Williams and Meck 1991), a behavior that is dependent on the integrity of the hippocampus (O'Keefe and Nadel 1978) and is thought to be evolutionarily homologous to human spatial cognition and memory (Gaulin and FitzGerald 1989; Gaulin and Hoffman 1991).

EFFECTS OF GONADAL STEROIDS ON HUMAN COGNITION

Behavioral effects of gonadal steroids are not restricted to nonhuman species. Mounting evidence indicates that sex steroid hormones may affect human cognitive, motor, and perceptual processes throughout development and into early and later adulthood. As with nonhuman species, some of the clearest effects of gonadal steroids on cognition have been observed on tasks that are performed differentially by men and women. Although there is considerable overlap in scores between the sexes on all cognitive measures, men and women excel on different aspects of cognitive processing. On average, women tend to outperform men on tests of verbal fluency and articulation, tests of perceptual speed, and some memory measures, whereas men tend to excel on tests of spatial and quantitative abilities and mathematical reasoning (Halpern 1986; Hampson and Kimura 1992; Linn and Petersen 1985; Maccoby and Jacklin 1974; Voyer et al. 1995).

Although direct experimental manipulations of steroid levels in humans are often not possible for ethical reasons, various research strategies allow assessment of the effect of the hormonal milieu on cognition. Organizational effects of excess androgenic hormones on human cognitive abilities have been investigated through assessment of individuals exposed prenatally to atypical hormonal environments caused by an endocrine disorder or by virilizing progestins ingested by the pregnant mother (Reinisch and Sanders 1992). For example, cognitive abilities have been studied in individuals with congenital adrenal hyperplasia who have an adrenal enzyme deficit characterized by reduced corticosteroid production and subsequent increases in adrenal androgens. Because these individuals typically receive a diagnosis and treatment early in life, the hormonal abnormality affects the prenatal and early postnatal period. Studies of cognitive abilities in congenital adrenal hyperplasia have found selective increases in spatial ability (Hampson et al. 1998; Resnick et al. 1986) in females with congenital adrenal hyperplasia compared with unaffected female relatives. These findings are consistent with early organizational effects of androgens on some cognitive functions.

Activational influences of hormones on cognition, the focus of this chapter, have been investigated through natural fluctuations in hormones over the menstrual cycle and, more recently, through the effects of hormone replacement therapy on postmenopausal women. Such studies provide a window to view the behavioral effects of gonadal steroids in humans.

EFFECTS OF OVARIAN STEROIDS ON COGNITION

Cognitive Fluctuations Across the Menstrual Cycle

Hormonal fluctuations over the menstrual cycle in women provide a convenient paradigm for investigating the effects of circulating levels of ovarian steroids on cognition. Estradiol and progesterone vary systematically over the normal spontaneous menstrual cycle such that both hormones are at a high level during the midluteal phase and at a low level during the menstrual phase of the cycle (see Figure 18–1). Several researchers have taken advantage of this fluctuation to investigate the effects of hormonal cyclicity on cognitive performance. For example, Hampson and Kimura (1988) administered a battery of spatial and motor tasks to women at high and low estradiol phases of the menstrual cycle. During the midluteal phase of the cycle, women performed better on tests of manual dexterity, a skill on which females obtain higher average scores, and performed more poorly on visuospatial tests, which typically show a male advantage.

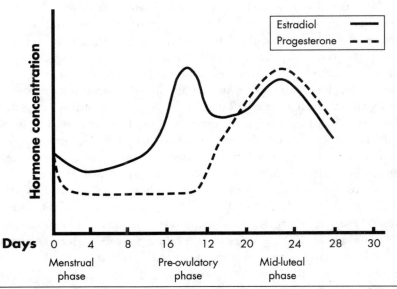

FIGURE 18–1. Fluctuations of estradiol and progesterone over the normal menstrual cycle. During the menstrual phase of the cycle, both estradiol and progesterone levels are low. Following a surge in luteinizing hormone concentration, estradiol levels increase sharply during the preovulatory phase. Both hormones are at relatively high concentrations during the midluteal phase of the cycle.

Consistent with the findings of Hampson and colleagues, Phillips and Silverman (1997) reported that performance on a three-dimensional mental rotation task, a cognitive measure on which males show superior performance, was better during the menstrual phase of the cycle than during the luteal phase. Phillips and Sherwin (1992a) reported significant reductions of visual memory performance during the menstrual phase of the cycle. Although sex differences in memory are not always found, higher memory scores in women have been reported for some memory tasks (Bleeker et al.

with a uterus are administered adjuvant progesterone therapy for protection against uterine cancer. Thus, observational studies include women taking combined estrogen and progesterone therapy and women taking estrogen alone. Another limitation of these studies is that women who choose to take ERT may be different in some way from nonusers (e.g., may be healthier, more highly educated, or more likely to use medical services).

In general, comparisons between ERT users and nonusers have indicated better cognitive performance in ERT users. ERT users obtained higher scores on tests of verbal memory (Kampen and Sherwin 1994; Maki et al. 2001), recall of proper names (Robinson et al. 1994), and short-term visual memory (Resnick et al. 1997) and had better cognitive abilities in general (Kimura 1995). In contrast to these positive findings, results of two large-scale observational studies indicated no cross-sectional differences between ERT users and nonusers (Barrett-Connor and Kritz-Silverstein 1993; Szklo et al. 1996). In these studies, verbal memory testing procedures required subjects to reach a criterion of performance before recall testing.

As Maki et al. (2001) recently reported, estradiol appears to have significant effects on initial encoding of verbal information. Thus, procedures that eliminate variability in initial encoding may mask potentially important differences between ERT groups.

In a third large-scale observational study (Grodstein et al. 2000), differences between women receiving ERT and nonusers were observed on tests of semantic memory (category fluency) but not on paragraph recall or word list memory. However, cognitive assessments in this study were conducted by telephone, and hormone status was based on information collected several years before the cognitive assessment.

In addition to cross-sectional comparisons of ERT users and nonusers, two studies have reported the effects of ERT on longitudinal decline in memory and cognition. In a subset of the women examined by Resnick et al. (1997), 18 women who began ERT use between two visual memory assessments—on average, 6 years apart—were compared with a group of never-treated women matched on age, education, intertest interval, and initial visual memory score. The results showed that visual memory performance of the women who were nonusers at the first test session but who subsequently began ERT before the second test session remained stable over time. In contrast, memory scores from women who remained off ERT for both sessions declined over the 6-year interval. This study provided an important complement to previous ERT studies in that it confirmed a protective effect on *longitudinal* memory decline. Moreover, whereas previous studies suggested that the possible beneficial effects of ERT may be restricted to verbal memory (Phillips and Sherwin 1992b), this study indicated that the effects also may extend to visual memory performance.

Jacobs et al. (1998) examined the cognitive effects of ERT history in a large cohort of women studied prospectively as part of a longitudinal cognitive aging study in New York City. They found that women who were previous or current users of ERT obtained higher scores on neuropsychological measures of memory, reasoning, and naming ability than did women who had never used estradiol. Moreover, longitudinal analysis indicated that women who had never used ERT showed mild decline on these cognitive measures over a 2-year interval, whereas women who used ERT showed a small improvement over time. Note that one limitation of this study was the low number of current as compared with past users.

Estrogen Replacement Therapy and Alzheimer's Disease

The incidence of AD may be as much as two- to threefold higher in women compared with men (Andersen et al. 1999). Moreover, evidence indicates that women with AD have lower serum estradiol levels than do women without dementia (Honjo et al. 1989). These observations, combined with the reports of effects of estradiol on specific cognitive abilities, have kindled interest in the possible protective effects of estradiol on the diagnosis of AD. Effects of estradiol on the risk for AD have been examined in several studies comparing rates of AD observed in groups of women who have been receiving ERT and in women with no history of ERT use.

A meta-analysis of the effects of ERT use on the risk of developing dementia reported a 29% reduction in the risk for AD among estradiol users (Yaffe et al. 1998). Several studies did not find significant effects of ERT on the development of dementia (Brenner et al. 1994; Broe et al. 1990; Graves et al. 1990), but other investigations yielded results consistent with a protective effect of ERT on the risk for AD. For example, in two case-control studies, patients with AD were less likely to have used ERT than were control subjects without dementia (Henderson et al. 1994; Mortel and Meyer 1995). However, a limitation of the case-control design is that the possibility of different estradiol prescribing practices in subjects with and without dementia cannot be excluded.

Two population-based studies also reported a reduced risk for AD in users of ERT (Paganini-Hill and Henderson 1994; Tang et al. 1996). Paganini-Hill and Henderson (1994) and Tang et al. (1996) reported relative risks for ERT users compared with nonusers of 0.46 for AD and related dementia and 0.40 for AD, respectively. Moreover, longer ERT duration (Paganini-Hill and Henderson 1994; Tang et al. 1996) and higher estradiol dosage (Paganini-Hill and Henderson 1994) were significantly associated with greater risk reduction for AD, suggesting a dose–response relation between ERT and the probability of developing AD. In a recent prospective study of postmenopausal women in the Baltimore Longitudinal Study of

Aging (Kawas et al. 1997), ERT use was associated with a decreased risk for a diagnosis of AD (relative risk for ERT users compared with nonusers = 0.46). However, duration of ERT was not related to disease outcome in this study.

Although the combined results across studies offer encouraging evidence of a beneficial effect of ERT on the risk for AD, more conclusive information awaits the results of several ongoing randomized clinical trials. If these findings are confirmed, they will represent an important public health advance in the study and prevention of AD.

In contrast to the possible beneficial effect of ERT in the prevention of AD, results of three recently completed randomized clinical trials did not support an effect of estrogen alone as a treatment in women who already have been given diagnoses of AD (Henderson et al. 2000; Mulnard et al. 2000; Wang et al. 2000).

EFFECTS OF ANDROGENS ON COGNITION

The existence of menstrual cyclicity and the widespread use of ERT in women provide convenient research paradigms to investigate the effects of ovarian steroids on cognition in women. Although comparable paradigms are not as readily available in men, several investigators have taken advantage of circadian and circannual variation in testosterone concentration to examine daily and seasonal fluctuations, respectively, in androgen in relation to cognitive variability. Moreover, although not as common as ERT, testosterone replacement is performed in some men, and studies of its effects on cognition are now being undertaken. Still another approach to investigating testosterone's effects on cognition has been to measure circulating androgen levels in blood or saliva and to relate these values to scores on standardized neuropsychological tests. Although considerable variability exists between studies, it could be tentatively suggested that in young adults, the relation between testosterone and spatial ability may be nonlinear, such that intermediate testosterone concentrations may be maximally beneficial to performance on measures of spatial ability (see Figure 18–2).

Direct Measurement of Androgens

Shute et al. (1983) administered a battery of spatial tasks and obtained blood plasma measures of androgen levels in a sample of healthy young adult males and females. When males and females were considered together, they reported that an inverted nonlinear function described the relation between circulating androgens and spatial performance. In a second study (Shute et al. 1983), the original findings were replicated; females with

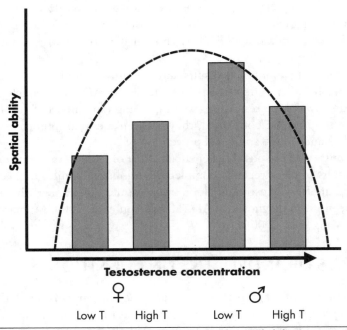

FIGURE 18–2. Relation between testosterone and spatial ability in young healthy adults. Moderate concentrations of testosterone, near the high end of the female range and near the low end of the male range, may be associated with optimum spatial performance.

higher androgen levels performed more accurately on a measure of spatial ability than did females with lower androgen levels, whereas males with higher androgen levels performed more poorly than did males with lower androgen concentrations. In these studies, nonspatial tests were not administered, raising the question of whether the observed relation is specific to spatial performance or whether it may generalize to other cognitive domains.

Subsequently, two other studies have replicated these findings with measures of salivary testosterone (Gouchie and Kimura 1991; Moffat and Hampson 1996). Gouchie and Kimura (1991) found that males with lower testosterone levels performed better on measures of spatial and mathematical abilities than did males with higher testosterone levels, whereas females with higher testosterone levels outperformed females with lower testosterone levels on the same measures. More recently, Moffat and Hampson (1996) reported an inverted quadratic relation between testosterone levels and a composite measure of spatial ability in healthy young adult males and females. In both studies (Gouchie and Kimura 1991; Moffat and Hampson

1996), no relation between testosterone and verbal performance was observed, providing evidence for the specificity of these findings to spatial performance.

It should be recognized, however, that not all studies investigating the relation between circulating testosterone and spatial ability observed nonlinear relations. Christiansen and Knussmann (1987), for example, reported a positive correlation between serum testosterone concentrations and spatial factor scores in a sample of healthy young men, whereas Mc-Keever et al. (1987) failed to find any relation between testosterone and spatial performance in a sample of male and female college students. Some of the inconsistencies between studies may be a result of the spatial measures that are used across studies. The tests differ considerably between studies, and different measures of spatial ability may load onto separate spatial processing factors (Borich and Bauman 1972; Ekstrom et al. 1976). Testosterone may be differentially related to these separate aspects of visuospatial processing. This possibility could be addressed in future studies including larger batteries of cognitive tests that load onto these separate spatial factors.

Two recent population-based epidemiological studies suggested that endogenous androgens may continue to influence cognitive function in elderly subjects. Barrett-Connor et al. (1999) measured androgen levels and neuropsychological performance in 547 men between ages 59 and 89 years. Higher total and bioavailable testosterone levels were associated with better performance on measures of short-term memory and concentration. Nonlinear relationships (inverted quadratic) also were found, in which moderately high testosterone levels predicted better mental control and long-term verbal memory among men. This finding of an optimal level of testosterone provides some convergence with the studies of young adult subjects. In a second study, the relation between endogenous gonadal steroid levels and cognition was investigated in 383 women aged 55–89 years (Barrett-Connor and Goldman-Gruen 1999). Women with higher mental status scores had significantly higher total and bioavailable testosterone levels. Higher endogenous estrogen levels were not associated with improved cognitive function in this sample of women. These data suggest that testosterone levels may modulate neuropsychological performance in elderly women and underscore the importance of undertaking androgen intervention studies in women as well as men.

Circadian and Circannual Variation in Testosterone

Circulating testosterone concentrations follow a marked circadian rhythm, with the daily peak occurring in early morning hours (~8:00 A.M.) and the nadir approximately 12 hours later (Dabbs 1990; Nieschlag 1974). Although the circadian rhythm in testosterone provides a convenient paradigm to investigate testosterone effects on cognitive ability, very few studies have attempted to capitalize on this diurnal variation (Mackenberg et al. 1974). In one recent study (Moffat and Hampson 1996), young adult male and female subjects were administered a battery of verbal and spatial cognitive tests either early in the morning or later in the day. The presence of a circadian rhythm in testosterone concentrations was confirmed by radioimmunoassay. A significant interaction between sex and time of testing was found; males tested in early-morning sessions, when testosterone concentrations were highest, performed more poorly on the spatial tests than did males tested late in the morning, when testosterone concentrations were lower. Among females, the reverse pattern was observed; females tested in the early-morning sessions outperformed females tested in the later session. These findings were specific to the spatial cognitive tests because verbal performance showed no diurnal fluctuation. These findings require replication, but they suggest that spatial performance may change dynamically over a relatively short time span, in association with the diurnal fluctuation in testosterone. Although some other hormonal and nonhormonal factors change as a function of time of day, the fact that the findings were specific to the spatial cognitive tests and that the pattern of results was opposite in male and female subjects makes an explanation based on nonspecific factors such as fatigue, motivation, or general biorhythms less likely.

Although the presence of a profound circadian rhythm in testosterone concentrations is firmly established, the possibility that human testosterone concentrations may fluctuate over the seasons is more controversial. Several researchers have reported that in the Northern Hemisphere, male testosterone concentrations are highest in the fall (Bellastella et al. 1986; Meriggiola et al. 1996; Reinberg et al. 1978), a possible consequence of the ecological advantages associated with fall conception and summer births (Sherry and Hampson 1997). Kimura and Hampson (1994) reported that in men, spatial performance was better in the spring, when testosterone concentrations were lower, than in the fall, when testosterone levels were higher. Once again, this effect was specific to the spatial tasks. In contrast to the significant seasonal variation observed in men, women showed no seasonal fluctuation in cognitive scores.

Testosterone Replacement Therapy

As noted earlier in this chapter, a drawback of studies that capitalize on circadian or circannual testosterone variations is the inability to confirm whether fluctuating testosterone concentration per se caused the observed cognitive effects. Age-associated declines in testosterone concentrations are well established, with testosterone decreasing by as much as 50% from age 30 to age 80 (Lamberts et al. 1997). The recent, albeit infrequent, use of testosterone replacement therapy provides a more powerful paradigm to investigate the effects of testosterone on later-life cognitive changes.

In a double-blind, placebo-controlled study, Janowsky et al. (1994) investigated cognitive performance in older androgen-deficient men who were given testosterone replacement therapy. They found that men who received testosterone had selectively enhanced Wechsler Adult Intelligence Scale—Revised block design scores compared with control subjects who received placebo, suggesting that testosterone replacement therapy in older men may enhance spatial-constructional abilities. At first glance, this study may appear inconsistent with prior investigations reporting that higher testosterone levels among men may be detrimental to spatial performance. However, as noted by Janowsky et al. (1994), testosterone levels were increased in these androgen-deficient men to approximately those observed in healthy young men, possibly increasing testosterone concentrations to a more optimal range.

In another testosterone replacement therapy study, Sih et al. (1997) reported no effect of testosterone supplementation on verbal or visual memory in a small sample of elderly men, although measures of spatial ability were not included in the cognitive test battery. In a more recent study, Janowsky et al. (2000) performed a randomized, placebo-controlled study investigating the effects of testosterone replacement therapy on working memory performance in men. Testosterone supplementation lasted for 1 month, and working memory measures were obtained both before and after treatment. Janowsky et al. (2000) found that men who received testosterone supplementation showed a marked reduction in working memory errors after testosterone treatment compared with men who received placebo. This suggests that testosterone supplementation may have beneficial effects on working memory in older men.

Although relatively few studies have investigated androgenic effects on human cognitive ability, the results from a variety of studies that used diverse approaches provide support for androgenic effects on cognition in both men and women. Cumulatively, these studies suggest that in young adults, moderate levels of testosterone may be optimal for performance on spatial cognitive tests. Although the neural mechanisms underlying this curvilinear function are not well understood, it is noteworthy that similar results have been obtained in nonhuman species (Roof and Havens 1992). In older men who have already experienced age-related decline in testosterone concentrations, testosterone replacement therapy may be beneficial to spatial performance. These studies are consistent in reporting significant effects on spatial processing and not on the other cognitive behaviors, including verbal abilities (Gouchie and Kimura 1991; Moffat and Hampson 1996), that have been assessed to date. However, recent epidemiological studies in both elderly men and women and one clinical trial in men reported that memory functions also may be affected by testosterone. Because this body of research is in a relatively preliminary stage, the delineation of the cognitive domains affected and a more precise description of possible differential effects in men and women await further study. Carefully conducted randomized, placebo-controlled intervention studies will no doubt help resolve these remaining issues.

PHYSIOLOGICAL MECHANISMS

Although the neural mechanisms by which steroids might modulate human cognition are poorly understood, studies in nonhuman species offer several putative physiological mechanisms that may underlie the behavioral effects of gonadal steroids.

For example, estradiol administration increases cerebral glucose metabolism (Namba and Sokoloff 1984) and attenuates oxidative and β-amyloid peptide toxicity in the central nervous system (Goodman et al. 1996). Estrogens also are known to modulate the efficacy of several neurotransmitter systems, including acetylcholine. Degeneration of cholinergic neurons and their projections emanating from the basal forebrain is one of the most significant neuropathological changes in AD (Coyle et al. 1983). Estradiol administration to ovariectomized rats increases choline acetyltransferase activity in the neocortex and hippocampus (Luine 1985). Moreover, estradiol administration reverses the deleterious cognitive effects of the cholinergic antagonist scopolamine (Dohanich et al. 1994) and may promote the survival of cholinergic neurons (Honjo et al. 1992). Estradiol receptors colocalize with nerve growth factor (NGF) receptors in cholinergic neurons, implying some survival-promoting mechanism on cholinergic cells (Toran-Allerand et al. 1992). Interestingly, estradiol administration in humans may potentiate the beneficial effects of tacrine, an acetylcholine agonist used for the treatment of AD (Schneider and Farlow 1997), suggesting that estradiol may have similar cholinergic-enhancing effects in humans. Estradiol also increases noradrenergic activity through the inhibition of monoamine oxidase activity (Luine et al. 1975) and may regulate dopaminergic activation in the striatum (Becker and Beer 1986).

Because of its putative role in spatial learning in nonhuman species (Morris et al. 1982; O'Keefe and Nadel 1978), the hippocampus has been the focus of considerable research attention. In humans, the hippocampal formation is thought to play a prominent role in some aspects of memory (Squire and Knowlton 1994). It is a primary site of neuronal degeneration in AD (de Leon et al. 1997; Jack et al. 1997; Morrison and Hof 1997), and some cell layers show age-associated neuronal loss in nondemented individuals (West 1993). Interestingly, Gould et al. (1990) reported that the dendritic spine density of hippocampal CA1 pyramidal cells was dependent on circulating concentrations of gonadal steroids in the adult female rat. These authors found that ovariectomy produced a reduction in spine density, whereas estradiol replacement prevented the reduction. Woolley et al. (1990) reported that dendritic spine density varied systematically across the rat estrous cycle, with increases in spine densities when estradiol and progesterone levels were high compared with the estrous phase, when estradiol and progesterone concentrations were low. The effect of estradiol on hippocampal CA1 spine density appears to be mediated by activation of N-methyl-D-aspartate (NMDA) (Woolley and McEwen 1994). These studies found that estrogen is capable of facilitating structural neuroanatomical changes in adult animals and raises the possibility of similar effects in humans.

There is also considerable evidence for significant androgenic effects on the neural substrate in nonhuman species. An important element in understanding the effects of testosterone on the nervous system is that many of its behavioral and anatomical effects occur after it has been converted to its metabolically active derivatives estradiol or dihydrotestosterone by the enzymes aromatase and 5α-reductase, respectively. Thus, testosterone may interact not only with androgen receptors but also with estradiol receptors, and, hence, testosterone administration may in some circumstances parallel the effects of estradiol throughout the nervous system (DeVoogd and Nottebohm 1981; Dorner et al. 1971).

In addition to testosterone exerting an early organizational effect on the development of the hypothalamus (Jacobson et al. 1981), the cerebral cortex (Diamond 1991), the hippocampus (Roof and Havens 1992), and many other cerebral structures, several observations suggest that testosterone is capable of modulating neural systems in adult animals. In adult animals, androgen receptors have been found in high concentration in hippocampal CA1 pyramidal cells (Kerr et al. 1995). Androgen treatment may prevent NMDA excitotoxicity in hippocampal CA1 neurons (Pouliot et al. 1996) and may facilitate recovery after injury by promoting fiber outgrowth and sprouting in hippocampal neurons (Morse et al. 1992). Moreover, testosterone administration increases NGF levels in the hippocampus, septum, and neocortex and induces an upregulation of NGF receptors in the forebrain (Tirassa et al. 1997).

An additional important influence of testosterone on hippocampal morphology involves its possible regulatory influence on glucocorticoids. It is now well established that chronic exposure to glucocorticoid hormones produced by the adrenal glands or exposure to chronic stress may cause cell death in hippocampal neurons, particularly in aged animals (McEwen and Sapolsky 1995; Sapolsky et al. 1990; Uno et al. 1989). Recent observations suggest that androgen treatment may counteract the deleterious effects of glucocorticoid exposure. This suggestion is supported by the observation that hippocampal cell death following chronic stress is greater in gonadectomized animals than in gonadally intact or androgen-treated males (Mizoguchi et al. 1992), suggesting a possible mechanism whereby androgens might suppress the neurotoxic effects of glucocorticoids on the hippocampus.

APPLICATION OF NEUROIMAGING IN HUMANS

Although the biochemical techniques used to investigate steroidal effects in animal models are not available to researchers investigating humans, the recent application of functional neuroimaging provides an opportunity to investigate the possible neural mechanisms in humans. For example, Berman et al. (1997) examined positron-emission tomography regional cerebral blood flow (rCBF) following pharmacological suppression of estradiol and progesterone. They found that suppression of estradiol and progesterone resulted in attenuation of the prefrontal cortex activation typically observed during performance on a test of executive function and perseveration. Administration of estradiol or progesterone restored the rCBF activation pattern in the prefrontal cortex, whereas estradiol increased parietal and temporal lobe activation. Resnick et al. (1998) investigated positron-emission tomography rCBF during verbal and figural memory processing in women who were using ERT compared with women who were not using ERT. Rather than showing consistently greater activation in one group than in the other, ERT users and nonusers differed in regionally specific patterns of relative activation and deactivation of brain regions thought to subserve performance on the positron-emission tomography memory tasks. Similarly, Shaywitz et al. (1999) used functional magnetic resonance imaging and a double-blind crossover trial with 21 days of estrogen treatment to show that estrogen modulated brain activation patterns during verbal and visual working memory tasks.

At least one study examined brain activation patterns over the menstrual cycle. Reiman et al. (1996) investigated positron-emission tomography glucose metabolism over the menstrual cycle in a sample of healthy young women. High levels of estradiol and progesterone were associated with significantly higher glucose metabolism in superior temporal, anterior temporal, occipital, cerebellar, cingulate, and anterior insular regions, whereas low levels of estradiol and progesterone were associated with significantly higher glucose metabolism in thalamic, prefrontal, temporoparietal, and inferior temporal regions. As far as we are aware, there are no studies relating androgen levels to measures of functional brain activation.

SUMMARY AND CONCLUSION

In summary, gonadal steroids are known to exert profound behavioral and physiological effects in nonhuman species, and evidence continues to accumulate that similar effects may occur in humans. The natural hormonal fluctuations that occur over the menstrual cycle may exert a detectable effect on cognition in young women. In postmenopausal women, estradiol may slow the normal cognitive decline associated with aging and may exert a protective effect on the development of AD. Moreover, testosterone appears to modulate cognitive performance in men and women throughout the life span, and testosterone replacement therapy may enhance spatial performance in elderly, androgen-deficient men. Investigations conducted in humans to date are either observational studies or placebo-controlled trials on small samples. Large-scale randomized clinical trials are needed to definitively assess the effect and magnitude of steroid hormone effects on human cognition. Studies in nonhuman species provide a plausible biological foundation for understanding the neurophysiology of steroid hormones. However, understanding the precise biological mechanisms by which these steroids modulate human behavior remains elusive. Studies investigating steroidal effects on functional brain activation will undoubtedly provide new insight into the neuroanatomical loci and physiological mechanisms that underlie the cognitive and behavioral effects of gonadal steroids in humans.

REFERENCES

Andersen K, Launer L, Dewey M, et al: Gender differences in the incidence of AD and vascular dementia. Neurology 53:1992–1997, 1999

Arnold AP, Breedlove SM: Organizational and activational effects of sex steroids on brain and behavior: a reanalysis. Horm Behav 19:469–498, 1985

Barrett-Connor E, Goodman-Gruen D: Cognitive function and endogenous sex hormones in older women. J Am Geriatr Soc 47:1289–1293, 1999

Barrett-Conner E, Kritz-Silverstein D: Estrogen replacement therapy and cognitive function in older women. JAMA 269:2637–2641, 1993

Barrett-Connor E, Goodman-Gruen D, Patay B: Endogenous sex hormones and cognitive function in older men. J Clin Endocrinol Metab 84:3681–3685, 1999

Beatty WW: Gonadal hormones and sex differences in nonreproductive behaviors, in Handbook of Behavioral Neurology, Vol II: Sexual Differentiation. Edited by Gerall AA, Moltz H, Ward IL. New York, Plenum, 1992, pp 85–128

Becker JB, Beer ME: The influence of estrogen on nigrostriatal dopamine activity: behavioral and neurochemical evidence for both pre- and postsynaptic components. Behav Brain Res 19:27–33, 1986

Becker JB, Breedlove SM, Crews D: Behavioral Endocrinology. Cambridge, MA, MIT Press, 1992

Bellastella A, Criscuolo T, Sinisi AA, et al: Circannual variations of plasma testosterone, luteinizing hormone, follicle-stimulating hormone and prolactin in Klinefelter's syndrome. Neuroendocrinology 42:153–157, 1986

Berman KF, Schmidt PJ, Rubinow DR, et al: Modulation of cognition-specific cortical activity by gonadal steroids: a positron-emission tomography study in women. Proc Natl Acad Sci U S A 94:8836–8841, 1997

Bleeker ML, Bolla-Wilson K, Agnew J, et al: Age-related sex differences in verbal memory. J Clin Psychol 44:403–411, 1988

Borich GD, Bauman PM: Convergent and discriminant validation of the French and Guilford-Zimmerman spatial orientation and spatial visualization factors. Educational and Psychological Measurement 32:1029–1033, 1972

Breedlove SM: Sexual differentiation of the brain and behavior, in Behavioral Endocrinology. Edited by Becker JB, Breedlove SM, Crews D. Cambridge, MA, MIT Press, 1992a, pp 3–37

Breedlove SM: Sexual dimorphism in the vertebrate nervous system. J Neurosci 12:4133–4142, 1992b

Brenner DE, Kukull WA, Stergachis A, et al: Postmenopausal estrogen replacement therapy and the risk of Alzheimer's disease: a population-based case-control study. Am J Epidemiol 140:262–267, 1994

Broe GA, Henderson AS, Creasey H, et al: A case-control study of Alzheimer's disease in Australia. Neurology 40:1698–1707, 1990

Campbell S, Whitehead M: Oestrogen therapy and the menopausal syndrome. Clin Obstet Gynecol 4:31–47, 1977

Christiansen K, Knussmann R: Sex hormones and cognitive functioning in men. Neuropsychobiology 18:27–36, 1987

Coyle JT, Price DL, DeLong MR: Alzheimer's disease: a disorder of cortical cholinergic innervation. Science 219:1184–1190, 1983

Craik FIM, Salthouse T: The Handbook of Aging and Cognition. Hillsdale, NJ, Lawrence Erlbaum, 1992

Dabbs JM: Salivary testosterone measurements: reliability across hours, days, and weeks. Physiol Behav 48:83–86, 1990

de Leon MJ, Convit A, DeSanti S, et al: Contribution of structural neuroimaging to the early diagnosis of Alzheimer's disease. Int Psychogeriatr 9:183–190; discussion 247–252, 1997

DeVoogd T, Nottebohm F: Gonadal hormones induce dendritic growth in the adult avian brain. Science 214:202–204, 1981

Diamond MC: Hormonal effects on the development of cerebral lateralization. Psychoneuroendocrinology 16:121–129, 1991

Ditkoff EC, Crary WG, Cristo M, et al: Estrogen improves psychological function in asymptomatic postmenopausal women. Obstet Gynecol 78:991–995, 1991

Dohanich GP, Fader AJ, Javorsky DJ: Estrogen and estrogen-progesterone treatments counteract the effect of scopolamine on reinforced T-maze alternation in female rats. Behav Neurosci 108:988–992, 1994

Dorner G, Docke F, Hinz G: Paradoxical effects of estrogen on brain differentiation. Neuroendocrinology 7:146–155, 1971

Duka T, Tasker R, McGowan JF: The effects of 3-week estrogen hormone replacement on cognition in elderly healthy females. Psychopharmacology 149:129–139, 2000

Ekstrom RB, French J, Harman HH, et al: Kit of Factor Referenced Tests. Princeton, NJ, Educational Testing Service, 1976

Fedor-Freybergh P: The influence of oestrogens on the wellbeing and mental performance in climacteric and postmenopausal women. Acta Obstet Gynecol Scand Suppl 64:1–91, 1977

Gaulin SJC, FitzGerald RW: Sexual selection for spatial-learning ability. Animal Behavior 37:322–331, 1989

Gaulin SJC, Hoffman HA: Evolution and development of sex differences in spatial ability, in Human Reproductive Behavior: A Darwinian Perspective. Edited by Betzig L, Borgerhof-Mulder M, Turke P. Cambridge, MA, Cambridge University Press, 1991, pp 129–152

Giambra LM, Zonderman AB, Kawas C, et al: Adult life span changes in immediate visual memory and verbal intelligence. Psychol Aging 10:123–139, 1995

Goodman Y, Bruce AJ, Cheng B, et al: Estrogens attenuate and corticosterone exacerbates excitotoxicity, oxidative injury, and amyloid beta-peptide toxicity in hippocampal neurons. J Neurochem 66:1836–1844, 1996

Gouchie C, Kimura D: The relationship between testosterone levels and cognitive ability patterns. Psychoneuroendocrinology 16:323–334, 1991

Gould E, Woolley CS, Frankfurt M, et al: Gonadal steroids regulate dendritic spine density in hippocampal pyramidal cells in adulthood. J Neurosci 10:1286–1291, 1990

Goy RW, McEwen BS: Sexual Differentiation of the Brain. Cambridge, MA, MIT Press, 1980

Graves AB, White E, Koepsell TD, et al: A case-control study of Alzheimer's disease. Ann Neurol 28:766–774, 1990

Grodstein F, Chen J, Pollen D, et al: Postmenopausal hormone therapy and cognitive function in healthy older women. J Am Geriatr Soc 48:746–752, 2000

Hackman BW, Galbraith D: Replacement therapy and piperazine oestrone sulphate ('Harmogen') and its effect on memory. Curr Med Res Opin 4:303–306, 1976

Halpern DF: Sex Difference in Cognitive Abilities. Hillsdale, NJ, Lawrence Erlbaum, 1986

Hampson E: Estrogen-related variations in human spatial and articulatory-motor skills. Psychoneuroendocrinology 15:97–111, 1990

Hampson E, Kimura D: Reciprocal effects of hormonal fluctuations on human motor and perceptual-spatial skills. Behav Neurosci 102:456–459, 1988

Hampson E, Kimura D: Sex differences and hormonal influences on cognitive function in humans, in Behavioral Endocrinology. Edited by Becker JB, Breedlove SM, Crews D. Cambridge, MA, MIT Press, 1992, pp 357–398

Hampson E, Rovet JF, Altman D: Spatial reasoning in children with congenital adrenal hyperplasia due to 21-hydroxylase deficiency. Dev Psychol 14:299–320, 1998

Henderson VW: The epidemiology of estrogen replacement therapy and Alzheimer's disease. Neurology 48:S27–S35, 1997

Henderson VW: Oestrogens and dementia, in Novartis Foundation. Edited by Chadwick DJ, Goode JA. London, England, Wiley, 2000, pp 254–265

Henderson VW, Paganini-Hill A, Emanuel CK, et al: Estrogen replacement therapy in older women: comparisons between Alzheimer's disease cases and non-demented control subjects. Arch Neurol 51:896–900, 1994

Henderson VW, Paganini-Hill A, Miller BL, et al: Estrogen for Alzheimer's disease in women: randomized, double-blind, placebo-controlled trial. Neurology 54:295–301, 2000

Herlitz A, Nilsson LG, Backman L: Gender differences in episodic memory. Mem Cognit 25:801–811, 1997

Honjo H, Ogino Y, Naitoh K, et al: In vivo effects by estrone sulfate on the central nervous system-senile dementia (Alzheimer's type). J Steroid Biochem Mol Biol 34:521–525, 1989

Honjo H, Tamura T, Matsumoto Y, et al: Estrogen as a growth factor to central nervous cells: estrogen treatment promotes development of acetylcholinesterase-positive basal forebrain neurons transplanted in the anterior eye chamber. J Steroid Biochem Mol Biol 41:633–635, 1992

Jack CR Jr, Petersen RC, Xu YC, et al: Medial temporal atrophy on MRI in normal aging and very mild Alzheimer's disease. Neurology 49:786–794, 1997

Jacobs DM, Tang MX, Stern Y, et al: Cognitive function in nondemented older women who took estrogen after menopause. Neurology 50:368–373, 1998

Jacobson CD, Csernus J, Shryne JE, et al: The influence of gonadectomy, androgen exposure, or a gonadal graft in the neonatal rat on the volume of the sexually dimorphic nucleus of the preoptic area. J Neurosci 1:1142–1147, 1981

Janowsky JS, Oviatt SK, Orwoll ES: Testosterone influences spatial cognition in older men. Behav Neurosci 108:325–332, 1994

Janowsky JS, Chavez B, Orwoll E: Sex steroids modify working memory. J Cogn Neurosci 12:407–414, 2000

Kampen DL, Sherwin BB: Estrogen use and verbal memory in healthy postmenopausal women. Obstet Gynecol 83:979–983, 1994

Kawas C, Resnick S, Morrison A, et al: A prospective study of estrogen replacement therapy and the risk of developing Alzheimer's disease: the Baltimore Longitudinal Study of Aging. Neurology 48:1517–1521, 1997

Kerr JE, Allore RJ, Beck SG, et al: Distribution and hormonal regulation of androgen receptor (AR) and AR messenger ribonucleic acid in the rat hippocampus. Endocrinology 136:3213–3221, 1995

Kimura D: Estrogen replacement therapy may protect against intellectual decline in postmenopausal women. Horm Behav 29:312–321, 1995

Kimura D, Hampson E: Cognitive pattern in men and women is influenced by fluctuations in sex hormones. Current Directions in Psychological Science 3:57–61, 1994

Lamberts SW, van den Beld AW, van der Lely AJ: The endocrinology of aging. Science 278:419–424, 1997

Linn MC, Petersen AC: Emergence and characterization of sex differences in spatial ability: a meta-analysis. Child Dev 56:1479–1498, 1985

Luine VN: Estradiol increases choline acetyltransferase activity in specific basal forebrain nuclei and projection areas of female rats. Exp Neurol 89:484–490, 1985

Luine VN, Khylchevskaya RI, McEwen BS: Effect of gonadal steroids on activities of monoamine oxidase and choline acetylase in rat brain. Brain Res 86:293–306, 1975

Maccoby EE, Jacklin CN: The Psychology of Sex Differences. Stanford, CA, Stanford University Press, 1974

Mackenberg EJ, Broverman DM, Vogel W, et al: Morning-to-afternoon changes in cognitive performances and in the electroencephalogram. Journal of Education Psychology 66:238–246, 1974

MacLusky NJ, McEwen BS: Oestrogen modulates progestin receptor concentrations in some rat brain regions but not others. Nature 274:276–278, 1978

Maki PM, Zonderman AB, Resnick SM: Enhanced verbal memory in nondemented elderly estrogen users. Am J Psychiatry 158:227–233, 2001

McEwen BS: Neural gonadal steroid actions. Science 211:1303–1311, 1981

McEwen BS: Non-genomic and genomic effects of steroids on neural activity. Trends Pharmacol Sci 12:141–147, 1991

McEwen BS, Sapolsky RM: Stress and cognitive function. Curr Opin Neurobiol 5:205–216, 1995

McKeever WF, Rich DA, Deyo RA, et al: Androgens and spatial ability: failure to find a relationship between testosterone and ability measures. Bulletin of the Psychonomic Society 25:438–440, 1987

Meriggiola MC, Noonan EA, Paulsen CA, et al: Annual patterns of luteinizing hormone, follicle stimulating hormone, testosterone and inhibin in normal men. Hum Reprod 11:248–252, 1996

Mizoguchi K, Kunishita T, Chui D, et al: Stress induces neuronal death in the hippocampus of castrated rats. Neurosci Lett 138:157–160, 1992

Moffat SD, Hampson E: A curvilinear relationship between testosterone and spatial cognition in humans: possible influence of hand preference. Psychoneuroendocrinology 21:323–337, 1996

Morris RG, Garrud P, Rawlins JN, et al: Place navigation impaired in rats with hippocampal lesions. Nature 297:681–683, 1982

Morrison JH, Hof PR: Life and death of neurons in the aging brain. Science 278:412–419, 1997

Morse JK, DeKosky ST, Scheff SW: Neurotrophic effects of steroids on lesion-induced growth in the hippocampus, II: hormone replacement. Exp Neurol 118:47–52, 1992

Mortel KF, Meyer JS: Lack of postmenopausal estrogen replacement therapy and the risk of dementia. J Neuropsychiatry Clin Neurosci 7:334–337, 1995

Mulnard RA, Cotman CW, Kawas C, et al: Estrogen replacement therapy for treatment of mild to moderate Alzheimer disease: a randomized controlled trial. JAMA 283:1007–1015, 2000

Namba H, Sokoloff L: Acute administration of high doses of estrogen increases glucose utilization throughout brain. Brain Res 291:391–394, 1984

Nieschlag E: Circadian rhythm of plasma testosterone, in Chronobiological Aspects of Endocrinology. Edited by Aschoff J, Ceresa F, Halberg F. Stuttgart, Germany, Schattauer, 1974, pp 117–128

O'Keefe J, Nadel L: The Hippocampus as a Cognitive Map. Oxford, England, Oxford University Press, 1978

Paganini-Hill A, Henderson VW: Estrogen deficiency and risk of Alzheimer's disease in women. Am J Epidemiol 140:256–261, 1994

Phillips K, Silverman I: Differences in the relationship of menstrual cycle phase to spatial performance on two- and three-dimensional tasks. Horm Behav 32:167–175, 1997

Phillips SM, Sherwin BB: Effects of estrogen on memory function in surgically menopausal women. Psychoneuroendocrinology 17:485–495, 1992a

Phillips SM, Sherwin BB: Variations in memory function and sex steroid hormones across the menstrual cycle. Psychoneuroendocrinology 17:497–506, 1992b

Phoenix CH, Goy RW, Gerall AA, et al: Organizing action of prenatally administered testosterone propionate on the tissues mediating mating behavior in the female guinea pig. Endocrinology 65:369–382, 1959

Polo-Kantola P, Portin R, Polo O, et al: The effect of short-term estrogen replacement therapy on cognition: a randomized double-blind, cross-over trial in postmenopausal women. Obstet Gynecol 91:459–466, 1998

Pouliot WA, Handa RJ, Beck SG: Androgen modulates N-methyl-D-aspartate-mediated depolarization in CA1 hippocampal pyramidal cells. Synapse 23:10–19, 1996

Reiman EM, Armstrong SM, Matt KS, et al: The application of positron emission tomography to the study of the normal menstrual cycle. Hum Reprod 11:2799–2805, 1996

Reinberg A, Lagoguey M, Cesselin F, et al: Circadian and circannual rhythms in plasma hormones and other variables of five healthy young human males. Acta Endocrinologica 88:417–427, 1978

Reinisch JM, Sanders SA: Effects of prenatal exposure to diethylstilbesterol (DES) on hemispheric laterality and spatial ability in human males. Horm Behav 26:62–75, 1992

Resnick SM, Berenbaum SA, Gottesman II, et al: Early hormonal influences on cognitive functioning in congenital adrenal hyperplasia. Dev Psychol 22:191–198, 1986

Resnick SM, Metter EJ, Zonderman AB: Estrogen replacement therapy and longitudinal decline in visual memory: a possible protective effect? Neurology 49:1491–1497, 1997

Resnick SM, Maki PM, Golski S, et al: Effects of estrogen replacement therapy on PET cerebral blood flow and neuropsychological performance. Horm Behav 34:171–182, 1998

Robinson D, Friedman L, Marcus R, et al: Estrogen replacement therapy and memory in older women. J Am Geriatr Soc 42:919–922, 1994

Roof RL, Havens MD: Testosterone improves maze performance and induces development of a male hippocampus in females. Brain Res 572:310–313, 1992

Sapolsky RM, Uno H, Rebert CS, et al: Hippocampal damage associated with prolonged glucocorticoid exposure in primates. J Neurosci 10:2897–2902, 1990

Schneider LS, Farlow M: Combined tacrine and estrogen replacement therapy in patients with Alzheimer's disease. Ann N Y Acad Sci 826:317–322, 1997

Shaywitz S, Shaywitz B, Pugh K, et al.: Effect of estrogen on brain activation patterns in postmenopausal women during working memory tasks. JAMA 281:1197–1202, 1999

Sherry DF, Hampson E: Evolution and the hormonal control of sexually dimorphic spatial abilities in humans. Trends in Cognitive Sciences 1:50–56, 1997

Sherwin BB: Estrogen and/or androgen replacement therapy and cognitive functioning in surgically menopausal women. Psychoneuroendocrinology 13:345–357, 1988

Sherwin BB: Estrogen effects on cognition in menopausal women. Neurology 48:S21–S26, 1997

Shute VJ, Pellegrino JW, Hubert L, et al: The relationship between androgen levels and human spatial abilities. Bulletin of the Psychonomic Society 21:465–468, 1983

Sih R, Morley JE, Kaiser FE, et al: Testosterone replacement in older hypogonadal men: a 12-month randomized controlled trial. J Clin Endocrinol Metab 82:1661–1667, 1997

Squire LR, Knowlton BJ: Memory, hippocampus, and brain systems, in The Cognitive Neurosciences. Edited by Gazzaniga MS. Cambridge, MA, MIT Press, 1994, pp 825–837

Stewart J, Skvarenina A, Pottier J: Effects of neonatal androgens on open-field behavior and maze learning in the prepubescent and adult rat. Psychology and Behavior 14:291–295, 1975

Szklo M, Cerhan J, Diez-Roux AV, et al: Estrogen replacement therapy and cognitive functioning in the Atherosclerosis Risk in Communities (ARIC) study. Am J Epidemiol 144:1048–1057, 1996

Tang MX, Jacobs D, Stern Y, et al: Effect of oestrogen during menopause on risk and age at onset of Alzheimer's disease. Lancet 348:429–432, 1996

Tirassa P, Thiblin I, Agren G, et al: High-dose anabolic androgenic steroids modulate concentrations of nerve growth factor and expression of its low affinity receptor (p75-NGFr) in male rat brain. J Neurosci Res 47:198–207, 1997

Toran-Allerand CD, Miranda RC, Bentham WD, et al: Estrogen receptors colocalize with low-affinity nerve growth factor receptors in cholinergic neurons of the basal forebrain. Proc Natl Acad Sci U S A 89:4668–4672, 1992

Uno H, Tarara R, Else JG, et al: Hippocampal damage associated with prolonged and fatal stress in primates. J Neurosci 9:1705–1711, 1989

Voyer D, Voyer A, Bryden MP: Magnitude of sex differences in spatial abilities: a meta-analysis and consideration of critical variables. Psychol Bull 117:250–270, 1995

Wang PN, Liao SQ, Liu RS, et al: Effects of estrogen on cognition, mood, and cerebral blood flow in AD: a controlled study. Neurology 54:2061–2066, 2000

West M: Regionally specific cell loss in the ageing human hippocampus. Neurobiol Aging 14:287–293, 1993

Whalen RE: Differentiation of the neural mechanisms which control gonadotrophin secretion and sexual behavior, in Reproduction and Sexual Behavior. Edited by Diamond M. Lafayette, IN, Indiana University Press, 1968, pp 303–340

Williams CL, Meck WH: The organizational effects of gonadal steroids on sexually dimorphic spatial ability. Psychoneuroendocrinology 16:155–176, 1991

Woolley CS, McEwen BS: Estradiol regulates hippocampal dendritic spine density via an N-methyl-D-aspartate receptor-dependent mechanism. J Neurosci 14:7680–7687, 1994

Woolley CS, Gould E, Frankfurt M, et al: Naturally occurring fluctuation in dendritic spine density on adult hippocampal pyramidal neurons. J Neurosci 10:4035–4039, 1990

Yaffe K, Sawaya G, Lieberburg I, et al: Estrogen therapy in postmenopausal women: effects on cognitive function and dementia. JAMA 279:688–695, 1998

19

Women as Caregivers for Patients With Alzheimer's Disease

Elaine McParland, M.D., J.D.
Judith Neugroschl, M.D.
Deborah Marin, M.D.

*D*isability in the elderly encompasses a wide range of deficits; however, dementing illness is one of the most prevalent and debilitating deficits in the aged. Alzheimer's disease (AD) is the most common cause of dementia, the principal characteristic of which is the gradual onset of memory impairment (McCann et al. 1997). Progressive impairments in language, behavior, and other areas of cognition gradually ensue (McCann et al. 1997). Behavior and personality changes are also an integral part of AD, and these behavior problems may make the care of the patient with AD especially difficult (Motenko 1989).

Estimates of the prevalence of AD vary, depending on one's definition of severe disease. In the United States alone, more than 4 million people are thought to be affected (McCann et al. 1997). The incidence of AD increases dramatically with age; the prevalence of AD has been estimated to be about 3% for persons aged 65–74, 19% for those aged 75–84, and up to 47% for those 85 years and older (McCann et al. 1997). Over the next 50 years, the number of people with AD is expected to double as the proportion of individuals older than 85 increases (Rabins et al. 1982). Approximately two-thirds of these persons with dementia reside at home; it is estimated that between 2.4 and 3.1 million caregivers for patients with AD currently live in the United States (Pett et al. 1988).

Caring for patients with dementia has been said to pose some of the most extreme challenges faced by caregivers, in part because of the chronicity of the disease and its relentlessly progressive impairments. Furthermore, caregivers spend substantial amounts of time in caring for patients with dementia (Schulz et al. 1995).

The variable rate of AD progression, and its associated behavioral disturbances, requires flexible emotional responses and caregiving plans. The caregiver's ability to effectively cope with the vicissitudes of the illness varies and cannot necessarily be predicted. A great deal of family conflict may be engendered in coming to terms with the illness. In some cases, the primary caregiver may not receive adequate support and may be resented by others in the family who may be in denial regarding the nature and extent of a patient's problems (Chenoweth and Spencer 1986).

ALZHEIMER'S DISEASE AS A WOMEN'S ISSUE

AD has been described as a women's health issue, in large part because of the enormous public health implications of this disease and its effect on multiple generations of women. Women constitute approximately 72% of the United States population older than 85; thus, AD directly affects a far greater proportion of women than men (McCann et al. 1997). However, AD is also very much a women's issue because the vast majority of informal community caregiving for those with AD is provided by women. It has been estimated that more than 70%–80% of the caregivers are women, primarily wives and daughters (McCann et al. 1997). Because women generally live longer than men and usually are younger than their husbands to begin with, women are significantly more likely to be caregivers for their husbands (Brody 1981). Similarly, daughters are more likely than sons to predominate as primary family caregivers and to provide in-home care to an aging parent.

Thus, in most families, a predictable pattern of selection of the caregiver emerges in which the initial family member to assume the burden of care for an elderly relative is the wife. It has been estimated that up to 46% of widows cared for their husbands at home before their deaths (Crossman et al. 1981). If a wife is not available, an adult daughter is the next most likely to assume caregiver responsibility. It has been estimated that a daughter's lifetime chance of providing parental care ranges from 55% to 75% (Farkas and Himes 1997). In the absence of a wife or a daughter, another relative assumes the major responsibility for care, often a daughter-in-law. Finally, if no family members are available, neighbors or friends are enlisted for assistance (Stone et al. 1987).

This caregiving role usually is undertaken voluntarily. Traditional values of familial responsibility for aged parents are accepted and embraced by many generations of women (Lang and Brody 1983). Families generally are reluctant to place elderly family members in institutions, and many intergenerational studies have established the willingness and commitment of multiple generations of women toward caring for aged relatives (Stoller 1983). Children generally expect to eventually care for their elderly parents, and most elderly individuals express a distinct preference for being cared for by relatives (Ory et al. 1985). However, the realities of coping with these filial responsibilities are complex and difficult. An enhanced understanding of the sociocultural, economic, and demographic characteristics of the typical caregiver as well as of the benefits and disadvantages of the informal caregiving system are necessary to minimize the difficulties experienced by caregivers in the future and to facilitate future planning for community-based long-term care.

Several factors are hypothesized to explain why women have dominated the primary caregiver role. Discrepancies in caregiver sex may be reflective of societal sex-role norms that emphasize the female role as interdependent with family and reinforce the notion of women as the family caregivers (Moen et al. 1995). Whether a result of social acculturation or innate sex-based traits, women may place a stronger emphasis on personal relationships and thus have stronger emotional ties to their families of origin than men do (Fitting et al. 1986). Caregiving also may have traditionally fallen to women because of the more flexible free time afforded by their role as homemakers (Fitting et al. 1986).

The dynamics and demographics of caregiving are bound to change in the coming decades, however, as a result of several factors. Declining family size and prolonged survival of the population means that there will be more individuals to care for and fewer caregivers to care for them. The growing numbers of elderly people and their increasing life expectancies will cause subsequent generations to delegate greater portions of their time to caregiving. The rising divorce rate and the increasing proportion of women entering the workplace make it likely that more men, particularly husbands, will be assuming the caregiving role (Allen 1994).

Notwithstanding the advent of these shifts, it is clear that, at present, women still compose the significant majority of caregivers for the elderly. The background and personal circumstances of these female caregivers vary widely. Given the heterogeneity of the demographic and circumstantial makeup of these female caregivers, the issues that are provoked in the context of caregiving are numerous and complex. The issues range from the gender dynamics of caregiving to differential coping mechanisms used by various caregivers to the effect of caregiving on the caregiver/patient relationship. Exploration of some of the pertinent controversies may help to advance effective planning and implementation of health care policies that reflect the increasing demands on family members to provide supportive care to the frail elderly.

Age

Female caregivers have a wide range of ages. It is important to view each age group as distinct because very different caregiving issues become prevalent as the age of the caregiver progresses. Caregivers for spouses are, on average, older than those caring for parents (Farkas and Himes 1997). The average age of a female caregiver is 57, but 36% are 65 years or older, and 10% are 75 and older caring for spouses or surviving parents (Brody 1981).

Women in the middle has been the prototype term often used to describe adult children or even wives who assume care of a parent or husband with dementia at a time in their lives when they have children or even grandchildren of their own (Brody 1981). However, the phenomenon of women in the middle encompasses a wide range of women with differing life circumstances. Older women in the middle must struggle with increasing parent care responsibilities at a time when age-related circumstances make coping with caregiving demands all the more difficult (Brody 1981). This subgroup of caregivers, representing the "young-old" (i.e., those aged 50 or older), have, in fact, a larger proportion of parent care responsibilities than do younger middle-aged caregivers (i.e., those in their 40s) (Lang and Brody 1983). This is because the probability of an adult child becoming a caregiver increases as the child ages because of the increasing physical and mental impairments of their family members (Dwyer and Coward 1991). For these women, mental and physical impairments and other health-related difficulties, interpersonal losses, and other changes attendant to the aging process are increasingly more likely to interfere with their ability to provide care to relatives with dementia (Lang and Brody 1983). This refilling of empty nests with impaired older family members also may operate to deprive the caregiver of plans to become more autonomous and self-sufficient and to devote larger amounts of time to activities that are more personally fulfilling in their retirement years (Lang and Brody 1983).

Younger caregivers may feel more stressed than older caregivers because caring for a chronic illness is an unexpected event occurring at a time when many caregivers either have recurring work and family responsibilities or have recently emptied their nest of dependents and are anticipating returning to the labor force (Fitting et al. 1986). These younger caregivers also may feel that they lack sufficient resources and personal time or energy to fulfill the obligations of all of their demanding and often competing roles.

Different Patterns of Care Provided by Women and Men

Definitions of *caregiving* differ greatly. The range of activities that fall within the rubric of caregiving includes diverse tasks such as personal care activities, providing emotional support, managing household tasks, providing transportation, and managing financial responsibilities (Farkas and Himes 1997). Caregiving can vary not only in the types of assistance provided but also in the duration and level of involvement of that assistance (Farkas and Himes 1997). The patient's dementia severity and availability of other supports in large part determine the intensity of the caregiving tasks. Thus, for some caregivers, caregiving may not be all-consuming and may consist of providing more episodic, as-needed care. In this type of caregiving situation, the stresses and burdens of caregiving may be significantly reduced or distinct from those of a full-time caregiver.

The apportionment of caregiving tasks is often consistent with a sex-based division of labor, and thus actual task allocation differs markedly between men and women (Neal et al. 1997). Women, as a whole, contribute higher levels of total assistance than do men (Stone et al. 1987). In addition, women are much more likely than men to provide direct services to the care recipient. They engage in a greater number of personal care tasks, such as bathing, dressing, and other personal hygiene needs of the care recipient, and provide considerably more assistance with household tasks and meal preparation. Daughters are more likely than sons to assume the caregiving role as the need for assistance evolves from less personal, instrumental tasks to personal needs (Dwyer and Coward 1991).

In contrast, male caregivers typically play a more substantial role in problem solving, providing financial assistance and transportation, and helping the older person with home repairs and yard work (Horowitz 1985). Men may be better able to delegate tasks that require more physical direct care and are more willing to obtain outside help in accomplishing these tasks. Men are, in general, more willing both to obtain additional help from relatives and friends and to use resources from the formal service sector, and they do not experience significant role strain or guilt in doing so (Allen 1994). Men experience greater role incongruence when undertaking tasks traditionally performed by women and thus feel more comfortable relegating these responsibilities to others (Allen 1994). Women may have more difficulty delegating these tasks because they believe that they should be able to manage both the patient and the household (Ory et al. 1985).

Some researchers have studied time allocation decisions within households as a means of offering some insights into the differential way care is provided by females and males to needy parents (Stoller 1983). These studies suggested that men traditionally devote a greater proportion of their attention to the labor market, whereas women, in effect, specialize in domestic undertakings; both sexes feel more comfortable in roles consistent with this pattern (Stoller 1983). Although professed attitudes about the respective responsibilities of males and females may be changing, in practice, these time-allocation decisions continue to dictate the allocation of care responsibilities (Brody 1981). Finally, some studies suggested that although female caregivers may be more likely than male caregivers to carry out personal care and household tasks, there may be no significant sex differences in total caregiver involvement (Horowitz 1985).

CAREGIVER BURDEN AND STRESS

The degree of stress reported by caregivers varies greatly. *Caregiver burden* is now a widely recognized term describing numerous dimensions, including the psychological, social, financial, and physical responses experienced by caregivers (George and Gwyther 1986). The outcomes include mental stress and exhaustion, depression, social isolation, family conflict, restrictions on time and freedom, financial hardships, and physical strain (Kosberg and Cairl 1986). The range of feelings most frequently experienced by caregivers as a result of these burdens includes helplessness, guilt, and anger. In general, caregiving is associated with decreases in life satisfaction and general physical and mental well-being. Caregivers have been found to be significantly more depressed and anxious and to have a greater tendency to alcohol and drug abuse compared with noncaregivers (George and Gwyther 1986).

Much research has been done to ascertain the underlying causes of caregiver stress. Although it may seem self-evident that caregiver burden is directly related to the severity of a patient's disabilities or, alternatively, to actual caregiver workload, this assumption may not be correct. The extent of burden endured by caregivers instead may be due to the subjective experience of the caregiver and his or her ability to handle the demands associated with caregiving. In fact, some studies have determined that for some caregivers, the ability to tolerate problem behavior may actually increase as the disease progresses because of the caregiver's growing familiarity with the behaviors associated with the disease (Zarit et al. 1986). Thus, caregivers may learn to manage problems more effectively as they spend more time coping with the illness (Zarit et al. 1986).

Another significant predictor of caregiver burden is the availability of resources for obtaining assistance, whether formal or informal, and the ability to obtain periodic respite from the demands of the caregiver role (Zarit et al. 1986). Thus, interventions such as day-care centers and visiting home care may affect the extent of burden for some caregivers.

A third significant predictor of stress may be the relationship between the caregiver and the elderly individual in need of care. The type of relationship between caregiver and patient appears to affect the level of negative consequences experienced by the caregiver. Those individuals in a filial relationship with the elderly person, such as children who are caregivers for parents, tend to feel more stress than do spousal caregivers (Fitting et al. 1986). Researchers have hypothesized that this may be a result of the difference in expectations accorded to spouses and children. For example, the more intimate emotional relationship that often exists between mother and daughter and the attendant desire to recapitulate the infant–caregiver relationship are thought to result in increased stress for the daughter in the caregiving role (Pett et al. 1988).

Sex Differences in Caregiver Burden

The degree of stress reported by caregivers varies extensively, depending on their sex (Collins and Jones 1997). When either subjective or objective measurements are used, caregiver burden is more prevalent in women than in men, and female caregivers of relatives with dementia show significantly more adverse physical and psychological effects than do male caregivers (Irvin and Acton 1997).

Some have hypothesized that this difference in perceptions of stress and burden may be due to different life trajectories experienced by women and men (Fitting et al. 1986). Women, at the time they assume their caregiving role, may be at the close of their child-rearing years and may have expectations that their middle years will be more personally fulfilling. Thus, they may resent being thrust back into the caregiving role. Men, on the contrary, have spent most of their working lives in the labor market and may perceive caregiving as an opportunity to adopt a new, more reciprocative relationship with their wives (Fitting et al. 1986).

Also, perceptions of the caregiving role may differ between women and men, such that men may feel that their caregiving responsibilities are fulfilled by problem solving and delegating the more personal and difficult tasks. Thus, their caregiving duties may feel less onerous to them (Lutzky and Knight 1994).

Explanations for these sex differences in caregiving are complex. Several overlapping factors may account for these differences. One theory is that men and women may be exposed to different types and levels of stressors. For example, wives may experience more stress from struggling with dementia symptoms that affect specific personality characteristics of their spouse, such as uncharacteristic onset of aggressive behavior and changes in personality, whereas husbands are particularly strained by the decreased interaction and support from their wives (Abel 1990).

Alternatively, women may be more willing to express burdens and stresses than men are and may, in fact, have greater awareness of emotional responses to stress (Lutzky and Knight 1994). Thus, women may tend to recognize and report emotional states more than men do. Men may simply be reporting less burden because they are unwilling to recognize the amount of stress that they are experiencing (Lutzky and Knight 1994).

Other researchers have hypothesized that women are more likely to apperceive stress because they have internalized stronger affiliative behaviors pursuant to ongoing social and cultural reinforcement (Abel 1990). Consequently, women as a sex may feel more constrained in limit setting, have greater competing family obligations, and feel more responsible for maintaining the highest possible quality of life for their impaired relative (Abel 1990). The existence of sex differences in appraisal of caregiver stress is an area that deserves further investigation.

Different Coping Mechanisms Based on Sex

Closely related to the experience of burden are methods for coping with the demands of caregiving. Women may be more negatively affected by their caregiving demands because they use coping mechanisms that are less effective than the strategies used by men (Lutzky and Knight 1994). An individual's response to stressful events is mediated by both the events and the stress responses. For example, *escape-avoidance* is a specific coping style, used much more frequently by women than by men, that uses avoidant behavior and personal blame as a means of coping with conflicting feelings toward the demands of the caregiving role. This style may be ineffective because it may result in behavior that makes effective limit setting and efficient task delegation more difficult (Lutzky and Knight 1994). This results in higher levels of burden and decreased life satisfaction. In contrast, men may use coping strategies that are more solution oriented and "problem focused" (Lutzky and Knight 1994). These more efficacious coping styles may translate to reduced caregiver stress and burden.

CARING FOR THE RELATIVE AT HOME VERSUS OUTSIDE THE HOME

It is also important to distinguish between intrahousehold caregiving and caregiving arrangements in which assistance is provided across households. Caregivers who co-reside with dependent elderly often have more demanding caregiving responsibilities than those who live separately (Lang and Brody 1983). Often, caregivers must, out of necessity, reside with the relative whose illness has become so debilitating that he or she can no longer live alone.

The number of caregivers who share a single household with a demented older person increases as the age of the caregiver increases. This is because of the parallel aging of family members. The tendency toward cohabitation also increases as the age of the caregiver increases. As people grow older, they are more likely to live with or close to their children and receive more help from them (Lang and Brody 1983).

The caregiving activities of an out-of-household caregiver usually are less demanding than those of an intrahousehold caregiver and require less intensive involvement with the patient (Soldo and Myllyluoma 1983). Thus, the effects of stress-related problems may not be so apparent with caregivers who do not reside with the impaired individual.

EMPLOYMENT

The increasing proportion of women participating in the paid labor force has contributed a new dimension to the caregiving issue. The proportion of women who work outside the home will have a significant effect on the available labor source for caregiving. The number of women who work outside the home has increased fourfold in the past half century; three-quarters of these women are employed on a full-time basis (Lang and Brody 1983). Currently, 58% of all American women aged 16 and older are employed, and an additional 5% are projected to be in the labor force by the year 2005 (Neal et al. 1997).

A large proportion of this increase is a result of the influx of middle-aged women into the employment market. Women in their peak employment years (i.e., between ages 35 and 64) account for the largest influx into the employment market in recent decades (Brody 1981). Thus, most women are now employed at the age when the demands of parental caregiving become manifest.

The effect of employment on caregiving is controversial. Numerous studies have shown that employment does not have a significant effect on the number of hours of assistance provided by wives or daughters (Neal et al. 1997). However, employment may have an effect on the type of care provided by the caregiver. Employed and unemployed women provide approximately equivalent amounts of assistance with respect to tasks such as shopping and transportation, managing the household, and providing emotional sustenance (Brody 1981). However, employed women may be more willing and able to delegate certain tasks and, instead, purchase help from the formal service sector. The tasks more likely to be delegated are personal care tasks, such as bathing, cooking, and toileting (Neal et al. 1997). This is similar to the pattern of task allocation between sexes. Working women also may be somewhat more likely to purchase care in an institution than are nonworking caregivers (Lang and Brody 1983).

Employment in the paid labor market also has the potential to influence the community, personal, or volunteer activities of women. Employed women may limit or restrict participation in personal, family, and community activities as a result of caregiving demands. Thus, women often perform their caregiving tasks at the expense of leisure or recreational activities. These activities might otherwise have been useful in reducing their stress and burden (Farkas and Himes 1997).

The effect of caregiving on employment, both to the individual and to the societal market forces, is generally negative. Caregivers who are employed experience greater job stress, have more absenteeism, and require greater flexibility on the part of the employer (Farkas and Himes 1997). Caregiving also may operate to prevent many individuals from being employed at all in that actual labor force. Participation may be deterred completely or in part by the need to devote extensive amounts of time to caregiving activities (Brody et al. 1987).

Some research has suggested that the employment status of a caregiver may differentially affect the pattern of caregiving, depending on the *sex* of the caregiver. Thus, employment may not significantly affect the amount of time that employed women engage in caregiving, but participation in the labor force does appear to have a negative effect on the time that men are able to devote to caregiving (Dwyer and Coward 1991). Also, the stress of caregiving may affect working women to a greater extent than working men. For example, caregiving daughters have been found to experience more difficulties with their employers than caregiving sons (Dwyer and Coward 1991). However, other studies have suggested that employment does not significantly influence either the style of caregiving or the stress experienced by the caregiver. Some have even theorized that employment actually improves the outlook and performance by the caregiver because employment provides a welcome respite from caregiving and provides needed funds for support from the formal service sector (Pett et al. 1988).

The extent to which employment and caregiving are successfully combined, of course, depends on much more than simply the existence of concomitant demands. The extent to which the disabled elderly person needs help, the level of the caregivers' earnings from their jobs, and other competing demands, such as the presence of young children or a disabled or an unsupportive spouse, all affect the ability to coordinate these dual roles.

CLASS AND RACE DIVISIONS AMONG WOMEN

Dementia occurs in at least the same proportion in elderly minorities (black, Hispanic, Asian, and Native American) as in elderly whites (Wykle and Segal 1990). Thus, because life expectancy is increasing in minorities in much the same way as it is for whites, a significant increase in elderly persons with dementia is expected in the minority population in the coming decades (Wykle and Segal 1990).

Although the vast majority of the caregiving literature addresses the experience of the white, middle-class caregiver, some significant differences exist between minority and nonminority caregivers. For example, coping strategies appear to differ to a great extent. Minorities are more likely to use prayer and religion as coping mechanisms, whereas nonminorities are more prone to seek the support of professional therapists or friends (Wykle and Segal 1990). Also, perceptions of the difficulties caused by caregiving differ. Inadequate respite and relief from the demands of caregiving has been cited as the most difficult problem encountered by African American caregivers, whereas a comparison group of Caucasian caregivers cited feelings of guilt, impatience, and lack of control as more prevailing concerns (Wykle and Segal 1990). Thus, planning for appropriate interventions to relieve caregiver burden may differ depending on the population of caregivers.

MARITAL STATUS

When adult children are the caregivers, marital status often plays an important role in determining who will provide assistance to an elderly parent and the intensity of stress experienced by the caregiver (Dwyer and Coward 1991). Caregiving responsibilities fall disproportionately to children who have never married, particularly daughters (Lang and Brody 1983). Elderly parents with more than one child tend to rely for help on the one with fewest competing demands; thus, women with no children or spousal responsibilities are more likely to be designated as family caregivers (Lang and Brody 1983). The demands of marriage create less opportunity to devote time to parent care (Lang and Brody 1983). Also, never-married women are more likely to co-reside with parents, resulting in greater participation in caregiving activities. Marital disruption and divorce also have a negative effect on caregiving involvement. Adult children with disrupted marriages provide less assistance to elderly parents than do adult children in intact marriages (Dwyer and Coward 1991).

Most of the caregivers for relatives with dementia are, in fact, married (Horowitz 1985). Furthermore, most married caregivers tend to depend, to some extent, on their spouses for assistance in their caregiving role. Men are significantly more likely than women to depend on their spouses for providing additional care. Men also perceive their spouses to have more supportive attitudes toward their caregiving activities and have greater expectations of their spouses, as compared with caregiving wives (Horowitz 1985).

The marital status of the recipient of care is also important and also reflects a significant sex difference. Although spouses are the first individuals to whom impaired elders turn for assistance, women (particularly as their age increases) are less likely to have a spouse available and, therefore, are more likely to be dependent on adult children. Men, on the other hand, are more likely to receive assistance from their wives and are more likely to have them available throughout their lives (Allen 1994).

CONFIGURATION OF THE SIBLING NETWORK

Family structure is a very important determinant of care provision. Some research has indicated that only children or children who are part of a single-sex sibling network are more likely to engage in a wider variety of caregiving tasks than are children from mixed-sex families (Dwyer and Coward 1991). Also, sibling networks that are larger or composed of a greater proportion of male siblings are more likely to have some siblings in that family who provided little or no care. Finally, eldest children tend to become caregivers more frequently than do younger siblings (Dwyer and Coward 1991).

ECONOMICS OF CAREGIVING

The economics of caregiving is a significant impetus behind the efforts to understand and improve the caregiving process as experienced by family caregivers. Quantifying the cost of institutional care compared with informal care is a very important component of this goal because of the prevalent assumption that informal care engenders considerable health care dollar savings. Thus, it is important for policymakers to understand specifics about the costs of formal and informal care for patients with dementia and the circumstances that influence those costs.

The costs of institutional care in general are substantial. Patients with dementia who are in the institutional setting may be significantly more costly than elderly patients without dementia because of the need for increased supervision and attendance. Ancillary personnel, physician, and drug and medical supply expenses all have been found to increase considerably when dementia care is required (Holmes et al. 1994). Because up to three-quarters of nursing home patients have some form of dementing illness, with AD being the most prevalent, the costs associated with care for the institutionalized elderly are considerable.

Family caregiving costs are much more difficult to quantify and include the direct costs of provision of personal care, transportation, and medical costs and the indirect costs of opportunities fand employment forgone (Huang et al. 1988). Quantification of the economic consequences of caregiving to women who might otherwise be reentering the workforce is especially difficult because of the lack of prior recent employment history and available data regarding compensation for these women.

Achieving an enhanced understanding of the economics of caregiving will have a particularly important effect on female caregivers because women bear the economic burdens of caregiving to a greater extent than do men. This discrepancy is the result of several factors. As noted earlier in this chapter, women often forgo employment altogether because of the demands of caregiving. Consequently, their standard of living is lower than it might otherwise be. Women who choose to remain in the labor force often have lower average annual incomes than do their male counterparts (McCann et al. 1997). Women also have a significantly higher incidence of poverty than do men and may not be able to provide appropriate quantity and quality of care (McCann et al. 1997). Economics thus may play a significant role in the amount of burden experienced by women as they struggle to cope with their caregiving demands.

INTERVENTION PROGRAMS

There have been numerous attempts to delineate means of improving caregiver burden and alleviate the stress of caregiving. Policymakers and health professionals are concerned that the ability of families to provide the level of caregiving required in today's economic climate may be jeopardized if the burdens and stresses of these tasks are not mitigated (Motenko 1989). They are particularly concerned that families, in order to avoid the extreme frustrations and burnout of caregiving, will resort more frequently to institutional care for their relatives (Motenko 1989). Because institutionalization is not economically or emotionally desirable as the major resource for provision of long-term care for many families, a substantial amount of research has been dedicated to ascertaining the types of interventions that might reduce caregiver burden and better facilitate families' abilities to provide long-term community-based care.

A great deal of controversy has been generated regarding the appropriate interventions to be used. Several services have been hypothesized as effective ways of reducing caregiver burden, including educational programs; respite services; support groups for either the family, the caregiver, or the patient; and individual or family counseling. All of these interventions have their potential benefits.

Psychoeducational programs may work by simply educating caregivers and/or their spouses about the course of the disease and the types of behaviors that they may encounter, or these programs may actively train caregivers in the use of problem-solving or other behavioral skills to help them cope more effectively with their caregiving tasks (Lovett and Gallagher 1988). Alternatively, such programs may train caregivers to facilitate development of a better social support network through social skills training or interpersonal problem-solving strategies (Lovett and Gallagher 1988).

Simply educating caregivers about the progression of AD, providing anticipatory guidance for the foreseeable demands of changing family roles, and shaping reasonable expectations of the patient and his or her abilities may help caregivers better cope with present changes and more effectively plan for future care. Many caregivers for patients with AD have expressed considerable frustration and disappointment that the physicians diagnosing AD in their family members do not apprise them adequately of the expectations that they should have regarding the progression of the disease, possible treatment interventions, and measures that they can adopt to reduce caregiver strain. Thus, sometimes, education about the nature of the disease may be all some caregivers need to cope more effectively.

Some caregiver intervention programs have offered training programs designed to increase caregivers' ability to mobilize social support (Robinson 1988). Social isolation is a common sequela of caregiving for patients with AD and is a major contributor to the stress experienced by the family caregiver. Reducing isolation through training programs designed to enhance interpersonal skills and improve social functioning is a possible means of increasing the capacity of caregivers to fulfill the caregiving role.

Alternatively, hands-on case management training with the goal of improving the level of competence experienced by the caregiver has been proffered as a means of empowering the caregiver to feel more in control

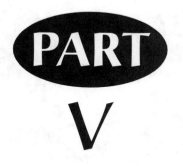

PART

V

Other Psychiatric Illnesses and Special Topics

TABLE 20–1.   Prevalence of victimization/posttraumatic stress disorder (PTSD) in individuals with substance use disorders

Study	Population	% With trauma	% With lifetime PTSD
Cohen and Densen-Gerber 1982	Treatment-seeking women	84	NA
Dansky et al. 1995	Treatment-seeking men and women	89	50
Grice et al. 1995	Treatment-seeking men and women	78	52
Ladwig and Andersen 1989	Treatment-seeking women	27	NA
Rohsenow et al. 1988	Treatment-seeking women	67	NA
Triffleman et al. 1995	Treatment-seeking men	58	50

have lifetime PTSD and 20%–40% have current PTSD. In the work conducted at our site, more than 90% of the women seeking treatment for cocaine dependence reported a history of sexual and/or physical assault (Dansky et al. 1994). Despite this, the history of victimization was often not documented in the clinical chart, and the assessment and treatment of PTSD symptoms often were not addressed (Dansky et al. 1997).

Women seeking treatment for substance use disorders have high rates of victimization and PTSD; in addition, women seeking services as a result of victimization experiences have high rates of alcohol and drug use. Studies have clearly documented a relation between alcohol use in particular and intimate violence. Alcohol was used by one or both parties involved in domestic violence in 56% of the cases of domestic violence reported to the police (Zacker and Bard 1977). Leonard and Senchak (1996) studied newlywed couples from a community sample and found that the husband's level of drinking was significantly and uniquely associated with marital aggression, even after premarital levels of aggression were factored out of the equation. Furthermore, a systematic review of medical examiner reports indicated that the risk of violent death from homicide was 28 times higher if a woman's family member used illicit drugs than among women who resided in households where drug use did not occur (Bailey et al. 1997).

Alcohol use by women appears to be a risk factor for becoming a victim of intimate violence. Specifically, Eberle (1982) documented that individuals who used alcohol were significantly more likely to be beaten by intimates who abused alcohol than were persons who did not use alcohol. Miller et al. (1993) conducted several studies on alcohol abuse by victims of intimate violence. They found that alcoholic women experienced higher levels of intimate violence than did nonalcoholic women, even after controlling for socioeconomic status, family history of alcoholism, family history of violence in the husband's family, and the husband's problems with alcohol. Women in treatment for problems associated with alcohol reported significantly more severe incidents of intimate violence than did women in treatment at mental health centers, women in a first-time driving-under-intoxication program, or women randomly selected from the community (Miller and Veltkamp 1989).

VICTIMIZATION, POSTTRAUMATIC STRESS DISORDER, AND OTHER COMORBIDITIES

In addition to the association between PTSD and substance use disorders, the prevalence rates of victimization have been significantly higher among women with eating disorders, somatization disorders, Axis II disorders, major depression, and other anxiety disorders when compared with individuals without such disorders (Brady 1997; Fergusson et al. 1996; Kessler et al. 1995). In the NCS, Kessler et al. (1997) found that 88% of the men and 79% of the women with PTSD met criteria for another psychiatric disorder. In fact, the odds ratios for all other anxiety and mood disorders were increased in individuals with PTSD, although a large sex difference was not apparent in these comorbidities.

In terms of disorders more likely to be found in women, the prevalence rates of victimization and PTSD have been significantly higher among women with a lifetime diagnosis of bulimia nervosa than among those without the disorder (Dansky et al. 1997). Somatization also is common in women with PTSD. In a sample of 77 female psychiatric outpatients with somatic complaints, more than 90% of the women with Briquet's syndrome (somatization disorder) reported some form of abuse (Pribor et al. 1993). Similarly, Walker et al. (1992) found a history of childhood abuse in 18 of 22 (82%) women with chronic pelvic pain compared with 9 of 22 (41%) randomly selected women without pain. This particularly high predominance of eating disorders and somatization disorders in women with PTSD may be connected to prescription drug abuse in these individuals. This area warrants further exploration.

In summary, the comorbidity of PTSD with other Axis I and II disorders in both men and women is quite common. Of particular interest for women is the predominance of trauma and victimization in individuals with eating disorders and somatization disorders. Because of the complex comorbidity and heterogeneity of the clinical presentation of women with PTSD, it is particularly important to screen individuals with multiple psychiatric symptoms and treatment resistance for victimization and PTSD.

Etiological Explanations for High Comorbidity Rates

Although a plethora of studies has documented the high rates of victimization and PTSD among women in treatment for substance use disorders, only recently have etiological explanations for the high rate of comorbidity been investigated. Some of the central themes in this investigation include the parental history of substance use disorder and victimization as risk factors for both genetic loading and early traumatization, substance use as self-medication for PTSD symptoms and substance-using lifestyles placing individuals at risk for traumatization, and finally, common neurobiological pathways between PTSD and substance use disorders. It is important to note that these theories are not mutually exclusive, and in any individual, causal pathways and the relation between the substance use, PTSD, and trauma may vary.

Parental History of Substance Use Disorder and Victimization

Miller et al. (1987) studied a sample of women with and without ethanol use and found that 67% of the women in the ethanol group reported a history of childhood sexual abuse compared with 28% of the women in the nonethanol group. Parental alcohol misuse was more common in the ethanol group. These researchers proposed that women with parents who misuse alcohol are more likely to have a history of sexual abuse and subsequently become more at risk for misusing alcohol. The parents' alcohol misuse leads to environmental and psychological vulnerabilities, which increase the likelihood that the children in the household will be sexually abused. Therefore, the children from these families will be vulnerable to alcohol misuse as a result of their family history of alcohol misuse and their history of childhood sexual abuse.

Cavaiola and Schiff (1988) also proposed that the parents' history may constitute a risk factor for an adolescent with a substance use disorder. They examined these relations in a sample of 500 adolescents with substance use disorders. They observed (but did not empirically test) that adolescents whose parents had divorced or who had a parent with a psychiatric disorder or a substance use disorder seemed to have a greater risk for becoming victims of physical or sexual abuse than did adolescents with a substance use disorder without such family characteristics.

Deykin and Buka (1997) also found that the adolescents with a history of trauma and those with a mother who abused drugs or a father who had received treatment for a psychiatric disorder were more vulnerable to developing PTSD than were adolescents whose parents did not have such problems.

These studies suggested that vulnerability to the development of comorbid PTSD and substance use disorders may be, in part, the result of a family history of substance use disorder (genetic loading) combined with victimization during childhood. Substance misuse in the home probably makes childhood victimization more likely to occur. Of particular interest in this regard is the finding by Breslau et al. (1991) that traumatization before age 15 was particularly likely to result in PTSD in women as compared with men. Hence, there may be some sex-specific issues in the relation of early trauma to the development of both PTSD and substance use disorders.

Self-Medication Hypothesis

The high co-occurrence of PTSD and substance use disorder does not necessarily imply any causal relation. In addition to the possibility that alcohol and drug abuse develop as an attempt to alleviate symptoms of PTSD (self-medication), lifestyles associated with substance use probably place an individual at risk for trauma and, thus, PTSD. One way to tease apart these causal pathways is to examine the order of onset of disorders.

Several studies have examined order of onset of PTSD relative to substance use disorders as an approach to investigating the self-medication hypothesis, and some interesting sex differences have been noted. Wasserman et al. (1997) sampled 450 individuals with a lifetime diagnosis of cocaine dependence and observed that two-thirds had been exposed to a traumatic event and that 50% of the women and 18% of the men met lifetime criteria for PTSD. They found that 61% developed PTSD before the cocaine dependence, 32% developed the cocaine dependence before the PTSD, and 7% developed both at the same time. The authors interpreted their data as indicating three processes: 1) PTSD leads to thoughts about the abuse, which leads to stress, which leads to substance use disorders; 2) cocaine use leads to increased risk of victimization, which leads to PTSD; and 3) cocaine use leads to neurochemical changes, which causes stress, which leads to PTSD. Sex differences in these relations were not explored.

Deykin and Buka (1997) documented in a sample of adolescents in treatment for substance use disorders that 40% of the girls and 12% of the boys met criteria for current PTSD. The odds ratio for risk of developing PTSD was 1.7 times higher for girls than for boys. There was a sex difference in the order of onset of PTSD relative to the substance use disorder, with 58% of the girls experiencing the trauma before the onset of the substance use disorder and only 28% of the boys experiencing the trauma first.

Sex differences in order of onset also were observed in a study conducted at our site with individuals seeking treatment for cocaine dependence. Among individuals with comorbid PTSD and cocaine dependence, women were significantly more likely than men to develop the PTSD before developing the cocaine dependence (Brady et al. 1998). Women also were significantly more likely to report a childhood victimization, and the time frame between age at victimization and the development of PTSD was significantly longer for women than for men. Men, in contrast, were significantly more likely to have their target victimization event occur as a result of their involvement with drugs.

Recently (Chilcoat and Breslau 1998), the temporal relation between PTSD and drug dependence was studied in a longitudinal assessment of individuals. PTSD signaled an increased risk for drug abuse or dependence. This risk for abuse or dependence was highest for prescribed psychoactive drugs. A preexisting substance use disorder did not increase the risk for subsequent exposure to traumatic events or the risk for developing PTSD. Sex differences in these risks were not explored. This study suggested that, in many cases, substance use disorders may develop as a result of self-medication.

Breslau et al. (1997) studied the risk for first-onset major depression, anxiety, and substance use disorders after PTSD in women. PTSD signaled increased risk for the subsequent development of both major depression (hazard ratio=2.1:1) and alcohol use disorder (hazard ratio=3.0:1). Of interest, illicit drug use, but not alcohol use, signaled an increased risk for exposure to traumatic events.

In fact, the relation between victimization and substance use disorder is complex, with many women experiencing a vicious circle of childhood victimization and subsequent addictive disorders, followed by revictimization. In the National Women's Study, victimization history was a risk factor for substance use, and substance use was associated with an increased risk for new assault, even after controlling for a history of assault (Kilpatrick et al. 1997). Similarly, Cottler et al. (1992) documented that the risk of assault was more than five times greater in individuals who used "hard drugs" than in nonusers. In fact, in the ECA study, female sex and cocaine or alcohol use were associated with the highest risk for developing PTSD (Cottler et al. 1992), and most individuals had used substances of abuse before the onset of PTSD symptoms. Other researchers (e.g., Breslau et al. 1991; Kessler et al. 1995) also reported an increased risk of victimization among people who used drugs. Finally, a study conducted at our site indicated that in individuals seeking treatment for cocaine dependence, those meeting criteria for current PTSD on entering the study were significantly more likely to experience a new assault in the next 4 months than those participants who did not have current PTSD at baseline (Dansky et al. 1998). Thus, as documented by other researchers (Briere et al. 1987; Wolfe and Kimerling 1997), having current PTSD also appears to be a risk factor for future victimization. The findings taken together indicate that a dangerous reciprocal relationship exists between drug use, victimization, and PTSD.

Biological Underpinnings

Of particular interest to this chapter, however, is whether sex differences exist in this reciprocal relationship. The fact that several studies among treatment-seeking samples found that PTSD was more likely to precede substance use disorder in women as compared with men is intriguing (Brady et al. 1998; Deykin and Buka 1997). The finding that women are more likely to develop PTSD as a result of childhood trauma when compared with men also lends credibility to this notion. Finally, in the NCS, PTSD was estimated to be primary more often than not with respect to substance use disorders in both men and women, but this finding was more robust in women than in men (Kessler et al. 1994).

Several common neurobiological systems are implicated in the pathophysiology of substance use disorders and PTSD (Kosten and Krystal 1988). In particular, the catecholaminergic, endogenous opioid, and serotonergic systems, as well as the hypothalamic-pituitary-adrenal (HPA) axis, are targets of investigation in the pathophysiology and treatment of both of these disorders. Some commonalties in neurobiology may, therefore, in part, explain the relation of PTSD to substance use disorders. Specifically, many drug withdrawal states (opiate, benzodiazepine, and alcohol withdrawal) are associated with central noradrenergic activation. Subjective alarm states, similar to those hypothesized for PTSD, are also associated with central noradrenergic activation (Charney et al. 1993). Many drugs of abuse, such as the opiates, benzodiazepines, and sedative-hypnotics, temporarily decrease stress-induced activation of central noradrenergic systems (S.J. Grant and Redmond 1981; Redmond and Krystal 1984), but drug withdrawal states are associated with activation of these systems. Thus, drug use may be an attempt to self-medicate PTSD symptoms, but withdrawal states are likely to have additive effects with PTSD on central noradrenergic function and therefore worsen the clinical presentation.

The HPA axis is one of the neuroendocrine systems known to be intimately involved in the response of the organism to stress. Chronic stress leads to dysfunction in HPA axis functioning, which may be related to some of the symptoms seen with PTSD (Charney et al. 1993). It has been shown in some laboratory settings that stressful experiences increase drug administration. The changes in the levels of glucocorticoid hormones seen with chronic stress (final step of the HPA axis) may be one link between stress and increased drug administration. The glucocorticoid hormones, through their action on dopamine, increase the behavioral responses to drugs of abuse (Piazza and Le Moal 1998). As such, stress, both acute and chronic, may modify, at the neurobiological level, the motivational and reinforcing properties of drugs of abuse.

Finally, accumulating evidence supports an integral role for serotonergic systems in PTSD (Connor and Davidson 1998). Sustained stress has been associated with serotonin depletion in animal models (Hensman et al. 1991). Similarly, serotonin depletion has been associated with both alcohol (Sellers et al. 1992) and cocaine (Ritz et al. 1990) use disorders. Of interest, as is discussed in the next section, the selective serotonin reuptake inhibitors (SSRIs) are one of the most promising classes of medication in the treatment of PTSD. These agents also have a potential role in the treatment of substance use disorder, particularly in individuals with comorbid anxiety and mood disorders.

In conclusion, several neurobiological systems are similarly involved in both PTSD and substance use disorders. As such, the notion of attempts at self-medication for PTSD symptoms may have an explanation at the neurobiological level. Similarly, substance withdrawal exacerbating PTSD symptoms also may be explained by the neurobiological underpinnings of both disorders. Although the sex-specific nature of these relations remains unexplored, the fact that this specific comorbidity is both likely to occur and likely to come to clinical attention because of the negative effect of each disorder on the other has major implications for the treatment of substance use disorders in women.

TREATMENT OF COMORBID POSTTRAUMATIC STRESS DISORDER AND SUBSTANCE USE DISORDERS

Despite the widely acknowledged prevalence of PTSD and victimization among substance abusers, little is known about effective treatment of comorbid PTSD and substance use disorders. One treatment approach often suggested in the literature (Nace 1988; Schnitt and Nocks 1984) is to treat the substance use disorder first and to defer treatment of trauma-related issues. Rationales for this approach include the premise that unchecked substance use disorder will impede therapeutic efforts directed at other problems (Nace 1988) and that some of the behavioral therapies known to be effective in the treatment of PTSD, such as imaginal flooding or implosive therapy, can be stressful and therefore may interfere with recovery as an individual attempts to self-medicate the negative emotional arousal induced by the treatment (Pitman et al. 1991). Because of these widely held views, there has been no systematic exploration of treatment of PTSD in individuals with substance use disorders. In this section, we describe several promising ongoing intervention trials, but questions about both the appropriate type and the appropriate timing of treatment intervention remain unanswered.

Seeking Safety

One promising new therapy for comorbid PTSD and substance use disorder in women is called *seeking safety:* cognitive-behavioral psychotherapy for PTSD and substance use disorder (Najavits et al. 1998). This manual-based therapy consists of 24 sessions. The treatment targets "safety," which is defined in terms of management of trauma-related symptoms, self-care, abstinence from substance use, prevention of self-harm, and development of healthy, supportive relationships with others. In a pilot study, Najavits et al. (1998) observed significant improvements on measures of both alcohol and drug use, as well as decreased substance use disorder severity. Psychological symptoms, such as suicide and dysfunctional attitudes about substance use, also were significantly improved over the course of treatment. Both PTSD and depressive symptoms decreased from pre- to posttreatment. These authors are currently conducting an investigation to compare the seeking safety treatment with a treatment-as-usual control.

Exposure Therapy

Another concurrent treatment designed to target both substance use disorder and PTSD is one developed at our site and involves the use of exposure therapy. Although there is a general admonition against using exposure therapy to treat PTSD in individuals who also are in early recovery from a substance use disorder, no systematic investigation has been conducted to determine the tolerability of this procedure. The combined treatment, referred to as *concurrent treatment of PTSD and cocaine dependence* (CTPCD), includes both in vivo exposure and prolonged imaginal exposure techniques, which are initiated after five sessions of cognitive-behavioral therapy (CBT) targeting cocaine dependence. CTPCD is an integration of a CBT manual designed by Carroll et al. (1988) for the treatment of cocaine dependence and a CBT manual developed by Foa and Rothbaum (1998) for the treatment of PTSD. Preliminary pretreatment to posttreatment comparisons indicated that individuals who completed treatment with CTPCD had significant reductions in their cocaine use, symptoms of PTSD, and general distress (Dansky et al. 1998).

Pharmacological Interventions

Treatment of PTSD is multimodal, but pharmacotherapy is playing an increasingly important role. Several agents have shown promise in uncontrolled case report studies, but only the antidepressant agents have been shown to be efficacious in placebo-controlled clinical trials. Specifically, trials of monoamine oxidase inhibitors, tricyclic antidepressants, and SSRIs have all been positive (Friedman 1998). Of particular interest in treating comorbid substance use disorders are issues concerning safety of the agents to be used should overdose occur, as well as potential interactions with drugs of abuse. For these reasons, work with the SSRIs is of particular importance. This class of agents has the benefit of being relatively safe in overdose and having low toxicity in combination with drugs of abuse. In addition, some evidence indicates that these agents may decrease consumatory behaviors in general (Sellers et al. 1992), particularly alcohol consumption.

One open-label pilot study (Brady et al. 1995) of sertraline treatment in a group of individuals with comorbid alcohol dependence and PTSD indicated that the medication treatment was useful in decreasing symptoms of PTSD as well as in decreasing alcohol consumption. A controlled trial has been completed (results not yet published). In a related study, Cornelius et al. (1997) found that fluoxetine treatment of comorbid depression and alcohol dependence decreased symptoms of both depression and alcohol consumption. Thus, the notion of targeting both disorders with one pharmacological treatment may have clinical utility.

Another issue of particular concern for women with PTSD is evidence that premenopausal women have a particularly robust response to SSRIs (Keller et al. 1996). The reasons for this preferential response are not clear, but the interaction of the SSRIs with the hormonal influences on disease states may be implicated.

As other agents are explored for utility in the treatment of PTSD, their use in the large subgroup of women with both PTSD and substance use disorders will be of interest. In particular, issues of safety, tolerability, and preferential efficacy will be of importance.

CONCLUSION

In conclusion, for women in particular, the relation between substance use disorders, victimization, and PTSD appears to be important. Data from epidemiological and treatment-seeking samples indicate that PTSD is common in women and, in particular, women with substance use disorders. Theoretical explanations for the high comorbidity and interaction of these disorders are complex but include self-medication of PTSD symptoms by substances of abuse as well as neurobiological and developmental issues.

Some evidence suggests sex-specific differences in the relation between PTSD and substance use disorder. Specifically, several studies indicated that for women, trauma and PTSD were more likely to precede the development of substance use as compared with men. These findings warrant further exploration because they may have treatment implications. Research in both pharmacological and psychotherapeutic treatments for PTSD is expanding. Unfortunately, substance users are often excluded from research studies, and the issue of both the timing and the type of treatment of PTSD in individuals with substance use disorders remains relatively underexplored. There are, however, ongoing projects with promising preliminary results for both pharmacological and psychotherapeutic treatments. Sex-specific elements of these treatments warrant a more thorough investigation. In particular, the notion of sex-specific pharmacological response is intriguing. Further work in this important area should prove extremely valuable and have enormous clinical utility.

REFERENCES

Abbott J, Johnson R, Koziol-McLain J, et al: Domestic violence against women: incidence and prevalence in an emergency department population [see comments]. JAMA 273:1763–1767, 1995

Bachman R: Violence Against Women: A National Crime Victimization Survey Report. Washington, DC, U.S. Department of Justice, Bureau of Justice Statistics, 1994

Bailey JE, Kellermann AL, Somes GW, et al: Risk factors for violent death of women in the home. Arch Intern Med 157:777–782, 1997

Brady K: Posttraumatic stress disorder and comorbidity: recognizing the many faces of PTSD. J Clin Psychiatry 58:12–15, 1997

Brady KT, Grice DE, Dustan L, et al: Gender differences in substance use disorders. Am J Psychiatry 150:1707–1711, 1993

Brady KT, Sonne SC, Roberts JM: Sertraline treatment of comorbid posttraumatic stress disorder and alcohol dependence. J Clin Psychiatry 56:502–505, 1995

Brady KT, Dansky BS, Sonne SC, et al: Posttraumatic stress disorder and cocaine dependence: order of onset. Am J Addict 7:128–135, 1998

Branson SL, Porter BK, Packer LE, et al: National Household Survey on Drug Abuse: Population Estimates 1996. Rockville, MD, Substance Abuse and Mental Health Services Administration, Office of Applied Studies, 1997

Breslau N, Davis GC, Andreski P, et al: Traumatic events and posttraumatic stress disorder in an urban population of young adults. Arch Gen Psychiatry 48:216–222, 1991

Breslau N, Davis GC, Peterson EL, et al: Psychiatric sequelae of posttraumatic stress disorder in women. Arch Gen Psychiatry 54:81–87, 1997

Briere R, Diop L, Gottberg E, et al: Stereospecific binding of a new benzazepine, [3H]SCH23390, in cortex and neostriatum. Can J Physiol Pharmacol 65:1507–1511, 1987

Burnam MA, Stein JA, Golding JM, et al: Sexual assault and mental disorders in a community population. J Consult Clin Psychol 56:843–850, 1988

Carroll KM, Rounsaville BJ, Gawin FH: A comparative trial of psychotherapies for ambulatory cocaine abusers: relapse prevention and interpersonal psychotherapy. Am J Drug Alcohol Abuse 17:181–188, 1988

Cavaiola AA, Schiff M: Behavioral sequelae of physical and/or sexual abuse in adolescents. Child Abuse Negl 12:181–188, 1988

Charney DS, Deutch AY, Krystal JH, et al: Psychobiologic mechanisms of posttraumatic stress disorder. Arch Gen Psychiatry 50:295–305, 1993

Chilcoat HD, Breslau N: Posttraumatic stress disorder and drug disorders: testing causal pathways. Arch Gen Psychiatry 55:913–917, 1998

Cohen FS, Densen-Gerber J: A study of the relationship between child abuse and drug addiction in 178 patients: preliminary results. Child Abuse Negl 6:383–387, 1982

Connor KM, Davidson JR: The role of serotonin in posttraumatic stress disorder: neurobiology and pharmacotherapy. CNS Spectrums 3:43–51, 1998

Cornelius JR, Salloum IM, Ehler JG, et al: Fluoxetine in depressed alcoholics: a double-blind, placebo-controlled trial [see comments]. Arch Gen Psychiatry 54:700–705, 1997

Cottler LB, Compton WM 3rd, Mager D, et al: Posttraumatic stress disorder among substance users from the general population. Am J Psychiatry 149:664–670, 1992

Dansky BS, Brady KT, Saladin ME: Untreated symptoms of PTSD among cocaine dependent individuals: changes over time. J Subst Abuse 15:1–6, 1998

Dansky BS, Brady KT, Roberts JT: Post-traumatic stress disorder and substance abuse: empirical findings and clinical issues. Substance Abuse 15:247–257, 1994

Dansky BS, Saladin ME, Brady KT, et al: Prevalence of victimization and posttraumatic stress disorder among women with substance use disorders: comparison of telephone and in-person assessment samples. International Journal of the Addictions 30:1079–1099, 1995

Dansky BS, Roitzsch JC, Brady KT, et al: Posttraumatic stress disorder and substance abuse: use of research in a clinical setting. J Trauma Stress 10:141–148, 1997

Davidson JR, Hughes D, Blazer DG, et al: Post-traumatic stress disorder in the community: an epidemiological study. Psychol Med 21:713–721, 1991

Deykin EY, Buka SL: Prevalence and risk factors for posttraumatic stress disorder among chemically dependent adolescents. Am J Psychiatry 154:752–757, 1997

Dunne FJ, Galatopoulos C, Schipperheijn JM: Gender differences in psychiatric morbidity among alcohol misusers. Compr Psychiatry 34:95–101, 1993

Eberle PA: Alcohol abusers and non-users: a discriminant analysis of differences between two subgroups of batterers. J Health Soc Behav 23:260–271, 1982

Fergusson DM, Lynskey MT, Horwood LJ: Origins of comorbidity between conduct and affective disorders. J Am Acad Child Adolesc Psychiatry 35:451–460, 1996

Foa EB, Rothbaum BO: Treating the Trauma of Rape: Cognitive-Behavioral Therapy for PTSD. New York, Guilford, 1998

Friedman MJ: Current and future drug treatment for posttraumatic stress disorder patients. Psychiatric Annals 28:461–468, 1998

Grant BF, Harford TC, Dawson DA, et al: Prevalence of DSM-IV alcohol abuse and dependence. Alcohol Health Res World 18:243–248, 1994

Grant SJ, Redmond DE Jr: The neuroanatomy and pharmacology of the nucleus locus coeruleus. Prog Clin Biol Res 71:5–27, 1981

Grice DE, Brady KT, Dustan LR, et al: Sexual and physical assault history and post-traumatic stress disorder in substance-dependent individuals. Am J Addict 4:1–9, 1995

Helzer JE, Robins LN, McEvoy L: Post-traumatic stress disorder in the general population: findings of the Epidemiologic Catchment Area survey. N Engl J Med 317:1630–1634, 1987

Hensman R, Guimaraes FS, Wang M, et al: Effects of ritanserin on aversive classical conditioning in humans. Psychopharmacology 104:220–224, 1991

Keller MB, Kocsis JH, McCullough JP, et al: Sertraline maintenance therapy in chronic depression (NR417), in 1996 New Research Program and Abstracts, American Psychiatric Association 149th Annual Meeting, New York, May 4–9, 1996. Washington, DC, American Psychiatric Association, 1996, p 181

Kessler RC, McGonagle KA, Zhao S, et al: Lifetime and 12-month prevalence of DSM-III-R psychiatric disorders in the United States: results from the National Comorbidity Survey. Arch Gen Psychiatry 51:8–19, 1994

Kessler RC, Sonnega A, Bromet E, et al: Posttraumatic stress disorder in the National Comorbidity Survey. Arch Gen Psychiatry 52:1048–1060, 1995

Kessler RC, Crum RM, Warner LA, et al: Lifetime co-occurrence of DSM-III-R alcohol abuse and dependence with other psychiatric disorders in the National Comorbidity Survey. Arch Gen Psychiatry 54:313–321, 1997

Kilpatrick DG, Best CL, Veronen LJ, et al: Mental health correlates of criminal victimization: a random community survey. J Consult Clin Psychol 53:866–873, 1985

Kilpatrick DG, Acierno R, Resnick HS, et al: A 2-year longitudinal analysis of the relationships between violent assault and substance use in women. J Consult Clin Psychol 65:834–837, 1997

Koop CE, Lundberg GB: Violence in America: a public health emergency: time to bite the bullet back (editorial) [see comments] [published errata appear in JAMA 268:3074, 1992, and 271:1404, 1994]. JAMA 267:3075–3076, 1992

Kosten TR, Krystal J: Biological mechanisms in posttraumatic stress disorder: relevance for substance abuse. Recent Dev Alcohol 6:49–68, 1988

Ladwig GB, Andersen MD: Substance abuse in women: relationship between chemical dependency of women and past reports of physical and/or sexual abuse. International Journal of the Addictions 24:739–754, 1989

Leonard KE, Senchak M: Prospective prediction of husband marital aggression within newlywed couples. J Abnorm Psychol 105:369–380, 1996

Luthar SS, Cushing G, Rounsaville BJ: Gender differences among opioid abusers: pathways to disorder and profiles of psychopathology. Drug Alcohol Depend 43:179–189, 1996

McLeer SV, Anwar R: A study of battered women presenting in an emergency department. Am J Public Health 79:65–66, 1989

Miller BA, Downs WR, Gondoli DM, et al: The role of childhood sexual abuse in the development of alcoholism in women. Violence Vict 2:157–172, 1987

Miller BA, Downs WR, Testa M: Interrelationships between victimization experiences and women's alcohol use. J Stud Alcohol Suppl 11:109–117, 1993

Miller TW, Veltkamp LJ: The adult nonsurvivor of child abuse. J Ky Med Assoc 87:120–124, 1989

Nace EP: Posttraumatic stress disorder and substance abuse: clinical issues. Recent Dev Alcohol 6:9–26, 1988

Najavits LM, Weiss RD, Shaw SR, et al: "Seeking safety": outcome of a new cognitive-behavioral psychotherapy for women with posttraumatic stress disorder and substance dependence. J Trauma Stress 11:437–456, 1998

Norris FH: Epidemiology of trauma: frequency and impact of different potentially traumatic events on different demographic groups. J Consult Clin Psychol 60:409–418, 1992

Piazza PV, Le Moal M: Stress as a factor in addiction, in Principles of Addiction Medicine. Edited by Graham AW, Schultz TK. Chevy Chase, MD, American Society of Addiction Medicine, 1998, pp 83–95

Pitman RK, Altman B, Greenwald E, et al: Psychiatric complications during flooding therapy for posttraumatic stress disorder. J Clin Psychiatry 52:17–20, 1991

Pribor EF, Yutzy SH, Dean JT, et al: Briquet's syndrome, dissociation, and abuse. Am J Psychiatry 150:1507–1511, 1993

Redmond DE Jr, Krystal JH: Multiple mechanisms of withdrawal from opioid drugs. Annu Rev Neurosci 7:443–478, 1984

Regier DA, Farmer ME, Rae DS, et al: Comorbidity of mental disorders with alcohol and other drug abuse. JAMA 264:2511–2518, 1990

Resnick HS, Kilpatrick DG, Dansky BS, et al: Prevalence of civilian trauma and posttraumatic stress disorder in a representative national sample of women. J Consult Clin Psychol 61:984–991, 1993

Ritz M, Cohen E, Kuhar M: Cocaine inhibition of ligand binding at dopamine, norepinephrine and serotonin transporters: a structure-activity study. Life Sci 46:635–645, 1990

Rohsenow DJ, Corbett R, Devine D: Molested as children: a hidden contribution to substance abuse? [published erratum appears in J Subst Abuse Treat 5:129, 1988]. J Subst Abuse Treat 5:13–18, 1988

Schnitt JM, Nocks JJ: Alcoholism treatment of Vietnam veterans with posttraumatic stress disorder. J Subst Abuse Treat 1:179–189, 1984

Sellers EM, Higgins GA, Sobell MB: 5-HT and alcohol abuse. Trends Pharmacol Sci 13:69–75, 1992

Triffleman EG, Marmar CR, Delucchi KL, et al: Childhood trauma and posttraumatic stress disorder in substance abuse patients. J Nerv Ment Dis 183:172–176, 1995

Walker EA, Katon WJ, Neraas K, et al: Dissociation in women with chronic pelvic pain [see comments]. Am J Psychiatry 149:534–537, 1992

Wasserman DA, Havassy BE, Boles SM: Traumatic events and post-traumatic stress disorder in cocaine users entering private treatment. Drug Alcohol Depend 46:1–8, 1997

Weisner C, Schmidt L: Gender disparities in treatment for alcohol problems. JAMA 268:1872–1876, 1992

Wolfe J, Kimerling R: Gender issues and assessment of posttraumatic stress disorder, in Assessing Psychological Trauma and PTSD. Edited by Wilson JP, Keane TM. New York, Guilford, 1997, pp 78–91

Zacker J, Bard M: Further findings on assaultiveness and alcohol use in interpersonal disputes. Am J Community Psychol 5:373–383, 1977

21

Sex Differences in Substance Use Disorders

Shelly F. Greenfield, M.D., M.P.H.
Grace O'Leary, M.D.

Recent studies have declared substance abuse and dependence a growing health problem among women in the United States (Center on Addiction and Substance Abuse at Columbia University 1996), including increasing prevalence of substance use disorders, more severe health consequences of substance abuse, and lower rates of treatment utilization. In this chapter, we review the current literature on sex differences in the epidemiology,

This work was supported by grants DA 00407 (S.F.G.), DA 07252 (S.F.G.), and DA 09400 (S.F.G.) from the National Institute on Drug Abuse; grants AA 09881 (S.F.G.) and AA 11756 (S.F.G.) from the National Institute on Alcohol Abuse and Alcoholism; and the Dr. Ralph and Marian C. Falk Research Trust (S.F.G. and G.O.).

Portions of this chapter are based on Greenfield SF: "Women and Substance Use Disorders," in *Psychopharmacology and Women*. Edited by Jensvold MP, Halbreich U, Hamilton JA. Washington, DC, American Psychiatric Press, 1996; and Greenfield SF, O'Leary G: "Sex Differences in Marijuana Use in the United States." *Harvard Review of Psychiatry* (in press).

The authors wish to thank Dawn Sugarman, B.S., for her help with preparation of this chapter.

course of illness, medical consequences, psychiatric comorbidity, and treatment outcome for alcohol, cocaine, opioids, marijuana, and tobacco.

ALCOHOL

Epidemiology

In 1994, the National Comorbidity Survey (NCS), a population-based survey of psychiatric disorders in the United States, reported a 14.1% prevalence of lifetime alcohol use disorders (Kessler et al. 1994). The lifetime prevalence was 20.1% for males and 8.2% for females, yielding a male-to-female ratio of lifetime prevalence of alcohol use disorders in the United States of approximately 2.5:1. In contrast, an earlier population-based survey, the Epidemiologic Catchment Area (ECA) survey (Helzer et al. 1991), reported a similar lifetime prevalence of alcohol use disorders of 13.6% but cited a male-to-female ratio of lifetime alcohol use disorders of 5:1. There are two possible explanations for this disparity between the two surveys. One is that certain methodological differences contributed to the greater male-to-female ratio in the ECA survey. Alternatively, the prevalence of these disorders in women may truly have increased relative to men, thereby decreasing the sex gap in alcohol-related disorders. It is likely that both of these factors contributed to the disparity between the NCS and ECA estimates of prevalence.

The results of a third epidemiologic study conducted in the early 1990s yielded a ratio similar to that of the NCS. In the National Longitudinal Alcohol Epidemiologic Survey (NLAES), which took place in 1992 (Grant et al. 1994), direct face-to-face interviews were conducted with 42,862 respondents age 18 years or older who resided in the community in the 48 contiguous states and the District of Columbia. This study found that 13.3% of all respondents had a lifetime history of alcohol dependence, with 18.6% prevalence among men and 8.4% prevalence among women, yielding a male-to-female ratio of 2.2:1 (Grant et al. 1997).

Although the lifetime prevalence of alcohol abuse and dependence is greater in men than in women, women with alcohol dependence appear to be at greater risk for death than are men with alcohol dependence when each is compared with a same-sex, nonalcoholic population (Gomberg 1989; Kilbey and Sobeck 1988). In addition, women appear to advance more rapidly from initial onset of problem drinking to the development of adverse medical consequences than do men (Ashley et al. 1977; Crawford and Ryder 1986; Orford and Keddie 1985; Piazza et al. 1989; Smith et al. 1983).

In one prospective study of 100 alcohol-dependent women admitted to psychiatric hospitals, 31% of the sample were deceased at 11-year follow-up, which was four times as many deaths as expected in the general population. Most of these women died of alcohol-related causes, and their life spans were shortened by an average of 15 years (Smith et al. 1983). These mortality rates are similar to those in a 20-year follow-up study of 4,872 male and female hospitalized alcoholic patients in Stockholm, Sweden, which found that when compared with the general population, alcoholic women had a fivefold greater risk of death, whereas alcoholic men had a threefold risk of death (Lindberg and Agren 1988).

Sex differences in predictors of mortality were reported by Lewis et al. (1995) in a 20-year follow-up study of 156 male and 193 female alcoholic patients admitted to a public or private psychiatric hospital. For alcohol-dependent men and women, marital status, liver cirrhosis, delirium tremens (DTs), and comorbidity other than antisocial personality disorder were independent predictors of death at 20-year follow-up. When these factors were analyzed by sex, marital disruption was a stronger predictor of mortality in men, and DTs were a stronger predictor of mortality in women. In addition, a comorbid diagnosis of depression lowered the mortality rate in alcohol-dependent women more than in alcohol-dependent men. Increased contact with mental health professionals after discharge from the inpatient facility was thought to contribute to the longer time to death in the dually diagnosed women.

Evidence shows that alcohol dependence has increased among younger members of the population, with the greatest increases among women (Penniman and Agnew 1989; Reich et al. 1988). Since 1961, the percentage of females who initiated alcohol use between ages 10 and 14 years increased more than fourfold—from 7.0% in 1961 to 30.9% in 1995 (Substance Abuse and Mental Health Services Administration 1998). The percentage of males who initiated alcohol use between ages 10 and 14 years also increased but less dramatically—from 20.2% to 35.4%. In the 2000 National Household Survey on Drug Abuse (NHSDA), the percentage of males ages 18 and older who reported any alcohol use in the past month was greater than for females in the same age group (Substance Abuse and Mental Health Services Administration 2001). However, in the youngest age group, 12- to 17-year-olds, the percentages of females and males who had used alcohol in the past month were essentially equivalent (no statistically significant difference): 16.5% of females and 16.2% of males reported past-month use. These data suggest that the numbers of very young female alcohol initiates are growing, and their numbers soon may equal those of young males. Because of women's heightened vulnerability to alcohol and more rapid development of adverse consequences, the decreasing age at initiation of alcohol use among girls is particularly disturbing.

Course of Illness

Several studies have found sex differences in the course of illness of alcohol use disorders (Beckman and Amaro 1986; Crawford and Ryder 1986; Hesselbrock et al. 1982; Lex 1991; Orford and Keddie 1985; Parrella and Filstead 1988; Schuckit et al. 1998; Wanberg and Horn 1970). In the 1970s and 1980s, studies indicated that women began to drink and to develop alcohol problems at a later age than did men (Beckman and Amaro 1986; Crawford and Ryder 1986; Hesselbrock et al. 1982; Lex 1991; Orford and Keddie 1985; Parrella and Filstead 1988; Wanberg and Horn 1970). For example, in a 1988 study of 1,940 alcoholic men and women, women were significantly older when regular drunkenness began, when they realized that alcohol gave relief from withdrawal symptoms, when their alcohol problem was identified by a significant other, and when they first tried to stop drinking (Parrella and Filstead 1988). For each age at first occurrence of drinking problems, women were significantly older; men met any of five different criteria, on average, between ages 28 and 34, whereas women met these same criteria between ages 34 and 42 (Parrella and Filstead 1988).

Compared with alcohol-dependent men, women are also thought to drink smaller quantities (Beckman and Amaro 1986; Schuckit et al. 1998; Wanberg and Horn 1970), to drink alone more often (Lex 1992), and to have more regular drinking patterns with less frequent binge drinking (Parrella and Filstead 1988). Even though women consume less alcohol than men do in general, they are also more likely to progress more rapidly from onset of drinking to the late stages of alcohol dependence, with its associated severe medical sequelae—the so-called telescoping course of illness (Piazza et al. 1989).

A study (Randall et al. 1999) of 1,307 men and 419 women with alcohol dependence demonstrated that women generally began getting drunk regularly (26.6 vs. 22.7 years, $P \leq 0.001$), began experiencing their first drinking problems (27.5 vs. 25.0 years, $P \leq 0.001$), and exhibited loss of control over their drinking (29.8 vs. 27.2 years, $P \leq 0.001$) at a later average age than men. However, these sex differences were more pronounced for older than for younger individuals. In addition, in this study, as in the earlier study by Piazza et al. (1989), women exhibited a telescoping course of illness, progressing more rapidly than men between first getting drunk regularly and first developing drinking problems (0.9 vs. 2.3 years, $P \leq 0.001$) and between first loss of control over their drinking and onset of worst drinking problems (5.5 vs. 7.8 years, $P \leq 0.001$). The interval between first regular drunkenness and first seeking treatment was similarly shorter for women than for men (11.6 vs. 15.8 years, $P \leq 0.001$).

Because of this accelerated course, it is of particular concern that epidemiological data from the 1990s indicate that a greater proportion of females are initiating their alcohol use at even younger ages (Substance Abuse and Mental Health Services Administration 1998). This raises the possibility that now and in the future, women may present themselves with the adverse consequences of alcohol abuse and dependence at earlier ages than in previous decades.

Some evidence indicates that certain adverse consequences of alcohol consumption may be disproportionately increasing in women compared with men. For example, a study by Popkin et al. (1988) reported that negative consequences of alcohol use, such as accidents and arrests from drunk driving, may be disproportionately greater in women than in men. During the 1980s, males constituted the majority of convicted drunk drivers (Yu et al. 1992). Women offenders, however, increased sharply from 9% in 1980 to a steady 13% by the middle and late 1980s. The Centers for Disease Control (1992) reported that the estimated alcohol involvement rate in fatal automobile crashes from 1982 to 1989 declined for both males and females, but the decline for male drivers (21%) was greater than that for female drivers (8%). Possible explanations for these changing trends offered by the authors of both studies (Centers for Disease Control 1992; Yu et al. 1992) included the increased acceptability of women as alcohol drinkers and as automobile drivers as well as the drunk-driving prevention programs that have targeted male drivers more than female drivers.

Sex differences also may exist in the psychosocial correlates of alcohol dependence. In one study of 50 alcoholic women, employment status, number of children, and parental alcohol use had the strongest relation with length of time from first intoxication to loss of control over drinking (Fortin and Evans 1983). A separate study found that employment within or outside the home did not predict outcome for alcoholic women but that women working within the home drank more at baseline (Herr and Pettinati 1984).

Several studies have found that childhood histories of experienced or witnessed domestic violence are correlated with adulthood alcohol use disorders and poorer treatment outcomes in women (Haver 1987; Hurley 1991; Miller et al. 1987; Root 1989). Of 117 alcoholic women subjects sampled from Alcoholics Anonymous, 28% reported childhood incest histories, as compared with estimated rates between 5% and 15% in the general population (Burnham et al. 1988; Winfield et al. 1990). These women were more likely than those without the incest history to have drinking problems at an earlier age and higher levels of anxiety (Kovach 1986). Women with these histories may represent a large subgroup with worse outcomes (Root 1989).

Investigators have examined female-specific factors, such as the phase of a woman's menstrual cycle, and alcohol intake (Allen 1996; Griffin et al. 1987; Lex et al. 1989; Mello et al. 1990). In one prospective inpatient study of 14 women, increased drinking during the premenstruum was associated with higher scores on the Premenstrual Assessment Form (Mello et al. 1990). A retrospective study conducted by Allen (1996) of 48 women attending a treatment center for alcoholic patients in England yielded similar results. Sixteen (one-third) of the women admitted to increased alcohol consumption premenstrually and had higher scores on the Premenstrual Assessment Form than did those women who did not increase their alcohol consumption premenstrually. A study of alcohol use across the menstrual cycle among marijuana users found that in the absence of severe premenstrual distress, menstrual cycle phase is not a good predictor of alcohol use among female social drinkers (Griffin et al. 1987).

Medical Consequences

Alcohol is metabolized differently by men and women (Frezza et al. 1990; Van Thiel and Gavaler 1988). Alcohol is water soluble and is metabolized primarily by alcohol dehydrogenase in the liver and gastric mucosa. After drinking comparable amounts of alcohol, women have been noted to have higher blood alcohol concentrations than men, even with allowance for differences in size and body weight (Jones and Jones 1976), although some evidence contradicts this (Goldstein 1992). Explanations for women's higher blood alcohol levels include smaller total volume of distribution in women (Marshall et al. 1983), decreased alcohol metabolism by the gastric mucosa in women (so-called first-pass metabolism) (Ammon et al. 1996; Frezza et al. 1990), and influence of hormones such as estrogen (Van Thiel and Gavaler 1988). These may be some of the same mechanisms that account for the increased vulnerability of women to alcoholic liver disease (Morgan and Sherlock 1977). When compared with men, women consume smaller quantities of alcohol or consume excessive quantities for shorter periods, but they are nevertheless twice as likely to develop cirrhosis of the liver (Lex 1991). Two studies reported a similar prevalence of cardiomyopathy in male and female alcoholic patients (Fernández-Solà et al. 1997; Urbano-Márquez et al. 1995). Women, however, developed cardiomyopathy with a lower total lifetime dose of ethanol than did men with the same disease. Similarly, although alcoholic women show a pattern of cognitive impairment similar to that of men, this occurs after a markedly shorter period of drinking smaller quantities of alcohol (Crawford and Ryder 1986).

A review of the literature between 1980 and 1996 on the medical risks of women who drink alcohol demonstrated that women develop many alcohol-related problems at lower levels of consumption than men (Bradley 1998). Breast cancer and mortality appear to be increased among women who report drinking more than two drinks daily, and higher levels of alcohol consumption by women are associated with increased menstrual symptoms, hypertension, and stroke (Bradley 1998).

Alcohol dependence is associated with severe disruption in reproductive function in men, such as impotence, low testosterone levels, testicular atrophy, gynecomastia, and diminished sexual interest (Lex 1991). Similarly, alcoholism in women is associated with amenorrhea, anovulation, and luteal phase dysfunction and also may increase the risk of early menopause (Lex 1991).

Effects of Alcohol on Pregnancy and Neonates

Fetal alcohol syndrome (FAS) is the most well-defined and well-established adverse effect of alcohol on the developing fetus. In 1973, Jones et al. first described several congenital abnormalities in infants born to women who abused alcohol during pregnancy. These abnormalities included delayed prenatal and postnatal growth, microcephaly, short palpebral fissures, epicanthic folds, maxillary hypoplasia, abnormal palmar creases, cardiac anomalies, and capillary hemangiomas. FAS occurs in 33% of the infants born to women who drink more than 150 g/day of alcohol during pregnancy (approximately 10 beers or the equivalent per day), another 33% of the infants without clear FAS are mentally retarded, and the perinatal mortality rate is 17% (Greenfield et al. 1997).

Other possible effects of alcohol on the outcome of pregnancy remain controversial. Several studies have reported an increase in spontaneous abortion (Kline et al. 1980; Windham et al. 1997) and low birthweight (Lazzaroni et al. 1993), but other studies have found weak (Faden and Graubard 1994) or no associations (Cavallo et al. 1995; Savitz et al. 1992) between alcohol consumption and these outcomes.

Psychiatric Comorbidity

Some studies have reported sex differences in the co-occurrence of psychiatric disorders in alcohol-dependent patients. For example, women with alcohol use disorders have been found to have concurrent mood (Cornelius et al. 1995; Hesselbrock et al. 1985; Rounsaville et al. 1987; Weiss et al. 1993), anxiety (Cornelius et al. 1995; Ross et al. 1988; Weiss et al. 1993), eating, and psychosexual disorders (Ross et al. 1988) more frequently than do men. Men more frequently have concurrent antisocial personality disorder (Cornelius et al. 1995; M.N. Hesselbrock et al. 1985; V.M. Hesselbrock et al. 1986; Rounsaville et al. 1987; Weiss et al. 1993).

However, evidence is inconsistent about the course and prognostic significance of concurrent psychiatric diagnoses and symptoms for alcohol-dependent men and women. In the early 1980s, two prospective studies of treatment-seeking alcohol-dependent men and women found that depressive symptoms were correlated with poorer prognoses in both women and men (Finney et al. 1980; Pettinati et al. 1982). However, more recent research has found that depressive symptoms in and of themselves are not predictive of poor drinking outcomes; rather, a concurrent or lifetime diagnosis of depression may be correlated with drinking outcomes. For example, a prospective study of treatment-seeking men and women with alcohol dependence found that a lifetime diagnosis of depression predicted a poor prognosis in men compared with nondepressed men and a better prognosis in women when compared with nondepressed women, whereas antisocial personality and drug abuse predicted poor outcomes in both (Rounsaville et al. 1987). However, at the 3-year follow-up of this cohort, both men and women who had a lifetime diagnosis of major depression at baseline had improved drinking outcomes compared with those without this history (Kranzler et al. 1996).

A more recent study by Greenfield et al. (1998) found that a current diagnosis of major depression was significantly related to time to first drink and time to relapse in alcohol-dependent men and women in the year following inpatient detoxification. The authors hypothesized that the difference between their findings and those of the Rounsaville and Kranzler groups might have resulted from their use of *current* diagnosis of depression rather than the *lifetime* diagnosis used in the previous studies. They also pointed out that their results were consistent with those of the National Institute of Mental Health–funded 5-year longitudinal study of depression (Hasin et al. 1996) as well as promising results of several small clinical trials of antidepressant treatment of concurrent depression and alcohol dependence (Mason et al. 1996; McGrath et al. 1996).

Fewer studies have reported on the prognostic effect of anxiety symptoms and diagnoses on the course of alcohol dependence. A study by Schuckit et al. (1990) showed the course and importance of anxiety symptoms in alcohol-dependent patients, but this study used an all-male sample and could not assess the importance of these symptoms in women.

Other substance use disorders have a significant correlation with the diagnosis of alcohol abuse or dependence. According to the ECA survey, 47.3% of the individuals with alcohol abuse or dependence in the community will in the course of their lifetime have a diagnosis of another drug dependence (Regier et al. 1990). In the United States, alcohol dependence thereby confers a sevenfold increased risk of other drug dependence. Of those individuals with alcohol dependence who are seen in alcohol, drug, or mental health treatment settings, 34% will have met criteria for another drug disorder in the 6 months before treatment (Glassman et al. 1990).

With respect to sex, alcohol dependence increases the risk of drug abuse and dependence in women more than in men (Robins and Regier 1991). The NCS (Kessler et al. 1997) reported that more females with the diagnosis of alcohol dependence had a lifetime co-occurrence of substance use disorder than did men (47.1% vs. 40.6%, respectively). According to Weisner (1993), however, important questions remain regarding the role of gender in the prevalence and natural histories of comorbid alcohol and drug dependence. In her comprehensive study of 685 individuals in all alcohol and drug treatment programs in one northern California county, Weisner (1993) found important distinctions between the women being treated in alcohol programs and the women in drug treatment. Women in drug treatment reported more criminal behavior than did women in alcohol treatment, and women in alcohol treatment reported heavier drinking and attributed their difficulties to their comorbid drug dependence more frequently than did women in drug treatment. The study also found that the differences between the women in the two treatment systems were greater than the differences between men and women within each system (Weisner 1993). These findings suggest that caution should be used in making assumptions about the homogeneity of women with alcohol and drug use disorders and that greater information is needed about the diversity of this population.

Treatment Outcome

Outcome studies of alcohol dependence treatment are limited (Finney and Moos 1986), frequently because of multiple methodological problems, including lack of randomization and control groups, lack of prospective design, and lack of adequate outcome measures and follow-up (Goldstein et al. 1984). Many of these studies have used all male samples (Kilbey and Sobeck 1988), and information on sex differences in treatment outcome is, therefore, even more limited.

Potentially significant predictors of recovery in men are 1) engagement in a continuing care program, 2) ongoing counseling, 3) use of self-help groups, 4) crisis intervention, and 5) use of family treatment (Mumme 1991). Vaillant et al. (1983) described four additional factors that may be important in men's recovery from alcohol dependence: 1) a positive substitute dependence (such as involvement in religion, exercise, or a hobby), 2) external reminders that alcohol is aversive, 3) increased unambiguous social support, and 4) a source of inspiration, hope, or enhanced self-esteem. It is not clear whether these same factors enhance recovery in women.

Women use alcohol treatment services less frequently than men do (Duckert 1987; Weisner and Schmidt 1992) but are more likely to seek treatment for marital problems, physical illness, and emotional problems (Duckert 1987). This underuse of alcohol treatment by women may be due to women's perception of society's harsher judgment of alcohol dependence (Sandmeier 1980); perception of greater social costs of treatment (Beckman and Amaro 1986); deficient training of health care, social service, and law enforcement professionals in identification and referral of women with alcoholism (Kilbey and Sobeck 1988); and lower utilization of services by women for disorders considered incongruous with sex-role stereotypes (Beckman and Amaro 1984). In one study by Thom (1986), women were more likely than men to believe that alcohol treatment was appropriate for those who drank for the sake of drinking. However, these same women described their own drinking as a legitimate response to their personal problems and therefore thought that they did not need specific alcohol treatment.

In their follow-up study of 592 persons with alcoholism (412 males and 180 females) discharged from a treatment program lasting 22–30 days, Schneider et al. (1995b) noted a sex difference in inpatient treatment outcome. Women who stayed for the full 30-day treatment program had higher relapse rates than did men who remained in treatment for the same length of time. The authors commented that the women who stayed for the full treatment may have felt less confident about their ability to remain sober after discharge and therefore remained longer. Additionally, the program's focus on group rather than individual therapy may not have served the treatment needs of the women as well and may have contributed to relapse after discharge.

In one treatment outcome study of 112 men and women in a community treatment center staffed by volunteers, women were more likely than men to drop out of treatment after the first visit (35% vs. 21%); no women were still attending the clinic 6 months later (Allan and Phil 1987). One explanation given by the investigators for this discrepancy was that self-referred patients dropped out of treatment more frequently than did patients who were referred by shelters, employers, or the courts. In this study's sample, more women than men were self-referred, and more men than women were referred by "coercive sources" (i.e., employers, shelters, or the courts).

In a more recent study of 41 men and 41 women with DSM-IV (American Psychiatric Association) alcohol dependence admitted for inpatient alcohol detoxification, assessments of subjects were performed at baseline and at 12 weeks after discharge. The women in this study were more likely to be in a higher social class, drink fewer units of alcohol in a typical week, and have a higher level of psychiatric symptoms than the men. However, no significant sex differences were found in relapse rates or in time taken to relapse (Foster et al. 2000). These results are similar to those of an earlier study of 60 men and 41 women with alcohol dependence who were followed for 1 year after discharge from inpatient alcohol dependence treatment (Greenfield et al. 1998). In this study as well there were no significant sex differences in relapse rates or in time to relapse in the year following discharge from inpatient treatment.

One important predictor of poor treatment outcome is a history of childhood or recent sexual or physical assault, which appears to be more prevalent in women than in men (Haver 1987; Hurley 1991; Miller et al. 1987; Root 1989; Thom 1986). According to Thom (1986), more women than men in her sample reported having been physically assaulted in the year before treatment. In a multiple regression analysis of predictors of outcome in 44 Norwegian alcoholic women, Haver (1987) found that 11% of the variance in outcome was explained by childhood violence; an additional 14% was explained by having a violent partner; and another 9% was explained by having a concurrent personality disorder. The likelihood of having a violent partner and having a concurrent personality disorder was increased in those with childhood exposure to violence. Therefore, fully 34% of the variance in outcome in these 44 alcoholic women may have been explained by the direct and indirect effects of childhood exposure to violence. These results are supported by other studies (Hurley 1991; Miller et al. 1987; Root 1989).

Duckert (1987) found that treatment programs for women had improvement rates that ranged from 20% to 60%, but it is unclear whether specific women's treatment programs have a greater success rate than traditional programs that treat men and women together. Some authors suggested that women might do better within same-sex treatment groups (Lex 1992) and that alcoholic women would benefit most from interactions with women staff members and other recovering women whom they might identify as role models (Connor and Babcock 1980). According to Underhill (1994), because of the social stigma associated with women's alcohol problems, alcoholic women tend to have decreased self-esteem, thus making confrontational techniques in individual and group therapy settings less likely to be productive. These and other issues of treatment techniques and efficacy deserve additional consideration and evaluation.

In spite of these issues, there are several clear guidelines in the evaluation and treatment of alcohol-dependent women. Women who seek treatment for alcohol dependence are often in a poor state of health and require a complete review of their physical health status as well as assessment of their family, work, and social environment (Popour 1983). Kilbey and

Sobeck (1988) recommend a complete physical evaluation, including 1) physical examination, vital signs, and appropriate blood chemistries; 2) assessment of obstetrical and gynecological status, including hormonal status, yearly Papanicolaou's test, breast examination and instruction in breast self-examination, and contraception; 3) review of HIV risk factors; 4) evaluation of psychiatric status, including other co-occurring diagnoses and suicidality; and 5) assessment of neuropsychiatric function. In addition, given the high prevalence of histories of childhood sexual abuse and later sexual assault in this population, it is important to assess the presence of these factors in each woman's history (Underhill 1994). Conversely, because more women with alcohol problems are seen in nonalcohol treatment settings, physical and mental health caregivers who see women must take a careful alcohol history from all of their patients and must be prepared to refer these patients to appropriate treatment settings when needed.

Greenfield et al. (1998) highlighted the importance of antidepressant treatment in alcohol-dependent populations in their naturalistic study of the effect of depression on return to drinking. Although the diagnosis of current major depression predicted a shorter time to first drink and first relapse in all alcohol-dependent patients admitted to an inpatient facility, those who were depressed and were discharged with antidepressant medications had a longer time to relapse than their untreated counterparts. Subjects who were depressed and received no pharmacological treatment had all relapsed by 100 days after discharge, whereas 20% of the antidepressant-treated subjects remained abstinent 1 year after inpatient admission. These findings are similar to those of two earlier pharmacotherapy studies (Mason et al. 1996; McGrath et al. 1996); these studies reported improvement in depression and in relapse risk in alcohol-dependent subjects with depression treated with tricyclic antidepressants. Although sex differences associated with antidepressant treatment and subsequent relapse have not been cited, these studies underscore the importance of detecting depression in alcohol-dependent men and women in order to provide appropriate treatment that may help prevent future relapses.

Finally, several pharmacological agents have been shown to be efficacious in the treatment of alcohol use disorders. Disulfiram (Wright and Moore 1990), naltrexone (Davidson et al. 1996; O'Malley et al. 1992; Volpicelli et al. 1992), and most recently acamprosate (Wilde and Wagstaff 1997) have been effective as adjunctive treatments to other modalities such as psychotherapies or group treatment. To date, no studies have specifically examined sex differences in treatment outcome with these agents.

COCAINE

Epidemiology

Cocaine, or benzoylmethylecgonine, is an alkaloid derived from the coca plant, *Erythroxylon coca*. In the United States, the most common routes of administration are intranasal "snorting" of cocaine hydrochloride, intravenous administration of cocaine hydrochloride dissolved in water, and smoking of alkaloidal cocaine, known as "freebase" or "crack."

The 1996 NHSDA (Substance Abuse and Mental Health Services Administration 1998) reported that 10.3% (12.8% males and 8.0% females) of the population aged 12 and older had lifetime cocaine use. Lifetime crack use was reported by 2.2% of the population aged 12 and older (2.8% of males and 1.6% of females). For all adults aged 18 and older, lifetime cocaine and crack use by men exceeded lifetime cocaine and crack use by women. However, this trend was reversed in the youngest cohort of 12- to 17-year-olds.

An analysis of the relationship between sex and age groups reporting cocaine use was included in the 1997 NHSDA (Substance Abuse and Mental Health Services Administration 1999). This survey reported that 10.5% (13.2% males and 7.9% females) of the population age 12 or older had lifetime cocaine use. Lifetime crack use was reported by 1.9% of the population age 12 or older (2.5% of males and 1.6% of females). For all adults age 18 or older, lifetime cocaine and crack use by men exceeded that by women. However, this trend was reversed in the youngest cohort, 12- to 17-year-olds. In 1997, 2.7% and 1.1% of males ages 12–17 years reported lifetime cocaine and lifetime crack use, respectively, whereas 3.3% and 1.0% of females ages 12–17 years reported lifetime cocaine and lifetime crack use, respectively.

Interestingly, compared with the 1996 NHSDA data, these results represent a slight increase in lifetime use of cocaine and crack among males and females in the 12–17 age group. In 1996, 1.6% and 0.5% of the males ages 12–17 years reported lifetime cocaine use and lifetime crack use, respectively, whereas 2.3% and 1.0% of the females age 12–17 years reported lifetime cocaine use and lifetime crack use, respectively. The 2000 NHSDA (Substance Abuse and Mental Health Services Administration 2001) reported that 11.2% of the population age 12 years or older reported lifetime cocaine use and that 2.4% reported lifetime crack use. Although sex-specific data are not available for 2000, there has been an overall decrease in the percentage of people age 12 years and older reporting lifetime cocaine and crack use. In 1999, of the population age 12 years or older, 11.5% reported lifetime cocaine use and 2.7% reported lifetime crack use.

This represents a 0.3% decrease for both lifetime cocaine and crack use, suggesting a trend toward a decreased number of people who use this substance. However, the sex-specific findings from 1996 and 1997 suggest that a somewhat greater proportion of females than males in this youngest age cohort have used cocaine and crack. This trend may mean a greater vulnerability of females to increased rates of syphilis, HIV infection, and other sexually transmitted diseases associated with cocaine use (Guinan 1989) at increasingly younger ages.

Course of Illness

The course of illness in cocaine-dependent individuals has been the focus of many research studies. In their study of 153 cocaine-dependent men, Khalsa et al. (1992) found that the mean age at first use was 15 years, and in the year prior to first cocaine use, 33% of the group used marijuana and alcohol. Sixty-nine percent of the men said that their main reason for first cocaine use was curiosity. In this sample of cocaine-dependent men, the average time from first cocaine use to entry into treatment was 11 years.

Sex differences in the course of illness among crack users were examined by Dudish and Hatsukami (1996) in their study of 176 crack smokers (88 men and 88 women) recruited from a community-based sample to participate in a research study on addiction. On average, both men and women first used cocaine at age 24 and currently smoked crack 5 days per week. Women were more likely than men to smoke cigarettes, to have physical problems such as headaches after smoking crack, and to present to emergency departments after smoking crack. Although both men and women reported involvement in the exchange of sex for crack, women traded sex for crack, whereas men traded crack for sex. Criminal activity was prevalent in both men and women, but men were more likely to engage in violent crimes; women frequently reported forgery, shoplifting, and prostitution.

Several researchers have investigated the natural history of cocaine dependence (Griffin et al. 1989; Kosten et al. 1993; McCance-Katz et al. 1999; Weiss et al. 1997). Griffin et al. (1989) found that when compared with men, women had earlier initial use, younger age at first treatment, more rapid development of dependence, more frequent involvement with an addicted partner, poorer social and occupational functioning, more premorbid depression, and slower recovery from depressive symptoms during the first month of abstinence. Women most commonly reported four reasons for initiating drug use: depression, feeling unsociable, family and job pressures, and health problems (Griffin et al. 1989).

McCance-Katz et al. (1999) studied sex differences in 1-year outcomes for 29 female and 65 male cocaine-dependent patients. The researchers found that, compared with the men, the women consumed similar quantities of cocaine, but by more addictive routes, and experienced more rapid progression of drug dependence. This accelerated progression of dependence was also demonstrated in a study of 118 male and 42 female polysubstance-abusing individuals admitted to two Florida drug court programs (Haas and Peters 2000). In this study, female and male offenders differed in the trajectory of their substance dependence. More specifically, compared with the men, the women began using cocaine earlier in the course of their drug use and reported more problems related to cocaine use and significantly more prior-treatment episodes. They were also found to have a shorter latency from first use of cocaine to cocaine abuse (Haas and Peters 2000).

In their study of 19 women and 53 men who abused cocaine, Kosten et al. (1993) supported some of these findings. Although they found that the women had used cocaine for more years than did the men, this was not statistically significant. Women had histories of more years of heroin use, whereas men used alcohol for more years and had longer periods of abstinence from cocaine. In this study group, a greater proportion of the men's cocaine use was intranasal than was that of the women.

In their recent 6-month follow-up study of 64 male and 37 female treatment seeking cocaine-dependent subjects, Weiss et al. (1997) found that both men and women reported cocaine use for a mean of 9 years. Women were more likely to be single (51.4% vs. 37.5%) and less likely to be employed (51.4% vs. 60.9%) than men. A greater proportion of women than men used cocaine intranasally (56.8% vs. 39.1%), whereas more men than women smoked cocaine (46.9 vs. 32.4%) and used intravenous cocaine (12.5% vs. 10.8%). Additional research investigating sex differences in the natural history of cocaine dependence and examining whether men and women differ with respect to age at initiation of use, time elapsed between first use and dependence, and the process of recovery will extend the findings of these studies.

Medical Consequences

Cocaine exerts direct stimulatory effects on the cerebral cortex and produces feelings of excitation, restlessness, euphoria, decreased social inhibition, increased energy, and enhanced strength and mental ability. It also causes central and peripheral sympathomimetic effects, such as vasoconstriction, tachycardia, increased blood pressure and temperature, and dilated pupils (Greenfield et al. 1997). The half-life of cocaine is approximately 1 hour; the drug is metabolized by plasma and liver cholinesterases to the metabolite benzoylecgonine, which is then excreted into the urine.

No clear information is currently available about sex differences in the metabolism of cocaine, but other sex differences in physiological response to cocaine have been elucidated. For example, Lukas et al. (1996) examined the question of sex-related differences in plasma cocaine levels and subjective effects of cocaine after acute administration. In this study, 14 cocaine users (7 male and 7 female) received an equivalent dose (0.9 mg/kg) of intranasal cocaine. Men achieved higher peak plasma levels and experienced the subjective effects of cocaine more rapidly and more intensely than did women. Among the female subjects, variations within the menstrual cycle also were seen; the follicular phase was associated with higher plasma levels than was the luteal phase, although no significant differences in subjective cocaine effects were associated with cycle phase. Possible explanations offered by the authors for these sex differences included increased viscosity of the nasal mucosa of women during the luteal phase, resulting in decreased cocaine absorption and increased cocaine metabolism by cholinesterases in women. More research is needed to clarify sex differences in plasma levels, metabolism, and subjective effects after cocaine administration.

Many medical complications are associated with cocaine use. Cocaine may adversely affect most organ systems, including the cardiovascular, gastrointestinal, pulmonary, and central nervous systems (Brown et al. 1992; Endress et al. 1992; Perper and Van Thiel 1992; Tannenbaum and Miller 1992). Few studies have investigated sex differences in the effects of cocaine on these organ systems.

A recent study investigated sex differences in the persistent neurochemical changes in the frontal lobes of subjects with a history of crack cocaine dependence (Chang et al. 1999). Using proton magnetic resonance spectroscopy, the researchers compared the frontal gray and white matter of 64 young asymptomatic and abstinent cocaine users with that of 58 healthy, non-drug-using individuals. Interaction effects of cocaine and sex were observed for creatine, N-acetyl/creatine ratio, and myoinositol/creatine ratio in frontal white matter. The authors concluded that cocaine use is associated with neuronal injury and that in the frontal lobe, the effect of cocaine on male users is different from its effect on female users.

Another study found sex-specific differences in the electroencephalograms (EEGs) of 20 currently abstinent cocaine-abusing men and 20 currently abstinent cocaine-abusing women (King et al. 2000). Males had elevated EEG beta and reduced alpha compared with females, suggesting that the EEGs of cocaine-abusing women may be more normal than those of cocaine-abusing men.

Cocaine has sex-specific effects on neuroendocrine function (Mendelson et al. 1988). Men with chronic cocaine abuse have been reported to have impotence and gynecomastia as well as persistent abnormalities in reproductive function, even after cessation of cocaine use (Cocores et al. 1986; Mendelson et al. 1988).

Cocaine-dependent women may manifest derangements in menstrual cycle function, galactorrhea, amenorrhea, and infertility (Cocores et al. 1986; Siegel 1982). One possible factor implicated in these abnormalities in reproductive function is derangement in plasma prolactin levels. One study (Gawin et al. 1985) found decreased plasma prolactin levels in men and women cocaine abusers, whereas three other studies found elevated plasma prolactin levels (Cocores et al. 1986; Dackis and Gold 1985; Mendelson et al. 1988). In one study of 14 men and 2 women with cocaine abuse, 86% of the men and both of the women had hyperprolactinemia at the time of admission (Mendelson et al. 1988). In all of the patients, plasma luteinizing hormone, cortisol, and testosterone levels in the men were within normal limits. Dopaminergic derangements caused by cocaine may be responsible for the selectively elevated prolactin levels in these patients.

Effects of Cocaine on Pregnancy and Neonates

In the 1980s, the concern about the rising number of infants born to women addicted to cocaine—the so-called crack babies—led to numerous stories in the media about the negative fate of these children (Griffith et al. 1994). Many of these stories, however, were based on anecdotal information, and the worst-case scenario was presented as the norm (Lyons and Rittner 1998). However, the issue of multiple toxin exposure, including cigarettes and alcohol, and environmental factors that also may have contributed to the complications seen in infants born to cocaine-addicted mothers were largely ignored (Lyons and Rittner 1998).

Despite the media's focus on the relation between cocaine-dependent women and negative outcomes in their offspring, there is some controversy about the effects of cocaine on the pregnant female, the developing fetus, and the neonate. In some studies, cocaine use during pregnancy has been associated with increased risk of placental abruption (Chasnoff et al. 1987; Dusick et al. 1993; Hulse et al. 1997c; Miller et al. 1995), placenta previa (Macones et al. 1997), premature rupture of membranes (Miller et al. 1995), and premature labor (Chasnoff et al. 1987). Cocaine may have direct stimulatory effects on the uterus, causing it to contract and thereby initiate labor prematurely.

With respect to potential fetal effects, cocaine crosses the placenta and may therefore cause vasoconstriction, increased heart rate, and decreased oxygen levels in the fetus. Some studies have indicated that cocaine causes physiological derangements in uterine blood flow, and this could potentially have an adverse effect on the fetus (Woods et al. 1987).

A study of the level of in utero cocaine exposure and neonatal cranial ultrasound findings compared neonatal ultrasounds from 241 well, full-term infants who were categorized as having no exposure, heavy exposure, or light exposure to cocaine in utero (Frank et al. 1999). The researchers found that the infants with lighter exposure were no different from those with no exposure; however, the infants with heavier exposure were more likely than unexposed infants to show subependymal hemorrhage in the caudothalamic groove. Thus, ultrasound findings suggestive of vascular injury in the neonatal central nervous system may be related to the level of prenatal cocaine exposure (Frank et al. 1999).

Animal models have shown that in utero exposure to cocaine caused cognitive impairment selectively in male rat offspring (Choi et al. 1998a), altered postnatal dopaminergic function in rats (Choi et al. 1998b) and in rabbits (Friedman and Wang 1998; Simansky et al. 1998), persistent behavioral deficits in a blocking paradigm in mice (Kosofsky and Wilkins 1998), impairments in rat brain serotonin (Battaglia et al. 1998), and other findings (Gabriel and Taylor 1998). However, studies of human infants and children who were exposed to cocaine in utero have had conflicting findings. In some studies, infants born to cocaine-using women have had low birthweight (Chiriboga et al. 1993; Hulse et al. 1997b; Slutsker 1992; Sprauve et al. 1997), genitourinary malformations (Chasnoff et al. 1988; Slutsker 1992), and neurological problems such as hypertonia, plantar extension, and coarse tremor (Chiriboga et al. 1993). Other studies have reported no difference in birthweight between infants born to cocaine-using women and control infants (Chasnoff et al. 1987, 1988). Others have found that after adjustments for potential confounders such as tobacco smoking and lack of prenatal care, birthweight did not differ between cocaine-exposed infants and control infants (Hurt et al. 1995; Miller et al. 1995).

One meta-analysis showed no increased developmental risk to the fetus (Koren and Graham 1992) exposed to cocaine in utero. A more recent meta-analysis of the effect of prenatal cocaine exposure on neurobehavioral outcomes found small but statistically significant differences between cocaine-exposed and nonexposed infants at birth and age 4 weeks on standard measures of motor performance and reflexes (Held et al. 1999).

Several longer-term prospective studies of prenatal exposure to cocaine have found several neurobehavioral effects often modified by environment (Chasnoff et al. 1998; Koren et al. 1998). One longitudinal prospective study of 95 children born to mothers who used cocaine and other drugs during pregnancy and 75 matched nonexposed children found that at age 6 years, prenatal exposure to cocaine and other drugs had no direct effect on IQ but had a direct effect on behavior (Chasnoff et al. 1998). In a similar study, teachers blinded to the in utero cocaine exposure status of 116 first graders

The last available household data analyzing the relationship between sex and age groups reporting heroin use is from 1997. The 1997 NHSDA reported that 0.9% of the household population older than 12 years had lifetime heroin use (Substance Abuse and Mental Health Services Administration 1999). This included 1.3% of males and 0.6% of females. Lifetime use was highest and equivalent among 18- to 25-year-olds, 26- to 34-year-olds, and those age 35 years or older (all 1.0%). In all age groups, lifetime use was also higher among those who were unemployed (2.0%) and those who had some college education (1.6%).

In the 2000 NHSDA (Substance Abuse and Mental Health Services Administration 2001), 1.2% of the population older than 12 years reported lifetime heroin use. This percentage represents a decrease from 1999 (Substance Abuse and Mental Health Services Administration 2001), when 1.4% of the population reported lifetime heroin use. Although the overall trend has been toward an increasing number of people reporting heroin use in their lifetimes, the most recent data show that this trend may be reversing itself.

Course of Illness

Studies of the antecedents of opioid dependence indicate that opioid abusers are a heterogeneous group. In their study of 276 male and 87 female opioid-dependent subjects in treatment, Rounsaville et al. (1982b) found three distinct subgroups based on antecedents to opioid dependence: 1) those with childhood trauma whose delinquent activity and drug abuse came only after substantial disruptive childhood events, 2) those with early delinquency whose initial illicit drug abuse came after the onset of regular antisocial and criminal activities, and 3) an initial drug use group for whom criminal activity and disruptive events happened after the initiation of illicit drug use. Men and women were equally represented in all three groups. Other studies have suggested that childhood sexual and physical abuse are highly prevalent among women drug abusers (Ladwig and Andersen 1989; Linn et al. 1983) and that heroin dependence is more often associated with early-life family problems in women than in men (Graeven and Schaef 1978). Sex differences in childhood characteristics of adult opiate users were the focus of a retrospective study of 95 opioid-dependent males and 106 opioid-dependent females by Luthar et al. (1996). They found that male heroin abusers reported more childhood behavior problems such as conduct problems at school, and female heroin users reported more childhood problems with psychological symptoms such as moodiness and anxiety.

Despite the range of possible antecedents to addiction, opioid dependence confers a relatively poor prognosis. In an 11-year follow-up study of a Danish cohort of 203 male and 97 female opioid-dependent subjects, 26% were deceased at 11-year follow-up, 10% had achieved some degree of unstable abstinence, and 24% could be classified as truly recovered (Haastrup and Jepsen 1988). In a similar study, Goldstein and Herrera (1995) performed a 22-year follow-up study of 1,019 heroin-dependent individuals who signed up for methadone maintenance treatment in Albuquerque, New Mexico, in 1969–1971. Thirty-four percent of the subjects were dead at the time of follow-up. A male with heroin dependence was four times as likely and a female with heroin dependence was 6.8 times as likely to die in any given year as a sex-matched non-heroin-dependent resident of New Mexico. Drug overdoses, violence, and chronic alcoholism accounted for most of the deaths; no sex differences were reported for the causes of death in these individuals.

Several sex differences have been found in the initiation of opioid use and development of dependence (Hser et al. 1987). In a study of 567 male and female heroin-dependent subjects in methadone maintenance treatment, Hser et al. (1987) found that initial heroin use by women was highly influenced by a man who was usually a sexual partner and frequently a daily heroin user. Women also were slightly younger than men at first use and were unskilled more often than men. Women most often reported using heroin because their partner used heroin or to decrease pain, whereas men reported initiating heroin use because of curiosity or to gain peer acceptance. Men more frequently had used alcohol and/or marijuana before initiation of narcotic use, but women reported more use of nonnarcotic drugs during the 12 months before treatment. Gossop et al. (1994) reported that, compared with male heroin abusers, women heroin abusers were more likely to be involved in a sexual relationship, to have a partner who was also a drug user, and to be living with another drug user.

Two studies investigated sex differences in the route of heroin administration (Gossop et al. 1994; Powis et al. 1996). In their study of 355 patients attending a London, England, community drug team, Gossop et al. (1994) found that women were less likely than men to use heroin by injection and were more likely to use heroin by inhalation. These findings were supported by Powis et al. (1996), who reported that a greater number of women used heroin via inhalation rather than via injection in a study of 253 male and 155 female heroin users. Among all subjects who used heroin intravenously in this study, female heroin users were more likely to have been given their first injection by a male sexual partner, whereas male heroin users were more likely to have been injected for the first time by a friend.

In a related study of the same population examined by Hser et al. (1987), Anglin et al. (1987a) found that although 25% of the subjects reported becoming addicted within 1 month after first heroin use, in general, women to increased μ receptor density in the central opioid neuronal pathways in women, as shown by positron-emission tomography scans. This increase in receptor density may lead to a better response to buprenorphine at lower doses in females but not in males.

In addition to noting sex differences in treatment-seeking patterns as well as treatment outcomes among opioid-dependent patients, a recent study indicated the need to consider also within-sex differences in the clinical presentation of drug-abusing women (McMahon and Luthar 2000). This study examined characteristics of 153 women in methadone maintenance treatment and defined four specific groups of women with different profiles of problem severity: unemployed, medically ill, psychiatrically distressed, and higher functioning. There were significant differences in the ethnic composition of the four groups as well as differences in psychiatric and medical status, vocational and educational histories, lifetime history of maltreatment, and perception of social support. The authors asserted that such within-sex differences ought not to be ignored in the development and evaluation of sex-sensitive treatment programs (McMahon and Luthar 2000).

Several specific factors seem to contribute to enhanced treatment outcome for women (Anglin et al. 1987b; Eldred and Washington 1976; Ladwig and Andersen 1989; Nurco et al. 1982; Stevens and Hollis 1989; Wiepert et al. 1979). Although later age at first use of marijuana and opioids and later termination of formal education appear to be predictive of better outcomes in men, this is generally not true for women. The most consistent factor reported for better treatment outcome in women is partner support for treatment (Anglin et al. 1987b; Eldred and Washington 1976) or absence of an addicted partner (Nurco et al. 1982). A lack of criminal involvement also appears to be associated with better treatment outcomes in women (Wiepert et al. 1979). Finally, evidence indicates that increasing the focus of treatment on concerns specific to women, such as adding women's treatment groups, increasing female staff, and increasing attention to women's sexual concerns including histories of abuse, may improve treatment outcomes in women (Ladwig and Andersen 1989; Stevens and Hollis 1989).

MARIJUANA

Epidemiology

Marijuana is derived from the leaves and flowering tops of the plant *Cannabis sativa*. The primary routes of administration are smoking through a cigarette or a water pipe, chewing (Adams and Martin 1996), and ingesting in food or tea (Leonard 1969). In 1995, 6.5% of females and 10.5% of males aged 12 and older reported marijuana use in the previous year (Substance Abuse and Mental Health Services Administration 1997). Although marijuana use was 4% greater for males than for females, the percentage of males using marijuana between 1994 and 1995 decreased by 0.8%. In contrast, marijuana use increased by 0.6% for females during that same period.

The 1997 NHSDA data reported sex differences in past-month marijuana use. That year, 5.1% of the household population age 12 and older reported marijuana use in the past month. This percentage included 3.5% of females and 7.0% of males (Substance Abuse and Mental Health Services Administration 1999). In 1996, however, 3.1% of females and 6.5% of males in the same cohort reported marijuana use in the previous month (Substance Abuse and Mental Health Services Administration 1998), indicating a trend toward increased substance use in both males and females during a 1-month period that year.

Although sex-specific data examining trends in marijuana use during the past month and the past year for the population age 12 years or older are not available for 2000, 4.8% of individuals age 12 years or older reported marijuana use in the past month, a 0.3% decrease from 1997 but a 0.1% increase from 1999 (Substance Abuse and Mental Health Services Administration 2001). The changes in marijuana use in the general population over the past several years suggest an overall tendency toward decreased marijuana use, but more research is needed to examine emerging trends.

The initiation of marijuana use occurred most frequently between the ages of 12 and 17, with a mean age of 17.0 years in 1999 (Substance Abuse and Mental Health Services Administration 2001). Recent data revealed a significant increase in the rate of initiation between the ages of 12 and 17. Between 1965 and 1999, the percentage of people initiating marijuana use in this age group increased from 9.2% to 73.0%, with a peak of 87.6% in 1996. Sex-specific data from 1995 (Substance Abuse and Mental Health Services Administration 1997), the last year in which initiation of marijuana use was analyzed by sex and age, showed that between 1961 and 1995, the percentage of male initiates between ages 10 and 14 almost doubled from 12.0% to 23.4%. The percentage of female initiates during that same period, however, increased more than fourfold from 5.4% of all female marijuana initiates in 1961 to 23.9% of all female marijuana initiates in 1995. These data suggest that the initiation of marijuana use among females has increased in this youngest age group at a rate twice that of males.

Course of Illness and Patterns of Use

In an analysis of data from the NHSDA, 1979–1994, Van Etten et al. (1997) reported that nearly one-half of all noninstitutionalized people age 12 and older have used marijuana at least once. The youngest cohort, 12-year-olds, was less likely to use marijuana in the 1-year period after initial opportunity as compared with an older cohort of 21-year-olds.

Over the past two decades, researchers have focused their attention on the use of marijuana, alcohol, and cigarettes as possible gateway drugs that lead to the use of other licit and illicit drugs (Adler and Kandel 1981; Kandel and Faust 1975; Warren et al. 1997; Yamaguchi and Kandel 1984a, 1984b). These researchers showed that adolescent involvement in legal and illegal drug use often follows a sequential pattern. Several studies that examined this pattern among high school students (Adler and Kandel 1981; Kandel and Faust 1975; Warren et al. 1997; Yamaguchi and Kandel 1984a, 1984b) found that alcohol or cigarette use most often preceded experimentation with marijuana. In 1992, a large cohort study of males and females aged 15–35 examined the progression of their use of substances (Kandel et al. 1992) and found that progression from use of alcohol or cigarettes to marijuana was similar to that in other studies; however, a sex difference in progression was also noted. For males, alcohol, in the absence of cigarettes, consistently preceded the use of marijuana. Among women, however, either cigarette *or* alcohol use was sufficient for progression to marijuana use.

Kandel (1984) also showed that once young adults have initiated use of marijuana, those who continued to use marijuana had specific characteristics that differentiated them from an age-matched group of nonusers. In a survey of 1,325 young adults aged 24–25, Kandel (1984) reported predictors associated with continued marijuana use. For both sexes, marijuana use was associated with a greater use of other illicit substances, a history of poor psychological health and psychiatric hospitalizations, employment instability, and involvement in delinquent behavior. Marijuana use in early adulthood was more common in males than in females; interpersonal factors such as use by spouse, partner, or friends played a more important role in continued marijuana use in women than in men. This finding of the importance of partner, friend, or spouse as a predictor of continued marijuana use is similar to findings for women with opioid use disorders (Greenfield 1996).

For those individuals who initiate marijuana use, it is possible to determine the proportion who eventually progress to having a problem with or being dependent on the substance. According to data obtained from the NCS, a large community-based survey of the prevalence of psychiatric and substance use disorders among individuals ages 15–54 in the United States, the lifetime prevalence marijuana use at least once is 47%, with a lifetime prevalence in males of 51.5% and in females of 42.5% (S.F. Greenfield and R. Kessler, unpublished manuscript). The lifetime prevalence of having a problem with marijuana (defined as a history of meeting a single criterion of the DSM-III-R [American Psychiatric Association 1987] diagnosis of dependence at any time in one's life) is 11.6%, with 15.6% prevalence in males and 8.3% prevalence in females, a male-to-female ratio of 1.8:1.0. The prevalence of lifetime dependence on marijuana is 4.2%, with 6.1% prevalence in males and 2.3% prevalence in females, a ratio of 2.7:1.0. Importantly, these data show that of all those who ever used marijuana, 27% develop a problem with the substance, and almost 9% develop dependence. A separate longitudinal study of a nationally representative sample of the United States general population found that the risk of cannabis abuse and dependence increased with the frequency of smoking occasions and slightly decreased with age. The strength of the association between cannabis use and abuse also increased as a function of the number of joints smoked among females but not among males (Grant and Pickering 1998).

Regarding the risk of marijuana initiation, one longitudinal prospective study of a national sample of 2,436 adolescents in Norway found that conduct problems that were closely related to a DSM-III-R diagnosis of conduct disorder were important precursors of early onset of marijuana use (Pedersen et al. 2001). Notably, conduct problems at a subclinical level appeared to have a significantly stronger effect in girls than in boys. Another study investigated the relation between genetic factors and the development of marijuana abuse and dependence. Kendler and Prescott (1998) interviewed 1,934 individual female twins selected from a population-based registry to examine the etiology of marijuana use, abuse, and dependence. Although environmental influences such as family and peers were important predictors for ever using marijuana, genetic factors had the strongest effect on the vulnerability to develop heavy marijuana use, marijuana abuse, or marijuana dependence in the female subjects. These data suggest that the risk of developing marijuana abuse and dependence in females may be heavily influenced by genetic determinants. To our knowledge, there are no similar published studies of these factors for male samples or in a mixed-sex sample.

Sex-specific patterns of marijuana use have been described by several researchers who investigated the relation between marijuana use and factors such as time of day and week, alcohol consumption, and menstrual cycle (Griffin et al. 1986; Lex et al. 1986; Mello and Mendelson 1985). For example, Lex et al. (1986) followed up 30 adult female marijuana users without dependence for approximately 90 days and examined their patterns of alcohol and marijuana consumption. Marijuana smoking occurred earlier in the day compared with alcohol ingestion; the use of both substances increased as the week progressed, with the heaviest consumption on weekends. Most of the subjects involved in this study were employed or were enrolled in school. The authors commented that the observed temporal variations in substance use patterns were primarily determined by the responsibilities of work or school.

In a 35-day study of 21 women, Mello and Mendelson (1985) found no consistent covariation between marijuana use and menstrual cycle phase. However, an important relation was found between premenstrual dysphoria and marijuana consumption. Women who increased their use of marijuana during the premenstrual phase reported significantly greater depression, mood lability, anxiety, anger, and impaired social function. These findings were supported in a study by Griffin et al. (1986), who reported no consistent relation between menstrual cycle phase and marijuana smoking in the absence of severe premenstrual dysphoria.

Medical Consequences

Marijuana contains more than 60 different cannabinoids. Δ^9-Tetrahydrocannabinol (THC) produces the primary pharmacological effects (Grinspoon and Bakalar 1997). Cannabinoid receptors are distributed in various regions of the brain, including the basal ganglia, the cerebellum, the hippocampus, and the cerebral cortex (Herkenham et al. 1990).

After marijuana is smoked, the average user will absorb approximately one-half the total dose into the bloodstream. The effects of marijuana are experienced almost immediately, and peak intensity is reached within 30 minutes. Plasma levels begin to decline after 1 hour; subjective effects disappear 3 hours after the last dose (Greenfield et al. 1997).

Marijuana intoxication initially causes a period of anxiety that is then followed by a feeling of calm and mild euphoria (Grinspoon and Bakalar 1997). Perceptual changes such as a distorted sense of time and an increased sensitivity to stimuli also have been described.

In a study of 1,000 New Zealanders, Thomas (1996) examined adverse effects associated with marijuana use. Of the 197 subjects (102 males and 95 females) who had used marijuana, the most commonly cited health consequences were acute anxiety or panic attacks, psychotic symptoms, and memory loss following marijuana use. Significantly more female subjects (32%) reported panic attacks compared with male subjects (13%). This was the only sex difference in adverse effects of marijuana use reported in this study.

Several clinical studies have examined the residual effects of marijuana on neuropsychological functioning (Block and Ghoneim 1993; Mendhiratta et al. 1988; Varma et al. 1988). Heavy marijuana use was associated with impairment in perceptual-motor tasks such as pencil tapping, time estimation, and size estimation (Varma et al. 1988). In a 10-year follow-up study of long-term marijuana users, Mendhiratta et al. (1988) found significantly poorer performance in marijuana users as compared with nonusers on various neuropsychological tests, including reaction time, speed and accuracy tests, digit span, and Bender Visual Motor Gestalt Test. When the investigators compared the current test results with the test results from the index study 10 years earlier, marijuana users had a greater deterioration in performance over time than did the nonusers. Selective memory impairment in retrieval processes as well as deficits in mathematical skills and verbal expression also have been associated with heavy marijuana use (Block and Ghoneim 1993).

Sex differences in neuropsychological functioning have been reported in two recent studies. Pope and Yurgelun-Todd (1996) compared 65 heavy marijuana users (38 males and 27 females) and 64 light marijuana users (31 males and 33 females) on a battery of neuropsychological tests after a supervised period of abstinence from marijuana. Heavy users had significantly greater impairment than did light users on attentional and executive functions; in particular, they showed greater perseveration on card sorting tasks and reduced learning of word lists. The impairments were somewhat more prominent among men than women despite similar lifetime marijuana use among the male and the female heavy users.

In a related study, Pope et al. (1997) compared 25 heavy marijuana smokers (16 males and 9 females) and 30 light smokers (15 males and 15 females) to assess residual cognitive impairment. A computerized battery of attentional tests was administered after a supervised period of abstinence from marijuana. On a subtest examining visuospatial memory, female heavy marijuana smokers performed significantly worse than did female infrequent smokers. Men, regardless of smoking history, showed no impairment on visuospatial memory. The authors suggested that marijuana may have a sex-specific effect on visuospatial recall that may be a result of multiple factors. These include a persisting effect of marijuana on the brain even after a period of abstinence, a direct neurotoxic effect of marijuana, or a withdrawal effect from the abrupt discontinuation of marijuana.

Because marijuana is most frequently administered by inhalation, many studies examining the medical consequences of marijuana use have focused on marijuana's effects on the respiratory tract. Compared with tobacco smoking, marijuana smoking is associated with a larger puff volume, a greater depth on inhalation, and a fourfold increase in breath-holding time (Wu et al. 1988). The prolonged exposure to particulate matter, also known as tar, and other irritants in marijuana cigarettes appears to account for the histological changes (Gong et al. 1987) and airway inflammation (Roth et al. 1998) seen in chronic marijuana smokers. Gong et al. (1987) reported more cellular disorganization on histological examination of lung biopsies from marijuana users compared with lung biopsies from tobacco smokers. Roth et al. (1998) found no difference in airway inflammation in the lungs of marijuana smokers when compared with the lungs of tobacco smokers. Sex differences in respiratory consequences of marijuana use have not been reported.

The relation between marijuana smoking and the development of cancer is unclear. Taylor (1988) reported 10 cases (6 male and 4 female) of carcinoma of the upper and/or lower respiratory tract in regular marijuana smokers younger than 40. Although most subjects had other risk factors, such as tobacco and/or alcohol use, they developed carcinomas an average of three decades earlier than subjects who never used marijuana, raising the question of whether additional carcinogenic factors in marijuana lead to the early development of respiratory carcinomas. Caplan and Brigham (1990) reported two cases of carcinoma of the tongue in two men who smoked marijuana regularly but had no other risk factors.

In a retrospective study of 64,855 members of a large insurance plan in California, Sidney et al. (1997) examined the relation of exclusive marijuana use to cancer incidence. A threefold increased risk of prostate cancer was found in men who had used marijuana but never used tobacco. An increased risk of cervical cancer was documented for marijuana-smoking women, but this risk did not have statistical significance. For all other sites, no increased risk of cancer was found.

Several studies have examined the effects of marijuana on reproductive functioning in males and females (Block et al. 1991; Kolodny et al. 1974; Mendelson et al. 1974, 1978, 1984, 1986). Low sperm counts and decreased sperm motility have been associated with heavy marijuana use in males (Kolodny et al. 1974). Kolodny et al. (1974) reported low plasma testosterone levels in male heavy marijuana users. This finding, however, has not been supported by the work of other researchers (Block et al. 1991; Mendelson et al. 1974, 1978) and remains controversial. Plasma levels of prolactin and luteinizing hormone in males also have not been altered by marijuana use (Block et al. 1991; Kolodny et al. 1974; Mendelson et al. 1978).

In contrast, marijuana appears to exert effects on female reproductive hormones. Mendelson et al. (1984, 1986) reported a suppression of plasma luteinizing hormone levels and plasma prolactin levels after administration of a single marijuana cigarette during the luteal phase of the menstrual cycle. Block et al. (1991), however, found no changes in luteinizing hormone or prolactin in chronic marijuana smokers. Marijuana may exert its effects on reproductive hormones by more acutely causing transient decreases in prolactin and luteinizing hormone in the immediate period after its use. A period of abstinence of even a few hours may allow for hormone levels to return to stable levels.

Marijuana use can lead to physical dependence, as evidenced by the onset of an abstinence syndrome on discontinuation of use (Bensusan 1971; Kaymakcalan 1981; Mendelson et al. 1984; Wiesbeck et al. 1996). The symptoms of marijuana withdrawal include anxiety, sleep disturbance, changes in appetite (Bensusan 1971; Kaymakcalan 1981; Wiesbeck et al. 1996), aggressiveness, tremors, hallucinations, and marijuana cravings (Kaymakcalan 1981). Mendelson et al. (1984) described a marijuana abstinence syndrome in one woman on a research study ward for 21 days. The subject smoked a mean of 9.53 marijuana cigarettes per day, with a marked increase in use on the last 3 days of the study (18, 19, and 25 marijuana cigarettes smoked on days 19, 20, and 21, respectively). Her withdrawal symptoms included anxiety, insomnia, dysphoria, anorexia, tremors, and sweating. These symptoms started 10 hours after cessation of smoking and peaked within 48 hours. The researchers thought that the intensity of her abstinence syndrome may have been associated with the greater concentration of THC in the study's marijuana cigarettes compared with the marijuana cigarettes she smoked before the study. It is, therefore, unclear to what extent the withdrawal syndrome described in this study of one subject would be generalizable to other individuals dependent on marijuana.

Effects of Marijuana on Pregnancy and Neonates

Marijuana use during pregnancy may adversely affect the health of the pregnant woman, the course of pregnancy, the development of the fetus, and early childhood development. In animal models, the main active ingredient of marijuana, THC, crosses the placenta more during early pregnancy than during late pregnancy (Idänpään-Heikkilä et al. 1969). Marijuana is highly lipophilic and is stored in the adipose tissue, where it may remain for 2–3 weeks (Greenfield et al. 1997). THC can be measured in the plasma for up to 6 days after a single episode of use (Greenfield et al. 1997). A single dose of marijuana early in pregnancy may lead to a prolonged exposure of the fetus to the drug (Zuckerman et al. 1989).

Several authors examined the effect of marijuana on the course of pregnancy (Fried et al. 1984; Gibson et al. 1983; Williams et al. 1991). For example, Williams et al. (1991) reported an increased risk of abruptio placentae in pregnant mothers who smoked marijuana at least daily. A significant reduction of 0.8 weeks in gestation length was associated with marijuana use six or more times per week during pregnancy (Fried et al. 1984). Finally, Gibson et al. (1983) found an association between regular marijuana use (at least twice a week) and an increased risk of giving birth to a premature infant.

The effects of marijuana smoking on neonates also have been reported (Fried 1982; Hingson et al. 1982; Linn et al. 1983; Zuckerman et al. 1989). Zuckerman et al. (1989) reported a significant decrease in birthweight and a significant decrease in body length in infants born to mothers who used marijuana during their pregnancy. Infants exposed to marijuana in utero also have been reported to have a greater incidence of congenital malformations (Hingson et al. 1982; Linn et al. 1983). Neurological disturbances such as marked tremors, startles, and altered visual responses have been observed in neonates whose mothers smoked marijuana regularly during pregnancy (Fried 1982). One recent review of this literature reported data from two cohort studies demonstrating that global IQ is not affected by prenatal marijuana exposure but that other cognitive functions (i.e., attentional behavior and visual analysis/hypothesis testing) may be negatively affected beyond the toddler age (Fried and Smith 2001).

A review of long-term effects of prenatal marijuana exposure on further childhood development is beyond the scope of this chapter. The reader is referred to a review (Fried 1995) for an in-depth discussion of this topic.

Psychiatric Comorbidity

Several studies have investigated the relation between marijuana use and comorbid psychiatric illness (Halikas et al. 1972; Kouri et al. 1995; Weller and Halikas 1985). Halikas et al. (1972) found that marijuana use was associated with a statistically significant greater incidence of antisocial personality disorder in a community-based sample of 100 regular marijuana smokers compared with 50 nonsmoking control subjects. Depression and alcohol abuse were common in the marijuana-smoking group, but the rates of these disorders were not significantly different from those in the nonsmoking control subjects.

Ninety-seven of the original 100 subjects in the marijuana-smoking group and all 50 of the nonsmoking control subjects described by Halikas et al. (1972) were reevaluated 7 years later (Weller and Halikas 1985). Antisocial personality disorder was still more prevalent among the users as compared with the nonusers. Statistically significant increases in antisocial personality disorder, depression, and alcohol abuse in the users as well as the nonusers occurred during the 7 years between the initial interview and follow-up evaluation. No new psychiatric problems were identified in the marijuana users, but the authors suggested that preexisting psychiatric problems did not improve and may have been worsened by the continued use of marijuana.

In a study of 45 heavy marijuana users and 44 occasional marijuana users drawn from a cohort of college students, Kouri et al. (1995) administered the Structured Clinical Interview for DSM-III-R (SCID) to assess for co-morbid Axis I and Axis II diagnoses. Among the heavy smokers, the most frequently diagnosed disorders were marijuana abuse or dependence (100%), alcohol abuse or dependence (24%), cocaine dependence (13%), and passive-aggressive personality disorder (11%). Among occasional users, alcohol abuse or dependence, major depression, and passive-aggressive personality disorder (all 11%) were the most commonly diagnosed disorders.

Some evidence indicates that among individuals with psychiatric disorders, marijuana use may be an attempt to self-medicate psychiatric symptoms (Dixon et al. 1991; Gruber et al. 1996; Peralta and Cuesta 1992). Marijuana use in individuals with schizophrenia has been associated with self-reported decreases in anxiety symptoms, increased energy (Dixon et al. 1991), and fewer negative symptoms, especially alogia (Peralta and Cuesta 1992). Gruber et al. (1996) presented five cases of individuals with major depression and concomitant marijuana use. In all five cases, the patients reported greater reduction in their depressive symptoms after marijuana use than they experienced when treated with traditional antidepressants. These studies highlight the importance of asking patients with psychiatric disorders about their use of marijuana. Conversely, it is also important to screen individuals with marijuana use, abuse, and dependence for concurrent mood, anxiety, and psychotic disorders.

Treatment Outcome

In a representative community sample of 706 marijuana users followed up from ages 15–16 to ages 34–35, event history analysis was applied to investigate the factors associated with cessation of marijuana use from adolescence to adulthood (Chen and Kandel 1998). The authors of the study found that frequent users who started using early and those who used other illicit drugs as well were more likely to continue their marijuana use. They also found that becoming pregnant and a parent was the most important social role leading to marijuana cessation among women (Chen and Kandel 1998).

The characteristics of individuals who seek treatment for marijuana dependence have been described (Budney et al. 1998; Copeland et al. 2001; Stephens et al. 1993). One study reported that among 382 adults seeking treatment for marijuana use, most (76%) were male, were not currently using other substances, and reported many negative consequences of their use (Stephens et al. 1993). Another study of 62 adults seeking treatment for marijuana use (Budney et al 1998) also found the majority (87%) of these adults to be male and to report similar marijuana-related negative consequences. A recent study of 238 individuals seeking treatment for marijuana dependence found clinically relevant sex differences within the study group (Copeland et al. 2001). Women were more likely than men to have a marijuana-using partner and were less likely to have a heavy marijuana-using social network. Despite these descriptions of the characteristics of individuals seeking treatment, treatment outcome studies for marijuana dependence are limited because most of the literature is directed at substance abuse treatment in general and not at marijuana abuse or dependence treatment in particular (Gruber and Pope 1997). To our knowledge, no published studies have examined sex differences in treatment outcome for marijuana dependence, and information in this area is, therefore, even more limited.

As with other substance use disorders, the overall goal of treatment for marijuana dependence is abstinence (Galanter and Kleber 1994). Severe withdrawal symptoms associated with discontinuation of marijuana use can be treated with long-acting benzodiazepines (Miller et al. 1989); pharmacological agents for mild marijuana withdrawal usually are not necessary. Twelve-step groups such as Narcotics Anonymous and Alcoholics Anonymous, individual psychotherapy, family therapy, group therapy, and behavioral therapy are all recognized treatment modalities for marijuana dependence (Miller et al. 1989; Millman and Beeder 1994; Zweben and O'Connell 1988). Urine monitoring programs also can be clinically useful in helping patients and clinicians monitor abstinence or detect relapse (Greenfield et al. 1997; Zweben and O'Connell 1988).

One study examined treatment outcome among marijuana-dependent patients. Roffman et al. (1988) randomized 84 males and 26 females into one of two behavioral treatment groups for 10 weeks. The relapse prevention group was based on a cognitive-behavioral approach focusing on coping behaviors and building necessary skills to prevent relapse. The social support group concentrated on accessing and using social supports to prevent relapse. At a follow-up interview 1-month posttreatment, the relapse prevention group had significantly fewer days of marijuana use in the preceding 30 days compared with the social support group (8.18 days vs. 12.96 days). Sex differences in treatment outcome for the two groups were not examined. The authors concluded that more research was needed to seek variables that predict treatment outcome and that highlight specific treatments for marijuana dependence.

There are reports of two randomized trials of cognitive-behavioral therapy (CBT) for marijuana dependence (Copeland et al. 2001; Stephens et al. 1994), one of which included a control group. These studies compared CBT with a basic skills training approach; both methods were tailored to meet the unique demands of marijuana-dependent patients. Future research is needed to verify the effectiveness of these approaches as well as to explore any potential sex differences in response to treatment.

TOBACCO

Epidemiology

The compulsive use of tobacco is observed in almost all cultures (Benowitz 1988). Nicotine, a powerful addictive substance, is the psychoactive agent in tobacco (Schmitz et al. 1997). In 1998, an estimated 47 million adults in the United States were current smokers (American Cancer Society 2001). This number included 25 million males and 22 million females. Cigarette smoking is the most prevalent form of nicotine addiction (Schmitz et al. 1997).

The 2000 NHSDA found that 71.9% of the males and 61.4% of the females age 12 and older reported lifetime cigarette use. In addition, 31.6% of the males and 26.6% of the females reported use in the past year, and 26.9% of the males and 23.1% of the females reported use in the past month (Substance Abuse and Mental Health Services Administration 2001). Although smoking among men was greater than for women for all groups age 18 and older, the prevalence of cigarette smoking in adolescent females ages 12–17 (14.1%) was greater than that for adolescent males (12.8%). These data suggest that among the youngest cohorts, females are initiating tobacco use at a greater rate than males. As the youngest cohorts age, prevalence rates for females of all age groups may someday equal and potentially exceed prevalence rates for males.

Course of Illness

Cigarette smoking begins most frequently in adolescence. The Centers for Disease Control and Prevention (1998) estimated that 80% of tobacco use occurs for the first time among persons younger than 18 years. In an analysis of smoking prevalence in the United States between 1974 and 1985 to project smoking trends for the year 2000, Pierce et al. (1989) estimated that 1 million new young people became regular smokers in the early 1980s. This figure is approximately equivalent to 3,000 new smokers each day.

With such large numbers of adolescents taking up cigarette smoking each year, research has focused on identifying variables associated with smoking initiation in youth. In a study of 1,125 boys and 1,213 girls aged 12 and 13 years old, Charlton and Blair (1989) examined social variables and their influence on cigarette smoking. No variable had a significant correlation with the initiation of smoking in boys, but several factors were significantly correlated with smoking in girls. In order of importance, these variables included having at least one parent who smoked, positive views on smoking, cigarette brand awareness, and a best friend who smoked. The most important predictor of smoking in boys was having a best friend who smoked, but this variable did not reach statistical significance. The authors recommended that educational efforts to prevent cigarette smoking in adolescents should focus not only on the health risks of cigarette smoking but also on these social factors and their important influence on smoking initiation.

The continued use of cigarettes in women is thought to be related to negative affect and an attempt to control body weight. For example, women are more inclined than men to use smoking as a means to reduce stress, tension, or emotional distress (Gritz et al. 1996). Kandel and Davies (1986) reported a correlation between depressed affect in female adolescents and heavy smoking in young adulthood. In her study of 16,000 students aged 9–19 in a school in England, Charlton (1984) found that girls who were the heaviest regular smokers also were most likely to agree that smoking controls weight. Gritz and Crane (1991) reported that use of amphetamines and diet pills was greatest among female high school seniors who also smoked cigarettes, suggesting a greater preoccupation with weight among females who smoke. Finally, fear of weight gain has been frequently cited as an obstacle to giving up cigarette smoking (Rigotti 1989).

Medical Consequences

A description of all the medical consequences associated with cigarette smoking is beyond the scope of this chapter. The primary focus of this section is an examination of the relation of gender and cigarette smoking to cardiovascular disease, lung cancer, breast cancer, ovarian cancer, and cervical cancer.

Cardiovascular disease is the leading cause of death among women in the United States, resulting in approximately 250,000 deaths annually (Wenger 1995). Cigarette smoking increases the risk of morbidity and mortality associated with cardiovascular disease in women (Brochier and Arwidson 1998; Hansen et al. 1993; Slone et al. 1978; Vriz et al. 1997; Willett et al. 1987). Kannel and Higgins (1990) reported a greater incremental increase in cardiovascular mortality in women (31%) than in men (18%) for each 10 cigarettes smoked per day.

The overall mortality rate for lung cancer increased nearly fourfold from 1950 to 1990 (Centers for Disease Control and Prevention 1993).

Over this same period, the rate of increase in lung cancer mortality for men began to slow during the early 1980s, whereas the rate for women continued to increase sharply. Although data for lung cancer death rates for the year 2000 are not available, a recent study examined differences in the incidence of lung cancer by comparing data from California with data from a combination of four states (Connecticut, Hawaii, Iowa, and New Mexico) and three metropolitan cities (Atlanta, Detroit, and Seattle-Puget Sound), called the SEER group (Centers for Disease Control and Prevention 2000). Sex-specific data showed that males had significant decreases in the incidence of lung cancer per 100,000 population when compared with females during the period of 1988 to 1997. In Californian males, the incidence decreased from 98.8 in 1988 to 74.9 in 1997, and in SEER males incidence decreased from 100.5 in 1987 to 84.9 in 1997. In contrast, incidences decreased from 52.6 in 1988 to 50.1 in 1997 among Californian females and increased from 44.5 to 50.1 among females in the SEER group. Although the overall incidence of lung cancer remains greater for males in both study groups, the incidence for Californian females has not decreased as significantly as for Californian males, and there is a disturbing trend toward increased incidence among females in the four states and three cities of the SEER group. It is unclear how the incidence of lung cancer will affect death rates from lung cancer, and more research is necessary to follow sex-specific trends in both incidence and death rates.

Several studies have reported that women may be more susceptible to tobacco carcinogens than men are (Brownson et al. 1992; McDuffie et al. 1987; Osann et al. 1993; Risch et al. 1993; Zang and Wynder 1992, 1996). Zang and Wynder (1996) recently reported that the higher susceptibility to tobacco carcinogens in women may be related to lower plasma clearance of nicotine in women, male–female variations in hepatic enzymes necessary for the metabolism of drugs, and potential effects of female-specific hormones on tumor growth.

Studies examining the relation between cigarette smoking and reproductive cancers have shown both positive and negative associations. Two large studies found an increased risk of developing breast cancer (Bennicke et al. 1995; Morabia et al. 1996); however, many studies reported no association between cigarette smoking and the development of breast cancer (Baron et al. 1996; Braga et al. 1996; Haile et al. 1996; Hiatt and Fireman 1986; Ranstam and Olsson 1995). Similarly, only one study (Purdie et al. 1995) showed a positive association between smoking and ovarian cancer. Most studies (Franks et al. 1987; Smith et al. 1984; Stockwell and Lyman 1987) found no correlation between cigarette smoking and the risk of developing ovarian cancer.

Several studies have identified a positive association between cigarette smoking and the development of cervical cancer (Clarke et al. 1982; Layde and Broste 1989; Nischan et al. 1988; Slattery et al. 1989; Trevathan et al. 1983). McCann et al. (1992) detected tobacco constituents in the cervical mucus of female smokers in a neoplasia clinic; the authors hypothesized that these constituents may play a causal role in the development of cervical cancer in women.

Effects of Tobacco on Pregnancy and Neonates

Cigarette smoking during pregnancy has been associated with a variety of health problems for the pregnant woman, the developing fetus, and the neonate. Maternal cigarette smoking is associated with a greater risk of ectopic pregnancy (Saraiya et al. 1998), spontaneous abortion (Armstrong et al. 1992; DiFranza and Lew 1995; Domínguez-Rojas et al. 1994), placenta previa (Ananth et al. 1996; Chelmow et al. 1996; Monica and Lilja 1995), placental abruption (Ananth et al. 1996), and preterm birth (Wright et al. 1998).

Neonates born to mothers who smoked cigarettes during pregnancy can have increased blood pressure (Beratis et al. 1996); reduced growth parameters, including weight and length (Roquer et al. 1995; Vik et al. 1996); and increased risk of sudden infant death syndrome (Kohlendorfer et al. 1998; Schlaud et al. 1996).

Psychiatric Comorbidity

Some investigators have reported that cigarette smoking is more common among individuals with psychiatric disorders. For example, Hughes et al. (1986) reported that the prevalence of smoking among psychiatric patients was 1.6 times that of population-based control subjects. Rates of cigarette smoking have been increased in individuals with schizophrenia (de Leon et al. 1995; Goff et al. 1992; Hughes et al. 1986; Lohr and Flynn 1992), major depression (Breslau et al. 1991; Glassman 1993; Glassman et al. 1988, 1990; Hughes et al. 1986), bipolar disorder (Gonzalez-Pinto et al. 1998; Hughes et al. 1986), and anxiety disorders (Breslau et al. 1991; Hughes et al. 1986). Experimentation with other illicit drugs is often preceded by cigarette use (Adler and Kandel 1981; Kandel and Faust 1975; Warren et al. 1997; Yamaguchi and Kandel 1984a, 1984b), and several studies have found a higher prevalence of cigarette smoking in subjects who also have other substance abuse or substance dependence (Breslau et al. 1991; Budney et al. 1993; DiFranza and Guerrera 1990).

Studies showing sex differences in rates of comorbid psychiatric disorders among individuals with tobacco use have focused on major depression.

Three large community-based studies found a significant association between depression and smoking in women but not in men (Frederick et al. 1988; Lee and Markides 1991; Perez-Stable et al. 1990). Kendler et al. (1993), in a study of 1,566 female twin pairs, reported a positive association between cigarette smoking and major depression; the authors suggested that genetic factors may have predisposed these women to the development of both major depression and tobacco use.

Treatment Outcome

Many studies have examined sex differences in smoking cessation. Several studies have found that women are more likely than men to relapse after quitting on their own or after quitting with the aid of a treatment program (Bjornson et al. 1995; Royce et al. 1997; Ward et al. 1997). Other studies, however, found no sex differences in relapse rates between women and men (Johnson and Karkut 1994; Matheny and Weatherman 1998; Nides et al. 1995; Pirie et al. 1991). A recent study by Hall et al. (1998) found that women with a history of major depression were less likely than nondepressed women to remain abstinent from smoking in a 64-week program involving psychological and pharmacological treatment. History of depression in men, however, did not affect abstinence. Major depression may confer a sex-specific disadvantage for women who attempt to quit smoking cigarettes.

A wide array of psychological and pharmacological treatments is available to aid in smoking cessation. CBT, aversive techniques, relaxation techniques, and hypnosis all have been recognized as treatments for nicotine dependence (Ockene and Kristeller 1994).

Pharmacological agents shown to be effective aids for smoking cessation include nicotine replacement systems, antihypertensives, and psychiatric medications. Nicotine gum (Hughes and Miller 1984; Hughes et al. 1984), transdermal nicotine patches (Fiore et al. 1994; Rose et al. 1985; Yudkin et al. 1996), nicotine nasal spray (Hjalmarson et al. 1994; Schneider et al. 1995a), and nicotine inhalers (Tonnesen et al. 1993) all have shown greater efficacy in smoking cessation compared with placebo. Clonidine, both oral (Glassman et al. 1988, 1993) and transdermal (Hilleman et al. 1993; Ornish et al. 1988); doxepin (Edwards et al. 1989; Murphy et al. 1990); buspirone (Cinciripini et al. 1995; Hilleman et al. 1992; West et al. 1991); and, most recently, bupropion (Goldstein 1998; Hurt et al. 1997) and nortriptyline (Hall et al. 1998) have been cited as pharmacological treatments for nicotine dependence. In two separate studies, Glassman et al. (1988, 1993) noted that oral clonidine was more effective for short-term smoking cessation in women than in men.

LEGAL IMPLICATIONS FOR PREGNANT AND PARENTING WOMEN WITH SUBSTANCE USE DISORDERS

There is no question that pregnant and parenting women with substance use disorders need treatment. However, clinicians have different views about the nature of this treatment and how it should be implemented. Criminal prosecution has been suggested as one way to deter future substance abuse in pregnant women known to use alcohol and other substances of abuse (Reed 1999). Although no state in the United States has a statute criminalizing substance use in pregnant women, more than 200 women in 30 states have been prosecuted for using drugs or alcohol during pregnancy (Greenfield and Sugarman 2001; Marshall and Nelson 1995; Reed 1999). However, fear of prosecution may do more harm than good. Women may delay obtaining necessary prenatal care because of fear of prosecution (Reed 1999). Howell and Chasnoff (1999) conducted a focus group with pregnant women in substance abuse treatment and the providers of that treatment to determine factors in women's lives that contributed to involvement and completion of treatment. Program staff noted that fear of prosecution after the discovery of addiction in pregnant women had hampered outreach efforts and led women to enter substance abuse treatment later in their pregnancy. In addition, the prison system does not routinely provide appropriate health care for pregnant women, including proper nutrition, prenatal diet and exercise, and necessary prenatal care (Greenfield and Sugarman 2001; Reed 1999).

Several researchers have offered alternatives to prosecution to help deter current and future substance abuse in pregnant and parenting women (Camp and Finkelstein 1997; McMurtrie et al. 1999; Schwartz and Schwartz 1998). Schwartz and Schwartz (1998) described the Rochester Drug Treatment Court, one of several such programs in the United States. In the drug treatment courts, women, including pregnant women, charged with drug-related and addiction-driven misdemeanor and felony charges are sent to a 2-year intensive drug treatment program that includes vocational and educational training. For pregnant women who are substance abusers, the program emphasizes areas such as family issues, parenting, housing assistance, medical and prenatal care, and job training. According to the authors, of the 800 women who entered the Rochester program over the first 2½ years of its implementation, 70% completed the program.

In 1999, McMurtrie et al. (1999) described the 5-year experience of the Parent and Child Enrichment (PACE) Project in New York City. The PACE Project offered a variety of programs for pregnant and parenting women with substance use disorders. For example, parenting classes were given to strengthen the skills of these women, who often lacked good parenting role models in their own lives. Similarly, Camp and Finkelstein (1997) described two urban residential treatment programs in Massachusetts for pregnant and parenting women with substance use disorders. During a 3-year period, 170 women completed the parenting skills training program while in the residential programs. Self-esteem was assessed at both the beginning and the completion of the program with the Hudson Index of Self-Esteem. Through the program, women learned about child development and were taught parenting skills such as behavior management, communication, and play activities. At the time of completion, the women made significant improvements in both their self-esteem and their parenting knowledge.

Although more research is needed to develop treatment programs for pregnant and parenting women with substance use disorders, the studies presented here show that effective and helpful treatment alternatives to prosecution are available.

CONCLUSION

Significant sex differences exist in the prevalence of substance use disorders in the United States as well as in the course of illness, medical consequences, psychiatric comorbidity, and treatment outcomes. This review of the literature showed that these sex differences vary from substance to substance; therefore, women with substance use disorders must be regarded as a heterogeneous group about which no single conclusion can be reached.

This review, however, does indicate certain themes and trends in the epidemiology and consequences of substance use disorders for females in the United States. First, an increasingly greater proportion of female alcohol, tobacco, and drug initiates are in the youngest age cohorts. The proportion of female initiates in these youngest cohorts for alcohol, tobacco, and many illicit drugs now equals that of males, indicating that girls are initiating their drug and alcohol use at increasingly younger ages. This appears to be true for alcohol, cocaine, marijuana, and tobacco. A heightened vulnerability to the medical and physical consequences in women has been clearly demonstrated for alcohol, opioids, marijuana, and tobacco. In addition, sex-specific effects are evident with alcohol, marijuana, tobacco, cocaine, and opioids, including cancer risks as well as effects on pregnancy and the neonate. The increasing vulnerability to these substances in women combined with the declining age at initiation presents a growing threat to women's health in the United States.

In general, treatment outcome studies find outcomes in women that are equivalent to, or sometimes better than, those in men. However, population-based studies report that women are less likely to avail themselves of alcohol and drug treatment services. These data, combined with growing use and abuse of as well as dependence on alcohol, tobacco, and illicit drugs among women, argue for increased investigation of effective ways to improve prevention, detection, and treatment of these disorders in women. This will probably necessitate broadening our methods of screening for these disorders in primary care health settings and investigating ways that screening and detection can be sex sensitive. In addition, more information is necessary on the specific methods that are most effective for boys and girls in preventing initiation of use of alcohol, tobacco, and illicit drugs. Finally, eliminating barriers and improving access to treatment is important for both men and women but is particularly important for women with substance use disorders whose use of treatment is significantly lower than that of men.

REFERENCES

Adams IB, Martin BR: Cannabis: pharmacology and toxicology in animals and humans. Addiction 91:1585–1614, 1996

Adler I, Kandel DB: Cross-cultural perspectives on developmental stages in adolescent drug use. J Stud Alcohol 42:701–715, 1981

Allan CA, Phil M: Seeking help for drinking problems from a community-based volunteer agency: patterns of compliance amongst men and women. British Journal of Addiction 82:1143–1147, 1987

Allen D: Are alcoholic women more likely to drink premenstrually? Alcohol 31:145–147, 1996

American Cancer Society: Cancer Facts and Figures 2001. Atlanta, GA, American Cancer Society, 2001

American Psychiatric Association: Diagnostic and Statistical Manual of Mental Disorders, 3rd Edition, Revised. Washington, DC, American Psychiatric Association, 1987

American Psychiatric Association: Diagnostic and Statistical Manual of Mental Disorders, 4th Edition. Washington, DC, American Psychiatric Association, 1994

Ammon E, Schäfer C, Hoffman U, et al: Disposition and first-pass metabolism of ethanol in humans: is it gastric or hepatic and does it depend on gender? Clin Pharmacol Ther 59:503–513, 1996

Ananth C, Savitz D, Luther E: Maternal cigarette smoking as a risk factor for placental abruption, placenta previa, and uterine bleeding in pregnancy. Am J Epidemiol 144:881–889, 1996

Anglin MD, Hser YI, McGlothlin WH: Sex differences in addict careers, II: becoming addicted. Am J Drug Alcohol Abuse 13:59–71, 1987a

Anglin MD, Hser Y, Booth MW: Sex differences in addict careers, IV: treatment. Am J Drug Alcohol Abuse 13:253–280, 1987b

Anthony JC, Helzer JE: Syndromes of drug abuse and dependence, in Psychiatric Disorders in America. Edited by Robins LN, Regier DA. New York, Free Press, 1991, pp 116–154

Armstrong B, McDonald A, Sloan M: Cigarette, alcohol, and coffee consumption and spontaneous abortion. Am J Public Health 82:85–87, 1992

Ashley M, Olin J, le Riche W, et al: Morbidity in alcoholics: evidence for accelerated development of physical disease in women. Arch Intern Med 137:883–887, 1977

Baron J, Newcomb P, Longnecker M, et al: Cigarette smoking and breast cancer. Cancer Epidemiol Biomarkers Prev 5:399–403, 1996

Battaglia G, Cabrera-Vera TM, Van de Kar LD, et al: Prenatal cocaine exposure produces long-term impairments in brain serotonin function in rat offspring. Ann N Y Acad Sci 846:355–357, 1998

Beckman LJ, Amaro H: Patterns of women's use of alcohol treatment agencies, in Alcohol Problems in Women. Edited by Wilsnack S, Beckman L. New York, Guilford, 1984, pp 319–348

Beckman LJ, Amaro H: Personal and social difficulties faced by women and men entering alcoholism treatment. J Stud Alcohol 47:135–145, 1986

Bennicke K, Conrad D, Sabroe S, et al: Cigarette smoking and breast cancer. BMJ 310:1431–1433, 1995

Benowitz N: Pharmacologic aspects of cigarette smoking and nicotine addiction. N Engl J Med 319:1318–1330, 1988

Bensusan AD: Marihuana withdrawal symptoms (letter to the editor). BMJ 3:112, 1971

Beratis N, Panagoulias D, Varvarigou A: Increased blood pressure in neonates and infants whose mothers smoked during pregnancy. J Pediatr 128:806–812, 1996

Bjornson W, Rand C, Connett J, et al: Gender differences in smoking cessation after 3 years in the Lung Health Study. Am J Public Health 85:223–230, 1995

Block RI, Ghoneim MM: Effects of chronic marijuana use on human cognition. Psychopharmacology 110:219–228, 1993

Block RI, Farinpour R, Schlechte JA: Effects of chronic marijuana use on testosterone, luteinizing hormone, follicle stimulating hormone, prolactin and cortisol in men and women. Drug Alcohol Depend 28:121–128, 1991

Bradley KA, Badrinath S, Bush K, et al: Medical risks for women who drink alcohol. J Gen Intern Med 13:627–639, 1998

Braga C, Negri E, La Vecchia C, et al: Cigarette smoking and the risk of breast cancer. Eur J Cancer Prev 5:159–164, 1996

Breslau N, Kilbey M, Andreski P: Nicotine dependence, major depression, and anxiety in young adults. Arch Gen Psychiatry 48:1069–1074, 1991

Brochier M, Arwidson P: Coronary heart disease risk factors in women. Eur Heart J 19:A45–A52, 1998

Brooner R, King V, Kidorf M, et al: Psychiatric and substance use comorbidity among treatment-seeking opioid abusers. Arch Gen Psychiatry 54:71–80, 1997

Brown E, Prager J, Lee H, et al: CNS complications of cocaine abuse: prevalence, pathophysiology, and neuroradiology. AJR Am J Roentgenol 159:137–147, 1992

Brownson R, Chang J, Davis J: Gender and histologic type variations in smoking-related risk of lung cancer. Epidemiology 3:61–64, 1992

Budney A, Higgins S, Hughes J, et al: Nicotine and caffeine use in cocaine-dependent individuals. J Subst Abuse 5:117–130, 1993

Budney AJ, Radonovich KJ, Higgins ST, et al: Adults seeking treatment for marijuana dependence: a comparison with cocaine-dependent treatment seekers. Experimental and Clinical Psychopathology 6:419–426, 1998

Burnham MA, Stein JA, Golding JM, et al: Sexual assault and mental disorders in a community population. J Consult Clin Psychol 56:843–850, 1988

Camp JM, Finkelstein N: Parenting training for women in residential substance abuse treatment: results of a demonstration project. J Subst Abuse Treat 14:411–422, 1997

Caplan GA, Brigham BA: Marijuana smoking and carcinoma of the tongue: is there an association? Cancer 66:1005–1006, 1990

Carroll KM, Rounsaville BJ, Keller DS: Relapse prevention strategies for the treatment of cocaine abuse. Am J Drug Alcohol Abuse 17:249–265, 1991

Cavallo F, Russo R, Zotti C, et al: Moderate alcohol consumption and spontaneous abortion. Alcohol 30:195–201, 1995

Center on Addiction and Substance Abuse at Columbia University: Substance Abuse and the American Woman. New York, Center on Addiction and Substance Abuse, 1996

Centers for Disease Control: Trends in alcohol-related traffic fatalities, by sex: United States. JAMA 268:313–314, 1992

Centers for Disease Control and Prevention: Mortality trends for selected smoking-related cancers and breast cancer: United States, 1950–1990. MMWR Morb Mortal Wkly Rep 42:857–866, 1993

Centers for Disease Control and Prevention: Cigarette smoking among adults: United States, 1995. MMWR Morb Mortal Wkly Rep 46:1217–1220, 1997

Centers for Disease Control and Prevention: Tobacco use among high school students: United States, 1997. JAMA 279:1250–1251, 1998

Centers for Disease Control and Prevention: Declines in Lung Cancer Rates: California, 1988–1997. MMWR Morb Mortal Wkly Rep 49:1066–1069, 2000

Chang L, Ernst T, Strickland T, et al: Gender effects on persistent cerebral metabolite changes in the frontal lobes of abstinent cocaine users. Am J Psychiatry 156:716–722, 1999

Charlton A: Smoking and weight control in teenagers. Public Health 98:277–281, 1984

Charlton A, Blair V: Predicting the onset of smoking in boys and girls. Soc Sci Med 29:813–818, 1989

Chasnoff I, Burns K, Burns W: Cocaine use in pregnancy: perinatal morbidity and mortality. Neurotoxicol Teratol 9:291–293, 1987

Chasnoff I, Chisum G, Kaplan W: Maternal cocaine use and genitourinary tract malformations. Teratology 37:201–204, 1988

Chasnoff IJ, Anson A, Hatcher R, et al: Prenatal exposure to cocaine and other drugs: outcomes at four to six years. Ann N Y Acad Sci 846:314–328, 1998

Chelmow D, Andrew D, Baker E: Maternal cigarette smoking and placenta previa. Obstet Gynecol 87:703–706, 1996

Chen K, Kandel DB: Predictors of cessation of marijuana use: an event history analysis. Drug Alcohol Depend 50:109–121, 1998

Chiriboga CA: Neurological correlates of fetal cocaine exposure. Ann N Y Acad Sci 846:109–125, 1998

Chiriboga C, Bateman D, Brust J, et al: Neurologic findings in neonates with intrauterine cocaine exposure. Pediatr Neurol 9:115–119, 1993

Choi SJ, Mazzio E, Soliman KF: The effects of gestational cocaine exposure on pregnancy outcome, postnatal development, cognition and locomotion in rats. Ann N Y Acad Sci 844:324–335, 1998a

Choi SJ, Mazzio E, Kolta MG, et al: Prenatal cocaine exposure affects postnatal dopaminergic systems in various regions of the rat brain. Ann N Y Acad Sci 844:293–302, 1998b

Cinciripini P, Lapitsky L, Seay S, et al: A placebo-controlled evaluation of the effects of buspirone on smoking cessation: differences between high- and low-anxiety smokers. J Clin Psychopharmacol 15:182–191, 1995

Clarke E, Morgan R, Newman A: Smoking as a risk factor in cancer of the cervix: additional evidence from a case-control study. Am J Epidemiol 115:59–66, 1982

Cocores J, Dackis C, Gold M: Sexual dysfunction secondary to cocaine abuse in two patients. J Clin Psychiatry 47:384–385, 1986

Connor B, Babcock M: The impact of feminist psychotherapy on the treatment of women alcoholics: focus on women. Journal of Addiction and Health 2:72–92, 1980

Copeland J, Swift W, Rees V: Clinical profile of participants in a brief intervention program for cannabis use disorder. J Subst Abuse Treatment 20:45–52, 2001

Cornelius J, Jarrett P, Thase M, et al: Gender effects on the clinical presentation of alcoholics at a psychiatric hospital. Compr Psychiatry 36:435–440, 1995

Cornish J, Maany I, Fudala P, et al: Carbamazepine treatment for cocaine dependence. Drug Alcohol Depend 38:221–227, 1995

Crawford S, Ryder D: A study of sex differences in cognitive impairment in alcoholics using traditional and computer-based tests. Drug Alcohol Depend 18:369–375, 1986

Crits-Christoph P, Siqueland L, Blaine J, et al: The National Institute on Drug Abuse Collaborative Cocaine Treatment Study: rationale and methods. Arch Gen Psychiatry 54:721–726, 1999

Cuskey W, Berger L, Densen-Gerber J: Issues in the treatment of female addiction: a review and critique of the literature. Contemporary Drug Problems 6:307–371, 1977

Dackis C, Gold M: New concepts in cocaine addiction: the dopamine depletion hypothesis. Neurosci Biobehav Rev 9:460–477, 1985

Dackis C, Gold M, Sweeney D, et al: Single-dose bromocriptine reverses cocaine craving. Psychiatry Res 20:261–264, 1987

Davidson D, Swift R, Fitz E: Naltrexone increases the latency to drink alcohol in social drinkers. Alcohol Clin Exp Res 20:732–739, 1996

de Leon J, Dadvand M, Canuso C, et al: Schizophrenia and smoking: an epidemiological survey in a state hospital. Am J Psychiatry 152:453–455, 1995

Delaney-Black V, Covington C, Templin T, et al: Prenatal cocaine exposure and child behavior. Pediatrics 102(4, Pt 1):945–950, 1998

Denier C, Thevos A, Latham P, et al: Psychosocial and psychopathology differences in hospitalized male and female cocaine abusers: a retrospective chart review. Addict Behav 16:489–496, 1991

DiFranza J, Guerrera M: Alcoholism and smoking. J Stud Alcohol 51:130–135, 1990

DiFranza J, Lew R: Effect of maternal cigarette smoking on pregnancy complications and sudden infant death syndrome. J Fam Pract 40:385–394, 1995

Dixon L, Haas G, Weiden PJ, et al: Drug abuse in schizophrenic patients: clinical correlates and reasons for use. Am J Psychiatry 148:224–230, 1991

Domínguez-Rojas V, de Juanes-Pardo J, Astasio-Arbiza P, et al: Spontaneous abortion in a hospital population: are tobacco and coffee intake risk factors? Eur J Epidemiol 10:665–668, 1994

Dorus W, Senay E: Depression, demographic dimensions, and drug abuse. Am J Psychiatry 137:669–704, 1980

Duckert F: Recruitment into treatment and effects of treatment for female problem drinkers. Addict Behav 12:137–150, 1987

Dudish S, Hatsukami D: Gender differences in crack users who are research volunteers. Drug Alcohol Depend 42:55–63, 1996

Dusick A, Covert R, Schreiber M, et al: Risk of intracranial hemorrhage and other adverse outcomes after cocaine exposure in a cohort of 323 very low birth weight infants. J Pediatr 122:438–445, 1993

Edwards N, Murphy J, Downs A, et al: Doxepin as an adjunct to smoking cessation: a double-blind pilot study. Am J Psychiatry 146:373–376, 1989

Eldred C, Washington M: Interpersonal relationships in heroin use by men and women and their role in treatment outcome. International Journal of the Addictions 11:117–130, 1976

Ellinwood E, Smith W, Vaillant G: Narcotic addictions in males and females: a comparison. International Journal of the Addictions 1:33–45, 1966

Endress C, Gray D, Wollschlaeger G: Bowel ischemia and perforation after cocaine use. AJR Am J Roentgenol 159:73–75, 1992

Faden V, Graubard B: Alcohol consumption during pregnancy and infant birth weight. Ann Epidemiol 4:279–284, 1994

Fernández-Solà J, Estruch R, Nicolás J, et al: Comparison of alcoholic cardiomyopathy in women versus men. Am J Cardiol 80:481–485, 1997

Finney J, Moos R: Matching patients with treatments: conceptual and methodological issues. J Stud Alcohol 47:122–134, 1986

Finney JW, Moos RH, Mewborn CR: Posttreatment experiences and treatment outcome of alcoholic patients six months and two years after hospitalization. J Consult Clin Psychol 48:17–29, 1980

Fiore M, Smith S, Jorenby D, et al: The effectiveness of the nicotine patch for smoking cessation: a meta-analysis. JAMA 271:1940–1947, 1994

Fischer G, Jagsch R, Eder H, et al: Comparison of methadone and slow-release morphine maintenance in pregnant addicts. Addiction 94:231–239, 1999

Fortin M, Evans S: Correlates of loss of control over drinking in women alcoholics. J Stud Alcohol 44:787–795, 1983

Foster JH, Peters TJ, Marshall EJ: Quality of life measures and outcome in alcohol-dependent men and women. Alcohol 22:45–52, 2000

Frank DA, McCarten KM, Robson CD, et al: Level of in utero cocaine exposure and neonatal ultrasound findings. Pediatrics 104(5, Pt 1):1101–1105, 1999

Franks A, Lee N, Kendrick J, et al: Cigarette smoking and the risk of epithelial ovarian cancer. Am J Epidemiol 126:112–117, 1987

Frederick T, Frerichs R, Clark V: Personal health habits and symptoms of depression at the community level. Prev Med 17:173–182, 1988

Frezza M, DiPadova C, Pozzato G, et al: High blood alcohol levels in women: the role of decreased gastric alcohol dehydrogenase activity and first-pass metabolism. N Engl J Med 322:95–99, 1990

Fried PA: Marihuana use by pregnant women and effects on offspring: an update. Neurobehavioral Toxicology and Teratology 4:451–454, 1982

Fried PA: Prenatal exposure to marihuana and tobacco during infancy, early and middle childhood: effects and an attempt at synthesis. Arch Toxicol 17:233–260, 1995

Fried PA, Smith AM: A literature review of the consequences of prenatal marijuana exposure: an emerging theme of a deficiency in aspects of executive function. Neurotoxicol Teratol 23:1–11, 2001

Fried PA, Watkinson B, Willan A: Marijuana use during pregnancy and decreased length of gestation. Am J Obstet Gynecol 150:23–27, 1984

Friedman E, Wang HY: Prenatal cocaine exposure alters signal transduction in the brain D1 dopamine receptor system. Ann N Y Acad Sci 846:238–247, 1998

Gabriel M, Taylor C: Prenatal exposure to cocaine impairs neuronal coding of attention and discriminative learning. Ann N Y Acad Sci 846:194–212, 1998

Galanter M, Kleber HD: The American Psychiatric Press Textbook of Substance Abuse Treatment. Washington, DC, American Psychiatric Press, 1994

Gawin F, Ricordan C, Kleber H: Methylphenidate treatment of cocaine abusers without attention-deficit disorder: a negative report. Am J Drug Alcohol Abuse 11:193–197, 1985

Gawin FH, Kleber HD, Byck R, et al: Desipramine facilitation of initial cocaine abstinence. Arch Gen Psychiatry 46:117–121, 1989

Gibson GT, Baghurst PA, Colley DP: Maternal alcohol, tobacco and cannabis consumption and the outcome of pregnancy. Aust N Z J Obstet Gynaecol 23:15–19, 1983

Glassman A: Cigarette smoking: implications for psychiatric illness. Am J Psychiatry 150:546–553, 1993

Glassman A, Stetner F, Walsh B, et al: Heavy smokers, smoking cessation, and clonidine. JAMA 259:2863–2866, 1988

Glassman A, Helzer J, Covey L, et al: Smoking, smoking cessation, and major depression. JAMA 264:1546–1549, 1990

Glassman A, Covey L, Dalack G, et al: Smoking cessation, clonidine, and vulnerability to nicotine among dependent smokers. Clin Pharmacol Ther 54:670–679, 1993

Goff D, Henderson D, Amico E: Cigarette smoking in schizophrenia: relationship to psychopathology and medication side effects. Am J Psychiatry 149:1189–1194, 1992

Goldstein A, Herrera J: Heroin addicts and methadone treatment in Albuquerque: a 22-year follow-up. Drug Alcohol Depend 40:139–150, 1995

Goldstein MJ: Psychosocial strategies for maximizing the effects of psychotropic medications for schizophrenia and mood disorder. Psychopharmacol Bull 28:237–240, 1992

Goldstein M: Bupropion sustained release and smoking cessation. J Clin Psychiatry 59(suppl):66–72, 1998

Goldstein M, Surber M, Wilner D: Outcome evaluations in substance abuse: a comparison of alcoholism, drug abuse, and other mental health interventions. International Journal of the Addictions 19:479–502, 1984

Gomberg ESL: Suicide risk among women with alcohol problems. Am J Public Health 79:1363–1365, 1989

Gong H, Fligiel S, Tashkin DP, et al: Tracheobronchial changes in habitual, heavy smokers of marijuana with and without tobacco. American Review of Respiratory Disease 136:142–149, 1987

Gonzalez-Pinto A, Gutierrez M, Ezcurra J, et al: Tobacco smoking and bipolar disorder. J Clin Psychiatry 59:225–228, 1998

Gorelick D: Alcohol and cocaine: clinical and pharmacological interactions, in Recent Developments in Alcoholism, Vol 10. Edited by Galanter M. New York, Plenum, 1992, pp 37–56

Gossop M, Griffiths P, Strang J: Sex differences in patterns of drug taking behaviour: a study at a London community drug team. Br J Psychiatry 164:101–104, 1994

Graeven D, Schaef R: Family life and levels of involvement in adolescent heroin epidemic. International Journal of the Addictions 13:747–771, 1978

Grant B: Prevalence and correlates of alcohol use and DSM-IV alcohol dependence in the United States: results from the National Longitudinal Alcohol Epidemiologic Survey. J Stud Alcohol 58:464–473, 1997

Grant BF, Pickering R: The relationship between cannabis use and DSM-IV cannabis abuse and dependence: results from the National Longitudinal Alcohol Epidemiologic Survey. J Subst Abuse 10:255–264, 1998

Grant B, Harford T, Dawson D, et al: Prevalence of DSM-IV alcohol abuse and dependence. Alcohol Health and Research World 18:243–248, 1994

Green SB, Byar DP: The effect of stratified randomization on size and power of statistical tests in clinical trials. Journal of Chronic Disease 31:445–454, 1978

Greenfield SF: Women and substance use disorders, in Psychopharmacology of Women: Sex, Gender, and Hormonal Considerations. Edited by Jensvold MF, Hamilton JA. Washington, DC, American Psychiatric Press, 1996, pp 299–321

Greenfield SF, Sugarman DE: Treatment and consequences of alcohol abuse and dependence during pregnancy, in Management of Psychiatric Disorders During Pregnancy. Edited by Yonkers KA, Little B. London, England, Edward Arnold Publishers, 2001, pp 213–227

Greenfield SF, Weiss RD, Mirin SM: Psychoactive substance use disorders, in The Practitioners Guide to Psychoactive Drugs, 4th Edition. Edited by Gelenberg AJ, Bassuk EL. New York, Plenum, 1997, pp 346–352

Greenfield SF, Weiss RD, Muenz LD, et al: The effect of depression on return to drinking: a prospective study. Arch Gen Psychiatry 55:259–265, 1998

Griffin ML, Mendelson JH, Mello NK, et al: Marihuana use across the menstrual cycle. Drug Alcohol Depend 18:213–224, 1986

Griffin ML, Weiss RD, Mirin SM, et al: The use of the Diagnostic Interview Schedule in drug dependent patients. Am J Drug Alcohol Abuse 13:281–291, 1987

Griffin ML, Weiss RD, Mirin SM: A comparison of male and female cocaine abusers. Arch Gen Psychiatry 46:122–126, 1989

Griffith DR, Azuma SD, Chasnoff IJ: Three-year outcome of children exposed prenatally to drugs. J Am Acad Child Adolesc Psychiatry 33:20–27, 1994

Grinspoon L, Bakalar JB: Marihuana, in Substance Abuse: A Comprehensive Textbook. Edited by Lowinson JH, Ruiz P, Millman RB, et al. Baltimore, MD, Williams & Willkins, 1997, pp 199–206

Gritz E, Crane L: Use of diet pills and amphetamines to lose weight among smoking and nonsmoking high school seniors. Health Psychol 10:330–335, 1991

Gritz E, Nielsen I, Brooks L: Smoking cessation and gender: the influence of physiological, psychological, and behavioral factors. J Am Med Womens Assoc 51:35–42, 1996

Gruber AJ, Pope HG: Cannabis-related disorders, in Psychiatry, Vol 1. Edited by Tasman A, Kay J, Lieberman JA. Philadelphia, PA, WB Saunders, 1997, pp 795–806

Gruber AJ, Pope HG, Brown ME: Do patients use marijuana as an antidepressant? Depression 4:77–80, 1996

Guinan M: Women and crack addiction. J Am Med Womens Assoc 44:129, 1989

Haas AL, Peters RH: Development of substance abuse problems among drug-involved offenders: evidence for the telescoping effect. J Subst Abuse 12:241–53, 2000

Haastrup S, Jepsen P: Eleven year follow-up of 300 young opioid addicts. Acta Psychiatr Scand 77:22–26, 1988

Haile R, Witte J, Ursin G, et al: A case-control study of reproductive variables, alcohol, and smoking in premenopausal bilateral breast cancer. Breast Cancer Res Treat 37:49–56, 1996

Halikas JA, Goodwin DW, Guze SB: Marihuana use and psychiatric illness. Arch Gen Psychiatry 27:162–165, 1972

Halikas J, Crosby R, Pearson V, et al: A randomized double-blind study of carbamazepine in the treatment of cocaine abuse. Clin Pharmacol Ther 62:89–105, 1997

Hall S, Reus V, Muñoz R, et al: Nortriptyline and cognitive-behavioral therapy in the treatment of cigarette smoking. Arch Gen Psychiatry 55:683–690, 1998

Hansen E, Andersen L, Von Eyben F: Cigarette smoking and age at first acute myocardial infarction, and influence of gender and extent of smoking. Am J Cardiol 71:1439–1442, 1993

Hasin D, Tsai W, Endicott J, et al: The effects of major depression on alcoholism. Am J Addict 5:144–155, 1996

Haver B: Female alcoholics, V: the relationship between family history of alcoholism and outcome 3–10 years after treatment. Acta Psychiatr Scand 76:21–27, 1987

Held JR, Riggs ML, Dorman C: The effect of prenatal cocaine exposure on neurobehavioral outcome: a meta-analysis. Neurotoxicol Teratol 21:619–625, 1999

Helzer JE, Burnam A, McEvoy LT: Alcohol abuse and dependence, in Psychiatric Disorders in America. Edited by Robins LN, Regier DA. New York, Free Press, 1991, pp 81–115

Herkenham M, Lynn AB, Little MD, et al: Cannabinoid receptor localization in brain. Neurobiology 87:1932–1936, 1990

Herr BM, Pettinati HM: Long term outcome in working and homemaking alcoholic women. Alcohol Clin Exp Res 8:576–579, 1984

Hesselbrock MN, Meyer RE, Keener JJ: Psychopathology in hospitalized alcoholics. Arch Gen Psychiatry 42:1050–1055, 1985

Hesselbrock V, Stabenau J, Hesselbrock M, et al: The nature of alcoholism in patients with different family histories for alcoholism. Prog Neuropsychopharmacol Biol Psychiatry 6:607–614, 1982

Hesselbrock VM, Hesselbrock MN, Workman-Daniels KL: Effect of major depression and antisocial personality on alcoholism: course and motivational patterns. J Stud Alcohol 47:207–212, 1986

Hiatt R, Fireman B: Smoking, menopause, and breast cancer. J Natl Cancer Inst 76:833–838, 1986

Higgins S, Delaney D, Budney A, et al: A behavioral approach to achieving initial cocaine abstinence. Am J Psychiatry 148:1218–1224, 1991

Hilleman D, Mohiuddin S, Del Core M, et al: Effect of buspirone on withdrawal symptoms associated with smoking cessation. Arch Intern Med 152:350–352, 1992

Hilleman D, Mohiuddin S, Delcore M, et al: Randomized, controlled trial of transdermal clonidine for smoking cessation. Ann Pharmacother 27:1025–1028, 1993

Hingson R, Alpert JJ, Day N, et al: Effects of maternal drinking and marijuana use on fetal growth and development. Pediatrics 70:539–546, 1982

Hjalmarson A, Franzon M, Westin A, et al: Effect of nicotine nasal spray on smoking cessation: a randomized, placebo-controlled, double-blind study. Arch Intern Med 154:2567–2572, 1994

Howell EM, Chasnoff IJ: Perinatal substance abuse treatment: findings from focus groups with clients and providers. J Subst Abuse Treat 17:139–148, 1999

Hser Y, Anglin M, McGlothin W: Sex differences in addict careers, I: initiation of use. Am J Drug Alcohol Abuse 13:33–57, 1987

Hughes J, Miller S: Nicotine gum to help stop smoking. JAMA 252:2855–2858, 1984

Hughes J, Hatsukami D, Pickens R, et al: Effect of nicotine on the tobacco withdrawal syndrome. Psychopharmacology 83:82–87, 1984

Hughes J, Hatsukami D, Mitchell J, et al: Prevalence of smoking among psychiatric outpatients. Am J Psychiatry 143:993–997, 1986

Hulse G, Milne E, English D, et al: Assessing the relationship between maternal cocaine use and abruptio placentae. Addiction 92:1547–1551, 1997a

Hulse G, English D, Milne E, et al: Maternal cocaine use and low birth weight newborns: a meta-analysis. Addiction 92:1561–1570, 1997b

Hulse G, Milne E, English D, et al: The relationship between maternal use of heroin and methadone and infant birth weight. Addiction 92:171–1579, 1997c

Hurley D: Women, alcohol and incest: an analytical view. J Stud Alcohol 52:253–268, 1991

Hurt H, Brodsky N, Braitman L, et al: Natal status of infants of cocaine users and control subjects: a prospective comparison. J Perinatol 15:297–304, 1995

Hurt R, Sachs D, Glover E, et al: A comparison of sustained-release bupropion and placebo for smoking cessation. N Engl J Med 337:1195–1202, 1997

Idänpään-Heikkilä J, Fritchie GE, Englert LF, et al: Placental transfer of tritiated-1-delta-9-tetrahydrocannabinol (letter to the editor). N Engl J Med 281:330, 1969

Johnson D, Karkut R: Performance by gender in a stop-smoking program combining hypnosis and aversion. Psychol Rep 75:851–857, 1994

Johnson R, Eissenberg T, Stitzer M, et al: A placebo controlled clinical trial of buprenorphine as a treatment for opioid dependence. Drug Alcohol Depend 40:17–25, 1995

Jones B, Jones M: Women and alcohol: intoxication, metabolism and the menstrual cycle, in Alcoholism Problems in Women and Children. Edited by Greenblatt M, Schuckit M. New York, Grune & Stratton, 1976, pp 103–136

Jones K, Smith D, Ulleland C, et al: Pattern of malformation in offspring of chronic alcoholic mothers. Lancet 1:1267–1271, 1973

Kampman K, Volpicelli J, Alterman A, et al: Amantadine in the early treatment of cocaine dependence: a double-blind, placebo-controlled trial. Drug Alcohol Depend 41:25–33, 1996

Kandall SR, Doberczak TM, Jantunen M, et al: The methadone-maintained pregnancy. Clin Perinatol 26:173–183, 1999

Kandel DB: Marijuana users in young adulthood. Arch Gen Psychiatry 41:200–209, 1984

Kandel D, Davies M: Adult sequelae of adolescent depressive symptoms. Arch Gen Psychiatry 43:255–262, 1986

Kandel D, Faust R: Sequence and stages in patterns of adolescent drug use. Arch Gen Psychiatry 32:923–932, 1975

Kandel DB, Yamaguchi K, Chen K: Stages of progression in drug involvement from adolescence to adulthood: further evidence for the gateway theory. J Stud Alcohol 53:447–457, 1992

Kannel W, Higgins M: Smoking and hypertension as predictors of cardiovascular risk in population studies. J Hypertens 8:S3–S8, 1990

Kaymakcalan S: The addictive potential of cannabis. Bull Narc 33:21–31, 1981

Kendler KS, Prescott CA: Cannabis use, abuse, and dependence in a population-based sample of female twins. Am J Psychiatry 155:1016–1022, 1998

Kendler K, Neale M, MacLean C, et al: Smoking and major depression: a causal analysis. Arch Gen Psychiatry 50:36–43, 1993

Kessler R, McGonagle K, Zhao S, et al: Lifetime and 12-month prevalence of DSM-III-R psychiatric disorders in the United States. Arch Gen Psychiatry 51:8–19, 1994

Kessler RC, Crum RM, Warner LA, et al: Lifetime co-occurrence of DSM-III-R alcohol abuse and dependence with other psychiatric disorders in the National Comorbidity Survey. Arch Gen Psychiatry 54:313–321, 1997

Khalsa H, Paredes A, Anglin MD: The role of alcohol in cocaine dependence, in Recent Developments in Alcoholism, Vol 10. Edited by Galanter M. New York, Plenum, 1992, pp 7–35

King DE, Herning RI, Gorelick DA, et al: Gender differences in the EEG of abstinent cocaine abusers. Neuropsychobiology 42:93–98, 2000

Kilbey MM, Sobeck JP: Epidemiology of alcoholism, in Women and Health Psychology. Edited by Travis CB. Hillsdale, NJ, Lawrence Erlbaum, 1988, pp 92–107

Kline J, Shrout P, Stein Z, et al: Drinking during pregnancy and spontaneous abortion. Lancet 2:176–180, 1980

Kohlendorfer U, Kiechl S, Sperl W: Sudden infant death syndrome: risk factor profiles for distinct subgroups. Am J Epidemiol 147:960–968, 1998

Kolodny RC, Masters WH, Kolodner RM, et al: Depression of plasma testosterone levels after chronic intensive marihuana use. N Engl J Med 290:872–874, 1974

Koren G, Graham K: Cocaine in pregnancy: analysis of fetal risk. Vet Hum Toxicol 34:263–264, 1992

Koren G, Nulman I, Rovet J, et al: Long-term neurodevelopmental risks in children exposed in utero to cocaine: the Toronto Adoption Study. Ann N Y Acad Sci 846:306–313, 1998

Kosofsky BE, Wilkins AS: A mouse model of transplacental cocaine exposure: clinical implications for exposed infants and children. Ann N Y Acad Sci 846:248–261, 1998

Kosten T, Rounsaville B: Psychopathology in opioid addicts. Psychiatr Clin North Am 9:515–532, 1986

Kosten TA, Gawin FH, Kosten TR, et al: Gender differences in cocaine use and treatment response. J Subst Abuse Treat 10:63–66, 1993

Kouri E, Pope HG, Yurgelun-Todd D, et al: Attributes of heavy vs. occasional marijuana smokers in a college population. Biol Psychiatry 38:475–481, 1995

Kovach J: Incest as a treatment issue for alcoholic women. Alcoholism Treatment Quarterly 3:1–15, 1986

Kranzler H, Bauer L, Hersh D, et al: Carbamazepine treatment of cocaine dependence: a placebo-controlled trial. Drug Alcohol Depend 38:203–211, 1995

Kranzler H, Del Boca F, Rounsaville B: Comorbid psychiatric diagnosis predicts three-year outcomes in alcoholics: a posttreatment natural history study. J Stud Alcohol 57:619–626, 1996

Ladwig G, Andersen M: Substance abuse in women: relationship between chemical dependency of women and past reports of physical and/or sexual abuse. International Journal of the Addictions 24:739–754, 1989

Lam S, To W, Duthie S, et al: Narcotic addiction in pregnancy with adverse maternal and perinatal outcome. Aust N Z J Obstet Gynaecol 32:216–221, 1992

Layde P, Broste S: Carcinoma of the cervix and smoking. Biomed Pharmacother 43:161–165, 1989

Lazzaroni F, Bonassi S, Magnani M, et al: Moderate maternal drinking and outcome of pregnancy. Eur J Epidemiol 9:599–606, 1993

Lee D, Markides K: Health behaviors, risk factors, and health indicators associated with cigarette use in Mexican Americans: results from the Hispanic HANES. Am J Public Health 81:859–864, 1991

Leonard BE: Cannabis: a short review of its effects and the possible dangers of its use. British Journal of Addiction to Alcohol and Other Drugs 64:121–130, 1969

Levy S, Doyle K: Attitudes to women in a drug treatment program. Journal of Drug Issues 4:423–434, 1974

Lewis C, Smith E, Kercher C, et al: Assessing gender interactions in the prediction of mortality in alcoholic men and women: a 20-year follow-up study. Alcohol Clin Exp Res 19:1162–1172, 1995

Lex B: Gender differences and substance abuse, in Advances in Substance Abuse: Behavioral and Biological Research, Vol 4. Edited by Mello N. London, England, Jessica Kingsley, 1991, pp 225–296

Lex BW: Alcohol problems in special populations, in Medical Diagnosis and Treatment of Alcoholism. Edited by Mendelson JH, Mello NK. New York, McGraw-Hill, 1992, pp 71–154

Lex BW, Griffin ML, Mello NK, et al: Concordant alcohol and marihuana use in women. Alcohol 3:193–200, 1986

Lex B, Griffin M, Mello N, et al: Alcohol, marijuana, and mood states in young women. International Journal of the Addictions 24:405–424, 1989

Lindberg S, Agren G: Mortality among male and female hospitalized alcoholics in Stockholm 1962–1983. British Journal of Addiction 83:1193–1200, 1988

Ling W, Charuvastra C, Collins J, et al: Buprenorphine maintenance treatment of opiate dependence: a multicenter, randomized clinical trial. Addiction 93:475–486, 1998

Linn S, Schoenbaum SC, Monson RR, et al: The association of marijuana use with outcome of pregnancy. Am J Public Health 73:1161–1164, 1983

Little B, Snell L, Klein V, et al: Maternal and fetal effects of heroin addiction during pregnancy. J Reprod Med 35:159–162, 1990

Lohr J, Flynn K: Smoking and schizophrenia. Schizophr Res 8:93–102, 1992

Lukas S, Sholar M, Lundahl L, et al: Sex differences in plasma cocaine levels and subjective effects after acute cocaine administration in human volunteers. Psychopharmacology 125:346–354, 1996

Luthar S, Cushing G, Rounsaville B: Gender differences among opioid abusers: pathways to disorder and profiles of psychopathology. Drug Alcohol Depend 43:179–189, 1996

Lyons P, Rittner B: The construction of the crack babies phenomenon as a social problem. Am J Orthopsychiatry 68:313–320, 1998

Macones G, Sehdev H, Parry S, et al: The association between maternal cocaine use and placenta previa. Am J Obstet Gynecol 177:1097–1100, 1997

Marsh K, Simpson D: Sex differences in opioid addiction careers. Am J Drug Alcohol Abuse 12:309–329, 1986

Marshall A, Kingstone D, Boss M, et al: Ethanol elimination in males and females: relationship to menstrual cycle and body composition. Hepatology 3:701–706, 1983

Marshall MF, Nelson LJ: Update on criminal prosecution of substance-abusing pregnant women. BioLaw 2:S17–S19, 1995

Martinez A, Kastner B, Taeusch HW: Hyperphagia in neonates withdrawing from methadone. Arch Dis Child Fetal Neonatal Ed 80:F178–F182, 1999

Mason B, Kocsis J, Ritvo E, et al: A double-blind, placebo-controlled trial of desipramine for primary alcohol dependence stratified on the presence or absence of major depression. JAMA 275:761–767, 1996

Matheny K, Weatherman K: Predictors of smoking cessation and maintenance. J Clin Psychol 54:223–235, 1998

McCance-Katz EF, Carroll KM, Rounsaville BJ: Gender differences in treatment-seeking cocaine abusers-implications for treatment and prognosis. Am J Addict 8:300–311, 1999

McCann M, Irwin D, Walton L, et al: Nicotine and cotinine in the cervical mucus of smokers, passive smokers, and nonsmokers. Cancer Epidemiol Biomarkers Prev 1:125–129, 1992

McDuffie H, Klaassen D, Dosman J: Female-male differences in patients with primary lung cancer. Cancer 59:1825–1830, 1987

McGrath P, Nunes E, Stewart J, et al: Imipramine treatment of alcoholics with primary depression: a placebo controlled clinical trial. Arch Gen Psychiatry 53:232–240, 1996

McKay J, Rutherford M, Cacciola J, et al: Gender differences in the relapse experiences of cocaine patients. J Nerv Ment Dis 184:616–622, 1996

McMahon TJ, Luthar SS: Women in treatment: within-gender differences in the clinical presentation of opioid-dependent women. J Nerv Ment Dis 188:679–687, 2000

McMurtrie C, Rosenberg KD, Kerker BD, et al: A unique drug treatment program for pregnant and postpartum substance-using women in New York City: results of a pilot project, 1990–1995. Am J Drug Alcohol Abuse 25:701–713, 1999

Mello N, Mendelson J: Buprenorphine suppresses heroin use by heroin addicts. Science 207:657–659, 1980

Mello NK, Mendelson JH: Operant acquisition of marihuana by women. J Pharmacol Exp Ther 235:162–171, 1985

Mello N, Mendelson J, Kuehnle J: Buprenorphine effects on human heroin self-administration: an operant analysis. J Pharmacol Exp Ther 223:30–39, 1982

Mello N, Mendelson J, Lex B: Alcohol use and premenstrual symptoms in social drinkers. Psychopharmacology 101:448–455, 1990

Mendelson JH, Kuehnle J, Ellingboe J, et al: Plasma testosterone levels before, during and after chronic marihuana smoking. N Engl J Med 291:1051–1055, 1974

Mendelson JH, Ellingboe J, Kuehnle JC, et al: Effects of chronic marihuana use on integrated plasma testosterone and luteinizing hormone levels. J Pharmacol Exp Ther 207:611–617, 1978

Mendelson JH, Mello NK, Lex BW, et al: Marijuana withdrawal syndrome in a woman. Am J Psychiatry 141:1289–1290, 1984

Mendelson JH, Mello NK, Ellingboe J, et al: Marihuana smoking suppresses luteinizing hormone in women. J Pharmacol Exp Ther 237:862–866, 1986

Mendelson J, Teoh S, Lange U, et al: Anterior pituitary, adrenal, and gonadal hormones during cocaine withdrawal. Am J Psychiatry 145:1094–1098, 1988

Mendhiratta SS, Varma VK, Dang R, et al: Cannabis and cognitive functions: a re-evaluation study. British Journal of Addiction 83:749–753, 1988

Miller B, Downs W, Gondoli D, et al: The role of childhood sexual abuse in the development of alcoholism in women. Violence Vict 2:157–172, 1987

Miller J, Boudreaux M, Regan F: A case-control study of cocaine use in pregnancy. Am J Obstet Gynecol 172:180–185, 1995

Miller NS, Gold MS, Pottash C: A 12-step treatment approach for marijuana (cannabis) dependence. J Subst Abuse Treat 6:241–250, 1989

Millman RB, Beeder AB: Cannabis, in The American Psychiatric Press Textbook of Substance Abuse Treatment. Edited by Galanter M, Kleber HD. Washington, DC, American Psychiatric Press, 1994, pp 91–109

Monica G, Lilja C: Placenta previa, maternal smoking and recurrence risk. Acta Obstet Gynecol Scand 74:341–345, 1995

Morabia A, Bernstein M, H'eritier S, et al: Relation of breast cancer with passive and active exposure to tobacco smoke. Am J Epidemiol 143:918–928, 1996

Morgan M, Sherlock S: Sex-related differences among 100 patients with alcoholic liver disease. BMJ 1:939–941, 1977

Mumme D: Aftercare: its role in primary and secondary recovery of women from alcohol and other drug dependence. International Journal of the Addictions 26:549–564, 1991

Murphy J, Edwards N, Downs A, et al: Effects of doxepin on withdrawal symptoms in smoking cessation. Am J Psychiatry 147:1353–1357, 1990

Najavits L, Gastfriend D, Barber J, et al: Cocaine dependence with and without PTSD among subjects in the National Institute on Drug Abuse Collaborative Cocaine Treatment Study. Am J Psychiatry 115:214–219, 1998

Nides M, Rakos R, Gonzales D, et al: Predictors of initial smoking cessation and relapse through the first 2 years of the Lung Health Study. J Consult Clin Psychol 63:60–69, 1995

Nischan P, Ebeling K, Schindler C: Smoking and invasive cervical cancer risk: results from a case-control study. Am J Epidemiol 128:74–77, 1988

Nurco D, Wegner N, Stephenson F: Female narcotic addicts: changing profiles. Journal on Addiction and Health 3:62–105, 1982

O'Brien CP: Recent developments in the pharmacotherapy of substance abuse. J Consult Clin Psychol 64:677–686, 1996

Ockene J, Kristeller J: Tobacco, in The American Psychiatric Press Textbook of Substance Abuse Treatment. Edited by Galanter M, Kleber H. Washington, DC, American Psychiatric Press, 1994, pp 157–177

O'Malley S, Jaffe A, Chang G, et al: Naltrexone and coping skills therapy for alcohol dependence: a controlled study. Arch Gen Psychiatry 49:881–887, 1992

Orford J, Keddie A: Gender differences in the functions and effects of moderate and excessive drinking. Br J Clin Psychol 24:265–279, 1985

Ornish S, Zisook S, McAdams L: Effects of transdermal clonidine treatment on withdrawal symptoms associated with smoking cessation: a randomized, controlled trial. Arch Intern Med 148:2027–2031, 1988

Osann K, Anton-Culver H, Kurosaki T, et al: Sex differences in lung-cancer risk associated with cigarette smoking. Int J Cancer 54:44–48, 1993

Parrella DP, Filstead WJ: Definition of onset in the development of onset-based alcoholism typologies. J Stud Alcohol 49:85–92, 1988

Pedersen W, Mastekaasa A, Wichstrom L: Conduct problems and early cannabis initiation: a longitudinal study of gender differences. Addiction 96:415–431, 2001

Penniman L, Agnew J: Women, work, and alcohol: occupational medicine, in Alcoholism and Chemical Dependency in the Workplace. Edited by Wright C. Philadelphia, PA, Hanley & Belfus, 1989, pp 264–273

Peralta V, Cuesta MJ: Influence of cannabis abuse on schizophrenic psychopathology. Acta Psychiatr Scand 85:127–130, 1992

Perez-Stable E, Marin G, Marin B, et al: Depressive symptoms and cigarette smoking among Latinos in San Francisco. Am J Public Health 80:1500–1502, 1990

Perper J, Van Thiel D: Respiratory complications of cocaine abuse. Recent Dev Alcohol 10:363–377, 1992

Pettinati H, Sugerman A, Maurer H: Four-year MMPI changes in abstinent and drinking alcoholics. Alcohol Clin Exp Res 6:487–494, 1982

Pettinati H, Cabezas R, Jensen J, et al: Incidence of personality disorders in cocaine vs. alcohol dependent females. NIDA Res Monogr 105:369–370, 1991

Piazza NJ, Vrbka JL, Yeager RD: Telescoping of alcoholism in women alcoholics. International Journal of the Addictions 24:19–28, 1989

Pierce J, Fiore M, Novotny T, et al: Trends in cigarette smoking in the United States: projections to the year 2000. JAMA 261:61–65, 1989

Pirie P, Murray D, Luepker R: Gender differences in cigarette smoking and quitting in a cohort of young adults. Am J Public Health 81:324–327, 1991

Pope HG, Yurgelun-Todd D: The residual cognitive effects of heavy marijuana use in college students. JAMA 275:521–527, 1996

Pope HG, Jacobs A, Mialet J-P, et al: Evidence for a sex-specific residual effect of cannabis on visuospatial memory. Psychother Psychosom 66:179–184, 1997

Popkin C, Rudisill L, Waller P, et al: Female drinking and driving: recent trends in North Carolina. Accid Anal Prev 20:219–255, 1988

Popour J: Planning Women's Alcohol and Drug Services in Michigan. Lansing, Michigan Department of Public Health, Office of Substance Abuse Services, 1983

Powis B, Griffiths P, Gossop M, et al: The differences between male and female drug users: community samples of heroin and cocaine users compared. Subst Use Misuse 31:529–543, 1996

Purdie D, Green A, Bain C, et al: Reproductive and other factors and risk of epithelial ovarian cancer: an Australian case-control study. Survey of Women's Health Study Group. Int J Cancer 62:678–684, 1995

Randall CL, Roberts JS, Del Boca FK, et al: Telescoping of landmark events associated with drinking: a gender comparison. J Stud Alcohol 60:252–60, 1999

Ranstam J, Olsson H: Alcohol, cigarette smoking, and the risk of breast cancer. Cancer Detect Prev 19:487–493, 1995

Rawson R, Obert J, McCann M, et al: Cocaine treatment outcome: cocaine use following inpatient, outpatient and no treatment, in Problems of Drug Dependence, 1985. Proceedings of the 47th Annual Scientific Meeting, The Committee on Problems of Drug Dependence (NIDA Res Monogr 67; DHHS Publ No ADM-86-1448). Edited by Harris LA. Washington, DC, U.S. Department of Health and Human Services, 1986, pp 111–120

Reed BG: Perinatal substance use, in The American Psychiatric Press Textbook of Substance Abuse Treatment, 2nd Edition. Edited by Galanter M, Kleber HD. Washington, DC, American Psychiatric Press, 1999, pp 491–501

Reed T: Outcome research on treatment and on the drug abuser: an exploration. International Journal of the Addictions 13:149–171, 1978

Regier DA, Farmer ME, Rae DS, et al: Comorbidity of mental disorders with alcohol and other drug abuse: results from the Epidemiologic Catchment Area (ECA) study. JAMA 264:2511–2518, 1990

Reich T, Cloninger R, Eerdewegh P, et al: Secular trends in familial transmission of alcoholism. Alcohol Clin Exp Res 12:458–464, 1988

Richardson GA: Prenatal cocaine exposure: a longitudinal study of development. Ann N Y Acad Sci 846:144–152, 1998

Rigotti N: Cigarette smoking and body weight. N Engl J Med 320:931–933, 1989

Risch H, Howe G, Jain M, et al: Are female smokers at higher risk for lung cancer than male smokers? A case-control analysis by histologic type. Am J Epidemiol 138:281–293, 1993

Robins LN, Regier DA: Psychiatric Disorders in America. New York, Free Press, 1991

Roffman RA, Stephens RS, Simpson EE, et al: Treatment of marijuana dependence: preliminary results. J Psychoactive Drugs 20:129–137, 1988

Rohsenow DJ, Monti PM, Martin RA, et al: Brief coping skills treatment for cocaine abuse: 12-month substance use outcomes. J Consult Clin Psychol 68:515–520, 2000

Root M: Treatment failures: the role of sexual victimization in women's addictive behavior. Am J Orthopsychiatry 59:542–549, 1989

Roquer J, Figueras J, Botet F, et al: Influence on fetal growth of exposure to tobacco smoke during pregnancy. Acta Paediatr 84:118–121, 1995

Rose J, Herskovic J, Trilling Y, et al: Transdermal nicotine reduces cigarette craving and nicotine preference. Clin Pharmacol Ther 38:450–456, 1985

Rosenbaum M: Becoming addicted: the woman addict. Contemporary Drug Problems 8:141–167, 1979

Rosenbaum M: Women on Heroin. New Brunswick, NJ, Rutgers University Press, 1981

Rosenthal B, Savoy M, Greene B, et al: Drug treatment outcomes: is sex a factor? International Journal of the Addictions 14:45–62, 1979

Ross HE, Glaser FB, Germanson T: The prevalence of psychiatric disorders in patients with alcohol and other drug problems. Arch Gen Psychiatry 45:1023–1031, 1988

Roth MD, Arora A, Barsky SH, et al: Airway inflammation in young marijuana and tobacco smokers. Am J Respir Crit Care Med 157:928–937, 1998

Rounsaville BJ, Kleber HD: Untreated opiate addicts: how do they differ from those seeking treatment? Arch Gen Psychiatry 42:1072–1077, 1985

Rounsaville B, Weissman M, Kleber H, et al: Heterogeneity of psychiatric diagnosis in treated opiate addicts. Arch Gen Psychiatry 39:161–166, 1982a

Rounsaville BJ, Weissman MM, Wilber CH, et al: Pathways to opiate addiction: an evaluation of differing antecedents. Br J Psychiatry 141:437–446, 1982b

Rounsaville BJ, Dolinsky ZS, Babor TF, et al: Psychopathology as a predictor of treatment outcome in alcoholics. Arch Gen Psychiatry 44:505–513, 1987

Rounsaville BJ, Anton SF, Carroll K, et al: Psychiatric diagnosis of treatment-seeking cocaine abusers. Arch Gen Psychiatry 48:43–51, 1991

Royce J, Corbett K, Sorensen G, et al: Gender, social pressure, and smoking cessations: the Community Intervention Trial for Smoking Cessation (COMMIT) at baseline. Soc Sci Med 44:359–370, 1997

Sandmeier M: The Invisible Alcoholics: Women and Alcohol Abuse in America. New York, McGraw-Hill, 1980

Saraiya M, Berg C, Kendrick J, et al: Cigarette smoking as a risk factor for ectopic pregnancy. Am J Obstet Gynecol 178:493–498, 1998

Savitz D, Zhang J, Schwingl P, et al: Association of paternal alcohol use with gestational age and birth weight. Teratology 46:465–471, 1992

Schlaud M, Kleemann W, Poets C, et al: Smoking during pregnancy and poor antenatal care: two major preventable risk factors for sudden infant death syndrome. Int J Epidemiol 25:959–965, 1996

Schmitz J, Schneider N, Jarvik M: Nicotine, in Substance Abuse: A Comprehensive Textbook, 3rd Edition. Edited by Lowinson J, Ruiz P, Millman R, et al. Baltimore, MD, Williams & Willkins, 1997, pp 276–293

Schneider R, Khantzian E: Psychotherapy and patient needs in treatment of alcohol and cocaine abuse. Recent Dev Alcohol 10:179–191, 1992

Schneider N, Olmstead R, Mody F, et al: Efficacy of a nicotine nasal spray in smoking cessation: a placebo-controlled, double-blind trial. Addiction 90:1671–1682, 1995a

Schneider K, Kviz F, Isola M, et al: Evaluating multiple outcomes and gender differences in alcoholism treatment. Addict Behav 20:1–21, 1995b

Schottenfeld R, Pakes J, Kosten T: Prognostic factors in buprenorphine- versus methadone-maintained patients. J Nerv Ment Dis 186:35–43, 1998

Schuckit MA, Irwin M, Brown SA: The history of anxiety symptoms among 171 primary alcoholics. J Stud Alcohol 51:34–41, 1990

Schuckit M, Daeppen J-B, Tipp J, et al: The clinical course of alcohol-related problems in alcohol dependent and nonalcohol dependent drinking women and men. J Stud Alcohol 59:581–590, 1998

Schwartz JR, Schwartz LP: The drug court: a new strategy for drug use prevention. Obstet Gynecol Clin North Am 25:255–268, 1998

Sidney S, Quesenberry CP, Friedman GD, et al: Marijuana use and cancer incidence (California, United States). Cancer Causes Control 8:722–728, 1997

Siegel R: Cocaine and sexual dysfunction: the curse of mama coca. J Psychoactive Drugs 14:71–74, 1982

Simansky KJ, Baker G, Kachelries WJ, et al: Prenatal exposure to cocaine reduces dopaminergic D1-mediated motor function but spares the enhancement of learning by amphetamine in rabbits. Ann N Y Acad Sci 846:375–378, 1998

Sinha C, Ohadike P, Carrick P, et al: Neonatal outcome following maternal opiate use in late pregnancy. Int J Gynaecol Obstet 74:241–6, 2001

Slattery M, Robison L, Schuman K, et al: Cigarette smoking and exposure to passive smoke are risk factors for cervical cancer. JAMA 261:1593–1598, 1989

Slone D, Shapiro S, Rosenberg L, et al: Relation of cigarette smoking to myocardial infarction in young women. N Engl J Med 298:1273–1276, 1978

Slutsker L: Risks associated with cocaine use during pregnancy. Obstet Gynecol 79:778–789, 1992

Smith E, Sowers M, Burns T: Effects of smoking on the development of female reproductive cancers. J Natl Cancer Inst 73:371–376, 1984

Smith EM, Cloninger CR, Bradford S: Predictors of mortality in alcoholic women: a prospective follow-up study. Alcohol Clin Exp Res 7:237–243, 1983

Sprauve M, Lindsay M, Herbert S, et al: Adverse perinatal outcome in patients who use crack cocaine. Obstet Gynecol 89:674–678, 1997

Stephens RS, Roffman RA, Simpson E: Adult marijuana users seeking treatment. J Consult Clin Psychol 62:92–99, 1993

Stephens RS, Roffman RA, Simpson E: Treating adult marijuana dependence: a test of the relapse prevention model. J Consult Clin Psychol 62:92–99, 1994

Stevens VJ, Hollis JF: Preventing smoking relapse using an individually tailored skills-training technique. J Consult Clin Psychol 57:420–424, 1989

Stockwell H, Lyman G: Cigarette smoking and the risk of female reproductive cancer. Am J Obstet Gynecol 157:35–40, 1987

Substance Abuse and Mental Health Services Administration: Substance Use Among Women in the United States. Rockville, MD, U.S. Department of Health and Human Services, 1997

Substance Abuse and Mental Health Services Administration: National Household Survey on Drug Abuse: Main Findings, 1996. Rockville, MD, U.S. Department of Health and Human Services, 1998

Substance Abuse and Mental Health Services Administration: National Household Survey on Drug Abuse: Main Findings 1997. Office of Applied Studies, NHSDA Series H-8. Rockville, MD, Department of Health and Human Services, 1999

Substance Abuse and Mental Health Services Administration: Summary of Findings from the 2000 National Household Survey on Drug Abuse. Office of Applied Studies, NHSDA Series H-13. Rockville, MD, Department of Health and Human Services, 2001

Tannenbaum J, Miller F: Electrocardiographic evidence of myocardial injury in psychiatrically hospitalized cocaine abusers. Gen Hosp Psychiatry 14:201–203, 1992

Taylor FM: Marijuana as a potential respiratory tract carcinogen. South Med J 81:1213–1216, 1988

Thom B: Sex differences in help-seeking for alcohol problems, I: the barriers to help-seeking. British Journal of Addiction 81:777–788, 1986

Thomas H: A community survey of adverse effects of cannabis use. Drug Alcohol Depend 42:201–207, 1996

Tonnesen P, Norregaard J, Mikkelsen K, et al: A double-blind trial of a nicotine inhaler for smoking cessation. JAMA 269:1268–1271, 1993

Trevathan E, Layde P, Webster L, et al: Cigarette smoking and dysplasia and carcinoma in situ of the uterine cervix. JAMA 250:499–502, 1983

Underhill B: Issues relevant to aftercare programs for women. Alcohol Health Res World 11:46–48, 1994

Urbano-Márquez A, Estruch R, Fernández-Solà J, et al: The greater risk of alcoholic cardiomyopathy and myopathy in women compared with men. JAMA 274:149–154, 1995

Vaillant GE, Clark W, Cyrus C, et al: Prospective study of alcoholism treatment: eight-year follow-up. Am J Med 75:455–463, 1983

Van Etten ML, Neumark YD, Anthony JC: Initial opportunity to use marijuana and the transition to first use: United States, 1979–1994. Drug Alcohol Depend 49:1–7, 1997

Van Thiel D, Gavaler J: Ethanol metabolism and hepatotoxicity: does sex make a difference?, in Recent Developments in Alcoholism, Vol 6. Edited by Galanter M. New York, Plenum, 1988, pp 291–304

Varma VK, Malhotra AK, Dang R, et al: Cannabis and cognitive functions: a prospective study. Drug Alcohol Depend 21:147–152, 1988

Vik T, Jacobsen G, Vatten L, et al: Pre- and post-natal growth in children of women who smoked in pregnancy. Early Hum Dev 45:245–255, 1996

Volpicelli J, Alterman A, Hayashida M, et al: Naltrexone in the treatment of alcohol dependence. Arch Gen Psychiatry 49:876–880, 1992

Vriz O, Nesbitt S, Krause L, et al: Smoking is associated with higher cardiovascular risk in young women than in men: the Tecumseh Blood Pressure Study. J Hypertens 15:127–134, 1997

Wanberg KW, Horn JL: Alcoholism symptom patterns of men and women: a comparative study. J Stud Alcohol 31:40–61, 1970

Wang ED: Methadone treatment during pregnancy. J Obstet Gynecol Neonatal Nurs 28:615–622, 1999

Ward K, Klesges R, Zbikowski S, et al: Gender differences in the outcome of an unaided smoking cessation attempt. Addict Behav 22:521–533, 1997

Warren CW, Kann L, Small ML, et al: Age of initiating selected health-risk behaviors among high school students in the United States. J Adolesc Health 21:225–231, 1997

Washton A: Nonpharmacologic treatment of cocaine abuse. Psychiatr Clin North Am 9:563–571, 1986

Wasserman GA, Kline JK, Bateman DA, et al: Prenatal cocaine exposure and school-age intelligence. Drug Alcohol Depend 50:203–210, 1998

Weddington W: Issues regarding short term abstinence in outpatient cocaine addicts. Am J Psychiatry 148:1759–1760, 1991

Weisner C: The epidemiology of combined alcohol and drug use within treatment agencies: a comparison by gender. J Stud Alcohol 54:268–274, 1993

Weisner C, Schmidt L: Gender disparities in treatment for alcohol treatment problems. JAMA 268:1872–1876, 1992

Weiss RD, Mirin SM, Michael JL, et al: Psychopathology in chronic cocaine abusers. Am J Drug Alcohol Abuse 12:17–29, 1986

Weiss RD, Mirin SM, Griffin ML, et al: Psychopathology in cocaine abusers: changing trends. J Nerv Ment Dis 176:719–725, 1988

Weiss RD, Mirin SM, Griffin ML, et al: Personality disorders in cocaine dependence. Compr Psychiatry 34:145–149, 1993

Weiss R, Martinez-Raga J, Griffin M, et al: Gender differences in cocaine dependent patients: a 6 month follow-up study. Drug Alcohol Depend 44:35–40, 1997

Weller RA, Halikas JA: Marijuana use and psychiatric illness: a follow-up study. Am J Psychiatry 142:848–850, 1985

Wenger N: Hypertension and other cardiovascular risk factors in women. Am J Hypertens 8:94S–99S, 1995

West R, Hajek P, McNeill A: Effect of buspirone on cigarette withdrawal symptoms and short-term abstinence rates in a smokers clinic. Psychopharmacology 104:91–96, 1991

Wiepert G, d'Orban P, Bewley T: Delinquency by opiate addicts treated at two London clinics. Br J Psychiatry 134:14–23, 1979

Wiesbeck GA, Schuckit MA, Kalmijn JA, et al: An evaluation of the history of a marijuana withdrawal syndrome in a large population. Addiction 91:1469–1478, 1996

Wilde M, Wagstaff A: Acamprosate: a review of its pharmacology and clinical potential in the management of alcohol dependence after detoxification. Drugs 53:1038–1053, 1997

Willett W, Green A, Stampfer M, et al: Relative and absolute excess risks of coronary heart disease among women who smoke cigarettes. N Engl J Med 317:1303–1309, 1987

Williams MA, Lieberman E, Mittendorf R, et al: Risk factors for abruptio placentae. Am J Epidemiol 134:965–972, 1991

Windham G, Von Behren J, Fenster L, et al: Moderate maternal alcohol consumption and risk of spontaneous abortion. Epidemiology 8:509–514, 1997

Winfield I, George L, Swarz M, et al: Sexual assault and psychiatric disorders among a community sample of women. Am J Psychiatry 147:335–341, 1990

Woods J, Plessinger M, Clark K: Effect of cocaine on uterine blood flow and fetal oxygenation. JAMA 257:957–961, 1987

Wright C, Moore R: Disulfiram treatment of alcoholism. Am J Med 88:647–655, 1990

Wright S, Mitchell E, Thompson J, et al: Risk factors for preterm birth: a New Zealand study. N Z Med J 111:14–16, 1998

Wu T-C, Tashkin DP, Djahed B, et al: Pulmonary hazards of smoking marijuana as compared with tobacco. N Engl J Med 318:347–351, 1988

Yamaguchi K, Kandel DB: Patterns of drug use from adolescence to young adulthood, II: sequences of progression. Am J Public Health 74:668–672, 1984a

Yamaguchi K, Kandel DB: Patterns of drug use from adolescence to young adulthood, III: predictors of progression. Am J Public Health 74:673–681, 1984b

Yu J, Essex D, Williford W: DWI/DWAI offenders and recidivism by gender in the eighties: a changing trend? International Journal of the Addictions 27:637–647, 1992

Yudkin P, Jones L, Lancaster T, et al: Which smokers are helped to give up smoking using transdermal nicotine patches? Results from a randomized, double-blind, placebo-controlled trial. Br J Gen Pract 46:145–148, 1996

Zang E, Wynder E: Cumulative tar exposure: a new index for estimating lung cancer risk among cigarette smokers. Cancer 70:69–76, 1992

Zang E, Wynder E: Differences in lung cancer risk between men and women: examination of the evidence. J Natl Cancer Inst 88:183–192, 1996

Zuckerman B, Frank DA, Hingson R, et al: Effects of maternal marijuana and cocaine use on fetal growth. N Engl J Med 320:762–768, 1989

Zweben JE, O'Connell K: Strategies for breaking marijuana dependence. J Psychoactive Drugs 20:121–127, 1988

22

Sex Composition and Sex Differences in the Dissociative Disorders

Relationship to Trauma and Abuse

Elizabeth S. Bowman, M.D.

*A*lthough dissociation has been described for many centuries, dissociative disorders were not so named until 1980 when DSM-III (American Psychiatric Association 1980) abandoned the term *hysteria* in favor of separate categories for somatoform and dissociative disorders. More than 90% of "hysteria" occurred in women (Robins et al. 1952), and most patients with somatoform disorders are female, so we might expect similar findings in the five dissociative disorders. In this chapter, I explore the sex ratios of one of the descendants of hysteria, the dissociative disorders, and consider their relation to the abuse of females.

DISSOCIATIVE IDENTITY DISORDER

Descriptions of the clinical characteristics of what we call *dissociative identity disorder* have been consistent for several centuries, but its name has fluctu-

535

ated wildly. Before DSM-III, it was called *exchanged personality*, *dual personality*, *alternating personalities*, *hysteria*, *dissociative reaction*, and *multiple personality disorder* (Greaves 1980; Kluft 1991). In DSM-III and DSM-III-R (American Psychiatric Association 1987), it was named *multiple personality disorder*, but in DSM-IV (American Psychiatric Association 1994), it was renamed *dissociative identity disorder* in recognition that its core pathology is splintering rather than multiplication of identity. The diagnostic criteria for multiple personality disorder and dissociative identity disorder in DSM-III, DSM-III-R, and DSM-IV all differ slightly from one another, so I use *multiple personality disorder* to refer to studies before DSM-IV and *dissociative identity disorder* to refer to studies thereafter and to the disorder in general.

Of all of the dissociative disorders, dissociative identity disorder has the most consistent data on sex distribution and the highest female preponderance. Table 22–1 shows the sex distribution of adult patients with multiple personality disorder or dissociative identity disorder in systematic case series (Bliss 1980, 1984; Boon and Draijer 1993; Coons et al. 1988; Martínez-Taboas 1991; Putnam et al. 1986; Ross et al. 1989a, 1990; Sar et al. 1996; Schultz et al. 1989). Table 22–1 does not include sex comparison studies, which intentionally overrepresent male patients. In 9 of the 11 studies, the proportion of females is between 88% and 96%. These sex data show good agreement across adult clinical populations on three continents.

Why are so many patients with dissociative identity disorder women? Most authors point to data on the strong association of dissociative identity disorder with severe prolonged childhood trauma, especially physical and sexual abuse (Coons 1986; Greaves 1980; Loewenstein and Putnam 1990; Putnam et al. 1986; Ross et al. 1989a). Except for Yuichi Hattori's report from Japan (personal communication, September 1996), which shows a 33% incidence of childhood physical and sexual abuse, these case series show astounding rates of childhood maltreatment: physical abuse, 60%–82%; sexual abuse, 57%–90%; physical and/or sexual abuse, 77%–97%; neglect, 22%–63%; emotional abuse, 10%–57%, and any childhood abuse, 94%–97%.

A popular explanation for sex differences in dissociative identity disorder lies in differential rates of childhood abuse. Generally, females report about twice the rate of childhood sexual abuse (16%–31%) (Russell 1983) as males (3%–16%) (Finkelhor 1987). Girls are significantly more likely than boys (35% vs. 11%) to be sexually assaulted by relatives (Siegel et al. 1987), a type of assault that may predispose to dissociative defenses (Freyd 1996). If incestual abuse were a major precipitant of dissociative identity disorder, then we would expect a 2:1 or 3:1 female-to-male sex ratio, not the 9:1 ratio seen in adult patients with dissociative identity disorder. Abuse data on patients with dissociative identity disorder indicate that both sexes experience multiple types of trauma at similar frequencies, suggesting that

TABLE 22–1. Sex distribution in case series of adult patients with dissociative identity disorder

Study	N	Male, n	Female, n	Female, %	Country studied
Bliss 1984	70	22	48	69	United States
Bliss 1980	14	0	14	100	United States
Boon and Draijer 1993	71	3	68	96	Netherlands
Coons et al. 1988	50	4	46	92	United States
Hattori 1996[a]	18	1	17	94	Japan
Martínez-Taboas 1991	15	1	14	93	Puerto Rico
Putnam et al. 1986	100	8	92	92	United States
Ross et al. 1989b	236	29	207	88	Canada and United States
Ross et al. 1990	102	10	92	90	Canada and United States
Sar et al. 1996	35	4	31	89	Turkey
Schultz et al. 1989	355	35	320	90	United States
All studies	1,066	117	949	89	

Note. [a]Y. Hattori, "Clinical Features of 18 Japanese Patients With Dissociative Identity Disorder" personal communication, 1996.

dissociative identity disorder in both sexes is strongly associated with multiple childhood traumas. It is possible that boys and girls are equally likely to create dissociative identity disorder in the face of prolonged, overwhelming abuse but that females' lifelong physical vulnerability vis-à-vis males may expose them to more years of a higher risk of physical and sexual abuse (Putnam 1989). In addition, females are culturally discouraged from responding physically against others and may perceive themselves as more helpless and trapped in the face of abuse. These factors provide the best explanation available to date for the sex imbalance in dissociative identity disorder, but they remain speculative. The exact reasons for the sex imbalance in dissociative identity disorder are unknown.

As evidenced in the above studies, the histories of dissociative identity disorder patients point to a childhood onset of dissociative identity disorder as a coping mechanism for surviving the emotional effect of childhood abuse or trauma. Adults with dissociative identity disorder invariably report the first creation of alter personalities in childhood, and dissociative identity disorder persists indefinitely without treatment (Kluft 1985). Childhood and adolescent cases of dissociative identity disorder show a 1:1 or 2:1

female-to-male ratio (Hornstein and Putnam 1992; Vincent and Pickering 1988). Because childhood dissociative identity disorder has rarely been treated, we could expect the same sex ratio in adult patients. However, as Table 22–1 indicates, this is not what occurs.

How can we explain the differences in sex proportions in childhood and adulthood dissociative identity disorder? Why are so many fewer males with dissociative identity disorder found in adult treatment settings than in childhood studies? Are there clinical differences between males and females with dissociative identity disorder that cause males to be underdiagnosed? The most commonly offered answer is that males with dissociative identity disorder tend to enter prison, whereas females enter treatment, but do data support this idea?

Sex Comparisons of Clinical Features of Dissociative Identity Disorder

Questions about the fate of males with dissociative identity disorder and sex differences in dissociative identity disorder have been addressed in three studies. Bliss (1986) studied 22 men and 48 women with DSM-III multiple personality disorder, and Ross and Norton (1989) reported on 28 men and 207 women with DSM-III or DSM-III-R multiple personality disorder. In a detailed sex comparison study, Loewenstein and Putnam (1990) compared 21 men with DSM-III and DSM-III-R multiple personality disorder with 92 women from another series of patients (Putnam et al. 1986).

The findings of these three studies were strikingly similar. They found that the clinical similarities between men and women with multiple personality disorder far outweigh the differences. Each study found that multiple personality disorder in both sexes presents with a highly polysymptomatic picture of affective, anxiety, somatic, substance abuse, dissociative, posttraumatic stress, and personality disorder symptoms. Men and women did not differ significantly in hypnotizability, the frequencies of presenting symptoms, age, socioeconomic status, marital status, number of personalities at initial diagnosis, ages or types of alter personalities (e.g., child, persecutor, opposite sex), the frequency of alter coconsciousness and switching, the number of previous diagnoses, the number of Schneiderian first-rank symptoms, specific dissociative symptoms, or Dissociative Experiences Scale (DES) scores (Bernstein and Putnam 1986).

Clinical sex differences in dissociative identity disorder tend to involve minor differences that reflect sex socialization. Examples include observations that females with dissociative identity disorder create opposite-sex child personalities more than males do, that both sexes tend to use adult male alters as protector personalities and adult female alters as nurturing parental alters, and that inter-alter differences in dress and elaboration of identity seem less marked in males than in females with dissociative identity disorder (Putnam 1989).

A few sex differences in dissociative identity disorder have emerged. Female subjects engaged in self-injury significantly more than did male subjects (58% vs. 40%) (Ross and Norton 1989). Men reported a slightly younger age when their first alter personality was formed (6.62 years vs. 7.85 years for females, $P<0.002$) (Loewenstein and Putnam 1990). Sex comparisons of childhood trauma reports in patients with dissociative identity disorder have not found significant differences in the likelihood of childhood abuse, the likelihood of repeated physical and sexual abuse, or the number of types of abuse, but they did not compare the duration of abuse (Loewenstein and Putnam 1990; Ross and Norton 1989). In one study, women with dissociative identity disorder (57%) were significantly more likely than men (17%) to report adulthood rapes (Loewenstein and Putnam 1990), but another study found that rates of lifetime rape were equal (~65%) in men and women with dissociative identity disorder (Ross et al. 1989a). Clinical and child abuse differences between men and women with dissociative identity disorder pale in comparison to their similarities, but women with dissociative identity disorder may endure more adult revictimization. In both sexes, the disorder is associated with overwhelming childhood trauma.

Comorbid Symptoms and Diagnoses

Adults with dissociative identity disorder have a mean of three to four lifetime comorbid psychiatric diagnoses that usually include major depression, posttraumatic stress disorder, panic disorder, phobias, eating disorders, substance use disorders, and personality disorders. Many of these patients also have been given misdiagnoses of schizophrenia or bipolar disorder (Coons et al. 1988; Putnam et al. 1986; Ross et al. 1989a). In general, men and women with dissociative identity disorder do not differ in the frequencies of their comorbid and prior diagnoses, but one study (Ross and Norton 1989) found that women were significantly more likely to have had a prior affective disorder diagnosis (65% vs. 48%), and another (Bliss 1986) found significantly more anxiety, phobias, and obsessive-compulsive symptoms in the female patients. These sex differences are similar to those observed in general psychiatric patients.

Hysteria, Dissociative Identity Disorder, and Somatoform Disorders

In DSM-III, the diagnosis of hysteria was abandoned, and its symptoms were split into two diagnostic sections: dissociative disorders and somatoform disorders (including conversion disorder). Hysteria has been considered a woman's disease since the days of Hippocrates, and the link between hysteria and women has been so strong that until the past 25 years, modern investigators generally have been unwilling to recognize hysteria in men (Robins et al. 1952). Like "hysterics," patients with dissociative identity disorder and those with a variety of somatoform disorders are overwhelmingly female and have markedly elevated rates of childhood sexual abuse compared with other psychiatric populations (Arnold and Privitera 1996; Boisset-Pioro et al. 1995; Bowman 1993; Loewenstein 1990; Walker et al. 1993, 1995). Patients with dissociative identity disorder surpass the general and psychiatric populations in their frequency of somatization disorder (18%–64%) and conversion disorder (Ross et al. 1989a, 1989b; Saxe et al. 1994). Likewise, patients with somatization disorder have elevated levels of dissociation (Pribor et al. 1993; Ross et al. 1989b; Saxe et al. 1994; Walker et al. 1992). These comorbidity findings suggest that the sex distribution of "hysteria" (somatization, conversion, and severe dissociative disorders) may reflect an association with trauma, especially childhood sexual abuse. I suspect that the sex imbalance and overlap of symptoms in pain disorder, somatization disorder, conversion disorder, and dissociative identity disorder are all related to higher rates of childhood sexual abuse in girls.

Although somatization disorder usually is a predominantly female diagnosis, one study found that the frequency of somatization disorder did not differ in men and women with multiple personality disorder (Ross and Norton 1989). This lack of a sex difference may be related to the similar abuse experiences of men and women with dissociative identity disorder. However, Bliss (1986) found more "hysteria" in women than men with multiple personality disorder, and Loewenstein and Putnam (1990) found a nonsignificant trend for women with dissociative identity disorder to report more conversion symptoms than do men (~60% vs. ~22%).

"Hysteria" did not die with DSM-III, but an awareness of childhood sexual abuse as a potential etiology for these symptoms has been born out of subsequent research on its descendants, including dissociative identity disorder. Such findings illustrate that hysteria likely reflected the socialization, victimization, and stereotyping of females rather than an inherent constitutional weakness (Lerner 1974).

Treatment History

Men and women with dissociative identity disorder do not differ in their frequency of hospitalization, attempted or completed suicide, or prior treatment with psychotherapy, antipsychotic medication, or electroconvulsive therapy. However, in one study, men spent significantly less time

(4.2±5.4 years) in the mental health system before diagnosis compared with women (7.1±6.2 years, $P<0.02$), and women had been prescribed antidepressants and benzodiazepines significantly more often than men were (Ross and Norton 1989). The shorter multiple personality disorder treatment history of men was noted by Loewenstein and Putnam (1990) as a probable reason for men reporting significantly fewer alter personalities compared with women (mean=7.2 vs. 19.1; $P<0.0001$). Men likely had not been in treatment long enough to have an opportunity for more alters to emerge.

Substance Use Disorders

Noting considerable rates of alcoholism in males with multiple personality disorder and the association of child abuse and adulthood alcohol abuse, several authors posited that males with multiple personality disorder may be found in substance abuse treatment settings rather than general psychiatric clinics (Kluft 1985; Loewenstein and Putnam 1990). Two studies of inpatients with substance abuse (Dunn et al. 1993; Ross et al. 1992), one of which used only male subjects (Dunn et al. 1993), found that approximately 40% have dissociative disorders or elevated scores on the DES. Other data support the concept that males with dissociative identity disorder might reside in the substance abuse treatment setting. Two studies found no significant sex differences in drug abuse (Loewenstein and Putnam 1990; Ross and Norton 1989), but two other studies found more alcoholism in males than in females with multiple personality disorder (46% vs. 19% [Bliss 1986] and ~68% vs. ~30% [Loewenstein and Putnam 1990]). Overall, studies indicate that males with dissociative identity disorder may abuse alcohol more than do females with dissociative identity disorder and may enter substance abuse treatment rather than another psychotherapy.

Sex Studies of Sociopathy in Dissociative Identity Disorder

A significant association between sociopathy and hysteria has been hypothesized because of observations of an increased prevalence of "hysteria" (including dissociative symptoms) among the relatives of male felons and of increased sociopathy and substance abuse in the relatives of women with "hysteria" (Cloninger and Guze 1970). This association, along with the popular myth that male multiple personality disorder is associated with violence, has resulted in studies of sociopathy and criminal behavior in males with multiple personality disorder. Popular fiction such as Stevenson's (1886) *The Strange Case of Dr. Jekyll and Mr. Hyde* and modern accounts of criminals with multiple personality disorder (Keyes 1981) have perpetuated the myth that males with multiple personality disorder are violent or criminal (Keyes 1981; Schultz et al. 1989). Sex comparison studies of multiple personality disorder have focused on criminal behavior to address this myth and determine whether males with multiple personality disorder go to jail rather than to treatment.

Allison (1981) was the first to report more criminal and antisocial behavior in males (62%) than in females (5%) with multiple personality disorder. All three sex comparison studies found that males with multiple personality disorder endorsed more sociopathic symptoms or committed more antisocial acts than did their female counterparts (Bliss 1986; Loewenstein and Putnam 1990; Ross and Norton 1989). Males with multiple personality disorder have higher rates of some, but not all, antisocial activities; one study found no difference in the proportion of each sex who had worked as prostitutes (Ross and Norton 1989), but two studies found that men had been incarcerated (28%–45%) more often than the women (10%–35%) (Loewenstein and Putnam 1990; Ross and Norton 1989). Sex differences in rates of criminal behavior in multiple personality disorder reached statistical significance only in the study by Ross and Norton (1989).

Loewenstein and Putnam (1990) studied interpersonal violence and found no significant difference between the proportion of men (90%) and women (74%) who reported having violent alters, having homicidal alters (one-third of each group), or having perpetrated a homicide (19% of men vs. 7% of women). Likewise, they found that intrapersonally directed violence (inter-alter violence and suicidal behavior) was equally common in men and women.

These studies found that antisocial behavior is reported more often by both sexes of patients with multiple personality disorder than in the general population but did not consistently find significant sex differences in interpersonal violence. One problem with most of these studies is that they involved patients with multiple personality disorder in treatment; if males with multiple personality disorder truly are more violent and tend to be found in the penal system, then clinical studies would have overlooked them.

There also appears to be an association between male dissociative identity disorder and criminal behavior when the problem is approached via studies of forensic populations. Bliss and Larson (1985) found that 7 of 33 (21%) convicted male sexual offenders had multiple personality disorder, and others had symptoms highly suggestive of multiple personality disorder. Their data suggest that males with multiple personality disorder may tend to be found in prison. Cloninger and Guze (1970) reported that many female felons whom they studied spontaneously mentioned having a "split personality," but no one has formally studied dissociative disorders in female felons. Overall, these studies hint at increased violence in persons with dissociative identity disorder, but data do not show definite sex differences in violence within the dissociative identity disorder population.

Conclusions About Sex and Dissociative Identity Disorder

The studies discussed in this section show that there are far more similarities than differences between men and women with dissociative identity disorder in their clinical presentation and abuse histories. Differences between men and women with dissociative identity disorder reflect the *frequency* rather than the *type* of symptoms and comorbidities. I agree with Ross and Norton (1989) that observed dissociative identity disorder sex differences are merely consistent with sex differences seen in our culture and in general psychiatric practice: women are diagnosed more often with depression, are prescribed more antidepressants and benzodiazepines, are more likely to self-injure, and are less likely to be convicted of crimes. Sex differences in the frequency of comorbid diagnoses usually involve sex-influenced diagnoses, such as increased alcoholism and sociopathy in males. Differences in the frequency of self-mutilation, conversion, and sociopathy seem to reflect the tendency of men to act out against others and women to act against themselves or to express somatic symptoms. However, the studies suggest that dissociative identity disorder patients of both sexes are more likely than the general population to express their distress by acting antisocially against others. This may be related to lack of control over dissociated rage related to their child abuse experiences. Dissociative identity disorder studies suggest that familial clustering of sociopathy, alcoholism, and "hysteria" (dissociation/somatization) could involve sex-influenced responses to a shared family environment of victimization. Dissociative identity disorder may be the result of social norms that encourage more sexual abuse of girls than boys and that prolong abuse in females by socializing submissive responses in females but sanctioning physically aggressive defenses in males.

Multiple personality disorder sex comparison studies are consistent with the conclusion that multiple personality disorder is a valid diagnostic category that shows good overlap between males and females in etiology, symptoms, and comorbid conditions (Loewenstein and Putnam 1990). Still, many questions remain unanswered about the different life pathways of males and females with dissociative identity disorder. These studies lend some support to the theory that males with dissociative identity disorder may avoid diagnosis by entering the penal system rather than treatment. However, the paucity of male patients with dissociative identity disorder in psychiatric treatment is not simply because they are in prison. Many males enter treatment after serving their sentences and returning to the community (Loewenstein and Putnam 1990).

Other reasons may exist for the sex imbalance of adults in treatment for dissociative identity disorder. The well-known female preponderance of patients with dissociative identity disorder may lead clinicians not to suspect dissociative identity disorder in men. The paucity of males in treatment may reflect the tendency for women to seek mental health care more than men do or to present more easily recognizable symptoms of dissociative identity disorder. Men with dissociative identity disorder tend to show less noticeable switching behaviors (Kluft 1986) and less elaboration of alternate identities. The female personalities in male patients with dissociative identity disorder are less obvious than the strikingly masculine male alters of females with dissociative identity disorder (Putnam 1989). These characteristics, combined with confusion between alcoholic and dissociative amnesia in men, may render the "average" male with dissociative identity disorder less recognizable to clinicians.

I suspect that a combination of factors (criminality, substance abuse, treatment-seeking patterns, more subtle symptoms, and the expectations of clinicians) may prevent men from being diagnosed with dissociative identity disorder as often as women are. The accuracy of the nearly equal sex ratios of children with dissociative identity disorder is unknown. Although the association of dissociative identity disorder with the abuse of children is certain, the actual lifetime sex distribution of dissociative identity disorder remains uncertain.

DISSOCIATIVE AMNESIA AND DISSOCIATIVE FUGUE

In DSM-IV, psychogenic amnesia and psychogenic fugue were renamed dissociative amnesia and dissociative fugue, respectively, but no information is given about their sex distribution. Amnesia for one's past or confusion of identity are part of the criteria for dissociative fugue, so all cases of fugue include the symptom of amnesia. Persons with dissociative amnesia can present with some elements of fuguelike travel, such as finding themselves in an adjacent part of their city of residence without remembering traveling there. These diagnoses are discussed together because of the overlap in their criteria and because older case series often contain an admixture of these diagnoses.

Table 22–2 shows the sex distribution of case series of dissociative amnesia (Abeles and Schilder 1935; Coons and Milstein 1992; Kanzer 1939;

TABLE 22–2. Sex distribution in case series of patients with dissociative amnesia

Study	N	Male, n	Female, n	Female, %	Population studied
Abeles and Schilder 1935	63	31	32	51	Psychiatric inpatients
Leavitt 1935	104	66	38	37	General hospital patients
Kanzer 1939	71	41	30	42	Psychiatric inpatients
Sargent and Slater 1941	144	144	0	0	Inpatient combat casualties
Parfitt and Gall 1944	30	30	0	0	Wartime military patients
Wilson et al. 1950	59	31	28	47	General hospital patients
Kennedy and Neville 1957	74	52	22	30	Emergency room patients
Kiersch 1962	98	92	6	6	Military general hospital
Kirshner 1973	30	23	7	23	Military general hospital
Coons and Milstein 1992	25	2	23	92	Psychiatric inpatients and outpatients
Nonmilitary studies[a]	396	223	173	44	
All studies	698	512	186	27	

Note. [a]Does not include Sargent and Slater 1941; Parfitt and Gall 1944; Kennedy and Neville 1957; Kiersch 1962; and Kirshner 1973.

Kennedy and Neville 1957; Kiersch 1962; Kirshner 1973; Leavitt 1935; Parfitt and Gall 1944; Sargent and Slater 1941; Wilson et al. 1950). Determining the true sex ratio of dissociative fugue and amnesia has been greatly complicated by imprecise diagnostic criteria and selection bias in case reporting. Generally, only the most dramatic cases of fugue and global amnesia are published. Except for the series by Coons and Milstein (1992), the studies in Table 22–2 contain cases of dramatic, sudden-onset, and rapidly resolving amnesia. These studies are sex biased by large studies drawn from solely male military populations. When military studies are included, approximately three-fourths of the dissociative amnesia cases are in men. When more general populations are studied, slightly more than half of the sudden-onset cases are in men.

The overwhelmingly female composition of the study by Coons and Milstein (1992) illustrates the critical role of subject selection and diagnostic criteria in dissociative amnesia studies. Most of the subjects in this study were inpatients in a longer-term psychiatric hospital, a group that is two-thirds female and excludes persons with acute, rapidly resolving amnesia. It is the only study conducted after the advent of clearly defined DSM criteria that differentiated between psychogenic amnesia and fugue and is the only study to systematically rule out dissociative disorder not otherwise specified (DDNOS) and dissociative identity disorder. It illustrated that 90% of the seriously ill people with chronic and stable dissociative amnesia are women and that they have elevated rates of childhood abuse. In contrast, the other case series, depicting persons with sudden-onset amnesia for identity (with or without fugue), reported that more than half were men.

These data suggest that chronic and stable amnesia may be quite common and has the sex distribution (about 90% female) seen in child-abuse-associated diagnoses such as dissociative identity disorder. Sudden amnesia for identity (outside of dissociative identity disorder patients) is much rarer and appears to afflict more men than women. Whether this presentation of amnesia is associated with a history of child abuse is unknown.

The occurrence of amnesia in response to a vast array of psychological traumas has been established beyond doubt (van der Kolk 1996). Persons with chronic and stable symptoms of dissociative amnesia are commonly identified by therapists while taking childhood histories from incest or childhood trauma survivors (Bowman 1993; Kirshner 1973). For this reason, dissociative amnesia is probably the most common dissociative disorder. These patients, who are overwhelmingly female, often report that they cannot recall significant periods of time during their youth. Amnesia is rarely their presenting complaint. The amnesia symptoms of child abuse survivors are often combined with other symptoms and classified as part of posttraumatic stress disorder or DDNOS. Thus, they do not show up in case series of "dissociative amnesia," even though many of these patients also meet DSM-IV-TR (American Psychiatric Association 2000) criteria for this disorder. Nearly all the dissociative amnesia cases that I have encountered have been chronic amnesia in women. I suspect that women may be underrepresented in literature reports of dissociative amnesia because women do not tend to present with sudden amnesia for their identity; instead, their amnesia involves long-past periods of their lives and is not their greatest concern.

Dissociative fugue is quite rare. As with amnesia studies, several studies of fugues have been performed in military settings and probably overrepresented male patients (Coons 2000; Loewenstein 1991). DSM-IV-TR criteria for both dissociative fugue and dissociative amnesia specify that the fugue or amnesia cannot be due to dissociative identity disorder. These exclusion criteria were inserted because dissociative fugue and amnesia are unique in being *disorders* as well as *symptoms* of other disorders (such as dissociative identity disorder) (Loewenstein 1991). The occurrence of the *symptom* of fugue in patients with dissociative identity disorder and

DDNOS may bias reports of the sex distribution of dissociative fugue. In case studies of fugue or sudden-onset amnesia, authors rarely mention having ruled out alter personality states. In some of the female patients, symptoms suggest the possibility of undetected complex dissociative disorders (Kirshner 1973; Loewenstein 1991). Because fugue states occur in approximately half of the adult patients with dissociative identity disorder (Coons and Milstein 1992; Putnam 1989), it is likely that some female cases of dissociative amnesia or fugue were actually undetected diagnoses of dissociative identity disorder or DDNOS. Patients with DDNOS also report past episodes of fuguelike behaviors that were brief, not accompanied by persistent autobiographical amnesia, and not reported to mental health personnel. For example, a patient I saw with DDNOS set out to visit her daughter in another town and ended up 3 hours away in the other direction with amnesia for the trip but awareness of her identity. She oriented herself, returned home, and only reported this and other fugue episodes months later when asked directly about them during an evaluation for conversion seizures.

If twentieth-century reports of more than a single case of fugue are considered (see Table 22–3) (Akhtar and Brenner 1979; Berrington et al. 1956; Fisher 1945; Fisher and Joseph 1949; Ford 1989; Kirshner 1973; Stengel 1941, 1943), males make up 65 (66%) of 99 cases. These reports include two small series (Fisher 1945; Kirshner 1973) from military settings in which more than 80% of the subjects were males. If these series were eliminated because of sampling bias, males still make up 54 (63%) of the 86 remaining cases. Thus, about two-thirds of the cases of dramatic or obvious presentations of fugue appear to occur in men. If some of the female cases include persons who actually had undetected dissociative identity disorder, then the male-to-female ratio of fugue cases may be even larger, but there is no way to accurately determine whether this is the case.

Reviews of dissociative fugue have agreed that fugue is a response to traumatic circumstances or severe inescapable psychological conflict (Coons 2000; Loewenstein 1991). Females (Loewenstein 1991) with fugues usually report a history of childhood abuse, but such histories also are reported by some men with fugues. It is not clear if men or women with a history of childhood abuse are more likely than persons without child abuse to have fugues, but abused persons are known to have a higher incidence of combat-related amnesia compared with nonabused persons (Loewenstein 1991).

Reports of amnesia and fugue in men increase during wartime and usually involve flight from combat. Of course, these reports are sex biased by exclusion of women from combat. The frequency of amnesia among soldiers in World War II rose with the severity of combat—from 6% in those

TABLE 22–3. Sex ratio in case series of patients with dissociative fugue

Study	N	Male, n	Female, n	Female, %	Comment
Akhtar and Brenner 1979	9	7	2	22	
Berrington et al. 1956	37	31	6	16	
Fisher 1945	6	5	1	17	Military population
Fisher and Joseph 1949	2	1	1	50	
Ford 1989	2	2	0	0	
Kirshner 1973	7	6	1	14	Military population
Stengel 1941	25	7	18	72	
Stengel 1943	11	6	5	45	
Nonmilitary studies	86	54	32	37	
All studies	99	65	34	34	

in "mild" combat to 35% in those in severe combat (Sargent and Slater 1941), but severity of combat experiences has not been studied in relation to fugues. In civilian populations, I and others have seen fugue states in men who were facing impending discovery of legal wrongdoing, embarrassing sexual behavior, marital dissolution, or bankruptcy (Coons 2000). In both sexes, investigators have noted the following causes of fugues: adult rape; threat of death or physical violence; bereavement; avoidance of suicidal, homicidal, or sexual urges; and the impending discovery of criminal behavior or sexual difficulties.

Do men and women with dissociative fugue flee from the same traumas and conflicts? Case series offer trends but no definitive answer. Both sexes tend to develop fugues in response to conflicts over shameful or unacceptable behaviors or threats to physical integrity. Sex differences exist in the latter category, with women showing fugues in response to rape, sexual abuse, or domestic violence and men showing fugues in response to combat. The underlying dynamic that produces fugues—a need to escape from overwhelming internal conflict or external horror—does not appear to differ between females and males (Abeles and Schilder 1935; Coons et al. 1997; Loewenstein 1991), but the types of external threat differ: men flee military combat, and women flee domestic "combat." The prevalence of fugue states in patients with dissociative identity disorder and the overwhelming number of females with dissociative identity disorder suggest that the *symptom* of fugue may occur more often in women and the *diagnosis* of dissociative fugue occurs more often in men. Data to test this hypothesis await further research and are unlikely until clinical skills in detecting dissociative identity disorder are more widespread.

DISSOCIATIVE DISORDER NOT OTHERWISE SPECIFIED

DDNOS is a diagnostic category that covers diverse presentations of dissociative symptoms that do not fit into the other four DSM-IV-TR dissociative disorders. Like depersonalization disorder, it has been poorly studied. Two sizable series include the study by Coons (1992) of 50 adult patients (86% female) and the study by Hornstein and Putnam (1992) of 20 children and adolescents with DDNOS (sex ratios not specified).

DDNOS is not a single disorder. Coons (1992) described diverse presentations of dissociation that qualify as DDNOS (e.g., nocturnal dissociation, "ego-state" disorder, derealization without depersonalization), but he did not comment on the sex distribution of the persons with these subtypes. The most common subgroup of DDNOS (52% of Coons's sample) is persons with ego-state disorder, a condition of ego division that is similar to dissociative identity disorder but with less overt switching between ego states and less clear-cut identity differentiation. The sex distribution and the trauma reports of Coons's subjects (96% reported child abuse or neglect) are similar to those in series of subjects with dissociative identity disorder. As in studies of patients with dissociative identity disorder, the study by Coons reported similar rates of child abuse in male and female subjects with DDNOS. It is unclear whether this single series is representative of the sex ratio of persons with DDNOS. The role of sex in the etiology of DDNOS is unclear, but it may be related to different rates of child abuse experiences in boys and girls.

DEPERSONALIZATION DISORDER

The *experience* of depersonalization is quite common and may rank behind anxiety and depression as the third most common psychiatric symptom (Dixon 1963). However, depersonalization *disorder*, consisting of persistent distressing depersonalization in the absence of another Axis I disorder or organic causes, is quite rare and poorly understood.

Two early series of patients with depersonalization included 70%–80% females (Mayer-Gross 1935; Shorvon 1946). In two sizeable studies of depersonalization disorder published since DSM-III, Simeon and colleagues reported 63% of 30 subjects were women (Simeon et al. 1997) but did not report gender composition of a study involving 49 subjects (Simeon et al. 2001). Of the six other smaller series reported in Table 22–4 (Ackner 1954; Chee and Wong 1990; Davison 1964; Hollander et al. 1990; Lehmann 1974; Shimizu and Sakamoto 1986), three reported more men than women. DSM-III-R reported a 1:1 sex ratio, DSM-IV did not comment on

TABLE 22–4.　Sex distribution in case series of patients with depersonalization disorder

Study	N	Male, n	Female, n	Female, %
Mayer-Gross 1935	25	5	20	80
Shorvon 1946	66	20	46	70
Ackner 1954	6	2	4	67
Davison 1964	7	5	2	29
Lehmann 1974	3	1	2	67
Shimizu and Sakamoto 1986	6	4	2	33
Hollander et al. 1990	8	3	5	63
Chee and Wong 1990	9	5	4	44
Simeon et al. 1997	30	11	19	63
All subjects	160	56	104	65

the sex distribution of depersonalization disorder, and DSM-IV-TR indicates that depersonalization disorder is diagnosed in clinical samples at a 2:1 (female to male) ratio. When all reported case series are combined, 84 of 135 cases (62%) are females. A review by Coons (1996) concluded that the sex ratio of depersonalization disorder is not clear.

Of all the dissociative disorders, depersonalization disorder is least associated with early physical and sexual abuse. Simeon et al. (1997) found that total trauma and physical abuse were each significantly higher in subjects with depersonalization disorder than in control subjects, but sexual abuse differences only approached significance. Later, Simeon et al. (2001) found that childhood interpersonal trauma as a whole is highly predictive of a diagnosis of depersonalization disorder and of symptoms of pathological dissociation, but that emotional abuse was the most significant factor predicting a diagnosis of depersonalization disorder and levels of depersonalization on the DES. In contrast, general dissociation scores were better predicted by a combination of emotional and sexual abuse.

Most authors cite a variety of life stresses and biological pathologies as the causes of depersonalization disorder. The nearly equal sex ratio of depersonalization disorder may be related to possibly organic causes that affect men and women nearly equally. In addition, it is possible that sex ratios in depersonalization disorder are less overwhelmingly female compared with those of dissociative identity disorder or dissociative amnesia because the type of trauma that produces depersonalization (emotional abuse) is directed more equally at boys and girls. In contrast, the childhood trauma prominently associated with dissociative disorder (sexual abuse) is disproportionately experienced by girls, producing overwhelmingly female clinical populations of dissociative identity disorder in adulthood.

CONCLUSION

The wide range of sex distributions in the dissociative disorders illustrates the effect of the abuse of females on development of some mental illnesses. The dissociative disorders with the strongest links to childhood abuse (i.e., dissociative identity disorder, DDNOS, chronic amnesia) show a strong female preponderance in adulthood and strong overlap with other descendants (conversion and other somatoform diagnoses) of the "female" illness of "hysteria." The male preponderance of dissociative fugue and sudden-onset dissociative amnesia hints that males dissociate when massively stressed in adulthood, but they seem to have less complex types of dissociative disorders, possibly because they have less exposure to the severe child abuse experiences that predispose to dissociative identity disorder and DDNOS. The association of various traumas with dissociative amnesia in both sexes is unquestionable. Females and males appear to show amnesia with equal frequency when traumatized, but their differential exposure to trauma appears to affect the dissociative symptoms that they develop. The different sex predominances in sudden global amnesia (males) and chronic circumscribed amnesia (females) suggest that sex-associated differences in the exposure to childhood and adulthood trauma affect the type of amnesia that develops. The diagnosis with little association to child abuse, depersonalization disorder, has a sex ratio that differs little from that of outpatient psychiatric populations (two-thirds female).

REFERENCES

Abeles M, Schilder P: Psychogenic loss of personal identity: amnesia. Arch Neurol Psychiatry 34:587–604, 1935

Ackner B: Depersonalization, II: clinical syndromes. Journal of Mental Science 100:854–872, 1954

Akhtar S, Brenner I: Differential diagnosis of fugue-like states. J Clin Psychiatry 40:381–385, 1979

Allison RB: Multiple personality and criminal behavior. American Journal of Forensic Psychiatry 82:181–192, 1981

American Psychiatric Association: Diagnostic and Statistical Manual of Mental Disorders, 3rd Edition. Washington, DC, American Psychiatric Association, 1980

American Psychiatric Association: Diagnostic and Statistical Manual of Mental Disorders, 3rd Edition, Revised. Washington, DC, American Psychiatric Association, 1987

American Psychiatric Association: Diagnostic and Statistical Manual of Mental Disorders, 4th Edition. Washington, DC, American Psychiatric Association, 1994

American Psychiatric Association: Diagnostic and Statistical Manual of Mental Disorders, 4th Edition, Text Revision. Washington, DC, American Psychiatric Association, 2000

Arnold LM, Privitera MD: Psychopathology and trauma in epileptic and psychogenic seizure patients. Psychosomatics 37:438–443, 1996

Bernstein EM, Putnam FW: Development, reliability, and validity of a dissociation scale. J Nerv Ment Dis 174:727–735, 1986

Berrington WP, Liddell DW, Foulds GA: A re-evaluation of the fugue. Journal of Mental Science 102:280–286, 1956

Bliss EL: Multiple personalities: a report of 14 cases with implications for schizophrenia and hysteria. Arch Gen Psychiatry 37:1388–1397, 1980

Bliss EL: A symptom profile of patients with multiple personalities, including MMPI results. J Nerv Ment Dis 172:197–202, 1984

Bliss EL: Multiple Personality, Allied Disorders and Hypnosis. New York, Oxford University Press, 1986, p 153

Bliss EL, Larson EM: Sexual criminality and hypnotizability. J Nerv Ment Dis 173:522–526, 1985

Boisset-Pioro MH, Esdaile JM, Fitzcharles MA: Sexual and physical abuse in women with fibromyalgia syndrome. Arthritis Rheum 2:235–241, 1995

Boon S, Draijer N: Multiple personality disorder in The Netherlands: a clinical investigation of 71 patients. Am J Psychiatry 150:489–494, 1993

Bowman ES: Etiology and clinical course of pseudoseizures: relationship to trauma, depression and dissociation. Psychosomatics 34:333–342, 1993

Chee KT, Wong KE: Depersonalization syndrome: a report of 9 cases. Singapore Med J 31:331–334, 1990

Cloninger CR, Guze SB: Psychiatric illness and female criminality: the role of sociopathy and hysteria in the antisocial woman. Am J Psychiatry 127:303–311, 1970

Coons PM: Child abuse and multiple personality disorder: review of the literature and suggestions for treatment. Child Abuse Negl 10:455–462, 1986

Coons PM: Dissociative disorder not otherwise specified: a clinical investigation of 50 cases with suggestions for typology and treatment. Dissociation 5:187–195, 1992

Coons PM: Depersonalization and derealization, in Handbook of Dissociation. Edited by Michelson LK, Ray WJ. New York, Plenum, 1996, pp 291–305

Coons PM: Dissociative fugue, in Kaplan and Saddock's Comprehensive Textbook of Psychiatry, Vol I, 7th Edition. Edited by Saddock BJ, Saddock VA. Philadelphia, PA, Lippincott Williams & Wilkins, 2000, pp 1548–1552

Coons PM, Milstein V: Psychogenic amnesia: a clinical investigation of 25 cases. Dissociation 5:73–79, 1992

Coons PM, Bowman ES, Milstein V: Multiple personality disorder: a clinical investigation of 50 cases. J Nerv Ment Dis 176:519–527, 1988

Coons PM, Bowman ES, Milstein V: Repressed memories in patients with dissociative disorder: literature review, controlled study and treatment recommendations, in American Psychiatric Press Review of Psychiatry, Vol 16. Edited by Dickstein LJ, Riba MB, Oldham JM. Washington, DC, American Psychiatric Press, 1997, pp II 153–II 172

Davison K: Episodic depersonalization: observations on 7 patients. Br J Psychiatry 110:505–513, 1964

Dixon JC: Depersonalization phenomenon in a sample population of college students. Br J Psychiatry 109:371–375, 1963

Dunn GE, Paolo AM, Ryan JJ, et al: Dissociative symptoms in a substance abuse population. Am J Psychiatry 150:1043–1047, 1993

Finkelhor D: The sexual abuse of children: current research reviewed. Psychiatric Annals 17:233–241, 1987

Fisher C: Amnesic states in war neuroses: the psychogenesis of fugues. Psychoanal Q 14:437–468, 1945

Fisher C, Joseph ED: Fugue with awareness of loss of personal identity. Psychoanal Q 18:480–493, 1949

Ford CV. Psychogenic fugue, in Treatments of Psychiatric Disorders, Vol 3. Edited by Karasu TB. Washington, DC, American Psychiatric Press, 1989, pp 2190–2196

Freyd JJ: Betrayal Trauma: The Logic of Forgetting Childhood Abuse. Cambridge, MA, Harvard University Press, 1996

Greaves GB: Multiple personality disorder: 165 years after Mary Reynolds. J Nerv Ment Dis 168:577–596, 1980

Hollander E, Liebowitz MR, DeCaria C, et al: Treatment of depersonalization with serotonin reuptake blockers. J Clin Psychopharmacol 10:200–203, 1990

Hornstein NL, Putnam FW: Clinical phenomenology of child and adolescent dissociative disorders. J Am Acad Child Adolesc Psychiatry 31:1077–1085, 1992

Kanzer M: Amnesia: a statistical study. Am J Psychiatry 96:711–716, 1939

Kennedy A, Neville J: Sudden loss of memory. BMJ 2:428–433, 1957

Keyes D: The Minds of Billy Milligan. New York, Random House, 1981

Kiersch TA: Amnesia: a clinical study of ninety-eight cases. Am J Psychiatry 119:57–60, 1962

Kirshner LA: Dissociative reactions: an historical review and clinical study. Acta Psychiatr Scand 49:698–711, 1973

Kluft RP: The natural history of multiple personality disorder, in Childhood Antecedents of Multiple Personality. Edited by Braun BG. Washington, DC, American Psychiatric Press, 1985, pp 197–238

Kluft RP: Personality unification in multiple personality disorder: a follow-up study, in The Treatment of Multiple Personality Disorder. Edited by Braun BG. Washington, DC, American Psychiatric Press, 1986, pp 29–60

Kluft RP: Multiple personality disorder, in American Psychiatric Press Review of Psychiatry, Vol 10. Edited by Tasman A, Goldfinger SM. Washington, DC, American Psychiatric Press, 1991, pp 161–188

Leavitt FH: The etiology of temporary amnesia. Am J Psychiatry 91:1079–1088, 1935

Lehmann LS: Depersonalization. Am J Psychiatry 131:1221–1224, 1974

Lerner HE: The hysterical personality: a "woman's disease." Compr Psychiatry 15:157–164, 1974

Loewenstein RJ: Somatoform disorders in victims of incest and child abuse, in Incest-Related Syndromes of Adult Psychopathology. Edited by Kluft RP. Washington, DC, American Psychiatric Press, 1990, pp 75–107

Loewenstein RJ: Psychogenic amnesia and psychogenic fugue: a comprehensive review, in American Psychiatric Press Review of Psychiatry, Vol 10. Edited by Tasman A, Goldfinger SM. Washington, DC, American Psychiatric Press, 1991, pp 189–223

Loewenstein RJ, Putnam FW: The clinical phenomenology of males with MPD: a report of 21 cases. Dissociation 3:135–143, 1990

Martínez-Taboas A: Multiple personality in Puerto Rico: analysis of 15 cases. Dissociation 4:189–192, 1991

Mayer-Gross W: On depersonalization. Br J Med Psychol 15:103–126, 1935

Parfitt DN, Gall CMC: Psychogenic amnesia: the refusal to remember. Journal of Mental Science 379:511–531, 1944

Pribor EF, Yutzy SH, Dean JT, et al: Briquet's syndrome, dissociation, and abuse. Am J Psychiatry 150:1507–1511, 1993

Putnam FW: Diagnosis and Treatment of Multiple Personality Disorder. New York, Guilford, 1989

Putnam FW, Guroff JJ, Silberman EK, et al: The clinical phenomenology of multiple personality disorder: a review of 100 recent cases. J Clin Psychiatry 47:285–293, 1986

Robins E, Purtell JJ, Cohen ME: "Hysteria" in men: a study of 38 patients so diagnosed and 194 control subjects. N Engl J Med 246:677–685, 1952

Ross CA, Norton GR: Differences between men and women with multiple personality disorder. Hosp Community Psychiatry 40:186–188, 1989

Ross CA, Norton GR, Wozney K: Multiple personality disorder: an analysis of 236 cases. Can J Psychiatry 34:413–418, 1989a

Ross CA, Heber S, Norton GR, et al: Somatic symptoms in multiple personality disorder. Psychosomatics 30:154–160, 1989b

Ross CA, Miller SD, Reagor P, et al: Structured interview data on 102 cases of multiple personality disorder from four centers. Am J Psychiatry 147:596–601, 1990

Ross CA, Dronson J, Koensgen S, et al: Dissociative comorbidity in 100 chemically dependent patients. Hosp Community Psychiatry 43:840–842, 1992

Russell DEH: The incidence and prevalence of intrafamilial and extrafamilial sexual abuse of female children. Child Abuse Negl 7:133–146, 1983

Sar V, Yargiç LI, Tutkun H: Structured interview data on 35 cases of dissociative identity disorder in Turkey. Am J Psychiatry 153:1329–1333, 1996

Sargent W, Slater E: Amnesic syndromes in war. Proceedings of the Royal Society of Medicine 34:757–764, 1941

Saxe GN, Chinman G, Berkowitz R, et al: Somatization in patients with dissociative disorders. Am J Psychiatry 151:1329–1334, 1994

Schultz R, Braun BG, Kluft RP: Multiple personality disorder: phenomenology of selected variables in comparison to major depression. Dissociation 2:45–51, 1989

Shimizu M, Sakamoto S: Depersonalization in early adolescence. Japanese Journal of Psychiatry 40:603–608, 1986

Shorvon HJ: The depersonalization syndrome. Proceedings of the Royal Society of Medicine 39:779–785, 1946

Siegel JM, Sorenson SB, Golding JM, et al: The prevalence of childhood sexual assault: the Los Angeles Epidemiologic Catchment Area Project. Am J Epidemiol 126:1141–1153, 1987

Simeon D, Gross S, Guralnik O, et al: Feeling unreal: 30 cases of DSM-III-R depersonalization disorder. Am J Psychiatry 154:1107–1113, 1997

Simeon D, Guralnik O, Schmeidler J, et al: The role of childhood interpersonal trauma in depersonalization disorder. Am J Psychiatry 158:1027–1033, 2001

Stengel E: On the aetiology of fugue states. Journal of Mental Science 87:572–599, 1941

Stengel E: Further studies on pathological wandering (fugues with the impulse to wander). Journal of Mental Science 89:224–241, 1943

Stevenson RL: The Strange Case of Dr. Jekyll and Mr. Hyde. London, England, Longmans, 1886

van der Kolk BA: Trauma and memory, in Traumatic Stress. Edited by van der Kolk BA, McFarlane AC, Weisaeth L. New York, Guilford, 1996, pp 279–302

Vincent M, Pickering MR: Multiple personality disorder in childhood. Can J Psychiatry 33:524–529, 1988

Walker EA, Katon WJ, Neraas K, et al: Dissociation in women with chronic pelvic pain. Am J Psychiatry 149:534–537, 1992

Walker EA, Katon WJ, Roy-Byrne PP, et al: Histories of sexual victimization in patients with irritable bowel syndrome or inflammatory bowel disease. Am J Psychiatry 150:1502–1506, 1993

Walker EA, Katon JW, Hansom J, et al: Psychiatric diagnoses and sexual victimization in women with chronic pelvic pain. Psychosomatics 36:531–540, 1995

Wilson G, Rupp C, Wilson WW: Amnesia. Am J Psychiatry 106:481–485, 1950

Serotonin Neuronal Function in Anorexia Nervosa and Bulimia Nervosa

Walter H. Kaye, M.D.
Michael Strober, Ph.D.
Kelly L. Klump, Ph.D.

*A*norexia nervosa (AN) and bulimia nervosa (BN) are disorders characterized by aberrant patterns of feeding behavior and weight regulation and disturbances in attitudes toward weight and in the perception of body shape. Patients with AN have an inexplicable fear of weight gain and unrelenting obsession with fatness, even in the face of increasing cachexia. BN usually emerges after a period of dieting, which may or may not have been associated with weight loss. Binge eating, which is the consumption of a large amount of food in an uncontrollable manner, is followed by either self-induced vomiting or some other means of compensation (e.g., misuse of laxatives, diuretics, or enemas or the use of excessive exercise or fasting) for the excess of food ingested. Most individuals with BN have irregular feeding patterns, and satiety may be impaired. Although abnormally low body weight is an exclusion for the diagnosis of BN, some 25%–30% of the patients with BN who present to treatment centers have a history of AN; however, all individuals with BN have pathological concern with weight and shape. Common to individuals with AN or BN are low self-esteem, depression, and anxiety.

In certain respects, both diagnostic labels are misleading. Individuals affected with AN rarely have the complete suppression of appetite that the name implies; rather, they show a volitional and, more often than not, ego-syntonic resistance to feeding drives, eventually becoming preoccupied with food and eating rituals to the point of obsession. Similarly, BN may not be associated with a primary pathological drive to overeat, as implied by the label; rather, like individuals with AN, those with BN have a seemingly relentless drive to restrain their food intake, an extreme fear of weight gain, and often a distorted view of their actual body shape. Loss of control with overeating usually occurs intermittently and typically only some time after the onset of dieting behavior. Episodes of binge eating ultimately develop in a significant proportion of the persons with AN (Halmi et al. 1991), whereas some 5% of those with BN will eventually develop AN (Hsu and Sobkiewicz 1989). Because restrained eating behavior and dysfunctional cognitions relating weight and shape to self-concept are shared by patients with both of these syndromes and because transitions between syndromes occur in many, some have argued (Schweiger and Fichter 1997) that AN and BN share at least some risk and liability factors.

The etiology of AN and BN is presumed to be complex and multiply influenced by developmental, social, and biological processes (Garner 1993; Treasure and Campbell 1994); however, the exact nature of these interactive processes remains incompletely understood. Certainly, cultural attitudes toward standards of physical attractiveness have relevance to the psychopathology of eating disorders, but cultural influences in pathogenesis are not likely to be very prominent. First, dieting behavior and the drive toward thinness are commonplace in industrialized countries throughout the world, yet AN and BN affect only an estimated 0.3%–0.7% and 1.7%–2.5%, respectively, of the females in the general population. Moreover, the fact that numerous clear descriptions of AN date from the middle of the nineteenth century (Treasure and Campbell 1994) suggests that factors other than our current culture play an etiological role. Second, both syndromes, AN in particular, have a relatively stereotypic clinical presentation, sex distribution, and age at onset, supporting the possibility of some biological vulnerability.

ILLNESS PHENOMENOLOGY AND COURSE

Illness Phenomenology

Variations in feeding behavior have been used to subdivide individuals with AN into two meaningful diagnostic subgroups that have been shown to differ in other psychopathological characteristics (Garner et al. 1985; Strober et al. 1982). In the *restricting* subtype of AN, subnormal body weight and an ongoing malnourished state are maintained by unremitting food avoidance; in the *binge-eating/purging* subtype of AN, comparable weight loss and malnutrition occur, yet the course of illness is marked by supervening episodes of binge eating, usually followed by some type of compensatory action, such as self-induced vomiting or laxative abuse. Individuals with the binge-eating/purging subtype of AN are also more likely to have histories of behavioral dyscontrol, substance abuse, and overt family conflict in comparison to those with the restricting subtype. Particularly common in individuals with AN are personality traits of marked perfectionism, conformity, obsessionality, constriction of affect and emotional expressiveness, and reduced social spontaneity. These traits typically appear in advance of the onset of illness and persist even after long-term weight recovery, indicating that they are not merely epiphenomena of acute malnutrition and disordered eating behavior (Casper 1990; O'Dwyer et al. 1996; Srinivasagam et al. 1995; Strober 1980; Von Ranson et al. 1999).

Individuals with BN remain at normal body weight, although many aspire to ideal weights far below the range of normalcy for their age and height. As mentioned earlier in this chapter, the core features of BN include repeated episodes of binge eating followed by compensatory self-induced vomiting, laxative abuse, or pathologically extreme exercise, as well as abnormal concern with weight and shape. DSM-IV-TR (American Psychiatric Association 2000) specifies a distinction within this group between those individuals with BN who engage in self-induced vomiting or laxative, diuretic, or enema abuse (*purging* type) and those who engage in other forms of compensatory action, such as fasting or excessive exercise (*nonpurging* type). Beyond these differences, it has been speculated (Vitousek and Manke 1994) that there are two clinically divergent subgroups of individuals with BN who differ significantly in psychopathological characteristics: 1) a so-called multi-impulsive type, in whom BN occurs in conjunction with more pervasive difficulties in behavioral self-regulation and affective instability; and 2) a type whose distinguishing features include self-effacing behaviors, dependence on external rewards, and extreme compliance. Patients with the multi-impulsive type of BN are far more likely to have histories of substance abuse and other impulse-control problems such as shoplifting and self-injurious behaviors. Considering these differences, it has been postulated that individuals with the multi-impulsive type of BN rely on binge eating and purging as a means of regulating intolerable states of tension, anger, and fragmentation; in contrast, individuals with BN who do not have this multi-impulsive type may have binge episodes precipitated by dietary restraint, with compensatory behaviors maintained through reduction of guilty feelings associated with fears of weight gain.

Illness Course

Most cases of AN emerge during adolescence, although the disorder can be observed in children. Whether prepubertal onset confers a more or less ominous prognosis is not known (Halmi et al. 1979; Theander 1985). Recovery from the illness tends to be protracted, but studies of long-term outcome indicate that the illness course is highly variable; approximately 50% of individuals will eventually have reasonably complete resolution of the illness, whereas another 30% will have lingering residual features that wax and wane in severity long into adulthood. Ten percent of patients with AN will pursue a chronic, unremitting course, and the remaining 10% of those affected will eventually die from the disease (Crisp et al. 1992; Isager et al. 1992; Strober et al. 1997b; Sullivan 1995).

BN usually is precipitated by dieting and weight loss, yet it can occur in the absence of apparent dietary restraint. The frequency and duration of binge episodes and the amount of food consumed during any one episode all vary considerably among patients. Age at onset is somewhat more variable in BN than in AN, with most cases developing during the period from mid to late adolescence through the mid 20s (Fairburn et al. 1997). Follow-up studies of clinic samples 5–10 years after presentation showed that 50% of the patients recovered, whereas nearly 20%–30% continued to meet full criteria for BN (Keel and Mitchell 1997; Keel et al. 1999). Following onset, disturbed eating behavior waxes and wanes over the course of several years in a high percentage of clinic patients. Approximately 30% of the remitted women experience relapse into bulimic symptoms.

SEROTONIN NEURONAL ACTIVITY

Evidence of Biological Influences

As noted earlier in this chapter, no convincing evidence shows that cultural factors are the primary or most formidable determinants of these disorders; however, the role of biology in the etiology of AN has been proposed for the past 60 years (Russell 1970). Emerging evidence suggests that both AN and BN are familial disorders with biological correlates. For example, family and twin studies have suggested significant genetic contributions to the etiology of both disorders (Lilenfeld et al. 1998; Strober 1991). Family studies have indicated that the prevalence of eating disorders is 7–12 times higher among relatives of AN and BN probands than among control subjects (Strober 1991; Strober et al. 1990, 2000). Significantly higher concordance rates among monozygotic relative to dizygotic AN and BN twins have suggested substantial genetic influence in the observed familiality (Fichter and Noegel

1990; Holland et al. 1984, 1988; Kendler et al. 1991). Indeed, heritability estimates have indicated that approximately 55%–80% of the variance in AN (Holland et al. 1988) and 55%–83% of the variance in BN (Bulik et al. 1998a; Kendler et al. 1991) are accounted for by genetic factors.

Earlier theories regarding the biological expression of the observed genetic liability raised the question of whether patients with AN had a pituitary or hypothalamic disturbance. More recently, a growing understanding of neurotransmitter modulation of appetitive behaviors has raised the question of whether some disturbance of neurotransmitter function causes AN and/or BN (Fava et al. 1989; Leibowitz 1986; Morley and Blundell 1988). Disturbances of brain neuropeptides and/or monoamines could contribute to other symptoms and behaviors, such as neuroendocrine or autonomic abnormalities or alterations of mood and behavior in patients with AN or BN. It is important to emphasize that monoamine or neuropeptide disturbances could be a consequence of dietary abnormalities or premorbid traits that contribute to a vulnerability to develop AN or BN. One way to tease apart cause and effect is to study patients with AN or BN at various stages in their illness—that is, while symptomatic and after recovery.

There has been considerable interest in the role that serotonin may play in AN and BN (Blundell 1992; Brewerton 1995; Jimerson et al. 1990; Kaye and Weltzin 1991; Treasure and Campbell 1994). A substantial number of studies have shown alterations in serotonin activity in the ill state. Although less well studied, serotonin disturbances appear to persist after recovery in both AN and BN (Kaye et al. 1991a, 1998). In addition, patients with AN and BN (see "Treatment" later in this chapter) respond to antidepressants in placebo-controlled trials.

Studies of Serotonergic Functioning

Serotonergic pathways play an important role in postprandial satiety. Treatments that increase intrasynaptic serotonin or directly activate serotonin receptors tend to reduce food consumption, whereas interventions that dampen serotonergic neurotransmission or block receptor activation reportedly increase food consumption and promote weight gain (Blundell 1984; Leibowitz 1986). Moreover, central nervous system serotonin pathways have been implicated in the modulation of mood, behavioral constraint, and obsessionality and affect a variety of neuroendocrine systems.

When underweight, patients with AN have a significant reduction in basal concentrations of the serotonin metabolite 5-hydroxyindoleacetic acid (5-HIAA) in the cerebrospinal fluid (CSF) compared with healthy control subjects (Demitrack et al. 1995; Kaye et al. 1988b), as well as blunted plasma prolactin response to drugs with serotonin activity (Hadigan et al. 1995) and reduced ^{3}H-imipramine binding (Weizman et al. 1986). Together, these findings suggest reduced serotonergic activity, which could be secondary to a diet-induced reduction of availability of the amino acid tryptophan, the precursor of serotonin. In contrast, CSF concentrations of 5-HIAA are reported to be elevated (Kaye et al. 1991a) and neuroendocrine responses to serotonin-stimulating drugs are normalized (O'Dwyer et al. 1996) in women with long-term weight recovery from AN. These contrasting findings of reduced and heightened serotonergic activity in acutely ill and long-term recovered AN individuals, respectively, may seem counterintuitive; however, because dieting lowers plasma tryptophan levels in otherwise healthy women (Anderson et al. 1990), resumption of normal eating in AN may unmask intrinsic abnormalities in serotonergic systems that mediate certain core behavioral or temperamental underpinnings of risk and vulnerability.

Considerable evidence also exists of dysregulation of serotonergic processes in patients with BN. This includes blunted prolactin response to the serotonin receptor agonists m-chlorophenylpiperazine (m-CPP) (Brewerton et al. 1992; Levitan et al. 1997), 5-hydroxytrytophan (Goldbloom et al. 1990a), and dl-fenfluramine (Jimerson et al. 1997; McBride et al. 1991); increased platelet serotonin uptake (Goldbloom et al. 1990b); reduced platelet imipramine binding capacity (Marazziti et al. 1988); and enhanced migrainelike headache response to m-CPP challenge (Brewerton et al. 1988). Moreover, acute perturbation of serotonergic tone by dietary depletion of tryptophan also has been linked to increased food intake and mood irritability in women with BN compared with healthy control subjects (Smith et al. 1999; Weltzin et al. 1994). Women with current BN have normal CSF 5-HIAA levels, but women who are long-term recovered from BN have elevated concentrations of 5-HIAA in the CSF (Kaye et al. 1998).

Together, these data show that women who have recovered from both AN and BN have elevated CSF 5-HIAA concentrations. Low levels of CSF 5-HIAA have been found to be associated with impulsive and nonpremeditated aggressive behaviors. Behaviors found after recovery from AN and BN, such as obsessions with symmetry, exactness, perfectionism, and negative affect, tend to be opposite in character to behaviors shown by people with low 5-HIAA levels. Together, these studies contribute to a growing literature suggesting that CSF 5-HIAA concentrations may correlate with a spectrum of behavior. These data support the hypothesis (Cloninger et al. 1993) that increased CSF 5-HIAA concentrations may be associated with exaggerated anticipatory overconcern with negative consequences (i.e., harm avoidance), whereas the lack of such concerns may explain impulsive, aggressive acts that are associated with low CSF 5-HIAA levels.

These findings raise the possibility that a disturbance of serotonin activity may create a vulnerability for the expression of a cluster of symptoms that are common to both AN and BN. The possibility of a common vulnerability for AN and BN may seem puzzling given well-recognized differences in behavior in these disorders; however, as described previously, studies suggest that AN and BN have a shared etiological vulnerability (Kendler et al. 1991; Strober et al. 1990; Walters and Kendler 1995). Other factors that are independent of a vulnerability for the development of an eating disorder may contribute to the development of eating disorder subgroups. For example, individuals with restricting-type AN have extraordinary self-restraint and self-control. The risk for obsessive-compulsive personality disorder is elevated only in this subgroup and their families, suggesting a shared transmission with restricting-type AN (Lilenfeld et al. 1998). In other words, an additional vulnerability for behavioral overcontrol and rigid and inflexible mood states, combined with a vulnerability for an eating disorder, may result in restricting-type AN.

The contribution of serotonin to specific human behaviors remains uncertain. Serotonin has been postulated to contribute to personality traits, such as harm avoidance (Cloninger 1987) and behavioral inhibition (Soubrie 1986); to categorical constructs, such as obsessive-compulsive disorder (Barr et al. 1992), anxiety and fear (Charney et al. 1990), and depression (Graheme-Smith 1992); and to satiety for food consumption. Importantly, these symptoms persist in AN and BN after recovery.

BN, the most common eating disorder, may be the prototypic expression of the disturbance of serotonin activity that contributes to the pathogenesis of eating disorders. Clinically, persons with BN have extremes of eating and behavior. They tend to eat few normal meals. They tend to either diet or overeat. Similarly, they tend to fluctuate between minimization and inhibition of mood states and extremes of mood and catastrophic overconcerns. These clinical observations, coupled with data from studies of ill and recovered women with BN, led to the speculation that the serotonin system in patients with BN is inherently unstable and poorly modulated. Certain traits, such as restricted eating, obsessive perfectionism and exactness, harm avoidance, and negative affect, might be consistent with increased serotonin transmission in a nondieting state. In contrast, a diet-induced decrease in synaptic serotonin release could result in a reduction of this dysphoric state but might lead, in turn, to extremes of unstable mood and binge eating. People with such an inherent modulatory defect in serotonin function may be prone to develop an eating disorder. Because of their modulatory serotonin defect, they can neither respond appropriately and precisely to stress or stimuli nor modulate their affective states. They may learn that extremes of dietary intake (by effects on plasma tryptophan) are a means by which they can crudely modulate their brain serotonin functional activity.

Several investigators (Jimerson et al. 1992; Kaye et al. 1988a) have proposed a model in which individuals with BN may restrict eating or overeat as a means of self-modulating serotonin activity. That is, dieting or binge episodes could alter the ratio of tryptophan to large neutral amino acids in plasma, which alters tryptophan availability to the brain, which results in changes in serotonin synthesis and release (Fernstrom and Faller 1978). In fact, studies (Smith et al. 1999; Weltzin et al. 1994) show that patients with BN, after tryptophan depletion, have an increase in labile and dysphoric mood and overeat compared with control women, supporting the possibility that women with BN have a fragile and dysregulated serotonin system that is vulnerable to dietary manipulations.

TREATMENT

Anorexia Nervosa

Patients with AN have responded less effectively to treatment than have patients with BN (Herzog et al. 1992). Extended hospitalizations can be lifesaving because such treatment can restore weight to emaciated people, which reverses medical complications; however, hospitalizations can be lengthy and expensive. In fact, the hospital utilization rate for patients with AN is higher than for any other psychiatric disorder, aside from schizophrenia and organic disorders (McKenzie and Joyce 1992). Moreover, relapse after hospitalization has been high (Russell et al. 1987).

The evaluation of the efficacy of medications in augmenting weight gain in AN is limited because most trials have been conducted in outpatients or inpatients participating in behavioral and nutritional eating disorders programs, which are themselves efficient in the short run. Nevertheless, in these settings, controlled trials have not provided consistent evidence for the efficacy of antidepressant medications in the treatment of AN (Attia et al. 1998; Biederman et al. 1985; Gross et al. 1981; Lacey and Crisp 1980). Cyproheptadine hydrochloride, a serotonin antagonist, may increase the rate of weight gain in patients with restricting-type AN (Halmi et al. 1986) but only in high doses (Goldberg et al. 1979; Vigersky and Loriaux 1977). Limited efficacy of pharmacological and psychological treatment in AN may be due, in part, to the fact that past treatments have mainly focused on attempts to increase the rate of weight gain of emaciated patients in a hospital setting. Inpatient treatment, consisting of nursing care, behavior modification, and supportive psychotherapy, succeeds in restoring the weight of most emaciated patients with AN. Thus, it is difficult to prove that an active medication is effective in such a setting.

Some, but not all (Strober et al. 1997a), recent studies that have focused on preventing relapse show more promise. Several psychotherapies specifically developed to treat AN appear to show reduced relapse at 1- to 2-year follow-up (Russell et al. 1987; Treasure et al. 1996). Our group (Kaye et al. 1991a, 1991b, 2001) found, in separate open and double-blind, placebo-controlled studies, that fluoxetine improved outcome and reduced relapse after weight restoration. That is, fluoxetine was associated with a significant reduction in core eating disorder symptoms, depression, anxiety, and obsessions and compulsions. In a recent double-blind, placebo-controlled study, our group found that fluoxetine, when given after weight restoration, significantly reduced the extremely high rate of relapse normally seen in AN. Subjects were started on fluoxetine ($n=16$) or placebo ($n=19$) after inpatient weight restoration, discharged from the hospital, and followed up for 1 year as outpatients. Ten of the 16 (63%) subjects receiving fluoxetine remained well over 1 year of outpatient follow-up, whereas only 3 of the 19 (16%) subjects receiving placebo remained well ($P=0.006$). Fluoxetine administration was associated with a significant weight gain and a significant reduction in obsessions and compulsions. Thus, fluoxetine improved outcome in AN by reducing symptoms and helping to maintain a healthy body weight in outpatient treatment.

Two studies (Attia et al. 1998; Ferguson et al. 1999) found that selective serotonin reuptake inhibitors (SSRIs) are not useful when patients with AN are malnourished and underweight. As noted by Tollefson (1995), SSRIs are dependent on neuronal release of serotonin for their action. If the release of serotonin from presynaptic neuronal storage sites were substantially compromised, and net synaptic serotonin concentration were negligible, a clinically meaningful response to an SSRI might not occur. In fact, malnourished individuals with AN have reduced CSF 5-HIAA, the major serotonin metabolite in the brain (Kaye et al. 1984), suggesting reduced synaptic serotonin. This could be a result of reduced availability of tryptophan, the essential amino acid precursor to serotonin (Schweiger et al. 1986).

This link between dietary intake and SSRI efficacy is supported by data that have repeatedly shown that dieting in healthy normal-weight and obese women reduces tryptophan availability, thereby limiting potential serotonergic production (Anderson et al. 1990; Gatti et al. 1993; Goodall 1990; Walsh et al. 1995; Wolfe et al. 1997). Moreover, studies in animals have shown that food restriction decreases serotonin and its synthesis rate in the brain (Haleem and Haider 1996) and downregulates the density of serotonin transporters (Heuther et al. 1997). In addition, depletion of tryptophan, the precursor of serotonin, reverses the effects of SSRI antidepressants in depressed patients (Barr et al. 1994; Bremner et al. 1997; Delgado et al. 1990). Finally, in the patients studied by Delgado et al. (1990), plasma tryptophan was inversely related to depression scores. In AN, weight restoration normalizes nutrition, and CSF 5-HIAA concentrations become elevated (Kaye et al. 1991a). These changes in nutrients and serotonin activity may explain why individuals with AN may become responsive to fluoxetine after weight restoration.

Bulimia Nervosa

It is fair to say that progress to date in establishing the efficacy of specific psychological and pharmacological therapies for eating disorders has been more dramatic for BN than for AN (Arnow 1997). With regard to psychotherapy, although few controlled clinical trials have been done, most indicate that cognitive-behavioral therapy (CBT) is an effective treatment for 60%–70% of the individuals with BN, with remission of binge eating and purging achieved in some 30%–50% of the patients (Bulik et al. 1998b; Connors et al. 1984; Fairburn et al. 1993; Kirkley et al. 1985; Wolf and Crowther 1992). Evidence for the efficacy of antidepressant pharmacotherapy in BN is impressive; however, the benefits may diminish over time in a significant proportion of individuals with BN who respond initially, and only a minority have complete suppression of their symptoms with antidepressant monotherapy (Agras et al. 1992; Crow and Mitchell 1996; Fluoxetine Bulimia Nervosa Collaborative Study Group 1992; Hoffman and Halmi 1993; Jimerson et al. 1996; Kaye et al. 2001; Mitchell and de Zwaan 1993; Mitchell et al. 1990, 1993; Russell 1988; Walsh 1991a).

The results of most double-blind, placebo-controlled randomized trials reported to date indicate that antidepressants show at least some superiority over placebo in reducing the frequency of binge-eating episodes (Walsh 1991b). In addition, some studies show a reduction in intensity of some other symptoms commonly seen in BN, such as preoccupation with food and depression (Goldbloom and Olmsted 1993). These findings have been reported with various antidepressant medications, including tricyclic agents (TCAs) (imipramine, desipramine, clomipramine, amitriptyline) (Agras et al. 1987; Barlow et al. 1988), monoamine oxidase inhibitors (phenelzine, isocarboxazid) (Walsh et al. 1984), and SSRIs (fluoxetine, fluvoxamine) (Goldstein et al. 1995). Patients participating in these trials typically reported from 8 to 10 episodes of binge eating per week at baseline. The "average" decrease in binge frequency for patients receiving the antidepressant medication was about 55%, with wide variation across studies. Placebo responses were similarly variable but generally were less than half the size of the response for the active treatment; however, only a minority of the patients actually achieved full abstinence from bingeing and purging behaviors (Mitchell et al. 1997). Most trials have shown no correlation between improvement in mood and reduction in BN symptoms. In addition, antidepressants suppress bulimic symptoms in nondepressed bulimic patients, suggesting a mode of action other than through their antidepressant effects (Blouin et al. 1989). In some studies, the patients receiving the antidepressant medication had a significant increase in dietary restraint and a reduction in the tendency for stressors to trigger binge eating.

There is little evidence for superiority of response to a single class of medication. Thus, differences in side effects may be a significant factor in the clinical choice of the antidepressant. The dosage level needed to achieve an effect appears to be similar to that required in major depression, with a tendency for higher dosages (e.g., 200–300 mg/day of the relevant TCA) to be more effective (Walsh 1991b). The time course of action of the medications also appears to be similar to that found in depression, with improvement occurring over the course of several weeks. Improvement in frequency of self-induced vomiting generally parallels the decrease in bingeing. Treatment failure should be considered only if adequate doses have been administered for 8–12 weeks. Fluoxetine 60 mg/day has proved significantly superior to 20 mg/day and to placebo in the reduction of binge eating and BN-related features (Fluoxetine Bulimia Nervosa Collaborative Study Group 1992). This dosage has been shown to be safe with minimal adverse effects, even over an extended treatment period. Other antidepressants have not been studied systematically in the treatment of BN. Bupropion is contraindicated in patients with BN because it has been associated with increased risk of seizures (Horne et al. 1988).

Information is limited on how long to continue antidepressant therapy in BN because most trials have incorporated only a relatively brief duration of treatment. A few follow-up studies extending from 4 to 24 months have found a high relapse rate on discontinuation of the antidepressant medication (Agras 1997; Beumont et al. 1997). In a recent large-scale, multicenter study of 150 subjects with BN, those who responded to 60 mg of fluoxetine in an 8-week open trial were randomized to fluoxetine or placebo and followed up for 1 year. Subjects who continued treatment with 60 mg of fluoxetine had a significantly lower relapse rate over 1 year compared with those taking placebo (Romano et al. 1998). These data support the notion that in BN, which often has a chronic course with a significant relapse rate, antidepressants may need to be continued for prolonged periods in patients responding well in the initial stages of treatment. It should be noted, however, that attenuation of the antibinge effect of the antidepressant has been noted over time.

Six studies (Agras et al. 1992; Fichter et al. 1991; Goldbloom et al. 1997; Leitenberg et al. 1994; Mitchell et al. 1990; Walsh et al. 1997) have been published or presented to date that have assessed the relative efficacy of combining psychotherapy (CBT in most trials) and antidepressants for the management of BN, compared with the isolated treatments themselves. Although differing in many respects, these studies suggested that the improvement in bulimic symptoms with CBT alone was greater than with the medication alone. Adding medication to the psychotherapy generally did not improve significantly the outcome over psychotherapy alone in terms of eating behaviors nor did it increase the speed of the therapeutic response; however, one prolonged follow-up evaluation found that combined treatment was more effective on several eating variables than CBT alone (Agras et al. 1992). Another study showed the superiority of combined therapy in reducing the rates of anxiety and depression (Mitchell et al. 1990).

SUMMARY

Emerging data support the possibility that substantial biological vulnerabilities contribute to the pathogenesis of AN and BN. The development of an eating disorder is often attributed to the effects of our cultural environment, as exemplified by messages conveyed by mass media about body image; however, all women in our society are exposed to cultural mores that value slimness, but only a small percentage of the women exposed to these messages develop an eating disorder. Thus, there may be an underlying biological, genetically transmitted diathesis that places someone at risk for developing BN. Studies of serotonergic functioning in individuals with AN and BN suggest that a dysregulation of this neurotransmitter system may contribute to this biological diathesis. Results from treatment studies corroborate these findings by indicating that SSRIs are effective for decreasing symptoms in individuals with BN and for possibly decreasing relapse rates in individuals with AN.

REFERENCES

Agras WS: Pharmacotherapy of bulimia nervosa and binge eating disorder: longer-term outcomes. Psychopharmacol Bull 33:433–436, 1997

Agras WS, Dorian B, Kirkley BG, et al: Imipramine in the treatment of bulimia: a double-blind controlled study. Int J Eat Disord 6:29–38, 1987

Agras WS, Rossiter EM, Arnow B, et al: Pharmacologic and cognitive-behavioral treatment for bulimia nervosa: a controlled comparison. Am J Psychiatry 149:82–87, 1992

American Psychiatric Association: Diagnostic and Statistical Manual of Mental Disorders, 4th Edition, Text Revision. Washington, DC, American Psychiatric Association, 2000

Anderson IM, Parry-Billings M, Newsholme EA, et al: Dieting reduces plasma tryptophan and alters brain 5-HT function in women. Psychol Med 20:785–791, 1990

Arnow B: Psychotherapy of anorexia and bulimia, in Balliére's Clinical Psychiatry. Edited by Jimerson DC, Kaye WH. London, England, Balliére Tindall Press, 1997, pp 235–257

Attia E, Haiman C, Walsh BT, et al: Does fluoxetine augment the inpatient treatment of anorexia nervosa? Am J Psychiatry 155:548–551, 1998

Barlow J, Blouin J, Blouin A, et al: Treatment of bulimia with desipramine: a double-blind crossover study. Can J Psychiatry 34:24–29, 1988

Barr LC, Goodman WK, Price LH, et al: The serotonin hypothesis of obsessive compulsive disorder: implications of pharmacologic studies. J Clin Psychiatry 53:17–28, 1992

Barr LC, Goodman WK, McDougle CJ, et al: Tryptophan depletion in patients with obsessive-compulsive disorder who respond to serotonin reuptake inhibitors. Arch Gen Psychiatry 51:309–317, 1994

Beumont PJ, Russell JD, Touyz SW, et al: Intensive nutritional counselling in bulimia nervosa: a role for supplementation with fluoxetine? Aust N Z J Psychiatry 31:514–524, 1997

Biederman J, Herzog DB, Rivinus TM, et al: Amitriptyline in the treatment of anorexia nervosa: a double-blind, placebo-controlled study. J Clin Psychopharmacol 5:10–16, 1985

Blouin J, Blouin A, Perez E: Bulimia: independence of antibulimic and antidepressant properties of desipramine. Can J Psychiatry 34:24–29, 1989

Blundell JE: Serotonin and appetite. Neuropharmacology 23:1537–1551, 1984

Blundell JE: Serotonin and the biology of feeding. Am J Clin Nutr 55:155S–159S, 1992

Bremner JD, Innis RB, Saloman EM, et al: Positron emission tomography measurement of cerebral metabolic correlates of tryptophan depletion-induced depressive relapse. Arch Gen Psychiatry 54:364–374, 1997

Brewerton TD: Toward a unified theory of serotonin dysregulation in eating and related disorders. Psychoneuroendocrinology 20:561–590, 1995

Brewerton TD, Murphy DL, Mueller EA, et al: The induction of migraine-like headaches by the serotonin agonist, *m*-chlorophenylpiperazine. Clin Pharmacol Ther 43:605–609, 1988

Brewerton TD, Mueller EA, Lesem MD, et al: Neuroendocrine responses to *m*-chlorophenylpiperazine and L-tryptophan in bulimia. Arch Gen Psychiatry 49:852–861, 1992

Bulik CM, Sullivan PF, Kendler KS: Heritability of binge eating and bulimia nervosa. Biol Psychiatry 44:1210–1218, 1998a

Bulik CM, Sullivan PF, Carter FA, et al: The role of exposure with response prevention in the cognitive-behavioral therapy for bulimia nervosa. Psychol Med 28:611–623, 1998b

Casper RC: Personality features of women with good outcome from restricting anorexia nervosa. Psychosom Med 52:156–170, 1990

Charney DS, Wood SW, Krystal JH, et al: Serotonin function and human anxiety disorders. Ann N Y Acad Sci 600:558–573, 1990

Cloninger CR: A systematic method for clinical description and classification of personality variants. Arch Gen Psychiatry 44:573–588, 1987

Cloninger CR, Svrakic DM, Przybeck TR: A psychobiological model of temperament and character. Arch Gen Psychiatry 50:975–990, 1993

Connors ME, Johnson CL, Stuckey MK: Treatment of bulimia with brief psychoeducational group therapy. Am J Psychiatry 141:1512–1516, 1984

Crisp AH, Callender JS, Halek C, et al: Long-term mortality in anorexia nervosa: a 20-year follow-up of the St George's and Aberdeen cohorts. Br J Psychiatry 161:104–107, 1992

Crow SJ, Mitchell JE: Integrating cognitive therapy and medications in treating bulimia nervosa. Psychiatr Clin North Am 19:755–760, 1996

Delgado PL, Price LH, Aghajanian GK, et al: Serotonin function and the mechanism of antidepressant action: reversal of antidepressant-induced remission by rapid depletion of plasma tryptophan. Arch Gen Psychiatry 47:411–418, 1990

Demitrack MA, Heyes MP, Altemus M, et al: Cerebrospinal fluid levels of kynurenine pathway metabolites in patients with eating disorders. Biol Psychiatry 37:512–520, 1995

Fairburn CG, Marcus MD, Wilson GT: Cognitive-behavioral therapy for binge eating and bulimia nervosa: a comprehensive treatment manual, in Binge Eating: Nature, Assessment and Treatment. Edited by Fairburn CG, Wilson GO. New York, Guilford, 1993, pp 361–404

Fairburn CG, Welch SL, Doll HA, et al: Risk factors for bulimia nervosa: a community-based case-control study. Arch Gen Psychiatry 54:509–517, 1997

Fava M, Copeland PM, Schweiger U, et al: Neurochemical abnormalities in anorexia nervosa and bulimia nervosa. Am J Psychiatry 146:963–971, 1989

Ferguson CP, La Via MC, Crossan PJ, et al: Are SSRI's effective in underweight anorexia nervosa? Int J Eat Disord 25:11–17, 1999

Fernstrom JD, Faller DV: Neutral amino acids in the brain: changes in response to food ingestion. J Neurochem 30:1531–1538, 1978

Fichter MM, Noegel R: Concordance for bulimia nervosa in twins. Int J Eat Disord 9:255–263, 1990

Fichter MM, Leibl K, Rief W, et al: Fluoxetine versus placebo: a double-blind study with bulimic inpatients undergoing intensive psychotherapy. Pharmacopsychiatry 24:1–7, 1991

Fluoxetine Bulimia Nervosa Collaborative Study Group: Fluoxetine in the treatment of bulimia nervosa. Arch Gen Psychiatry 49:139–147, 1992

Garner DM: Pathogenesis of anorexia nervosa. Lancet 341:1631–1635, 1993

Garner DM, Garfinkel PE, O'Shaughnessy M: The validity of the distinction between bulimia with and without anorexia nervosa. Am J Psychiatry 142:581–587, 1985

Gatti E, Porroni M, Noe D, et al: Plasma amino acids changes in obese patients on very low-calorie diets. Int J Vitam Nutr Res 63:81–85, 1993

Goldberg SC, Halmi KA, Eckert ED, et al: Cyproheptadine in anorexia nervosa. Br J Psychiatry 134:67–70, 1979

Goldbloom DS, Olmsted MP: Pharmacotherapy of bulimia nervosa and its associated attitudinal disturbances: the clinical significance of change. Am J Psychiatry 150:770–774, 1993

Goldbloom DS, Garfinkel PE, Katz R, et al: The neuroendocrine response to L-5-hydroxytryptophan in bulimia nervosa. Paper presented at the 47th annual meeting of the American Psychosomatic Society, Boston, MA, March 1990a

Goldbloom DS, Hicks LK, Garfinkel PE: Platelet serotonin uptake in bulimia nervosa. Biol Psychiatry 28:644–647, 1990b

Goldbloom DS, Olmsted M, Davis R, et al: A randomized controlled trial of fluoxetine and cognitive behavioral therapy for bulimia nervosa: short-term outcome. Behav Res Ther 35:803–811, 1997

Goldstein DJ, Wilson MG, Thompson VL, et al: Long-term fluoxetine treatment of bulimia nervosa. Br J Psychiatry 166:660–666, 1995

Goodall E: Dieting, tryptophan and mood. BNF Nutrition Bulletin 15:137–141, 1990

Graheme-Smith DG: Serotonin in affective disorders. Int J Clin Psychopharmacol 6:S5–S13, 1992

Gross HA, Ebert MH, Faden VB, et al: A double-blind controlled trial of lithium carbonate in primary anorexia nervosa. J Clin Psychopharmacol 1:376–381, 1981

Hadigan CM, Walsh TB, Buttinger C, et al: Behavioral and neuroendocrine responses to *meta*-CPP in anorexia nervosa. Biol Psychiatry 37:504–511, 1995

Haleem DJ, Haider S: Food restriction decreases serotonin and its synthesis rate in the hypothalamus. Neuroreport 7:1153–1156, 1996

Halmi KA, Casper RC, Eckert ED, et al: Unique features associated with age of onset of anorexia nervosa. Psychiatry Res 1:209–215, 1979

Halmi KA, Eckert E, LaDu TJ, et al: Anorexia nervosa: treatment efficacy of cyproheptadine and amitriptyline. Arch Gen Psychiatry 43:177–181, 1986

Halmi KA, Eckert E, Marchi P, et al: Comorbidity of psychiatric diagnoses in anorexia nervosa. Arch Gen Psychiatry 48:712–718, 1991

Herzog DB, Keller MB, Strober M, et al: The current status of treatment for anorexia nervosa and bulimia nervosa. Int J Eat Disord 12:215–220, 1992

Heuther G, Zhou D, Schmidt S, et al: Long-term food restriction down-regulates the density of serotonin transporters in the rat frontal cortex. Biol Psychiatry 41:1174–1180, 1997

Hoffman L, Halmi KA: Psychopharmacology in the treatment of anorexia and bulimia nervosa. Psychiatr Clin North Am 16:767–778, 1993

Holland AJ, Hall A, Murray R, et al: Anorexia nervosa: a study of 34 twin pairs. Br J Psychiatry 145:414–419, 1984

Holland AJ, Sicotte N, Treasure J: Anorexia nervosa: evidence for a genetic basis. J Psychosom Res 32:561–571, 1988

Horne RL, Ferguson JM, Pope HG, et al: Treatment of bulimia with bupropion: a multicenter controlled trial. J Clin Psychiatry 49:262–266, 1988

Hsu LKG, Sobkiewicz TA: Bulimia nervosa: a four- to six-year follow-up study. Psychol Med 19:1035–1038, 1989

Isager T, Brinch M, Kreiner S, et al: Death and relapse in anorexia nervosa: survival analysis of 151 cases. J Psychiatr Res 19:515–521, 1992

Jimerson DC, Lesem MD, Hegg AP, et al: Serotonin in human eating disorders. Ann N Y Acad Sci 600:532–544, 1990

Jimerson DC, Lesem MD, Kaye WH, et al: Low serotonin and dopamine metabolite concentrations in cerebrospinal fluid from bulimic patients with frequent binge episodes. Arch Gen Psychiatry 49:132–138, 1992

Jimerson DC, Wolfe BE, Brotman AW, et al: Medications in the treatment of eating disorders. Psychiatr Clin North Am 19:739–754, 1996

Jimerson DC, Wolfe BE, Metzger ED, et al: Decreased serotonin function in bulimia nervosa. Arch Gen Psychiatry 54:529–534, 1997

Kaye WH, Weltzin TE: Neurochemistry of bulimia nervosa. J Clin Psychiatry 52:21–28, 1991

Kaye WH, Ebert MH, Raleigh M, et al: Abnormalities in CNS monoamine metabolism in anorexia nervosa. Arch Gen Psychiatry 41:350–355, 1984

Kaye WH, Gwirtsman HE, Brewerton TD, et al: Bingeing behavior and plasma amino acids: a possible involvement of brain serotonin in bulimia nervosa. Psychiatry Res 3:31–43, 1988a

Kaye WH, Gwirtsman HE, George DT, et al: CSF-5HIAA concentrations in anorexia nervosa: reduced values in underweight subjects normalize after weight gain. Biol Psychiatry 23:102–105, 1988b

Kaye WH, Gwirtsman HE, George DT, et al: Altered serotonin activity in anorexia nervosa after long-term weight recovery. Arch Gen Psychiatry 48:556–562, 1991a

Kaye WH, Weltzin T, Hsu LKG, et al: An open trial of fluoxetine in patients with anorexia nervosa. J Clin Psychiatry 52:464–471, 1991b

Kaye WH, Greeno CG, Moss H, et al: Alterations in serotonin activity and psychiatric symptomatology after recovery from bulimia nervosa. Arch Gen Psychiatry 55:927–935, 1998

Kaye WH, Nagata T, Weltzin TE, et al: Double-blind placebo-controlled administration of fluoxetine in restricting- and restricting-purging-type anorexia nervosa. Biol Psychiatry 49:644–652, 2001

Keel PK, Mitchell JE: Outcome in bulimia nervosa. Am J Psychiatry 154:313–321, 1997

Keel PK, Mitchell JE, Miller KB, et al: Long-term outcome of bulimia nervosa. Arch Gen Psychiatry 56:63–69, 1999

Kendler KS, MacLean C, Neals M, et al: The genetic epidemiology of bulimia nervosa. Am J Psychiatry 148:1627–1637, 1991

Kirkley BG, Schneider JA, Agras WS, et al: Comparison of two group treatments for bulimia. J Consult Clin Psychol 53:43–48, 1985

Lacey JH, Crisp AH: Hunger, food intake and weight: the impact of clomipramine on a refeeding anorexia nervosa population. Postgrad Med J 56:S79–S85, 1980

Leibowitz SF: Brain monoamines and peptides: role in the control of eating behavior. Federation Proceedings 45:1396–1403, 1986

Leitenberg J, Rosen JC, Wolf J, et al: Comparison of cognitive-behavior therapy and desipramine in the treatment of bulimia nervosa. Behav Res Ther 32:37–45, 1994

24

Pharmacological Management of Psychiatric Illness During Pregnancy

Weighing the Risks

Adele C. Viguera, M.D.
Lee S. Cohen, M.D.

*T*he management of psychiatric illness during pregnancy raises several clinical challenges. Many psychiatric disorders, such as mood and anxiety disorders, tend to cluster in women during the childbearing years (Kessler et al. 1993). All psychotropic medications diffuse readily across the placenta, and no psychotropic drug has been approved by the U.S. Food and Drug Administration for use during pregnancy. Because a growing number of women are treated with psychotropic medications, concerns about prenatal exposure to these psychotropic agents and the potential risks of relapse if maintenance medication is discontinued are common reasons for consultation. Risks of psychotropic drug use during pregnancy include teratogenic effects, neonatal toxicity, and the potential for long-term neurobehavioral sequelae. Knowledge of the risks to the fetus of prenatal exposure to psychotropic medications is incomplete. Even less is known about the possible long-term neurobehavioral sequelae associated with prenatal exposure to psychotropics. The data are seriously limited and typically insufficient to determine absolute risk of organ dysgenesis. The potential negative sequelae of untreated psychiatric illness to both mother and fetus also represent an important and often overlooked risk. Thus, the clinical challenge in caring for these patients is to minimize the risk of fetal exposure to medications while limiting morbidity from untreated psychiatric illness.

RISK–BENEFIT ASSESSMENT OF WOMEN OF CHILDBEARING POTENTIAL

Any decisions about initiation, modification, or frank discontinuation of psychotropic medications during pregnancy are made only after the relative risks and benefits of pharmacological intervention are carefully weighed. As part of the informed consent process, physicians and their patients need to weigh three important risks in the overall risk–benefit analysis: 1) teratogenic risks of pharmacotherapy, 2) risk of untreated psychiatric illness, and 3) risk of relapse following discontinuation of maintenance treatments. A discussion of each of these risks should be documented in the patient's medical record. Clinicians must work collaboratively with patients to arrive at the safest decisions based on the available information. A patient's psychiatric history, current presenting symptoms, and attitude toward taking medications during pregnancy should be carefully assessed. The relative risks and benefits of drug therapy must be weighed with the patient. Both clinician and patient must acknowledge that no clinical decision is ever risk free. In general, the use of psychotropic medication during pregnancy should be reserved for those clinical situations in which the risk to the mother and fetus from the psychiatric disorder outweighs the risk of drug treatment.

Risk of Pharmacotherapy

The decision of whether to use a psychotropic medication should take into consideration three major risk factors: 1) teratogenic risk, 2) longer-term neurobehavioral sequelae (so-called behavioral teratogenesis), and 3) direct neonatal toxicity (Koren et al. 1998). A *teratogen* is defined as a drug that increases the risk of congenital malformation above the baseline incidence of congenital malformations with first-trimester exposure. Estimates of the baseline incidence of congenital malformations in the United States are 3%–4% (Fabro 1987). Exposure to a teratogen before 2 weeks' gestation is not typically teratogenic and is more likely to result in a nonviable blighted ovum (Langman 1985). Therefore, the date of treatment discontinuation and the range of half-lives of prescribed medication are important to determine.

Neurobehavioral risk refers to the potential for long-term neurobehavioral sequelae with fetal exposure to a particular drug. For example, are children who have been exposed to antidepressants in utero at risk for cognitive or behavior problems as they develop? Unfortunately, the area of neurobehavioral teratogenicity is understudied. Animal studies, however, show changes in behavior and neurotransmitter function after prenatal exposure to a variety of psychotropic agents (Coyle et al. 1976; Kellogg 1988; Lauer et al. 1989; Miller and Friedhoff 1987; Montero et al. 1990; Robertson et al. 1980).

The extent to which these findings are of consequence to humans has yet to be established. Behavioral outcomes after prenatal exposure to psychotropics, including tricyclic antidepressants (TCAs), benzodiazepines, lithium, and, more recently, fluoxetine, have been reported (Laegreid et al. 1992; Misri and Sivertz 1991; Nulman et al. 1997; Schou 1976). Except for the fluoxetine data, most data are extremely limited by retrospective design and by small sample size. Furthermore, relevant control groups with psychiatric disorders but no psychotropic exposure have not been included in the analysis.

Neonatal toxicity or perinatal syndromes refer to a spectrum of physical and behavioral symptoms observed in the acute neonatal period that frequently are attributed to drug exposure at or near the time of delivery. Several factors may contribute to the variability of adverse events from psychotropic exposure, including 1) immature central nervous system of the infant, 2) diminished hepatic microsomal enzyme activity, and 3) decreased plasma protein and protein-binding affinity, leading to greater amounts of free drug and theoretically increased risk for transient neonatal toxicity. Although case reports over the last two decades have described a wide range of transient neonatal distress syndromes associated with exposure to antidepressants, antipsychotics, and benzodiazepines, the incidence of these adverse events is low, and the significance of anecdotal reports that describe these syndromes must be cautiously interpreted (Athinarayanan et al. 1976; Eggermont 1973; Falterman and Richardson 1980; Fisher et al. 1985; Gillberg 1977; Hill et al. 1966; Mazzi 1977; Schimmell et al. 1991; Shearer et al. 1972; Tamer et al. 1969; Webster 1973; Whitelaw et al. 1981).

Risk of Untreated Psychiatric Illness

Not only absolute risk from in utero exposure to psychotropics but also the risks of untreated psychiatric disorder may be difficult to quantify. Consequences of untreated psychiatric disorder must be calculated against the risk of prenatal exposure to drug. To date, the effect of untreated psychiatric illness on the developing fetus and infant is unclear. Stress in pregnant animal models can lead to sustained dysfunction of the hypothalamic-pituitary-adrenal axis in their offspring (Glover 1997; Ladd et al. 1997; Plotsky and Meaney 1993). A clinical counterpart of such effects is not yet proved. Impaired self-care because of psychiatric symptoms may adversely affect the outcome of pregnancy. Antenatal depression and anxiety are linked to premature labor, low birthweight, lower Apgar scores, smaller head circumference, and inferior functional assessment in the newborn (Cutrona 1983; Istvan 1986; Orr and Miller 1995; Perkin et al. 1993; Sapolsky and Meaney 1986; Steer et al. 1992; Zuckerman et al. 1990). Suicidality associated with depressive illness and impulsivity seen in bipolar disorder are other examples of clinical risks that may drive the decision to institute or continue pharmacological treatment during pregnancy. Moreover, the potential risk for chronicity and treatment resistance with repeated relapse of psychiatric disorder is an important factor to consider when assessing the potential use of psychotropic medications during pregnancy (Post 1992; Tohen et al. 1990). Other risks include poor prenatal care and risk of injury to mother and fetus caused by disorganization, impulsivity, and suicidality.

Untreated maternal psychiatric illness almost certainly has a negative effect on infant development. Most studies have examined the effect of maternal unipolar depression on infant development (Downey and Coyne 1990; Field 1995; Murray 1992; Murray and Cooper 1997; Weinberg and Tronick 1998). Infants of mothers with untreated depression looked at their mothers less, had greater physiological reactivity, and made fewer vocalizations than did infants of mothers who were not affected by depression. Perhaps most concerning, these infants performed more poorly on developmental tasks at age 1 year compared with control infants (Downey and Coyne 1990; Field 1995; Murray 1992; Murray and Cooper 1997; Weinberg and Tronick 1998). These sobering findings emphasize the importance of reducing risk for recurrences of mood disorders during pregnancy and postpartum.

Risks of Discontinuing Maintenance Psychotropic Medications

New accumulating evidence for the increased risk of relapse associated with abrupt discontinuation of maintenance psychotropics and its attendant implications call for particular caution in the clinical management of patients, especially pregnant women. Data support the increased risk of relapse with abrupt discontinuation of maintenance mood stabilizers, antipsychotics, and antidepressants (Baldessarini and Tondo 1998; Baldessarini et al. 1996; Faedda et al. 1993; Suppes et al. 1991; Viguera and Baldessarini 1995; Viguera et al. 1998). Recurrences have averaged 50% within 6 months after discontinuing lithium in men and women with bipolar I or II disorders (Baldessarini and Tondo 1998; Baldessarini et al. 1996; Faedda et al. 1993; Suppes et al. 1991). Similar findings apply to abruptly stopping neuroleptics and antidepressants, with approximately 50% of patients relapsing within 24–30 weeks of abruptly discontinuing maintenance treatments (Viguera and Baldessarini 1995; Viguera et al. 1998). Rapid compared with more gradual discontinuation of lithium appears to increase the risk for relapse even further (Baldessarini and Tondo 1998; Baldessarini et al. 1996; Faedda et al. 1993). However, this risk may be modified by gradually discontinuing a maintenance medication over several weeks (i.e., >2 weeks).

In addition to the risk of recurrence of illness, stopping a medication abruptly may lead to serious morbidity from suicidal or self-injurious behaviors. Studies have shown that discontinuation of lithium is followed by sharply increased suicide risk, mainly in recurrences of bipolar depressive or mixed-dysphoric states (Tondo et al. 1998). Evidence also indicates that this phenomenon of early relapse with abrupt discontinuation of maintenance treatment may occur with other disorders and treatments, including neuroleptics in schizophrenia and antidepressants in recurrent major depression (Viguera and Baldessarini 1995; Viguera et al. 1998). Thus, not only the teratogenic risk of psychotropics but also the high risk of morbidity and mortality associated with stopping maintenance medication are of serious concern. Discontinuation of maintenance treatment is potentially dangerous, and such a decision should be made only after careful consideration.

ANTIDEPRESSANTS

Tricyclics

Although early case reports suggested a possible association between first-trimester exposure to TCAs and limb malformations (McBride 1972), the accumulated data on the teratogenic effects of TCAs show no significant association between in utero exposure to TCAs and major congenital anomalies. Three prospective and more than 10 retrospective studies have examined the risk for organ dysgenesis after first-trimester exposure to TCAs (Banister et al. 1972; Briggs et al. 1994; Crombie et al. 1972; Heinonen et al. 1977; Idanpaan-Heikkila and Saxen 1973; Jacobs 1972; Kuenssberg and Knox 1972; Morrow 1972; Pastuszak et al. 1993; Rachelefsky et al. 1972; Scanlon 1969; Sim 1972). A combined 500,000 births have been evaluated, and more than 400 cases of first-trimester exposure to TCAs have been documented. Although the estimates of risk are based on tricyclics of a class compared with a particular TCA, no single study or group of studies consistently supports an increased risk of congenital malformations after first-trimester exposure to TCAs. However, it is important to inform the patient that the long-term neurobehavioral effects are unknown. Data on behavioral teratogenicity are limited to one recent study that suggested no long-term negative sequelae to drug exposure (Nulman et al. 1997). Animal data show evidence of significant changes at the receptor level in animals exposed to TCAs prenatally, including decreased adrenergic receptor binding and decreased density of serotonin receptor binding (Ali et al. 1986; Auerbach et al. 1992; Coyle 1975; Del Rio et al. 1988; File and Tucker 1984; Jason et al. 1981). The implications of these findings for the developing human fetus are unclear and remain to be studied.

Various case reports have described perinatal withdrawal syndromes at delivery after exposure to TCAs in utero, including TCA withdrawal syndromes characterized by jitteriness, irritability, and seizures (Cowe et al. 1982; Eggermont 1973; Schimmell et al. 1991; Webster 1973). Case reports of anticholinergic effects of TCAs, including bowel obstruction and urinary retention, also have been published (Falterman and Richardson 1980; Shearer et al. 1972).

Although the longer history of use of TCAs during pregnancy is reassuring, these data become less practically helpful as most patients who have mood disorders receive treatment with newer agents such as the selective serotonin reuptake inhibitors (SSRIs).

Selective Serotonin Reuptake Inhibitors

Except for fluoxetine, the reproductive safety data on SSRIs are limited. Four prospective studies have evaluated rates of malformations in approximately 1,100 fluoxetine-exposed infants (Chambers et al. 1996; Goldstein 1995; Nulman and Koren 1996; Pastuszak et al. 1993). The postmarketing surveillance register established by the manufacturer of fluoxetine adds to this database. The accumulated data on the reproductive safety of fluoxetine consist of more than 3,000 cases. No increased risk of congenital malformations has been noted over baseline risk in the general population for either retrospectively or prospectively enrolled patients.

In one recent study by Chambers et al. (1996), no higher rates of major malformations were noted in a group of 228 pregnant women who used fluoxetine during the first trimester. However, an increase in multiple minor malformations was described in offspring of this sample, as compared with a control group. Minor anomalies were defined as structural defects that have no cosmetic or functional importance. In this study, no particular pattern of anomalies was noted. In addition, a greater frequency of admissions to special care nurseries was reported in children of the women who used fluoxetine during the later stages of pregnancy. Interpretation of these latter findings is limited by methodological difficulties. For example, raters were not blind to maternal treatment status, and only half of the sample of exposed children was examined for the presence of minor malformations, which raises the question of selection bias (Cohen and Rosenbaum 1997). Moreover, the fluoxetine-exposed women and control group differed significantly on important variables such as age, presence of psychiatric illness, and use of concomitant psychotropic medications. In this study, the incidence of prematurity was significantly greater for women who took fluoxetine throughout their pregnancy than for control subjects. To date, no other studies have replicated this finding. Although further data are needed to ensure clinical confidence, the data collected on fluoxetine thus far suggest that it is unlikely to be a significant human teratogen.

Information about the safety of sertraline and paroxetine use during pregnancy is gradually accumulating but, as compared with fluoxetine, lacks significantly in terms of sample size (Inman et al. 1993; Kulin et al. 1998; McElhatton et al. 1996). This is partially because of a lack of post-marketing surveillance of exposure to these agents. Recently, in a prospective, controlled cohort study, Kulin et al. (1998) reported on the rates of major congenital malformations in neonates who were exposed to fluvoxamine ($n=26$), paroxetine ($n=97$), and sertraline ($n=147$) compared with control subjects. One infant was exposed to both sertraline and fluoxetine, whereas two other infants were exposed to both paroxetine and sertraline when their mothers took these drugs during the first trimester. Of the total 267 women exposed to any one of these SSRIs, 49 used the drug throughout the pregnancy. Pregnancy outcomes did not differ between the two groups (exposed vs. not exposed) in terms of risk for major malformations or higher rates of miscarriage, stillbirth, or prematurity. Birthweights and gestational ages among SSRI users were similar to those among the control subjects. Among the women who took SSRIs, birth outcomes did not differ between those who had stopped taking SSRIs in the first trimester and those who continued to take these agents throughout pregnancy. One of the major limitations of this study was that the analysis grouped the three antidepressants together instead of analyzing each antidepressant individually for teratogenic potential.

Further retrospective data on paroxetine are available from another study involving 63 infants with histories of first-trimester exposure. They were not noted to develop any congenital malformations (Inman et al. 1993). However, prospective data on the use of mirtazapine, venlafaxine, nefazodone, bupropion, and trazodone are not available.

The extent to which prenatal exposure to SSRIs increases the risk of neonatal toxicity is unclear. Several case reports described neonatal toxicity, including central nervous system agitation (i.e., jitteriness), tachycardia, and bleeding abnormalities, after exposure to fluoxetine (Chambers et al. 1996; Spencer 1993). Other data regarding risk for neonatal toxicity have been inconsistent, with at least one study that described higher rates of perinatal complications. However, another prospective study did not suggest postnatal complications following in utero exposure to fluoxetine (Goldstein 1995).

With regard to long-term neurobehavioral sequelae in children exposed to either fluoxetine or TCAs, the data are limited but reassuring. In a landmark study describing long-term neurobehavioral sequelae of medication exposure in utero, Nulman et al. (1997) followed up a cohort of children up to age 7 years who had been exposed to either TCAs ($n=80$) or fluoxetine ($n=55$) in utero and compared them with a cohort of nonexposed control subjects ($n=84$). Results showed no significant differences in IQ, temperament, behavior, mood, reactivity, distractibility, or activity levels in any of the children, suggesting that these drugs are not behavioral teratogens in humans.

Other Antidepressants

Scant information is available about the reproductive safety of monoamine oxidase inhibitors (MAOIs). Thus, given the lack of data, they are typically avoided during pregnancy. Moreover, during labor and delivery, they may produce a hypertensive crisis should tocolytic medications such as terbutaline be used to forestall premature delivery. In addition, several animal studies have described fetal growth retardation after prenatal exposure to MAOIs (Poulson and Robson 1964). One study in humans also described an increase in congenital malformations after prenatal exposure to tranylcypromine and phenelzine, although the sample size was extremely small (Heinonen et al. 1977).

Psychostimulants such as amphetamines and methylphenidate are used frequently as adjuncts in treating mood disorders and as first-line therapy for attention-deficit disorder (Chiarello and Cole 1987). Data regarding stimulant use during pregnancy are difficult to interpret because populations sampled frequently have had substance abuse disorders as opposed to mood disorders. Whereas amphetamine abuse has been associated with growth retardation and premature delivery, use of amphetamines for other purposes in the medical setting has not appeared to increase the risk for organ dysgenesis in most, but not all, studies (Heinonen et al. 1977; Kalter and Warkany 1983; Milkovich and van den Berg 1976; Nora et al. 1967, 1970; Zierler 1985). For example, in one series, no overall increase in congenital malformations was noted after prenatal exposure to amphetamines, but an excess of oral clefts was noted in the offspring of mothers who used the drug in the first trimester (Milkovich and van den Berg 1977). Data regarding long-term behavioral sequelae after prenatal exposure to psychostimulants are lacking. Although symptoms of irritability, apnea, and jerking movements have been reported during the neonatal period in children whose mothers used amphetamines, these findings were limited to cases of amphetamine abuse and not to use of stimulants for medical reasons or for treating mood disorder (Oro and Dixon 1987; Ramer 1974).

BENZODIAZEPINES

The data on the reproductive safety of benzodiazepines are controversial. Early reports described an increased risk of oral clefts after first-trimester exposure to drugs such as diazepam (Aarskog 1975; Safra and Oakley 1975; Saxen 1975), but later studies did not support the association (Heinonen et al. 1977; McElhatton 1994; Rosenberg et al. 1983; Shiono and Mills 1984).

A recent meta-analysis pooling the available literature calculated a 0.7% risk of oral cleft associated with first-trimester exposure to benzodiazepines (Altshuler et al. 1996). This is approximately a 10-fold increase in risk for oral cleft over that observed in the general population (6 in 10,000 or 0.06%) (Altshuler et al. 1996; Czeizel and Racz 1990; Hartz et al. 1975; Heinonen et al. 1977; Rosenberg et al. 1983; Shiono and Mills 1984; St. Clair and Schirmer 1992). Methodological limitations inherent in the analysis include pooling of studies of different benzodiazepines administered at different doses for varying amounts of time in dissimilar populations. Nonetheless, the likelihood that a woman taking benzodiazepines during the first trimester will give birth to a child with this congenital anomaly, although significantly increased, remains less than 1%. This risk must be discussed with the patient and weighed against the likelihood of relapse after benzodiazepine discontinuation.

In terms of neonatal toxicity, benzodiazepine withdrawal syndromes in the infant have been described (Athinarayanan et al. 1976; Fisher et al. 1985; Gillberg 1977; Mazzi 1977; Rementeria and Bhatt 1977; Rowlatt 1978). Case reports have described impaired temperature regulation, apnea, depressed Apgar scores, muscular hypotonia, and failure to feed. In one recent prospective study of 39 pregnant women with panic disorder, clonazepam (0.5–3.5 mg/day) was given alone for varying periods (Weinstock 1996). No evidence of congenital malformations was noted, but the sample was quite small. The Apgar scores, however, were uniformly high, and no infants showed signs of neonatal withdrawal syndromes, hypotonia, temperature dysregulation, or other perinatal difficulties.

Systematically derived data on the long-term neurobehavioral effects of benzodiazepine exposure are sparse. Several studies have reported motor and developmental delays, although these studies have been criticized for having significant ascertainment biases (Laegreid et al. 1990; Milkovich and van den Berg 1974). Other studies have found no association between benzodiazepine exposure and developmental delay (Bergman et al. 1992; Hartz et al. 1975). Overall, the balance of the data, although limited, does not support a significant effect on neurobehavioral function.

Currently, no systematic data are available on the reproductive safety of nonbenzodiazepine agents such as buspirone and zolpidem; therefore, they are not recommended for use in pregnancy.

ANTIPSYCHOTIC AGENTS

An early case report describing limb malformations raised concerns about first-trimester exposure to haloperidol, but several studies have not shown increased teratogenic risk with high-potency neuroleptics (Hanson and Oakley 1975; Kopelman et al. 1975; van Waes and van de Velde 1969; Waldman and Safferman 1993). A recent meta-analysis of the available studies noted a higher risk of congenital malformations after first-trimester exposure to low-potency neuroleptics compared with the general population (Altshuler et al. 1996). However, these data are largely based on the use of these medications for nausea and hyperemesis gravidarum, in which neuroleptics are used at low doses for their antiemetic effects. In clinical practice, higher-potency neuroleptics such as haloperidol and trifluoperazine are recommended over the lower-potency neuroleptics in managing psychiatric illness in pregnant women.

Information on the reproductive safety of atypical antipsychotics is sparse. No data are available on olanzapine or risperidone use in pregnancy; however, Eli Lilly and Company has established a postmarketing surveillance registry for olanzapine. To date, five case reports of pregnant women maintained on clozapine in pregnancy with no evidence of major congenital malformations in the neonate have been published (Barnas et al. 1994; Dickson and Hogg 1998; Stoner et al. 1997; Waldman and Safferman 1993). In addition, the manufacturer of clozapine has collected outcome information on infants exposed to clozapine through their Drug

Monitoring Center. Of the 29 infants, 25 were noted to be healthy, and 4 showed a variety of abnormalities (neonatal convulsions, Turner's syndrome, collarbone fracture, deformities of the face and congenital hip dislocation, and congenital blindness). These outcome data, however, need to be interpreted cautiously because a larger sample size would be needed to support any causal relation between outcome and drug.

Clinically, typical neuroleptics, particularly higher-potency neuroleptics, are recommended over the use of atypical antipsychotics in the pregnant population. However, if a patient presents with symptoms that have only responded to an atypical agent premorbidly, a clinician may consider maintaining the patient on this medication despite sparse data. The rationale of such a decision is based on a clinical risk–benefit analysis; the risk of precipitating relapse with discontinuation of her maintenance neuroleptics may outweigh the unknown teratogenic risk of continuing an atypical agent (Viguera et al. 1997). Moreover, children born to unmedicated mothers with psychosis during pregnancy appear to have a twofold greater incidence of congenital anomalies. Electroconvulsive therapy always should be considered a reasonable treatment alternative in the setting of an acute psychotic episode.

A transient perinatal syndrome has been described in neonates exposed to neuroleptic drugs during pregnancy. Although no systematic study of the incidence of these perinatal syndromes has been conducted, several case reports have documented motor restlessness, tremor, difficulty with oral feeding, hypertonicity, dystonic movements, and parkinsonian-like effects in infants exposed to neuroleptics (Auerbach et al. 1992; Hill et al. 1966; Levy and Wisniewski 1974; Tamer et al. 1969). These symptoms are typically of short duration, and these infants have been noted to have normal motor development (Desmond et al. 1967).

Studies of the long-term neurobehavioral sequelae associated with prenatal exposure to neuroleptic agents are lacking. No controlled prospective study on neurobehavioral outcome of children exposed to antipsychotic agents has been performed. Although data from animal studies suggest a spectrum of behavioral abnormalities after fetal exposure to high- and low-potency neuroleptics, the applicability of these findings to humans is unclear (Cagiano et al. 1988; Clark et al. 1970; Golub and Kornetsky 1974; Robertson et al. 1980; Spear et al. 1980). In one longitudinal study of IQ and behavioral functioning in children exposed to low-potency neuroleptics, followed up until age 5 years, no significant abnormalities were noted (Slone et al. 1977).

Little information is available about reproductive safety of medications typically used to treat extrapyramidal side effects of neuroleptic medications.

A possible association has been described between exposure to benztropine and trihexyphenidyl and risk that has been linked to congenital malformations (Heinonen et al. 1977). This contrasts with reports that described outcome of fetal exposure to diphenhydramine, which failed to show heightened risk of organ malformation (Aselton et al. 1985; Nelson and Forfar 1971). Studies of propranolol and atenolol during pregnancy have found no increase in congenital anomalies or pregnancy complications (Rubin 1981).

MOOD STABILIZERS

At least six major mood stabilizers are used to treat bipolar disorder, including lithium, valproic acid, carbamazepine, lamotrigine, gabapentin, and verapamil. Most of the data with regard to the reproductive safety of mood stabilizers has been collected on lithium.

Concern about the extent to which prenatal exposure to lithium heightens the risk for congenital and specifically cardiovascular malformations dates back to the early 1970s and the first reports from the International Register of Lithium Babies (Schou et al. 1973; Weinstein 1976), which was based on a voluntary physician reporting system. Initial and subsequent reports from the register described increased rates of cardiovascular malformations—most notably Ebstein's anomaly, a cardiovascular malformation characterized by right ventricular hypoplasia and congenital downward displacement of the tricuspid valve into the right ventricle (Nora et al. 1974; Schou et al. 1973; Weinstein 1976). The relative risk of this rare malformation (baseline risk in the general population is 1 in 20,000 births) with first-trimester lithium exposure was determined to be 400 times the rate in the general population. However, the major methodological limitation of the register was an inherent bias toward overreporting of adverse outcome. Nonetheless, this increased teratogenic risk associated with first-trimester use of lithium dominated clinical practice for almost 20 years, and women with bipolar disorder were counseled frequently either to defer pregnancy or to terminate pregnancies (Cohen et al. 1994b).

More recent epidemiological studies suggested a more modest teratogenic risk associated with first-trimester exposure to lithium than proposed previously (Edmonds and Oakley 1990; Jacobson et al. 1992; Kallen 1988; Kallen and Tandberg 1983; Sipek 1989; Zalzstein et al. 1990). A pooled analysis of the data supports a revised risk for this congenital malformation (Cohen et al. 1994b). The new revised risk for this congenital malformation after first-trimester exposure lies between 1 in 2,000 (0.05%) and 1 in 1,000 (0.1%), or 10–20 times that noted in the general population. Hence, the relative risks for Ebstein's anomaly may be somewhat increased, but the absolute risk is particularly small.

Perinatal toxicity in offspring exposed to lithium at the time of labor and delivery has been reported, including a "floppy baby" syndrome characterized by cyanosis and hypotonicity (Ananth 1976; Schou and Amdisen 1975; Woody et al. 1971). One case of neonatal hypothyroidism and nephrogenic diabetes insipidus also has been described. A naturalistic study of bipolar women maintained on lithium treatment during pregnancy and the puerperium found no direct evidence of neonatal toxicity in newborns whose mothers were taking lithium during either pregnancy or labor and delivery (Cohen et al. 1994b). Limited data are available regarding behavioral outcome of older children who were exposed to lithium during pregnancy. A 5-year follow-up investigation of children exposed to lithium during the second and third trimester of pregnancy did not identify any significant behavior problems (Schou 1976).

ANTICONVULSANTS

Studies of the reproductive safety of anticonvulsants have focused on epileptic patients, not on pregnant women treated for psychiatric illness. Although children of epileptic women appear to have greater numbers of congenital malformations regardless of perinatal anticonvulsant exposure compared with the general population, malformations in offspring exposed to anticonvulsants in utero remain higher than in nonexposed control subjects, even after controlling for the effects of epilepsy (Koch et al. 1992).

In comparison to lithium, anticonvulsants may represent a more serious teratogenic threat. Rates of neural tube defects after in utero exposure to carbamazepine and valproic acid have been as high as 1% and 3%–5%, respectively (Omtzigt et al. 1992; Robert and Guibaud 1982). Combining anticonvulsants makes the risk higher, perhaps because of higher maternal plasma levels (Battino et al. 1992; Koch et al. 1992; Nakane et al. 1980). In addition to serious neural tube effects, fetal exposure to these agents is associated with craniofacial abnormalities, and possible cognitive dysfunction may follow even after exposure late in pregnancy (Koch et al. 1992; Omtzigt et al. 1992; Robert and Guibaud 1982; Rosa 1991). No systematic data on the reproductive safety of the newer anticonvulsants—gabapentin and lamotrigine—are available except for a few case reports (Briggs et al. 1998; White and Andrews 1999). With few data supporting their reproductive safety, it is difficult to justify their use in pregnancy.

TREATMENT GUIDELINES

Major Depression

The prevalence of depression during pregnancy is approximately 10% and appears to be comparable to rates of depression in matched nongravid women (Gotlib et al. 1989; O'Hara 1986). Data do not support the notion that pregnancy protects against the development of depression, as has been previously suggested (Kendell et al. 1976; Zajicek 1981). Women with a history of recurrent affective disorder who discontinue maintenance antidepressant treatment are especially at high risk for relapse during pregnancy (Cohen and Altshuler 1997).

Diagnosis of depression during pregnancy can be difficult. Depressive symptoms in pregnant women, such as sleep problems, change in appetite, fatigue, and changes in libido, can be difficult to distinguish from normative experiences of pregnancy. Further compounding the difficulty of recognizing depression in pregnancy is the failure to assess for medical disorders such as anemia, gestational diabetes, and thyroid dysfunction that could potentially contribute to depressive symptoms (Klein and Essex 1995). Given these potential confounds, better markers of mood disorder in pregnant women include a lack of interest in pregnancy, guilty ruminations, and profound anhedonia. Other potential predictors of depression during pregnancy include a history of mood disorder, a family history of depression, marital discord, poor psychosocial support, low levels of perceived emotional support, recent adverse life events, and unwanted pregnancy (Frank et al. 1987; Gotlib et al. 1989; O'Hara 1986).

Although management of depression during pregnancy remains largely empirical, with few definitive data and no controlled treatment studies of depression during pregnancy, the most appropriate treatment algorithm depends on the severity of the disorder. Use of antidepressants during pregnancy is generally indicated for those patients who have neurovegetative symptoms that interfere with maternal well-being or for those who experience the symptoms as intolerable.

Women who develop minor depressive symptoms during pregnancy may benefit from nonpharmacological treatments such as interpersonal psychotherapy or cognitive therapy (Beck et al. 1979; Klerman et al. 1984). These nonpharmacological strategies also may be appropriate for patients with histories of mild to moderate episodes of depression who become pregnant or who are taking antidepressants and wish to conceive. Gradual tapering followed by discontinuation of antidepressants may be appropriate for these patients when performed in conjunction with cognitive-behavioral strategies and may help eliminate the need for medication.

Preliminary data suggest that the majority of women (approximately 60%) will discontinue antidepressants proximate to conception or during pregnancy (Cohen and Altshuler 1997), and half of them will reintroduce antidepressant medications during pregnancy. However, it should be underscored that patients with histories of recurrent major depression who discontinue medications proximate to conception appear to be at high risk for relapse early in pregnancy (Cohen and Altshuler 1997).

Pharmacotherapeutic intervention is clearly appropriate for pregnant patients who have symptoms of severe depression, including diminished oral intake, suicidality, or psychosis. For women with histories of repeated episodes of recurrent major depression who have tried and failed to discontinue antidepressants, remaining on maintenance antidepressants may be the safest option. Among the TCAs, desipramine and nortriptyline are the preferred agents because they are less anticholinergic and the least likely to exacerbate orthostatic hypotension. With the most extensive literature supporting its reproductive safety, compared with other antidepressants, fluoxetine is also a good choice during pregnancy. Severely depressed patients with acute suicidality or psychosis require hospitalization, and electroconvulsive therapy is frequently the treatment of first choice. Two reviews of electroconvulsive therapy use during pregnancy noted efficacy and safety of the procedure (Ferrill et al. 1992; Miller 1994).

Data are not yet sufficient regarding teratogenic risk associated with sertraline or paroxetine. However, there is a growing literature on the reproductive safety of these antidepressants (Kulin et al. 1998). These agents may be appropriate in certain situations for women with mild to moderate depression who are trying to conceive, such as women undergoing infertility treatments or older women in whom it may take longer to become pregnant. If antidepressants are discontinued in these women, they may be left vulnerable to relapse for months as they try to conceive. In such a situation, one possible treatment strategy is to maintain these patients on sertraline or paroxetine and then taper them off after early documentation of pregnancy. Discontinuation of short half-life SSRIs after documentation of pregnancy (and prior to the missed period) would permit washout of drug and metabolite before the fetoplacental circulation is established, allowing for continued treatment before pregnancy with drug discontinuation after documentation of pregnancy. The one possible drawback of such a strategy is the possible early precipitation of relapse following a fairly rapid taper off drug (Baldessarini and Tondo 1998; Baldessarini et al. 1996). Even with a rapid washout, the use of short-acting agents proximate to conception means possible fetal exposure to drugs lacking sufficient data regarding reproductive safety.

Clinicians caring for patients who have a history of depression and have discontinued maintenance medications during pregnancy must consider the possibility that symptoms may re-emerge during the postpartum period. Several studies describe a strong association between a history of depression or depression during pregnancy and postpartum worsening of mood (Gotlib et al. 1989; O'Hara et al. 1983, 1984). Prophylactic reintroduction of antidepressants either during the latter portion of the third trimester or immediately after delivery may benefit those patients who have a history of severe depression, even though no abundant systematically derived data support this practice (Wisner and Wheeler 1994). Based on several anecdotal reports of toxicity in neonates born to mothers who were treated with antidepressants at the time of delivery, some early reports have recommended discontinuation of antidepressants several days before delivery to avoid neonatal toxicity (Cowe et al. 1982; Eggermont 1973; Schimmell et al. 1991; Webster 1973). Given the rarity of these perinatal syndromes, this practice needs reconsideration because it withdraws treatment from patients precisely as they enter a period of heightened risk for affective worsening.

Bipolar Disorder

The effect of pregnancy on the course of bipolar disorder is unclear. Case reports suggest that pregnancy is not associated with significantly altered risk of recurrences of bipolar illness, and some patients maintain euthymia during pregnancy despite medication discontinuation (Lier et al. 1989; Sharma and Persad 1995; Targum et al. 1979). However, growing clinical experience suggests that recurrences of mania and bipolar depression are, at least, not uncommon during pregnancy (Finnerty et al. 1996; Viguera et al. 1997). One recent study of pregnant bipolar women described relapse rates of approximately 50% within 6 months of lithium discontinuation (Viguera et al. 1997). In contrast to the sparse data on bipolar disorder during pregnancy, the postpartum period has received a more systematic study because it carries high risks of acute recurrences of mania and depression of about 30%–50% (Bratfos and Haug 1966; Brockington et al. 1981; Davidson and Robertson 1985; Dean et al. 1989; Kendell et al. 1987; Klompenhouwer and van Hulst 1991; Reich and Winokur 1970). Many women who acquire puerperal psychosis also have bipolar disorder, and these are responsive to standard treatments (Kendell et al. 1987). Postpartum affective and psychotic episodes can be very severe and often require emergency psychiatric intervention to avoid injury to or suicide in the mother and abuse or infanticide of the newborn (Davidson and Robertson 1985).

Clinical guidelines for the safe management of the pregnant woman with bipolar disorder are still emerging. Thus far, the data strongly support the use of lithium prophylaxis and possibly other mood stabilizers as bipolar women enter the postpartum period (Abou-Saleh and Coppen 1983; Austin 1992; Cohen et al. 1995; Stewart 1988; Stewart et al. 1991; Targum et al. 1979; van Gent and Verhoeven 1992). Women with bipolar disorder who are taking mood stabilizers need to attend carefully to family planning. Such patients should be made aware of the attendant teratogenic risks of lithium and the anticonvulsants and should be counseled to continue contraception unless they are willing to accept such risks.

The decision to use lithium during pregnancy depends on illness severity. Patients with histories of a single past episode of mania with sustained affective well-being may be able to gradually taper (>2 weeks) and discontinue lithium before conception. Bipolar women with more than one past episode of mania or depression offer a greater clinical challenge. The patient may choose to gradually discontinue lithium (and/or other mood stabilizer) before conception. If the patient becomes symptomatic during the taper, lithium may be easily resumed, and the feasibility of conceiving while not taking medication should be reassessed. Alternatively, lithium discontinuation could await early documentation of pregnancy. This strategy minimizes exposure and affords antimanic prophylaxis for the longest period while women try to conceive. However, this option involves a more abrupt discontinuation of lithium (i.e., taper<2weeks) and may actually provoke or hasten relapse, as has been previously reported in nonpregnant cohorts (Baldessarini and Tondo 1998; Baldessarini et al. 1996; Suppes et al. 1991).

Certainly, for women with the most severe forms of bipolar disorder, maintenance of lithium treatment before and during pregnancy is advisable. Accepting the relatively small absolute increase in teratogenic risk with first-trimester exposure to lithium seems particularly justified because these patients are at highest risk for clinical deterioration in the absence of treatment. A full relapse of bipolar disorder during pregnancy is potentially dangerous to mother and fetus and may require aggressive treatment, including hospitalization and exposure to multiple psychotropics (neuroleptics, benzodiazepines) at higher doses. Therefore, patients with brittle bipolar disorder may opt to continue taking lithium to maintain euthymia.

All women who use lithium during the first trimester of pregnancy should be counseled about the higher risk of cardiovascular malformations. A level II ultrasound at 16–18 weeks' gestation to detect cardiac anomalies is recommended (Cohen et al. 1994). Finally, pregnant women with bipolar disorder should be clearly informed of the high risk for relapse as they enter the postpartum period, and prophylaxis with a mood stabilizer (and/or neuroleptic) should be recommended strongly, especially for those who have not taken medication during the pregnancy. Clinically, this practice is often neglected, thus placing these pregnant women at significant risk for psychiatric morbidity. Prophylaxis with anticonvulsants may be considered; however, the risk of potential subtle cognitive sequelae remains even with late third-trimester exposure (Scolnik et al. 1994; Wisner 1998). Although neurogenesis is completed by 20 weeks of gestation, the brain continues to develop throughout pregnancy (Langman 1985). In addition, current practice is to reduce the lithium dose by 30% before delivery; this is done because of concerns about potential lithium toxicity due to changes in a woman's volume status as she enters the postpartum period. However, this practice may need to be reevaluated in light of data from nonpregnant patients that even rapid reductions in lithium serum concentration (especially from high to low serum concentrations) may precipitate relapse (Cohen et al. 1994b; Lapierre et al. 1980; Rosenbaum et al. 1994). In addition, reports linking lithium therapy during pregnancy to neonatal toxicity are extremely rare. Therefore, withholding lithium or use of relatively low doses in the early postpartum period may be particularly dangerous psychiatrically. Clinically, a more prudent option may be to measure serial serum levels during labor and delivery as well as the first few days postpartum and adjust the dose accordingly.

Anxiety Disorders

The course of panic disorder in pregnancy is variable. Pregnancy may ameliorate symptoms of panic in some patients and afford them a chance to discontinue medication for an interval during the course of their illness (Cohen et al. 1996; Cowley and Roy-Byrne 1989; George et al. 1987; Klein 1994; Villeponteaux et al. 1992; Wheeler et al. 1950).

However, some studies described persistence or worsening of panic symptoms during pregnancy (Cohen et al. 1996; Cowley and Roy-Byrne 1989; Northcott and Stein 1994). Predictors of relapse of panic disorder during pregnancy are not yet established. However, in one study, discontinuation of maintenance antipanic medications precipitated early relapse in remitted patients who either tapered or discontinued antipanic drugs during pregnancy.

The preferred approach to patients with panic disorder who wish to conceive is to taper these drugs gradually. Adjunctive cognitive-behavioral therapy may be of some benefit in helping patients discontinue antipanic agents and may increase the well interval before relapse (Robinson et al. 1992). If taper is unsuccessful and if symptoms recur, reinstitution of pharmacotherapy may be required. However, for those patients with severe disorder, maintenance medication may be a clinical necessity.

Given the reported increase in oral clefts with first-trimester benzodiazepine exposure, TCAs or fluoxetine represent a nonbenzodiazepine alternative for panic (Altshuler et al. 1996). However, the extent to which many patients with panic disorder do not respond to TCAs alone makes the use of benzodiazepines a reasonable alternative. Given the accumulated data regarding the reproductive safety of fluoxetine, the use of this medication also is a viable treatment alternative.

Some patients may conceive inadvertently while taking antipanic medications and may present for emergent consultation. Abrupt discontinuation of antipanic maintenance medication is not recommended. However, gradual taper (i.e., >2 weeks) with adjunctive cognitive-behavioral therapy may be pursued in an effort to minimize fetal exposure.

Obsessive-Compulsive Disorder

For patients with a premorbid obsessive-compulsive disorder (OCD), their symptoms appear to worsen during pregnancy and the postpartum period without treatment (Buttolph and Holland 1990; Sichel et al. 1993). In a prospective study of 14 patients who were not taking maintenance medications during pregnancy, 43% required a reinstitution of their medication because of relapse (Cohen et al. 1994a). Of those who remained off medications during pregnancy, all had a recurrence or an exacerbation of their symptoms in the postpartum period. Several studies have also documented an association between pregnancy and new onset of OCD (Buttolph and Holland 1990; Ingram 1961; Neziroglu et al. 1992). In one study, 52% of the women experienced the onset of OCD during their first pregnancy (Buttolph and Holland 1990).

Other studies have not confirmed this finding (Lo 1967). No known biological mechanism explains the high rates of OCD in pregnancy, and no systematic data are available that prospectively describe the course of OCD during pregnancy.

Behavioral techniques (cognitive-behavioral therapy) for OCD during the first trimester should be considered as an alternative to medication. For those patients with moderate to severe symptoms, maintenance medications throughout pregnancy are highly recommended given the potentially disabling sequelae of untreated OCD symptoms. Although postpartum prophylaxis in patients with OCD has never been systematically investigated, maintenance medications during pregnancy may protect against probable relapse during the postpartum period.

TCAs and fluoxetine represent a reasonable pharmacological approach during or after the first trimester. The TCA clomipramine may be used if previously successful. Although not considered teratogenic, it may aggravate orthostatic hypotension; thus, its use may be limited in pregnancy. It also has been associated with neonatal seizures at the time of labor and delivery (Cowe et al. 1982). This is based on anecdotal data; therefore, clomipramine is not an absolute contraindication for pregnant women who have severe OCD. As with any other psychotropic, close monitoring during labor and delivery is the most prudent course of action. Withdrawal of medication in women with active illness who require treatment during pregnancy may increase the risk for puerperal worsening of the disorder.

CONCLUSION

Pregnancy does not appear to be protective for women with psychiatric illness. Psychotropic medications may be used during pregnancy when the potential risk to the fetus from drug exposure is outweighed by the risk of untreated maternal psychiatric disorder. Although concern regarding the teratogenic effects of prenatal exposure to psychotropics has kindled appropriate vigilance, discontinuation of these maintenance medications may result in significant morbidity for the patient. Moreover, of growing concern is the risk of untreated psychiatric illness on fetal development. These risks must be weighed carefully on an individual basis, with particular attention to the history of severity of illness and rapidity of decompensation when relapse occurs.

In general, data support the relative reproductive safety of TCAs and fluoxetine as antidepressants. Emerging data on the other SSRIs are also reassuring. First-trimester exposure to some phenothiazines, lithium, benzodiazepines, and the anticonvulsants increases the relative risk of congenital malformation. However, this risk may translate clinically into a small absolute risk in light of an individual's illness history and current mental status.

The potential for long-term behavioral changes after prenatal exposure to psychotropics requires more systematic study. Animal studies suggest changes in brain receptor number and function after in utero exposure to various psychotropic medications. Large epidemiological follow-up studies of children exposed to medication in utero are needed. Pending such studies, the clinician must continue to act in a state of relative uncertainty, weighing partially calculated risks to manage clinical dilemmas. Coordinated care among patient, husband or partner, obstetrician, and psychiatrist is essential. For some patients, the decision to accept an increase in teratogenic risk may be appropriate to ensure stable maternal mental health during pregnancy.

REFERENCES

Aarskog D: Association between maternal intake of diazepam and oral clefts. Lancet 2:921, 1975

Abou-Saleh MT, Coppen A: The prognosis of depression in old age: the case for lithium therapy. Br J Psychiatry 143:527–528, 1983

Ali S, Buelke-Sam J, Newport GD, et al: Early neurobehavioral and neurochemical alterations in rats prenatally exposed to imipramine. Neurotoxicology 7:365–380, 1986

Altshuler LL, Cohen LS, Szuba MP, et al: Pharmacologic management of psychiatric illness during pregnancy: dilemmas and guidelines. Am J Psychiatry 153:592–606, 1996

Ananth J: Side effects on fetus and infant of psychotropic drug use during pregnancy. International Pharmacopsychiatry 11:246–260, 1976

Aselton P, Jick H, Milunsky A: First-trimester drug use and congenital disorders. Obstet Gynecol 65:451–455, 1985

Athinarayanan P, Peirog SH, Nigam SK, et al: Chlordiazepoxide withdrawal in the neonate. Am J Obstet Gynecol 124:212–213, 1976

Auerbach JG, Hans SL, Marcus J, et al: Maternal psychotropic medication and neonatal behavior. Neurotoxicol Teratol 14:399–406, 1992

Austin MP: Puerperal affective psychosis: is there a case for lithium prophylaxis? Br J Psychiatry 161:692–694, 1992

Baldessarini R, Tondo L: Effects of lithium treatment in bipolar disorders and post-treatment-discontinuation reoccurrence risk. Clinical Drug Investigation 15:337–351, 1998

Baldessarini RJ, Tondo L, Faedda GL, et al: Effects of the rate of discontinuing lithium maintenance treatment in bipolar disorders. J Clin Psychiatry 57:441–448, 1996

Banister P, Dafoe C, Smith ESO, et al: Possible teratogenicity of tricyclic antidepressants (letter). Lancet 1:838–839, 1972

Barnas C, Bergant A, Hummer M, et al: Clozapine concentrations in maternal and fetal plasma, amniotic fluid, and breast milk (letter). Am J Psychiatry 151:945, 1994

Battino D, Binelli S, Caccamo ML, et al: Malformation in offspring of 305 epileptic women: a prospective study. Acta Neurol Scand 85:204–207, 1992

Beck AT, Rush AJ, Shaw BF, et al: Cognitive Therapy of Depression. New York, Guilford, 1979

Bergman UF, Rosa FW, Baum C, et al: Effects of exposure to benzodiazepine during fetal life. Lancet 340:694–696, 1992

Bratfos O, Haug JO: Puerperal mental disorders in manic-depressive females. Acta Psychiatr Scand 42:285–294, 1966

Briggs GG, Freeman RK, Schofield EM: Drugs in Pregnancy and Lactation: A Reference Guide to Fetal and Neonatal Risk, 5th Edition. Baltimore, MD, Williams & Wilkins, 1994

Briggs G, Freeman R, Yaffe SJ: Drugs in Pregnancy and Lactation. Baltimore, MD, Williams & Wilkins, 1998

Brockington IF, Cernik KF, Schofield EM, et al: Puerperal psychosis: phenomena and diagnosis. Arch Gen Psychiatry 38:829–833, 1981

Buttolph ML, Holland A: Obsessive compulsive disorders in pregnancy and childbirth, in Obsessive Compulsive Disorders, Theory and Management. Edited by Jenike M, Baer L, Minichiello WE. Chicago, IL, Year Book Medical, 1990, pp 89–95

Cagiano R, Barfield RJ, White NR, et al: Subtle behavioural changes produced in rat pups by in utero exposure to haloperidol. Eur J Pharmacol 157:45–50, 1988

Chambers CD, Johnson KA, Dick LM, et al: Birth outcomes in pregnant women taking fluoxetine. N Engl J Med 335:1010–1015, 1996

Chiarello RJ, Cole JO: The use of psychostimulants in general psychiatry: a reconsideration. Arch Gen Psychiatry 44:286–295, 1987

Clark CV, Gorman D, Vernadakis A: Effects of prenatal administration of psychotropic drugs on behavior of developing rats. Dev Psychobiol 3:225–235, 1970

Cohen LS, Altshuler LL: Pharmacologic management of psychiatric illness during pregnancy and the postpartum period. Psychiatr Clin North Am 4:21–60, 1997

Cohen LS, Rosenbaum JF: Fluoxetine in pregnancy (letter). N Engl J Med 336:872, 1997

Cohen LS, Sichel DA, Dimmock JA, et al: Impact of pregnancy on panic disorder: a case series. J Clin Psychiatry 55:284–288, 1994a

Cohen LS, Friedman JM, Jefferson JW, et al: A reevaluation of risk of in utero exposure to lithium. JAMA 271:146–150, 1994b

Cohen LS, Sichel DA, Robertson LM, et al: Postpartum prophylaxis for women with bipolar disorder. Am J Psychiatry 152:1641–1645, 1995

Cohen LS, Sichel DA, et al: Prospective study of panic disorder during pregnancy. Paper presented at the 149th annual meeting of the American Psychiatric Association, New York, May 1996

Cowe L, Lloyd DJ, Dawling S: Neonatal convulsions caused by withdrawal from maternal clomipramine. BMJ 284:1837–1838, 1982

Cowley DS, Roy-Byrne PP: Panic disorder during pregnancy. J Psychosom Obstet Gynaecol 10:193–210, 1989

Coyle IR: Changes in developing behavior following prenatal administration of imipramine. Pharmacol Biochem Behav 3:799–807, 1975

Coyle I, Wayner MJ, Singer G: Behavioral teratogenesis: a critical evaluation. Pharmacol Biochem Behav 4:191–200, 1976

Crombie DL, Pinsent RJ, Fleming D: Imipramine in pregnancy (letter). BMJ 1:745, 1972

Cutrona CE: Causal attributions and perinatal depression. J Abnorm Psychol 92:161–172, 1983

Czeizel A, Racz J: Evaluation of drug intake during pregnancy in the Hungarian Case-Control Surveillance of Congenital Anomalies. Teratology 42:505–512, 1990

Davidson J, Robertson E: A follow-up study of postpartum illness 1946–1978. Acta Psychiatr Scand 71:451–457, 1985

Dean C, Williams RJ, Brockington IF: Is puerperal psychosis the same as bipolar manic-depressive disorder? A family study. Psychol Med 19:637–647, 1989

Del Rio J, Montero D, De Caballos ML: Long lasting changes after perinatal exposure to antidepressants. Prog Brain Res 73:173–187, 1988

Desmond MM, Rudolph AJ, Hill RM, et al: Behavioral alterations in infants born to mothers on psychoactive medication during pregnancy, in Congenital Mental Retardation. Edited by Farrell G. Austin, University of Texas, 1967, pp 235–245

Dickson RA, Hogg L: Pregnancy of a patient treated with clozapine. Psychiatr Serv 49:1081–1083, 1998

Downey G, Coyne JC: Children of depressed parents: an integrative review. Psychol Bull 108:50–76, 1990

Edmonds LD, Oakley GP: Ebstein's anomaly and maternal lithium exposure during pregnancy. Teratology 41:551–552, 1990

Eggermont E: Withdrawal symptoms in neonates associated with maternal imipramine therapy (letter). Lancet 2:680, 1973

Fabro SE: Clinical Obstetrics. New York, Wiley, 1987

Faedda GL, Tondo L, Baldessarini RJ, et al: Outcome after rapid vs gradual discontinuation of lithium treatment in bipolar disorders. Arch Gen Psychiatry 50:448–455, 1993

Falterman CG, Richardson CJ: Small left colon syndrome associated with maternal ingestion of psychotropic drugs. J Pediatr 97:308–310, 1980

Ferrill MJ, Kehoe WA, Jacisin JJ: ECT during pregnancy: physiologic and pharmacologic considerations. Convulsive Therapy 8:186–200, 1992

Field T: Infants of depressed mothers. Infant Behavior and Development 18:1–13, 1995

File SE, Tucker JC: Prenatal treatment with clomipramine: effects on the behaviour of male and female adolescent rats. Psychopharmacology 82:221–224, 1984

Finnerty M, Levin Z, Miller LJ: Acute manic episodes in pregnancy. Am J Psychiatry 153:261–263, 1996

Fisher J, Edgren B, Mammel MC, et al: Neonatal apnea associated with maternal clonazepam therapy. Obstet Gynecol 66:34–35, 1985

Frank E, Kupfer DJ, Jacob M, et al: Pregnancy-related affective episodes among women with recurrent depression. Am J Psychiatry 144:288–293, 1987

George DT, Ladenheim JA, Nutt DJ: Effect of pregnancy on panic attacks. Am J Psychiatry 144:1078–1079, 1987

Gillberg C: "Floppy infant syndrome" and maternal diazepam (letter). Lancet 2:244, 1977

Glover V: Maternal stress or anxiety in pregnancy and emotional development of the child. Br J Psychiatry 171:105–106, 1997

Goldstein DJ: Effects of third trimester fluoxetine exposure on the newborn. J Clin Psychopharmacol 15:417–420, 1995

Golub M, Kornetsky C: Seizure susceptibility and avoidance conditioning in adult rats treated prenatally with chlorpromazine. Dev Psychobiol 7:79–88, 1974

Gotlib IH, Whiffen VE, Mount JH, et al: Prevalence rates and demographic characteristics associated with depression in pregnancy and the postpartum. J Consult Clin Psychol 57:269–274, 1989

Hanson JW, Oakley GP Jr: Haloperidol and limb deformity (letter). JAMA 231:26, 1975

Hartz SC, Heinonen OP, Shapiro S, et al: Antenatal exposure to meprobamate and chlordiazepoxide in relation to malformations, mental development, and childhood mortality. N Engl J Med 292:726–728, 1975

Heinonen O, Sloan D, Shapiro S: Birth Defects and Drugs in Pregnancy. Littleton, MA, Publishing Services Group, 1977

Hill RM, Desmond MM, Kay JL: Extrapyramidal dysfunction in an infant of a schizophrenic mother. J Pediatr 69:589–595, 1966

Idanpaan-Heikkila J, Saxen L: Possible teratogenicity of imipramine-chloropyramine. Lancet 2:282–284, 1973

Ingram IM: Obsessional illness in mental hospital patients. Journal of Mental Science 107:382–402, 1961

Inman W, Kubota K, Pearce G, et al: Prescription event monitoring of paroxetine. PEM Reports PXL 1206:1–44, 1993

Istvan J: Stress, anxiety, and birth outcome: a critical review of the evidence. Psychol Bull 100:331–348, 1986

Jacobs D: Imipramine (tofranil) (letter). S Afr Med J 46:1023, 1972

Jacobson SJ, Jones K, Johnson K, et al: Prospective multicentre study of pregnancy outcome after lithium exposure during first trimester. Lancet 339:530–533, 1992

Jason KM, Cooper TB, Friedman E: Prenatal exposure to imipramine alters early behavioral development and beta adrenergic receptors in rats. J Pharmacol Exp Ther 217:461–466, 1981

Kallen B: Comments on teratogen update: lithium (letter). Teratology 38:597, 1988

Kallen B, Tandberg A: Lithium and pregnancy: a cohort study on manic-depressive women. Acta Psychiatr Scand 68:134–139, 1983

Kalter H, Warkany J: Congenital malformations. N Engl J Med 308:491–497, 1983

Kellogg CK: Benzodiazepines: influence on the developing brain. Prog Brain Res 73:207–228, 1988

Kendell RE, Wainwright S, Hailey A, et al: The influence of childbirth on psychiatric morbidity. Psychol Med 6:297–302, 1976

Kendell RE, Chalmers JC, Platz C: Epidemiology of puerperal psychoses. Br J Psychiatry 150:662–673, 1987

Kessler RC, McGonagle KA, Swartz M, et al: Sex and depression in the National Comorbidity Survey, I: lifetime prevalence, chronicity and recurrence. J Affect Disord 29:85–96, 1993

Klein DF: False suffocation alarms, spontaneous panics, and related conditions. Arch Gen Psychiatry 50:306–317, 1994

Klein MH, Essex MJ: Pregnant or depressed? The effects of overlap between symptoms of depression and somatic complaints of pregnancy on rates of major depression in the second trimester. Depression 2:308–314, 1995

Klerman GL, Weissman MM, Rounsaville B, et al: Interpersonal Psychotherapy of Depression. New York, Basic Books, 1984

Klompenhouwer JL, van Hulst AM: Classification of postpartum psychosis: a study of 250 mother and baby admissions in the Netherlands. Acta Psychiatr Scand 84:255–261, 1991

Koch S, Losche G, Jager-Roman E, et al: Major and minor birth malformations and antiepileptic drugs. Neurology 42(suppl 5):83–88, 1992

Kopelman AE, McCullar FW, Heggeness L: Limb malformations following maternal use of haloperidol. JAMA 231:62–64, 1975

Koren G, Pastuszak A, Ito S: Drugs in pregnancy. N Engl J Med 338:1128–1137, 1998

Kuenssberg EV, Knox JD: Imipramine in pregnancy (letter). BMJ 2:292, 1972

Kulin NA, Pastuszak A, Sage SA, et al: Pregnancy outcome following maternal use of the new selective serotonin reuptake inhibitors: a prospective controlled multicenter study. JAMA 279:609–610, 1998

Ladd CO, Owens MJ, Nemeroff CB: Persistent changes in corticotropin-releasing factor neuronal systems induced by maternal deprivation. Endocrinology 137:1212–1218, 1997

Laegreid L, Olegard R, Conradi N, et al: Congenital malformations and maternal consumption of benzodiazepines: a case control study. Dev Med Child Neurol 32:432–441, 1990

Laegreid L, Hagberg G, Lundberg A: The effect of benzodiazepines on the fetus and the newborn. Neuropediatrics 23:18–23, 1992

Langman J: Human development: normal and abnormals, in Medical Embryology. Edited by Langman J. Baltimore, MD, Williams & Wilkins, 1985, p 123

Lapierre YD, Gagnan A, Kokkinidis L: Rapid recurrence of mania following lithium withdrawal. Biol Psychiatry 15:859–864, 1980

Lauer JA, Adams PM, Johnson KM: Perinatal diazepam exposure: behavioral and neurochemical consequences. Neurotoxicol Teratol 9:213–219, 1989

Levy W, Wisniewski K: Chlorpromazine causing extrapyramidal dysfunction in newborn infant of psychotic mother. New York State Journal of Medicine 74:684–685, 1974

Lier L, Katru M, Rafaelsen OJ: Psychiatric illness in relation to pregnancy and childbirth, II: diagnostic profiles, psychosocial and perinatal aspects. Nordisk Psykiatrisk Tidsskrif 43:535–542, 1989

Lo WH: A follow-up study of obsessional neurotics in Hong Kong Chinese. Br J Psychiatry 113:823–832, 1967

Mazzi E: Possible neonatal diazepam withdrawal: a case report. Am J Obstet Gynecol 129:586–587, 1977

McBride WG: Limb deformities associated with iminodibenzyl hydrochloride (letter). Med J Aust 1:492, 1972

McElhatton PR: The effects of benzodiazepine use during pregnancy and lactation. Reprod Toxicol 8:461–475, 1994

McElhatton P, Garbis H, Elefant E, et al: The outcome of pregnancy in 689 women exposed to therapeutic doses of antidepressants: a collaborative study of the European Network of Teratology Information Services (ENTIS). Reprod Toxicol 10:285–294, 1996

Milkovich L, van den Berg BJ: Effects of prenatal meprobamate and chlordiazepoxide hydrochloride on human embryonic and fetal development. N Engl J Med 291:1268–1271, 1974

Milkovich L, van den Berg BJ: An evaluation of the teratogenicity of certain antinauseant drugs. Am J Obstet Gynecol 125:244–248, 1976

Milkovich L, van den Berg BJ: Effects of antenatal exposure to anorectic drugs. Am J Obstet Gynecol 121:637–642, 1977

Miller JC, Friedhoff AG: Prenatal neurotransmitter programming of postnatal receptor function. Prog Brain Res 2:509–522, 1987

Miller LJ: Use of electroconvulsive therapy during pregnancy. Hosp Community Psychiatry 45:444–450, 1994

Misri S, Sivertz K: Tricyclic drugs in pregnancy and lactation: a preliminary report. Int J Psychiatry Med 21:157–171, 1991

Montero D, DeCeballos ML, Del Rio J: Down-regulation of 3H-imipramine binding sites in rat cerebral cortex after prenatal exposure to antidepressants. Life Sci 46:1619–1626, 1990

Morrow AW: Imipramine and congenital abnormalities. N Z Med J 75:228–229, 1972

Murray L: The impact of postnatal depression on infant development. J Child Psychol Psychiatry 33:543–561, 1992

Murray L, Cooper P: Effects of postnatal depression on infant development. Arch Dis Child 77:99–101, 1997

Nakane Y, Okuma T, Takahashi R, et al: Multi-institutional study on the teratogenicity and fetal toxicity of antiepileptic drugs: a report of a collaborative study group in Japan. Epilepsia 21:663–680, 1980

Nelson MM, Forfar JO: Associations between drugs administered during pregnancy and congenital abnormalities in the fetus. BMJ 1:523–527, 1971

Neziroglu F, Anemone R, Yaryura-Tobias JA: Onset of obsessive-compulsive disorder in pregnancy. Am J Psychiatry 149:947–950, 1992

Nora J, McNamara D, Fraser FC: Dextroamphetamine sulphate and human malformations. Lancet 1:570–571, 1967

Nora JJ, Vargo TA, Nora AH, et al: Dexamphetamine: a possible environmental trigger in cardiovascular malformations. Lancet 1:1290–1291, 1970

Nora JJ, Nora AH, Toews WH: Lithium, Ebstein's anomaly and other congenital heart defects. Lancet 2:594–595, 1974

Northcott CJ, Stein MB: Panic disorder in pregnancy. J Clin Psychiatry 55:539–542, 1994

Nulman I, Koren G: The safety of fluoxetine during pregnancy and lactation. Teratology 53:304–308, 1996

Nulman I, Rovet J, Stewart DE, et al: Neurodevelopment of children exposed in utero to antidepressant drugs. N Engl J Med 336:258–262, 1997

O'Hara MW: Social support, life events, and depression during pregnancy and the puerperium. Arch Gen Psychiatry 43:569–573, 1986

O'Hara MW, Rehm LP, Campbell SB: Postpartum depression: a role for social network and life stress variables. J Nerv Ment Dis 171:335–341, 1983

O'Hara MW, Neunaber DJ, Zekoski EM: Prospective study of postpartum depression: prevalence, course, and predictive factors. J Abnorm Psychol 93:158–171, 1984

Omtzigt JG, Los FJ, Grobbee DE, et al: The risk of spina bifida aperta after first-trimester exposure to valproate in a prenatal cohort. Neurology 42(suppl 5):119–125, 1992

Oro AS, Dixon SD: Perinatal cocaine and methamphetamine exposure: maternal and neonatal correlates. J Pediatr 111:571–578, 1987

Orr ST, Miller CA: Maternal depressive symptoms and the risk of poor pregnancy outcome: review of the literature and preliminary findings. Epidemiol Rev 17:165–171, 1995

Pastuszak A, Schick-Boschetto B, Zuber C, et al: Pregnancy outcome following first-trimester exposure to fluoxetine (Prozac). JAMA 269:2246–2248, 1993

Perkin MR, Bland JM, Peacock JL, et al: The effect of anxiety and depression during pregnancy on obstetric complications. Br J Obstet Gynaecol 100:629–634, 1993

Plotsky PM, Meaney MJ: Early postnatal experience alters hypothalamic corticotropin-releasing factor (CRF) mRNA median eminence CRF content and stress-induced release in adult rats. Brain Res Mol Brain Res 18:195–200, 1993

Post RM: Transduction of psychosocial stress into the neurobiology of recurrent affective disorder. Am J Psychiatry 149:999–1010, 1992

Poulson E, Robson JM: Effect of phenelzine and some related compounds in pregnancy. J Endocrinol 30:205–215, 1964

Rachelefsky GS, Flynt JN Jr, Ebbin AJ, et al: Possible teratogenicity of tricyclic antidepressants (letter). Lancet 1:838, 1972

Ramer CM: The case history of an infant born to an amphetamine-addicted mother. Clin Pediatr 13:596–597, 1974

Reich T, Winokur G: Postpartum psychoses in patients with manic depressive disease. J Nerv Ment Dis 151:60–68, 1970

Rementeria JL, Bhatt K: Withdrawal symptoms in neonates from intrauterine exposure to diazepam. J Pediatr 90:123–126, 1977

Robert E, Guibaud P: Maternal valproic acid and congenital neural tube defects (letter). Lancet 2:937, 1982

Robertson RT, Majka JA, Peter CP, et al: Effects of prenatal exposure to chlorpromazine on postnatal development and behavior of rats. Toxicol Appl Pharmacol 53:541–549, 1980

Robinson L, Walker JR, Anderson D: Cognitive-behavioural treatment of panic disorder during pregnancy and lactation. Can J Psychiatry 37:623–626, 1992

Rosa FW: Spina bifida in infants of women treated with carbamazepine during pregnancy. N Engl J Med 324:674–677, 1991

Rosenbaum JF, Sachs GS, Lafer B: High rates of relapse in bipolar patients abruptly changed from standard to low serum lithium levels in a double-blind trial. Paper presented at the American College of Neuropsychopharmacology, San Juan, Puerto Rico, December 1994

Rosenberg L, Mitchell AA, Parsello JL, et al: Lack of relation of oral clefts to diazepam use during pregnancy. N Engl J Med 309:1282–1285, 1983

Rowlatt RJ: Effect of maternal diazepam on the newborn (letter). BMJ 1:985, 1978

Rubin PC: Current concepts: beta-blockers in pregnancy. N Engl J Med 305:1323–1326, 1981

Safra MJ, Oakley GP Jr: Association between cleft lip with or without cleft palate and prenatal exposure to diazepam. Lancet 2:478–480, 1975

Sapolsky RM, Meaney MJ: Maturation of the adrenocortical stress response: neuroendocrine control mechanisms and the stress hyporesponsive period. Brain Res 396:64–76, 1986

Saxen I: Association between oral clefts and drugs taken during pregnancy. Int J Epidemiol 4:37–44, 1975

Scanlon FJ: Use of antidepressant drugs first trimester (letter). Med J Aust 2:1077, 1969

Schimmell MS, Katz EZ, Shaag Y, et al: Toxic neonatal effects following maternal clomipramine therapy. J Toxicol Clin Toxicol 29:479–484, 1991

Schou M: What happened later to the lithium babies? A follow-up study of children born without malformations. Acta Psychiatr Scand 54:193–197, 1976

Schou M, Amdisen A: Lithium and the placenta (letter). Am J Obstet Gynecol 122:541, 1975

Schou M, Goldfield MD, Weinstein MR, et al: Lithium and pregnancy, I: report from the Register of Lithium Babies. BMJ 2:135–136, 1973

Scolnik D, Nulman I, Rovet J, et al: Neurodevelopment of children exposed in utero to phenytoin and carbamazepine monotherapy. JAMA 271:767–770, 1994

Sharma V, Persad E: Effect of pregnancy on three patients with bipolar disorder. Ann Clin Psychiatry 7:39–42, 1995

Shearer WT, Schreiner RL, Marshall RE: Urinary retention in a neonate secondary to maternal ingestion of nortriptyline. J Pediatr 81:570–572, 1972

Shiono PH, Mills IL: Oral clefts and diazepam use during pregnancy (letter). N Engl J Med 311:919–920, 1984

Sichel DA, Cohen LS, Dimmock JA, et al: Postpartum obsessive compulsive disorder: a case series. J Clin Psychiatry 54:156–159, 1993

Sim M: Imipramine and pregnancy (letter). BMJ 2:45, 1972

Sipek A: Lithium and Ebstein's anomaly. Cor et Vasa 31:149–156, 1989

Slone D, Siskind V, Heinonen OP, et al: Antenatal exposure to the phenothiazines in relation to congenital malformations, perinatal mortality rate, birth weight, and intelligence quotient score. Am J Obstet Gynecol 128:486–488, 1977

Spear LP, Shalaby IA, Brick J: Chronic administration of haloperidol during development: behavioral and psychopharmacological effects. Psychopharmacology (Berl) 70:47–58, 1980

Spencer MJ: Fluoxetine hydrochloride (Prozac) toxicity in the neonate. Pediatrics 92:721–722, 1993

St. Clair SM, Schirmer RG: First-trimester exposure to alprazolam. Obstet Gynecol 80:843–846, 1992

Steer RA, Scholl TO, Hediger ML, et al: Self-reported depression and negative pregnancy outcomes. J Clin Epidemiol 45:1093–1099, 1992

Stewart DE: Prophylactic lithium in postpartum affective psychosis. J Nerv Ment Dis 176:485–489, 1988

Stewart DE, Klompenhouwer JL, Kendell RE, et al: Prophylactic lithium in puerperal psychosis: the experience of three centres. Br J Psychiatry 158:393–397, 1991

Stoner SC, Sommi RW Jr, Marken PA, et al: Clozapine use in two full-term pregnancies (letter). J Clin Psychiatry 58:364–365, 1997

Suppes T, Baldessarini RJ, Faedda GL, et al: Risk of recurrence following discontinuation of lithium treatment in bipolar disorder. Arch Gen Psychiatry 48:1082–1088, 1991

Tamer A, McKey R, Arias D, et al: Phenothiazine-induced extrapyramidal dysfunction in the neonate. J Pediatr 75:479–480, 1969

Targum SD, Davenport YB, Webster MJ: Postpartum mania in bipolar manic-depressive patients withdrawn from lithium carbonate. J Nerv Ment Dis 167:572–574, 1979

Tohen M, Waternaux CM, Tsuang MT: Outcome in mania: a 4-year prospective follow-up of 75 patients utilizing survival analysis. Arch Gen Psychiatry 47:1106–1111, 1990

Tondo L, Baldessarini R, Hennen J, et al: Lithium treatment and risk of suicidal behavior in bipolar disorder patients. J Clin Psychiatry 59:405–414, 1998

van Gent EM, Verhoeven WM: Bipolar illness, lithium prophylaxis, and pregnancy. Pharmacopsychiatry 25:187–191, 1992

van Waes A, van de Velde E: Safety evaluation of haloperidol in the treatment of hyperemesis gravidum. J Clin Psychopharmacol 9:224–237, 1969

Viguera AC, Baldessarini RC: Neuroleptic withdrawal in schizophrenic patients. Arch Gen Psychiatry 52:189–192, 1995

Viguera A, Nonacs R, Cohen L, et al: Risks of discontinuing maintenance treatment in pregnant women with bipolar disorder, in 1997 New Research Program and Abstracts, American Psychiatric Association 150th Annual Meeting, San Diego, CA, May 17–22, 1997. Washington, DC, American Psychiatric Association, 1997

Viguera AC, Baldessarini RJ, Friedberg J: Discontinuing antidepressant treatment in major depression: risks of interrupting continuation or maintenance treatment with antidepressants in major depressive disorders. Harv Rev Psychiatry 5:293–306, 1998

Villeponteaux VA, Lydiard RB, Laraia MT, et al: The effects of pregnancy on pre-existing panic disorder. J Clin Psychiatry 53:201–203, 1992

Waldman MD, Safferman AZ: Pregnancy and clozapine. Am J Psychiatry 150:168–169, 1993

Webster PAC: Withdrawal symptoms in neonates associated with maternal antidepressant therapy. Lancet 2:318–319, 1973

Weinberg M, Tronick E: The impact of maternal psychiatric illness on infant development. J Clin Psychiatry 59(suppl 2):53–61, 1998

Weinstein MR: The international register of lithium babies. Drug Information Journal 50:81–86, 1976

Weinstock L: Clonazepam use during pregnancy. Paper presented at the 149th annual meeting of the American Psychiatric Association, New York, May 1996

Wheeler EO, White PD, Reed EW, et al: Neurocirculatory anthenia (anxiety neurosis, effort syndrome, neurasthenia): a twenty-year follow-up study of 173 patients. JAMA 142:878–890, 1950

White AD, Andrews EB: The Pregnancy Registry Program at Glaxo Wellcome Company. J Allergy Clin Immunol 103:S362–S363, 1999

Whitelaw A, Cummings A, McFadyen IR: Effect of maternal lorazepam on the neonate. BMJ 282:1106–1108, 1981

Wisner KL: Prevention of postpartum episodes in bipolar women, in Syllabus and Proceedings Summary, American Psychiatric Association Annual Meeting, Toronto, ON, Canada, May 30–June 4, 1998. Washington, DC, American Psychiatric Association, 1998

Wisner KL, Wheeler SB: Prevention of recurrent postpartum major depression. Hosp Community Psychiatry 45:1191–1196, 1994

Woody JN, London WL, Wilbanks GD Jr: Lithium toxicity in a newborn. Pediatrics 47:94–96, 1971

Zajicek E: Psychiatric problems during pregnancy, in Pregnancy: A Psychological and Social Study. Edited by Wolkind S, Zajicek E. London, England, Academic Press, 1981, pp 57–73

Zalzstein E, Koren G, Einarson T, et al: A case control study on the association between first-trimester exposure to lithium and Ebstein's anomaly. Am J Cardiol 65:817–818, 1990

Zierler S: Maternal drugs and congenital heart disease. Obstet Gynecol 65:155–165, 1985

Zuckerman B, Bauchner H, Parker S, et al: Maternal depressive symptoms during pregnancy, and newborn irritability. J Dev Behav Pediatr 11:190–194, 1990

25

Women, Ethnicity, and Psychopharmacology

David A. Ruskin, M.D.
Ricardo P. Mendoza, M.D.
Michael W. Smith, M.D.
Keh-Ming Lin, M.D., M.P.H.

*M*ultiple factors appear to be responsible for the characteristic differences between the sexes, as well as between distinct racial/ethnic groups, with respect to their ability to metabolize drugs or alcohol. Although gender has long been considered an important variable in pharmacological responsiveness, research into the determinants of gender disparity is still in its relative infancy. Fortunately, the mechanisms surrounding cross-ethnic differences in drug effectiveness have been under closer scrutiny in recent years. As a result, it is now generally accepted that mutations in the genetic code have given rise to the existence of multiple or *polymorphic* forms of certain drug-metabolizing enzymes. This polymorphic variability has been

From the Research Center on the Psychobiology of Ethnicity and the Department of Psychiatry, UCLA School of Medicine, Harbor-UCLA Medical Center. Supported in part by the Research Center on the Psychobiology of Ethnicity MH47193.

linked to several clearly identifiable mutations, each predominant in one or more ethnic populations. These mutated enzyme variants have been found to be responsible for the classic variations in drug responsiveness noted across distinct ethnic boundaries (Kalow 1991). Several of these have been studied extensively. Specific variants of cytochrome P450 enzymes and the alcohol-metabolizing enzymes have been reported (Kalow 1991).

Polymorphic changes also have been implicated in the differential binding of drugs to certain carrier proteins in the blood. Carrier proteins have no inherent enzymatic activity. However, they are extremely important to pharmacological response because they partially determine drug bioavailability. α_1-Glycoprotein, for example, is involved in the binding of many compounds that are used in the treatment of psychiatric disorders today (Baumann and Eap 1991). Genetically determined polymorphisms of this drug-binding protein have been identified, and ethnic specificity for this protein has been demonstrated (Baumann and Eap 1991).

Research suggests that sex may play a crucial role in the way drugs are metabolized. Those hormones that are unique to female physiology also may be important determinants of pharmacological response. A small but increasing body of evidence suggests that hormonally influenced female cycles, such as menstruation, pregnancy, and menopause, may each cause specific changes in drug-metabolizing enzymatic function. These sex-specific variations in drug responsiveness often appear to be mediated through their effect on certain cytochrome P450 enzymes and N-acetyltransferase (Kalow 1991). In addition, sex variability in the metabolism of alcohol has been reported (Kalow 1991).

Environmentally based factors also contribute to variability in drug response. Exposure to xenobiotics, alcohol, cigarette smoke, certain dietary ingredients, and medications such as oral contraceptives can markedly influence the way pharmacological agents are used and metabolized by the human body. In addition, some people tend to believe that over-the-counter herbal and homeopathic remedies are "natural" safe agents and not drugs. However, there is little understanding into how these herbal remedies affect overall drug metabolism. These agents are now ubiquitous in food and health food stores and are poorly regulated. At least some of these products likely affect the bioavailability or metabolism of more common pharmacological agents.

ALCOHOL METABOLISM

One of the longest and most intensely studied models serving to illustrate the differences in drug responsiveness across sex and ethnic boundaries is that of alcohol. For decades, it has been recognized that sex and ethnicity play a crucial role in the development and continuation of alcoholism. More than basic social and cultural determinants, they serve as meaningful *physiological* factors in the development of this disease (Mello 1980). Animal research indicates that a significant difference exists between males and females in the way they metabolize alcohol (C.J.P. Eriksson 1973; K. Eriksson and Malmstrom 1967; Wilson et al. 1984). Hormonal influences appear to be involved in this discrepancy (Collins et al. 1975; Rachamin et al. 1980). Although parallel research in humans has produced inconsistent data (Cole-Harding and Wilson 1987), hereditary and hormonal influences are thought to play important roles in the development of alcoholism in humans.

The general mechanism underlying alcohol metabolism is well understood. Ethanol is first oxidized by alcohol dehydrogenase (ADH) to acetaldehyde, which is a toxic substance. Acetaldehyde is then rapidly oxidized by aldehyde dehydrogenase (ALDH), producing nontoxic acetate. It is logical to assume that sex and ethnic differences in this process might be due to variations in function or structure of one or both of these enzymes. Indeed, *both* ADH and ALDH are enzyme systems that possess polymorphic variability.

Alcohol Dehydrogenase

ADH does not exist as one characteristic structure. Rather, this enzymatic *system* represents several "classes" of structurally similar enzymes or *isoenzymes*, each possessing its own structural distinctions (Yoshida et al. 1991). Class I ADH oxidizes ethanol at a rapid rate and thus plays a major role in alcohol metabolism. Its major site of action is in the liver, but sites also have been found in other tissues, such as the lung and kidney. Class II ADH is found primarily in the liver and stomach (Moreno and Parés 1991; Yin et al. 1990). Class III ADH has been found in all tissues. In humans, all known ADH genes are located on chromosome 4q21–25 (Yoshida 1983). This fact suggests that each of these genes began as a copy of some parent gene and later evolved, through the process of mutation, into its present form.

All humans possess these ADH isoenzymes. More recent research, however, has determined that various ethnic groups have an even greater variability in their ability to metabolize alcohol than can be explained by isoenzymes alone. It has long been known that certain ethnic groups show consistently higher rates of alcoholism than others. Although cultural factors surely have a role in alcoholic behavior, significant evidence now shows that genetic and physiological factors may be crucial to the development of this disease. Studies of alcohol metabolism were some of the first to evidence polymorphism in drug-metabolizing enzymes.

Three distinct ADH enzymes—ADH2 (β subunit), ADH3 (γ subunit), and ADH4 (π subunit)—are polymorphic and show both ethnic and sex variation. The frequency of the most common, or wild-type, *ADH21* gene is greater than 90% in Caucasians. In stark contrast, only 30% of Asians produce this particular enzyme, and virtually all other Asians possess the atypical *ADH22* genotype. Two other ADH genes, the wild-type *ADH31* and the atypical variant *ADH32*, are commonly found in Caucasians. In contrast, the frequency of the variant gene is low in Asian populations (Yoshida 1983; Yoshida et al. 1991). *ADH23* is another fairly uncommon variant, which is highly represented in black populations (Table 25–1). Research is currently in progress to determine whether certain polymorphic variants impart susceptibility to the development of alcoholism in specific ethnic populations.

Sex also appears to play an important role in alcohol metabolism. Women appear to be more susceptible to alcoholic liver injury than do men. In a direct comparison of ethanol metabolism, researchers reported that males metabolize a significantly larger proportion of ethanol in their stomachs than do females (Frezza et al. 1990). Males also were noted to have higher rates of ADH activity in their stomach mucous membranes (Frezza et al. 1990). Thus, if equal quantities of alcohol are given to men and women, women may have proportionally larger amounts available for absorption because of their lower rates of ADH activity. This increased alcohol absorption could potentially contribute to the higher peak blood alcohol levels classically observed in women. This may be a significant factor in their increased risk of alcoholic liver disease.

Aldehyde Dehydrogenase

Long before the polymorphism of metabolizing enzymes was understood, the phenomenon of "alcohol flushing" among Asians was well recognized. More recently, this phenomenon has been proven to be the result of ethnic-specific genetic variability at the *ALDH* gene locus. Specific mutations in the gene coding for ALDH have resulted in inefficient metabolism of acetaldehyde in those who are affected. When enough alcohol is administered, those possessing these ALDH variants will have significantly increased plasma concentrations of toxic acetaldehyde. Clinically, abnormally high concentrations of circulating acetaldehyde result in the well-known characteristic presentation, which may include tachycardia, anxiety, nausea, and the classic symptom of facial flushing. This syndrome is rare in Caucasians. However, approximately 50% of American Indians and as many as 80% of Asians possess the mutant variant (Wolff 1972, 1973), making the "alcohol flushing" syndrome quite common in these populations.

Research has identified several ALDH isoenzymes (Yoshida et al. 1991). Two of these enzyme systems, which are located in the liver, are considered the main players in acetaldehyde detoxification. ALDH1 exists in the cell

TABLE 25–1. Drugs subject to debrisoquine P450 enzyme metabolism

Cardiovascular	Psychotropics	Analgesics
Alprenolol	Amitriptyline*	Phenformin
Amiflamine	Chlorpromazine	Codeine*
Bufuralol	Clozapine*	Phenacetin
Encainide	Clomipramine	Dextromethorphan
Flecainide	Desipramine	
Guanoxan	Fluoxetine	
Indoramin	Fluvoxamine	
Methoxyphenamine	Haloperidol*	
Metiamide	Imipramine*	
Metoprolol	Methoxyamphetamine	
Perhexilene	Nortriptyline	
Propafenone	Olanzapine*	
Propranolol	Paroxetine	
Sparteine	Perphenazine	
Timolol	Risperidone	
	Sertraline	
	Thioridazine	

Note. *Partially metabolized through this pathway.

body, whereas ALDH2 is specific to the mitochondria. Both function as potent oxidizers of acetaldehyde. The ALDH2 system has been implicated in alcohol flushing. Indeed, approximately half of the total Asian population lacks ALDH2 activity. The problem lies in an ethnic-specific mutation at the *ALDH2* locus (Hsu et al. 1985; Yoshida et al. 1984). Although the frequency of this variant (*ALDH22*) is negligible in Caucasians, approximately 30% of Japanese carry the mutation in some form or another (Shibuya and Yoshida 1988). Because the mutant *ALDH22* is dominant, both homozygous and heterozygous individuals will have impaired acetaldehyde metabolism (see Table 25–2). In other words, individuals need only possess one copy of the mutant gene in order to be prone to alcohol flushing.

Of certain clinical significance, the same genotypes associated with alcohol flushing appear to furnish at least some protection against alcoholism. Indeed, most patients with alcoholic liver disease are homozygous for the wild-type gene (Yoshida 1983). Of course, it might be argued that the differential rates of alcoholism noted across various ethnic populations could be fully explained by cultural factors alone. However, several other studies that specifically evaluated Japanese and Chinese persons with alcoholism

TABLE 25–2.   Mephenytoin oxidation phenotypes

Country	Poor metabolizers, %
Studies in East Indians	
India	0.8
Studies in American Indians	
Panama	0.0
Studies in Asians	
Chinese	
China	17.4
Canada	5.0
Japanese	
Japan	22.0
Canada	23.0
Studies in Caucasians	
Denmark	2.5
Canada	2.4–4.2
France	6.0
Switzerland	5.0
United States	2.6–6.7
Sweden	2.8
Studies in Hispanics	
United States	4.8–14
Studies in African Americans	
United States	18.5

confirmed that these patients also were homozygous for the wild-type gene (Harada 1990; Thomasson et al. 1991). Whether this mutant gene acts directly as a modifier of alcoholic behavior or indirectly by punishing the alcohol drinker with an aversive environment (alcohol flush) remains unclear. At any rate, this research has provided a solid framework for understanding the role of ethnic and sex variability in the development and continuation of alcoholism. Moreover, it points to new and interesting avenues for future study, which could eventually lead to the identification of other genes implicated in this dreadful disease.

DRUG-METABOLIZING ENZYMES AND THE METABOLIC PROCESS

In the body, medications must be rendered water soluble to be excreted in the urine. Many psychotropic drugs used in the treatment of psychiatric illness are metabolized to this effect by a two-step process. Phase I, which is predominantly carried out by cytochrome P450 isoenzymes, involves the addition of a functional group into the substrate (Clark et al. 1988; Shen and Lin 1990). Phase II involves the conjugation of these agents by sulfation and glucuronidation. The function of the various drug-metabolizing enzymes can be significantly altered by mutations, resulting in changes in inherent enzymatic structure. Environmental factors also significantly alter enzymatic efficiency. Ethnic and sex-specific variations in drug responsiveness are thought to be dictated by an amalgamation of these factors.

Sex-Specific Variation of P450 Enzymes in Animals

Several sex-specific P450 enzyme systems have been identified through research conducted on rodents. Apparently, these particular enzymes are influenced by certain sex and pituitary hormones (Gonzalez and Nebert 1990; Gonzalez et al. 1988; Nebert and Gonzalez 1985). Several studies indicated, for example, that exposure to testosterone in the neonatal period is crucial to the expression of a particular male-specific P450 enzymatic form, termed P450h, found in both rats and mice (Dannan et al. 1986). Furthermore, P450h expression can be completely negated by castration during the neonatal period. In contrast, castration in adult rodents only partially reduces expression. In either case, castrated rats will have new or greater production of the male-specific P450h on administration of exogenous testosterone (Gonzalez and Nebert 1990; Gonzalez et al. 1988; Nebert and Gonzalez 1985). Research has evidenced some interesting data particular to female rodents as well. The female-specific P450i enzymatic form is present in both sexes at birth. With the onset of puberty, however, the presence of testosterone acts differentially on the sexes. In female rodents, the enzyme continues to be expressed. However, in males, a surge in testosterone production completely suppresses P450i expression (Dannan et al. 1986).

Several studies of growth hormone secretion in rodents also have elicited sex-specific characteristics in P450 activity. Sex-specific patterns of growth hormone secretion seem to be a very important regulator of sex-specific P450 production (Mode et al. 1981; Morgan et al. 1985; Pampori and Shapiro 1994). These secretion patterns are largely determined by neonatal and adult androgen exposure. In the pituitary glands of rodents, a pulsatile secretion pattern is observed in males, whereas a constant secretion pattern is observed in females (Jansson et al. 1985). When these patterns of excretion are artificially changed, however, impressive changes in the characteristic expression of the P450 system are also evidenced. In hypophysectomized rats, for example, a continuous versus pulsatile exogenous infusion of growth hormone will artificially induce the inappropriate expression of the female-specific P450i or male-specific P450h enzyme, respectively (Kato et al. 1986; Morgan et al. 1985; Pampori and Shapiro 1994). Analysis of the data from these animal studies clearly supports the assertion that hormonal influences play an important role in cytochrome P450 enzyme regulation.

Sex- and Ethnic-Specific Variation of P450 Enzymes in Humans

In humans, phenotypic analysis of the P450 system has successfully measured functional enzyme expression after administration of a probe drug. Sex- and ethnic-specific variations in the P450 enzyme system have been clearly shown with this methodology. Analysis of numerous populations has determined that the enzymatic responsiveness of two cytochrome P450 isoenzymes—CYP2D6 and CYP2C19—is bimodally distributed. More specifically, an individual in a given population can be classified as either an *extensive metabolizer* or a *poor metabolizer*, depending on the rate that he or she is able to metabolize a probe drug (Gonzalez 1989; Kalow 1991; Wilkinson et al. 1989; Wood and Zhou 1991). Extensive metabolizers are typically those individuals who show aggressive enzymatic activity, whereas poor metabolizer status indicates a total lack of enzymatic function. Both extensive and poor metabolizers generally possess homozygous status. However, whereas extensive metabolizers possess the wild-type genotype, poor metabolizers are generally homozygous for a specific nonfunctional mutation. Because the enzymes of heterozygous individuals typically have an intermediate or diminished metabolic capacity, such individuals have been termed *slow metabolizers*. In the specific case of CYP2D6, an additional mutation has been identified that results in the production of far greater numbers of that enzyme. These *superextensive metabolizers* rapidly metabolize drugs normally processed by CYP2D6 (Dahl et al. 1995). These individuals do not obtain therapeutic drug levels at standard doses because of the rapid rate of enzymatic activity and substrate clearance conferred by this mutation. Because phenotyping methodologies can be influenced by environmental factors, molecular analysis has been enlisted to link various enzymatic phenotypes to actual genetic structures. Both polymerase chain reaction (PCR) and restriction fragment length polymorphism (RFLP) have been used in this endeavor.

Studies that have incorporated both phenotyping and genotyping techniques have concluded that genetic mutations are the primary cause of the cross-ethnic variations observed in CYP2D6 and CYP2C19 activity. Although an abundance of data supports ethnic-specific enzymatic polymorphisms, human sex studies paralleling those in animals have not yet elicited any evidence supporting the existence of sex-specific variations in cytochrome P450 expression (George et al. 1995). At any rate, the ethnic- and sex-specific variations observed in CYP1A2 and CYP3A3/4 are inevitably related to multiple environmental factors, including diet, oral contraceptive therapy, menstrual fluctuations, and toxin exposure.

Cytochrome P450 2D6

CYP2D6 is responsible for metabolizing various medications, including antihypertensive agents, antidepressants, antipsychotics, and many other prescription and over-the-counter drugs (Bertilsson and Aberg-Wistedt 1983; Bertilsson et al. 1980; Dahl-Puustinen et al. 1989; Mellstrom et al. 1983; Skjelbo et al. 1991) (see Table 25–1). Because of its importance to the processing of so many common medications, CYP2D6 has been extensively studied.

Recent reports that have focused on pregnancy and its effect on cytochrome P450 enzymes have pointed to the importance of circulating hormones to determining functional CYP2D6 expression. In a 1997 study, pregnancy was shown to induce CYP2D6 activity (Wadelius et al. 1997). Although the sample size was small, both extensive metabolizers and slow metabolizers showed significant enzymatic induction. As expected, because of their inherent lack of significant enzymatic functioning, none of the poor metabolizers showed this induction. Both the extensive and the slow metabolizer females had CYP2D6 induction during pregnancy, presumably secondary to transient hormonal influences. The far greater induction, however, was noted in the slow metabolizers, who were heterozygous for the mutant variant *CYP2D6* gene. This study confirms the earlier finding that the antihypertensive agent metoprolol, a drug also metabolized by CYP2D6, is cleared at a rate four to five times faster in women who are pregnant as compared with women who delivered 3–6 months earlier (Hogstedt et al. 1985).

Although the reasons behind these prominent metabolic changes in pregnancy remain unclear, it is likely that endogenous substrates are responsible for this transient enzymatic induction. The available research data suggest, however, that the two most likely candidates for endogenous inducers are the female-specific steroid hormones estrogen and progesterone. For example, in the menstrual cycle, a 25% induction in CYP2D6 activity of debrisoquine was observed during the luteal phase, in which progesterone plays a particularly prominent role (Llerena et al. 1996). In another female-specific study, propranolol, a drug metabolized by CYP2D6 via ring oxidation, showed a significantly increased rate of clearance when administered in conjunction with ethinyl estradiol (Hogstedt et al. 1985).

In stark contrast to the sparse and inadequate data concerning sex-specific variation, data regarding cross-ethnic variations in the frequency of CYP2D6 poor metabolizers are quite extensive (see Table 25–3). The frequency of CYP2D6 poor metabolizers is less than 1% in Mexican Americans (Mendoza et al. 2001) and several Asian populations, including Chinese (Du and Lou 1990) and Japanese (Horai et al. 1990). This is significantly different from the rate of 3%–10% reported in Caucasians in Europe and North America. A greater variability in the frequency of poor metabolizers is seen across black populations. Poor metabolizers occur at rates of 19% in Sans Bushmen, up to 8% in Saharan Africans, and only 1.9% in African Americans (Lin et al. 1993). These data suggest that the greater the geographic distance between two potential interbreeding populations, the greater the disparity in the frequencies of certain mutational variants. Thus, genetic drift may play a role in this cross-ethnic variability.

Cytochrome P450 2C19

CYP2C19 is important to the metabolism of several psychotropic medications, including imipramine and several benzodiazepines (Bertilsson et al. 1989; Inaba et al. 1986; Meier et al. 1985) (see Table 25–3). CYP2C19 is inherited as an autosomal recessive trait (Inaba et al. 1986) and is another enzyme that shows cross-ethnic disparity in the incidence of poor metabolizers. The frequency of Caucasians possessing the CYP2C19 variant is low, but Asians tend to have a high frequency of poor metabolizers in their populations (Lin et al. 1993). African Americans tend to have an intermediate poor metabolizer rate that is significantly higher than that of Caucasians (Masimirembwa and Hasler 1997).

No direct evidence supports the existence of sex-specific CYP2C19 polymorphic enzymes. However, several indirect studies suggest that sex differences do exist. Female subjects, for example, show consistently lower rates of clearance of certain drugs when compared with males (Macleod et al. 1979; Walle et al. 1989). More specifically, this trend has been noted with drugs, such as propanolol (Walle et al. 1989), that are thought to undergo CYP2C19 metabolism.

CYP2C19 function may be significantly altered by the presence of circulating sex hormones. In some part, these alterations may be sex dependent. For example, researchers have noted a positive correlation between circulating testosterone levels and rates of propanolol clearances in males, but not in females (Walle et al. 1994). Females, on the other hand, show a reduction in CYP2C19 activity most prevalent in the age range between 18 and 40 years (Tamminga et al. 1999). Some of this variation is presumed to be secondary to the use of ethinyl estradiol and oral contraceptives (Hagg et al. 2001; Tamminga et al. 1999).

TABLE 25–3. Cytochrome P450 2D6 poor metabolizer frequency as determined by either debrisoquine/dextromethorphan or sparteine oxidation

Ethnic group	Poor metabolizers, %
Africans and African Americans	
African Americans	1.9
Sub-Saharan Africans	0–8
Sans Bushmen	19
Venda	0–4
American Indians and Hispanics	
United States Hispanics	1–4.5
Cuna	0
Ngawbe Guaymi	5.2
Asians	
Chinese	
China	32
Canada	31
Singapore	0
Japanese	
Japan	0–2.4
Malayans	
Thai	1.2
Caucasians	
Finland	
Finns	3.2
Lapps	8.6
Spain	6.6
Denmark	9.2

The fact that both CYP2D6 and CYP2C19 appear to be influenced by sex hormone regulation has additional clinical significance. A number of medications have been shown to be under the control of both of these cytochrome P450 pathways. In actuality, many drugs are metabolized simultaneously by multiple cytochrome P450 enzymes. Thus, exposure to circulating sex hormones can produce dramatic and opposite results in enzyme systems that normally work in parallel to clear a particular compound. Because of the multiplicity of enzymes involved in this process, inducing or inhibiting a specific pathway may not necessarily affect the overall clearance of a particular compound. However, because distinct enzyme systems process substrates in different ways, such hormonal alterations could radically shift the amount and type of metabolites produced. The possibility of significantly shifting metabolic pathways may have profound consequences on the side effect profile, toxic properties, drug–drug interactions, and even carcinogenicity of certain pharmacological agents.

Cytochrome P450 3A3/4

Accounting for more than half of the total complement of P450, the CYP3A3/4 enzyme system is probably the most important of the P450 enzymes. CYP3A3/4 is involved in the metabolism of many medications in use today. These include certain antibiotics, cardiac drugs, antihistamines, and multiple psychiatric medications (Ereshefsky 1996; Lown et al. 1994). Currently, no direct evidence supports the existence of ethnic-specific CYP3A3/4 polymorphisms. However, large interindividual variations have been noted within this enzyme system. One study showed that the amount of functional enzyme in the liver and intestines can vary immensely from individual to individual (Paine et al. 1997). Moreover, differential enzymatic rates have been noted between each of these organs (Paine et al. 1997). This could explain the disparity in metabolism that has been noted when a drug's route of entry into the body is varied between oral and parenteral administration (Ducharme et al. 1995).

In animals and humans, females consistently show more CYP3A3/4 activity than do males. Several sex studies on rats and dogs have supported this fact (Lin et al. 1996). The results of these studies suggested that the greater enzymatic rates noted in females of certain animal species may be a result of the tendency of these females to possess higher levels of several types of the CYP3A3/4 enzyme (Lin et al. 1996). In humans, women have been shown to have much greater CYP3A3/4 activity compared with men in both the liver and the gut (Gleiter and Gundert-Remy 1996; Harris et al. 1995). As with other cytochrome P450 systems, some studies have attempted to correlate the cross-sex disparity in CYP3A3/4 enzymatic function to sex-specific hormonal factors. One study, for example, observed that older women metabolized nefazodone, an antidepressant metabolized by CYP3A3/4, only half as fast as did younger women (Barbhaiya et al. 1996). This suggests that estrogen or progesterone, both of which are more abundant in younger women, may in some way facilitate CYP3A3/4 functioning. In contrast to this finding, however, other sex studies (Thummel et al. 1996) and recent studies examining the menstrual cycle and its effect on CYP3A3/4 metabolism (Kharasch et al. 1997) have failed to support this conclusion.

CYP3A3/4 has been shown to express cross-ethnic variability as well. Bimodal distribution in this enzymatic system has been noted within human kidneys (Haehner et al. 1996). Moreover, several authors have reported cross-ethnic differential rates in the metabolism of a drug actively metabolized by CYP3A3/4 (Ahsan et al. 1991; Kleinbloesem et al. 1984).

Mexican and East Asian populations, for example, have been reported to metabolize this drug more slowly than Caucasians do. These studies suggest that CYP3A3/4, like the other cytochrome P450 systems previously mentioned, exists in at least two distinct polymorphic forms. However, a subsequent study refuted this conclusion, arguing that earlier reports of polymorphic variation were products of either environmental influences or small sample size (von Moltke et al. 1996). Indeed, this study reported only a unimodal drug metabolism. Because of the conflicting nature of these data, more research must be completed before the true nature of CYP3A3/4 distribution in humans can be realized.

What is clear, however, is that CYP3A3/4 is significantly influenced by environmental factors. It has consistently been one of the most sensitive of the P450 systems to alterations in diet and interaction with other drugs. Seemingly benign environmental factors, such as using antifungal remedies or drinking grapefruit juice, can markedly inhibit this enzymatic system (Hukkinen et al. 1995; von Moltke et al. 1996). It is crucial that physicians be aware of the more recent literature concerning CYP3A3/4 and its prominent causative role in clinically significant drug–drug and drug–diet interactions (Greene and Barbhaiya 1997; Lown et al. 1994).

Cytochrome P450 1A2

CYP1A2 is important in that it also is highly sensitive to environmental factors. Cigarette smoking, for example, has been shown to increase the rate of clearance of certain medications metabolized by CYP1A2 by as much as 30% (Ereshefsky 1996). Nitrosamines, which are plentiful in cigarette tar, are potent inducers of CYP1A2. Nitrosamines also are found in certain vegetables, such as brussels sprouts and cabbage, and food that is cooked over charcoal (Kall and Clausen 1995). In contrast, certain substances can inhibit CYP1A2 activity. Oral contraceptives, for example, have been shown to decrease its rate of clearance (Balogh et al. 1995).

Few data are available concerning cross-ethnic and -sex differences in CYP1A2 metabolism. Some indirect evidence, however, supports sex-specific differential metabolism in this enzyme system. Multiple studies have noted consistently higher concentrations of certain probe drugs in females, sometimes by as much as 30% (Ereshefsky 1996; Preskorn 1997). This cross-sex disparity might again be explainable by sex-specific hormonal factors.

Phase II Metabolizing Enzymes

Many different pharmacological substances, including synthetic sex hormones and certain psychotropic drugs, are eventually cleared from the body during the second phase of drug metabolism (Kalow 1994). Unfortunately, little is known about cross-ethnic and -sex variation in this important enzymatic system. Studies that have focused on certain rodent species have noted definite sex differences in several classic phase II enzymes (Watanabe et al. 1997). However, similar findings have yet to be reported in humans.

N-Acetyltransferase

N-acetyltransferase is primarily located in the liver. The wild-type gene is inherited in an autosomal recessive manner. Like many of the compounds previously discussed, N-acetyltransferase has a bimodal distribution of enzymatic rates within the population. It functions by acetylation and provides a major route of metabolism for numerous pharmacological agents (Lin et al. 1991; Mendoza et al. 1991) (Table 25–4). The distribution of N-acetyltransferase enzymatic forms is extremely important because certain phenotypes directly correlate to certain significant risk factors for disease. The poor metabolizer phenotype, for example, imparts a significantly greater risk for developing drug-induced systemic lupus erythematosus, isoniazid polyneuropathy, and other important hypersensitivity reactions (Rieder et al. 1991). Moreover, poor metabolizers are at greater risk for developing certain types of cancer (Weber 1987). N-acetyltransferase poor metabolizers are quite common in the United States. In fact, their frequency ranges between 38% and 50% in most Western populations (Grant et al. 1990; Weber and Hein 1985). Asian populations, conversely, have a significantly greater proportion of extensive metabolizers in their populations (Catania et al. 1995; Grant et al. 1983).

Tuberculosis and, thus, isoniazid therapy are currently on the rise in the United States. Therefore, it is becoming increasingly important for physicians to be aware of these cross-ethnic differences and their importance to drug sensitivity and toxicity. Although very few studies have correlated sex with acetylation efficiency, certain women had higher overall isoniazid plasma levels (Iselius and Evans 1983) than did men. Moreover, certain women taking hydralazine appear to have an increased risk for developing drug-induced systemic lupus erythematosus (Batchelor et al. 1980). The acetylation process and its importance to many disease states are still under close scrutiny and remain intense areas of research (Weber 1987).

Glucuronidation

Glucuronidation is another enzymatic process that shows differential metabolic activity across various ethnic populations. Researchers have found what appears to be another bimodal distribution in enzymatic func-

TABLE 25–4. Drugs subject to acetylation

Aminoglutethimide	Inhibitor of adrenal steroid synthesis
Amrinone	Positive inotropic
Caffeine	Stimulant
Clonazepam	Antiepileptic
Dapsone	Antimicrobial
Dipyrone	Analgesic
Endralazine	Antihypertensive
Hydralazine	Antihypertensive
Isoniazid	Antimicrobial
Nitrazepam	Hypnotic
Phenelzine	Antidepressant
Prizidilol	Antihypertensive
Procainamide	Antiarrhythmic
Sulfadiazine	Antimicrobial
Sulfamerazine	Antimicrobial
Sulfamethazine	Antimicrobial
Sulfapyridine	Antimicrobial

tioning. Several studies noted a significant difference between Chinese and Caucasian individuals in their rate of glucuronidation of codeine (Yue et al. 1989a, 1989b, 1990, 1991). Indeed, Caucasian subjects consistently showed faster overall rates of metabolism by this method. As a consequence of their slower metabolic rate, Chinese subjects, in comparison with Caucasians in the study, had significantly higher concentrations of codeine in their plasma. These studies have far-reaching clinical implications. It is quite possible that Chinese and, perhaps, other Asian populations may achieve therapeutic analgesia at significantly lower doses of codeine as well as other important opiate medications.

Also, sufficient evidence in both animals and humans suggests that glucuronidation has sex-specific characteristics. One study reported that males of certain animal species had clearly higher metabolic rates than did females (Catania et al. 1995). A parallel study in humans produced similar results (Gleiter and Gundert-Remy 1996). Moreover, isolated reports of increased sex disparity during puberty (Capparelli 1994) hint that sex-specific steroid hormones may play a significant role in the variability noted in enzymatic activity.

Plasma Protein Binding

Medicines and other pharmacologically active compounds do not always act as independent units in plasma. In fact, only a small fraction of a drug's complement is free and, thus, biologically active. The rest remains bound to specialized carrier proteins in the plasma, effectively removed from circulation. Changes in the concentration and efficiency of these binding proteins can significantly alter the amount of drug available for biological effect. Albumin and α_1-acid glycoprotein (AAG) are generally considered to be the most important of the native plasma binding proteins (Baumann and Eap 1988; Kragh-Hansen 1981; Kremer et al. 1988). Only AAG, however, has been shown to exist as various distinct polymorphic forms.

Several studies have elicited sex-specific disparity in both the absolute levels and the genetic distribution of AAG (Eap and Bauman 1989; Fukuma et al. 1990; Juneja et al. 1988; Montiel et al. 1990; Umetsu et al. 1988; Zhou et al. 1990). These studies identified a bimodal distribution, defined by populations with either the S (slow) or the F (fast) variants of the glycoprotein. In general, Asians tend to express the S variant at a frequency only half that of blacks and whites in the United States and Europe. Eskimos, South American Indians, and North American Indians also show this ethnic-specific variation and have their own characteristic rates of S and F variant expression.

As might be expected, because of the overall lack of cross-sex studies of this nature, data on sex-specific variations in protein binding are incomplete. Several researchers have maintained, however, that protein binding of drugs can be decreased in certain circumstances (Wilkinson and Kurata 1974). In pregnancy, for example, many drugs have a decreased proportion of binding to plasma proteins (Dean et al. 1980). The greatest decrease generally was seen in the third trimester (Perucca and Crema 1982). Although these data appear to implicate sex hormones as a cause of the differential binding patterns, the decreased levels of bound drug, at least in part, may be secondary to decreased levels of albumin typically noted during pregnancy (Yoshikawa et al. 1984).

Several reports have suggested that one or more aspects specific to sex may influence the absolute levels of AAG within the circulation. One study reported, for example, that men have significantly higher concentrations of AAG than do women (Kishino et al. 1995). Other studies implicated sex-specific hormones in the noted differences in AAG concentrations. Variations in glycoprotein concentration, for example, have been successfully correlated to variations in the menstrual cycle (Parish and Spivey 1991). Moreover, pregnant women tend to show transient decreases in AAG concentration (Adams and Wacher 1968; Ganrot 1972). Whether oral contraceptive therapy affects AAG concentration remains unclear. The current data are limited and have produced conflicting results (Blain et al. 1985; Routledge 1986; Song et al. 1970; Walle et al. 1994). More data must be acquired before the true clinical importance of sex to AAG and other binding proteins can be fully realized.

CONCLUSION

The research into the molecular and genetic basis for pharmacological response is becoming progressively more sophisticated. Newer available search techniques, such as PCR and RFLP, have markedly improved researchers' ability to link clinically reported phenotypes to actual genetic structures. In the future, as the research into pharmacogenetics progresses, increasingly subtle refinements will be possible in the practice of pharmacotherapy. The current hotbed of pharmacogenetic research lies within the realm of the drug-metabolizing enzymes. Researchers have noted multiple genetic and environmental forces that can dramatically influence the distribution and efficiency of those enzymes that ultimately dictate pharmacological response.

The interethnic variability in drug responsiveness that has long been reported in the literature has now been clearly correlated to these same factors. Unfortunately, parallel research into cross-sex variations has been sorely lagging behind the available technology, and the data that have been acquired are scanty and often conflicting. Indeed, only recently have researchers begun to report that gender may play a role in pharmacological response.

Sex-specific variations in drug metabolism have been documented in several animal studies. Most of these studies have implicated sex-specific steroid hormones as the most likely determinants of the sex disparity. However, parallel studies in humans have thus far failed to produce similar convincing results. The indirect evidence supporting hormonal control, however, is impressive enough to demand further, more complex investigation.

Several statements can be made regarding the issue of hormonal control. First, hormonal regulation probably does play an important role in modulating the complex cytochrome P450 enzyme system as well as several other metabolizing enzyme systems. Second, steroid hormones do appear to have a part in determining the concentration of certain drug-binding plasma proteins. Third, results of several animal studies suggested that exposure to particular sex hormones during early stages of development may affect future enzyme expression. However, some of these conclusions have yet to be fully examined in human studies. Thus, more research is required before clinically significant conclusions can be addressed.

The environment may have an even greater importance to metabolic functioning than has yet been realized. Far from being simple modifiers of behavior, specific environmental factors have been shown to possess partial control over certain genetically determined enzymatic processes. The influences of diet, pollution, cigarette smoking, and various medications, including oral contraceptives, have each been implicated in the induction or inhibition of certain important drug-metabolizing enzymes. It is clear that these extraneous factors may have far-reaching implications when considering their possible influences on a drug's therapeutic dose, side effect spectrum, and toxic profile. Moreover, with so little known about the role of sex in drug metabolism, the differences in enzymatic functioning noted between the sexes may be due in part to other, more environmentally based factors.

Many important lessons have been learned from the psychopharmacological management of various distinct ethnic populations. Many of these same lessons must be applied when considering the administration of psychotropic medications to women. Women are moved by many of the same environmental forces that influence men. However, they are also confronted with several other important physiological variables that normally need not be considered when dealing only with men. The female physiology depends on a delicate balance of several distinct hormones, which are differentially secreted and, thus, constantly changing in their relative concentrations. The two most important of these—estrogen and progesterone—have been implicated in effecting significant changes in the various drug-metabolizing enzyme systems. Because of the dynamic nature of these hormones, women are at greater risk for developing clinically significant alterations in therapeutic drug levels, side effects, or toxic profiles. Because of the cyclical nature of female sex hormones, such potentially harmful alterations might not manifest for days or even weeks following the initiation of psychotropic therapy. Moreover, pregnancy and menopause are life-stage events that add even greater variability to hormonal balance. These potential risks may be compounded in women of color because certain ethnic-specific mutations may confer poor or absent enzymatic activity to a particular drug-metabolizing system. If estrogen or progesterone, for example, acts to inhibit a system that is already dysfunctional, an affected woman could develop hazardous side effects or toxic injury caused by inordinately high concentrations of nonmetabolized substrate.

As pharmacological agents become more complex, researchers will need to pay greater attention to ethnic, sex, environmental, and hormonal variables. If psychopharmacotherapy is to remain safe and effective, new lessons must be learned as physicians attempt to grapple with progressively sophisticated medications in a setting of rapidly increasing ethnic diversity.

REFERENCES

Adams JB, Wacher A: Specific changes in the glycoprotein components of seromucoid in pregnancy. Clin Chim Acta 21:155–157, 1968

Ahsan CH, Renwick AG, Macklin B, et al: Ethnic differences in the pharmacokinetics of oral nifedipine. Br J Clin Pharmacol 31:399–403, 1991

Balogh A, Klinger G, Henschel L, et al: Influence of ethinylestradiol-containing combination oral contraceptives with gestodene or levonorgestrel on caffeine elimination. Eur J Clin Pharmacol 48:161–166, 1995

Barbhaiya RH, Buch AB, Greene DS: A study of the effect of age and gender on the pharmacokinetics of nefazodone after single and multiple doses. J Clin Psychopharmacol 16:19–25, 1996

Batchelor JR, Welsh KI, Tinoco RM, et al: Hydralazine-induced systemic lupus erythematosus: influence of HLA-DR and sex on susceptibility. Lancet 1:1107–1109, 1980

Baumann P, Eap C: Alpha-Acid Glycoprotein Genetics, Biochemistry, Physiological Functions and Pharmacology. New York, Alan R Liss, 1988

Baumann P, Eap C: Plasma monitoring of antidepressants: clinical relevance of the pharmacogenetics of metabolism and of acid glycoprotein binding. Biol Psychiatry 29:75–95, 1991

Bertilsson L, Aberg-Wistedt A: The debrisoquine hydroxylation test predicts steady-state plasma levels of desipramine. Br J Clin Pharmacol 15:388–390, 1983

Bertilsson L, Eichelbaum M, Mellstrom B, et al: Nortryptiline and antipyrine clearance in relation to debrisoquine hydroxylation in man. Life Sci 27:1673–1677, 1980

Bertilsson L, Henthorn TK, Sanz E, et al: Importance of genetic factors in the regulation of diazepam metabolism: relationship to S-mephenytoin, but not debrisoquine, hydroxylation phenotype. Clin Pharmacol Ther 45:348–355, 1989

Blain PG, Mucklow JC, Rawlins MD, et al: Determinants of plasma alpha-1-acid glycoprotein (AAG) concentrations in health. Br J Clin Pharmacol 20:500–502, 1985

Capparelli EV: Pharmacokinetic considerations in the adolescent: non-cytochrome P450 metabolic pathways. J Adolesc Health 15:641–647, 1994

Catania VA, Dannenberg AJ, Luquita MG, et al: Gender-related differences in the amount and functional state of rat liver UDP-glucuronosyltransferase. Biochem Pharmacol 50:509–514, 1995

Clark W, Brater D, Johnson A: Goth's Medical Pharmacology, 12th Edition. St. Louis, MO, CV Mosby, 1988

Cole-Harding S, Wilson JR: Ethanol metabolism in men and women. J Stud Alcohol 48:380–387, 1987

Collins AC, Yeager TN, Leback ME, et al: Variations in alcohol metabolism: influence of sex and age. Pharmacol Biochem Behav 3:973–978, 1975

Dahl ML, Johansson I, Bertilsson L, et al: Ultrarapid hydroxylation of debrisoquine in a Swedish population: analysis of the molecular genetic basis. J Pharmacol Exp Ther 274:516–520, 1995

Dahl-Puustinen ML, Liden A, Alm C, et al: Disposition of perphenazine is related to polymorphic CYP2D6e hydroxylation in human beings. Clin Pharmacol Ther 46:78–81, 1989

Dannan GA, Guengerich FP, Waxman DJ: Hormonal regulation of rat liver microsomal enzymes: role of gonadal steroids in programming, maintenance, and suppression of delta 4-steroid 5 alpha-reductase, flavin-containing monooxygenase, and sex-specific cytochromes P-450. J Biol Chem 261:10728–10735, 1986

Dean M, Stock B, Patterson RJ, et al: Serum protein binding of drugs during and after pregnancy in humans. Clin Pharmacol Ther 28:253–261, 1980

Du YL, Lou YQ: Polymorphism of debrisoquine 4-hydroxylation and family studies of poor metabolizers in Chinese population. Acta Pharmacologica Sinica 11:7–10, 1990

Ducharme MP, Warbasse LH, Edwards DJ: Disposition of intravenous and oral cyclosporine after administration with grapefruit juice. Clin Pharmacol Ther 57:485–491, 1995

Eap CB, Bauman P: The genetic polymorphism of human alpha-1-acid glycoprotein: genetics, biochemistry, physiological functions, and pharmacology. Prog Clin Biol Res 300:111–125, 1989

Ereshefsky L: Pharmacokinetics and drug interactions: update for new antipsychotics. J Clin Psychiatry 57(suppl 11):12–25, 1996

Eriksson CJP: Ethanol and acetaldehyde metabolism in rat strains genetically selected for their ethanol preference. Biochem Pharmacol 22:2283–2292, 1973

Eriksson K, Malmstrom KK: Sex differences in consumption and elimination of alcohol in albino rats. Annales Medicinae Experimentalis Et Biologiae Fenniae 45:389–392, 1967

Frezza M, di Padova C, Pozzato G, et al: High blood alcohol levels in women: the role of decreased gastric alcohol dehydrogenase activity and first pass metabolism. N Engl J Med 322:95–99, 1990

Fukuma Y, Kashimimura S, Umetsu K, et al: Genetic variation of alpha-2-HS-glycoprotein in the Kyushu district of Japan: description of three new rare variants. Hum Hered 40:49–51, 1990

Ganrot PO: Variation of the concentrations of some plasma proteins in normal adults, in pregnant women and in newborns. Scand J Clin Lab Invest 29(suppl 24):83–88, 1972

George J, Byth K, Farrell GC: Age but not gender selectively affects expression of individual cytochrome P450 proteins in human liver. Biochem Pharmacol 50:727–730, 1995

Gleiter CH, Gundert-Remy U: Gender differences in pharmacokinetics. Eur J Drug Metab Pharmacokinet 21:123–128, 1996

Gonzalez F: The molecular biology of cytochrome P450s. Pharmacol Rev 40:243–288, 1989

Gonzalez F, Nebert D: Evolution of the P450 gene superfamily: animal-plant "warfare" molecular drive and human genetic differences in drug oxidation. Trends Genet 6:182–186, 1990

Gonzalez FJ, Skoda RC, Kimura S, et al: Characterization of the common genetic defect in humans deficient in debrisoquin metabolism. Nature 331:442–446, 1988

Grant DM, Tang BK, Kalow W: Polymorphic N-acetylation of a caffeine metabolite. Clin Pharmacol Ther 33:355–359, 1983

Grant DM, Morike K, Eichelbaum M, et al: Acetylation pharmacogenetics. J Clin Invest 85:968–972, 1990

Greene DS, Barbhaiya RH: Clinical pharmacokinetics of nefazodone. Clin Pharmacokinet 33:260–275, 1997

Haehner BD, Gorski JC, Vandenbranden M, et al: Bimodal distribution of renal cytochrome P450 3A activity in humans. Mol Pharmacol 50:52–59, 1996

Hagg S, Spigset O, dahlqvist R: Influence of gender and oral contraceptives on CYP2D6 and CYP2C19 activity in healthy volunteers. Br J Clin Pharmacol 51:169–173, 2001

Harada S: Genetic polymorphism of aldehyde dehydrogenase and its physiological significance to alcohol metabolism. Prog Clin Biol Res 344:289–291, 1990

Harris RZ, Benet LZ, Schwartz JB: Gender effects in pharmacokinetics and pharmacodynamics. Drugs 50:222–239, 1995

Hogstedt S, Lindberg B, Peng DR, et al: Pregnancy-induced increase in metoprolol metabolism. Clin Pharmacol Ther 37:688–692, 1985

Horai Y, Taga J, Ishizaki T, et al: Correlations among the metabolic ratios of three test probes (metoprolol, debrisoquine and sparteine) for genetically determined oxidation polymorphism in a Japanese population. Br J Clin Pharmacol 29:111–115, 1990

Hsu LC, Tani K, Fujiyoshi T, et al: Cloning of cDNAs for human aldehyde dehydrogenase 1 and 2. Proc Natl Acad Sci U S A 82:3771–3775, 1985

Hukkinen SK, Varhe A, Olkkola KT, et al: Plasma concentrations of triazolam are increased by concomitant ingestion of grapefruit juice. Clin Pharmacol Ther 58:127–131, 1995

Inaba T, Jurima M, Kalow W: Family studies of mephenytoin hydroxylation deficiency. Am J Hum Genet 38:768–772, 1986

Iselius L, Evans DAP: Formal genetics of isoniazid metabolism in man. Clin Pharmacokinet 8:541–544, 1983

Jansson JO, Ekberg S, Isaksson O, et al: Imprinting of growth hormone secretion, body growth, and hepatic steroid metabolism by neonatal testosterone. Endocrinology 117:1881–1889, 1985

Juneja R, Weitkamp L, Straitil A: Further studies of the plasma, alpha B-glycoprotein polymorphism: two new alleles and allele frequencies in Caucasians and in American Blacks. Hum Hered 38:267–272, 1988

Kall MA, Clausen J: Dietary effect on mixed function P450 1A2 activity assayed by estimation of caffeine metabolism in man. Hum Exp Toxicol 14:801–807, 1995

Kalow W: Interethnic variation of drug metabolism. Trends Pharmacol Sci 12:102–107, 1991

Kalow W: Pharmacogenetic variability in brain and muscle. J Pharm Pharmacol 46(suppl 1):425–432, 1994

Kato R, Yamazoe Y, Shimada M, et al: Effect of growth hormone and ectopic transplantation of pituitary gland on sex-specific forms of cytochrome P-450 and testosterone and drug oxidations in rat liver. J Biochem 100:895–902, 1986

Kharasch ED, Russell M, Mautz D, et al: The role of cytochrome P450 3A4 in alfentanil clearance: implications for interindividual variability in disposition and peri-operative drug interactions. Anesthesiology 87:36–50, 1997

Kishino S, Nomura A, Di ZS, et al: Alpha-1-acid glycoprotein concentration and the protein binding of disopyramide in healthy subjects. J Clin Pharmacol 35:510–514, 1995

Kleinbloesem CH, van Brummelen P, Faber H, et al: Variability of nifedipine pharmacokinetics and dynamics: a new oxidation polymorphism in man. Biochem Pharmacol 33:3721–3724, 1984

Kragh-Hansen U: Molecular aspects of ligand binding to serum albumin. Pharmacol Rev 33:17–53, 1981

Kremer J, Wilting J, Janssen L: Drug binding to human alpha-1-acid glycoprotein in health and disease. Pharmacol Rev 40:1–45, 1988

Lin JH, Chiba M, Balani SK, et al: Species differences in the pharmacokinetics and metabolism of indinavir, a potent human immunodeficiency virus protease inhibitor. Drug Metab Dispos 24:1111–1120, 1996

Lin K, Poland R, Smith M, et al: Pharmacokinetic and other related factors affecting psychotropic responses in Asians. Psychopharmacol Bull 27:427–439, 1991

Lin K, Poland R, Silver B: Overview: the interface between psychobiology and ethnicity, in Psychopharmacology and Psychobiology of Ethnicity. Edited by Lin K, Poland R, Nakasaki G. Washington, DC, American Psychiatric Press, 1993, pp 11–36

Llerena A, Cobaleda J, Martinez C, et al: Interethnic differences in drug metabolism: influence of genetic and environmental factors on debrisoquine hydroxylation phenotype. Eur J Drug Metab Pharmacokinet 21:129–138, 1996

Lown KS, Kolars JC, Thummel KE, et al: Interpatient heterogeneity in expression of CYP3A4 and CYP3A5 in small bowel: lack of prediction by the erythromycin breath test. Drug Metab Dispos 22:947–955, 1994

Macleod SM, Giles HG, Bengert B, et al: Age and gender related differences in diazepam pharmacokinetics. J Clin Pharmacol 1:15–19, 1979

Masimirembwa CM, Hasler JA: Genetic polymorphism of drug metabolizing enzymes in African populations: implications for the use of neuroleptics and antidepressants. Brain Res Bull 44:561–571, 1997

Meier UT, Dayer P, Male PJ, et al: Mephenytoin hydroxylation polymorphism: characterization of the enzymatic deficiency in liver microsomes of poor metabolizers phenotyped in vivo. Clin Pharmacol Ther 38:488–494, 1985

Mello NK: Some behavioral and biological aspects of alcohol problems in women, in Alcohol and Drug Problems in Women: Research Advances in Alcoholism and Drug Problems, Vol 5. Edited by Kalant OJ. New York, Plenum, 1980, pp 263–298

Mellstrom B, Bertilsson L, Lou YC, et al: Amitriptyline metabolism: relationship to polymorphic CYP2D6e hydroxylation. Clin Pharmacol Ther 34:516–520, 1983

Mendoza R, Smith MW, Poland RE, et al: Ethnic psychopharmacology: the Hispanic and Native American perspective. Psychopharmacol Bull 27:449–461, 1991

Mendoza R, Wan YJ, Poland RE, et al: CYP2D6 polymorphism in a Mexican American population. Clin Pharmacol Ther 70:552–560, 2001

Mode A, Norstedt G, Simic B, et al: Continuous infusion of growth hormone feminizes hepatic steroid metabolism in the rat. Endocrinology 108:2163–2168, 1981

Montiel MD, Carracedo A, Blazquez-Caeiro JL, et al: Orosomucoid (ORM1 and ORM2) types in the Spanish Basque Country, Galicia, and northern Portugal. Hum Hered 40:330–334, 1990

Moreno A, Parés X: Purification and characterization of a new alcohol dehydrogenase from human stomach. J Biol Chem 266:1128–1133, 1991

Morgan ET, MacGeoch C, Gustafsson JA: Hormonal and developmental regulation of expression of the hepatic microsomal steroid 16a-hydroxylase cytochrome P-450 apoprotein in the rat. J Biol Chem 260:11895–11898, 1985

Nebert DW, Gonzalez FJ: Cytochrome P450 gene expression and regulation. Trends Pharmacol Sci 6:160–164, 1985

Paine MF, Khalighi M, Fisher JM, et al: Characterization of interintestinal and intraintestinal variations in human CYP3A-dependent metabolism. J Pharmacol Exp Ther 283:1552–1562, 1997

Pampori NA, Shapiro BH: Over-expression of CYP2C11, the major male-specific form of hepatic cytochrome P450, in the presence of nominal pulses of circulating growth hormone in adult male rats neonatally exposed to low levels of monosodium glutamate. J Pharmacol Exp Ther 271:1067–1073, 1994

Parish RC, Spivey C: Influence of menstrual cycle phase on serum concentration of a-1-acid glycoprotein. Br J Clin Pharmacol 31:197–199, 1991

Perucca E, Crema A: Plasma protein binding of drugs in pregnancy. Clin Pharmacokinet 7:336–356, 1982

Preskorn SH: Clinically relevant pharmacology of selective serotonin reuptake inhibitors: an overview with emphasis on pharmacokinetics and effects on oxidative drug metabolism. Clin Pharmacokinet 32(suppl 1):1–21, 1997

Rachamin G, MacDonald JA, Wahid S, et al: Modulation of alcohol dehydrogenase and ethanol metabolism by sex hormones in the spontaneously hypertensive rat. Biochem J 186:483–490, 1980

Rieder MJ, Shear NH, Kanee A, et al: Prominence of slow acetylator phenotype among patients with sulfonamide hypersensitivity reactions. Clin Pharmacol Ther 49:13–17, 1991

Routledge P: The plasma protein binding of basic drugs. Br J Clin Pharmacol 22:499–506, 1986

Shen W, Lin K: Cytochrome P-450 monooxygenases and interactions of psychotropic drugs. Int J Psychiatry Med 21:21–30, 1990

Shibuya A, Yoshida A: Frequency of the atypical aldehyde dehydrogenase-2 gene (ALDH) in Japanese and Caucasians. Am J Hum Genet 43:744–748, 1988

Skjelbo E, Brosen K, Hallas J, et al: The mephenytoin oxidation polymorphism is partially responsible for the N-demethylation of imipramine. Clin Pharmacol Ther 49:18–23, 1991

Song CD, Merkatz IR, Rifkind AB, et al: The influence of pregnancy and oral contraceptive steroids on the concentration of plasma proteins. Am J Obstet Gynecol 108:227–231, 1970

Tamminga WJ, Wemer J, Oosterhuis B, et al: CYP2D6 and CYP2C19 activity in a large population of Dutch healthy volunteers: indications for oral contraceptive-related gender differences. Eur J Clin Pharmacol 55:177–184, 1999

Thomasson HR, Edenberg HJ, Crabb DW, et al: Alcohol and aldehyde dehydrogenase genotypes and alcoholism in Chinese men. Am J Hum Genet 48:677–681, 1991

Thummel KE, O'Shea D, Paine MF, et al: Oral first-pass elimination of midazolam involves both gastrointestinal and hepatic CYP3A-mediated metabolism. Clin Pharmacol Ther 59:491–502, 1996

Umetsu K, Yuasa I, Nishimura H: Genetic polymorphisms of orosomucoid and alpha-2-HS-glycoprotein in a Philippine population. Hum Hered 38:287–290, 1988

von Moltke LL, Greenblatt DJ, Harmatz JS, et al: Triazolam biotransformation by human liver microsomes in vitro: effects of metabolic inhibitors and clinical confirmation of a predicted interaction with ketoconazole. J Pharmacol Exp Ther 276:370–379, 1996

Wadelius M, Darj E, Frenne G, et al: Induction of CYP2D6 in pregnancy. Clin Pharmacol Ther 62:400–407, 1997

Walle T, Walle UK, Cowart TD, et al: Pathway-selective sex differences in the metabolic clearance of propanolol in human subjects. Clin Pharmacol Ther 46:257–263, 1989

Walle T, Walle UK, Fagan TC, et al: Influence of gender and sex steroid hormones on plasma binding of propranolol enantiomers. Br J Clin Pharmacol 37:21–25, 1994

Watanabe M, Tanaka M, Tateishi T, et al: Effects of the estrous cycle and the gender differences on hepatic drug-metabolising enzyme activities. Pharmacol Res 35:477–480, 1997

Weber WW: The Acetylator Genes and Drug Responses. New York, Oxford University Press, 1987

Weber WW, Hein DW: N-Acetylation pharmacogenetics. Pharmacol Rev 37:26–79, 1985

Wilkinson GR, Kurata D: The uptake of diphenylhydantoin by the human erythrocyte and its application to the estimation of plasma binding, in Drug Interactions. Edited by Mortselli PL, Garattini S, Cohen SN. New York, Raven, 1974, pp 289–297

Wilkinson GR, Guengerich FP, Branch RA: Genetic polymorphism of S-mephenytoin hydroxylation. Pharmacol Ther 43:53–76, 1989

Wilson JR, Erwin VG, DeFries JC, et al: Ethanol dependence in mice: direct and correlated responses to ten generations of selective breeding. Behav Genet 14:235–256, 1984

Wolff PH: Ethnic difference in alcohol sensitivity. Science 175:449–450, 1972

Wolff PH: Vasomotor sensitivity to alcohol in diverse Mongoloid population. Am J Hum Genet 25:193–199, 1973

Wood AJ, Zhou HH: Ethnic differences in drug disposition and responsiveness. Clin Pharmacokinet 20:1–24, 1991

Yin SJ, Wang MF, Liao CS, et al: Identification of a human stomach alcohol dehydrogenase with distinctive kinetic properties. Biochemistry International 22:829–835, 1990

Yoshida A: A possible structural variant of human cytosolic aldehyde dehydrogenase with diminished enzyme activity. Am J Hum Genet 35:1115–1116, 1983

Yoshida A, Huang IY, Ikawa M: Molecular abnormality of an inactive aldehyde dehydrogenase variant commonly found in Orientals. Proc Natl Acad Sci U S A 81:258–261, 1984

Yoshida A, Hsu LC, Yasunami M: Genetics of human alcohol-metabolizing enzymes. Prog Nucleic Acid Res Mol Biol 40:255–287, 1991

Yoshikawa T, Sugiyama Y, Sawada Y, et al: Effect of late pregnancy on salicylate, diazepam, warfarin, and propranolol binding: use of fluorescent probes. Clin Pharmacol Ther 36:201–208, 1984

Yue QY, Bertilsson L, Dahl-Puustinen ML, et al: Disassociation between debrisoquine hydroxylation phenotype and genotype among Chinese. Lancet 2:870, 1989a

Yue Q, Svensson JO, Alm C, et al: Interindividual and interethnic differences in the demethylation and glucuronidation of codeine. Br J Clin Pharmacol 28:629–637, 1989b

Yue QY, VonBahr C, Odar-Cederlof I, et al: Glucuronidation of codeine and morphine in human liver and kidney microsomes: effect of inhibitors. Pharmacol Toxicol 66:221–226, 1990

Yue QY, Hasselstrom J, Svensson JO, et al: Pharmacokinetics of codeine and its metabolites in Caucasian healthy volunteers: comparisons between extensive and poor hydroxylators of debrisoquine. Br J Clin Pharmacol 31:635–642, 1991

Zhou H, Adedoyin A, Wilkinson GR: Differences in plasma binding of drugs between Caucasian and Chinese subjects. Clin Pharmacol Ther 48:10–17, 1990

Concluding Remarks

*T*he overall awareness and importance of issues involving women's mental health and cognitive behaviors have been studied intensely and augmented over the past decade. The prevalence of these newly perceived sex differences in mental and cognitive disorders might result from interactions of many diverse causes, including environmental, hormonal, genetic, and social factors. These factors are believed to play an important role in the disorders that are perceived as being more commonly diagnosed in women, such as eating disorders, mood disorders, social phobia, panic disorder, generalized anxiety disorder, dissociative disorders, and obsessive-compulsive disorder.

Women experience stressors and hormonal changes that are very different from the stressors that men experience. Women must personally tolerate life events, such as menstruation, contraceptive use, pregnancy, childbirth, menopause, and premenstrual syndrome, that may influence disease pervasiveness and manipulate underlying response to treatment. These sex differences appear to exist not only in the etiology or progression of a disease but also in the response to intervention. Numerous studies have shown that women tend to seek out preventive measures and therapy more often than men do. Thus, because women more commonly use health care and more often request pharmacological treatment, physicians may more often overmedicate women.

With the above facts in mind, data obtained from new clinical trials could be beneficial in improving health, treating disorders, and controlling disease in women, especially because they are the major consumers of marketed medication. Previously, health policies traditionally excluded women from participating in clinical trials (in particular, in Phase I studies) with the intention of protecting them and their unborn children. These policies are now considered paternalistic and discriminatory because potential sex differences in response to treatment were ignored when the clinical data obtained from men were extrapolated to women. This bygone policy now violates current principles of clinical practice, which focus on individualizing treatment to optimize therapeutic benefit and minimize risk.

A clinical trial without appropriate numbers of women may be viewed as scientifically and clinically flawed; therefore, the inclusion of women as research subjects is viewed as an issue of scientific merit. Sufficient numbers of females should be included in early Phase I studies. In later trials, such as Phase II and III, data should be analyzed by sex to assess potential pharmacokinetic and pharmacodynamic differences. If preclinical findings indicate specific sex differences, then additional studies in women should be conducted during the clinical development of therapeutic agents to address specific concerns. This becomes particularly important for older women, who may respond differently than men or younger women do. In addition, consideration needs to be given to safety and effectiveness in women because these variables may differ because of age or hormonal status. Consequently, studies must analyze for potential sex differences for pre- and postmenopausal women. During a studies analysis, adverse events also should be examined carefully given that certain adverse events may be sex specific. To ensure valid results, prospective studies will need to control for factors such as comorbid psychiatric and medical disorders, concomitant psychotherapy, exogenous and endogenous hormones, and concomitant medications, all of which can affect the pharmacodynamics and pharmacokinetics of medications.

An extensive amount of research is still needed in the area of sex differences. As new studies are completed and results appear, clinicians will gain a more balanced and clearer view of the similarities and differences that may occur between the sexes. Clinicians should use this newfound knowledge about sex differences to take a broader approach to optimizing treatment outcomes and quality-of-life issues within mental and cognitive disorders because these disorders affect neurobiological, psychological, interpersonal, and social aspects of an individual. In addition to other individual factors, sex must be carefully considered by clinicians when formulating an optimum treatment regimen. This will help ensure a favorable drug response, patient compliance, and a decreased incidence of undesirable adverse events.

Clearly, we have made important strides in understanding sex issues, as evidenced by the diverse and excellent collection of scientific data and thought characterized in this text. Nevertheless, significant, well-focused, and well-thought-out research in all fields must continue and be nurtured to ensure that sex issues become a regular routine of scientific and clinical output.

Index

*Page numbers printed in **boldface** type refer to tables or figures.*